MDS 3.0
RAI User's Manual

ISBN: 978-1-61569-267-5

Melissa D'Amico, Associate Editor
James DeWolf, Publisher and Editorial Director
Mike Mirabello, Graphic Artist
Matt Sharpe, Senior Manager of Production
Shane Katz, Art Director
Jean St. Pierre, Vice President, Operations and Customer Relations

Arrangements can be made for quantity discounts. For more information, contact:

HCPro, Inc.
75 Sylvan Street, Suite A-101
Danvers, MA 01923
Telephone: 800/650-6787 or 781/639-1872
Fax: 800/639-8511
E-mail: customerservice@hcpro.com

Visit HCPro online at: *www.hcmarketplace.com* and *www.hcpro.com*

Contents

Downloadable Content

Thank you for purchasing the *MDS 3.0 RAI User's Manual.* You may download the item sub-set forms located in Appendix H at *www.hcpro.com/downloads/7292.*

CMS ACKNOWLEDGEMENTS

Contributions provided by the numerous people, organizations, and stakeholders listed below are very much acknowledged by CMS. Their collective hard work and dedication over the past several years in the development, testing, writing, formatting, and ongoing review and maintenance of the MDS 3.0 RAI Manual, MDS 3.0 Data Item Set, and MDS 3.0 Data Specifications have resulted in a new RAI process that increases clinical relevancy, data accuracy, clarity, and notably adds more of the resident voice to the assessment process. We wish to give thanks to all of the people that have contributed to making this manual possible. Thank you for the work you do to promote the care and services to individuals in nursing homes.

Experts in Long Term Care

- Elizabeth Ayello, PhD, RN
- Barbara Bates-Jensen, PhD, RN, CWOCN
- Robert P. Connolly, MSW
- Kate Dennison, RN, RAC-MT
- Linda Drummond, MSM
- Rosemary Dunn, RN
- Elaine Hickey, RN, MS
- Karen Hoffman, RN, MPH
- Christa Hojlo, PhD
- Carol Job, RN RAC-CT
- Sheri Kennedy, RN, BA, MSEd., RAC-MT
- Steve Levenson, MD, CMD
- Carol Maher, RN-BC, RAC-CT
- Michelle McDonald, RN, MPH
- Jan McCleary, MSA, RN
- Dann Milne, PhD
- Tracy Burger Montag, RN, BSN, RAC-CT
- Teresa M. Mota, BSN, RN, CALA, WCC, CPEHR
- John Morris, PhD, MSW
- Diane Newman, RNC MSN, CRNP, FAAN
- Jennifer Pettis, RN, BS, WCC
- Terry Raser, RN, CRNAC, RAC-CT
- Therese Rochon, RNP, MSN, MA
- Debra Saliba, MD, MPH
- Rena Shephard, MHA, RN, RAC-MT, C-NE
- Ann Spenard, MSN, RNC, WCC
- Pauline (Sue) Swalina, RN
- Mary Van de Kamp, MS/CCC-SLP
- Nancy Whittenberg

- Sheryl Zimmerman, PhD

Organizations and Stakeholders

- Academy of Nutrition and Dietetics
- American Association of Nurse Assessment Coordinators
- American Health Care Association
- American Health Information Management Association
- American Hospital Association
- American Medical Directors Association
- American Nurses Association
- Association of Health Facility Survey Agencies – RAI Panel
- Commonwealth Fund
- interRAI
- Kansas Department on Aging
- Leading Age
- National Association of Directors of Nursing Administration/Long Term Care
- National Association of Subacute and Post Acute Care
- The National Consumer Voice for Quality Long Term Care
- State Agency RAI Coordinators and RAI Automation Coordinators
- State Quality Improvement Organizations
- US Department of Veterans Affairs

Contractors

Abt Associates

- Rosanna Bertrand, PhD
- Donna Hurd, RN, MSN
- Terry Moore, BSN, MPH

IFMC

- Gloria Batts
- Debra Weiland, BSN, RN
- Jean Eby, BS
- Debra Cory, BS
- Kathy Langenberg, RN

RAND Corporation

- Joan Buchanan, PhD
- Malia Jones

RTI International

- Roberta Constantine, RN, PhD
- Rajiv Ramakrishnan, BA
- Karen Reilly, Sc.D.

Stepwise Systems, Inc

- Robert Godbout, PhD
- David Malitz, PhD

CMS

- Ellen M. Berry, PT
- CMS Regional Office RAI Coordinators
- Jemima Drake, RN
- Shelly Ray, RN
- Thomas Dudley, MS, RN
- Penny Gershman, MS, CCC-SLP
- Lori Grocholski, MSW, LCSW
- Renee Henry, MSN, RN
- Alice Hogan, PMP
- Alesia Hovatter, MPP
- Melissa Hulbert, Director—Division of Advocacy and Special Issues
- John Kane
- Jeanette Kranacs, Director - Division of Institutional Post-Acute Care
- Sheila Lambowitz, Director (Retired)—Division of Institutional Post Acute Care
- Shari Ling, MD
- Stella Mandl, BSW, BSN, PHN, RN
- Mary Pratt, MSN, RN, Director—Division of Chronic and Post-Acute Care
- MaryBeth Ribar, MSN, RN
- Karen Schoeneman, Director (Retired)—Division of Nursing Homes
- John E. V. Sorensen
- Christina Stillwell-Deaner, RN, MPH, PHP
- Michael Stoltz
- Daniel Timmel
- John Williams, Director—Division of National Systems
- Cheryl Wiseman, MPH, MS

Special Recognition for the development of the RAI Manual goes to Ellen Berry, PT and Stella Mandl, BSW, BSN, PHN, RN. Without their dedication, drive, and endless hours of work this manual would not have come to fruition.

Questions regarding information presented in this Manual should be directed to your State's RAI Coordinator. Please continue to check our web site for more information at: http://www.cms.gov/Medicare/Quality-Initiatives-Patient-Assessment-Instruments/NursingHomeQualityInits/Downloads/MDS30Appendix_B.pdf

CHAPTER 1: RESIDENT ASSESSMENT INSTRUMENT (RAI)

1.1 Overview

The purpose of this manual is to offer clear guidance about how to use the Resident Assessment Instrument (RAI) correctly and effectively to help provide appropriate care. Providing care to residents with post-hospital and long-term care needs is complex and challenging work. Clinical competence, observational, interviewing and critical thinking skills, and assessment expertise from all disciplines are required to develop individualized care plans. The RAI helps nursing home staff gather definitive information on a resident's strengths and needs, which must be addressed in an individualized care plan. It also assists staff with evaluating goal achievement and revising care plans accordingly by enabling the nursing home to track changes in the resident's status. As the process of problem identification is integrated with sound clinical interventions, the care plan becomes each resident's unique path toward achieving or maintaining his or her highest practical level of well-being.

The RAI helps nursing home staff look at residents holistically—as individuals for whom quality of life and quality of care are mutually significant and necessary. Interdisciplinary use of the RAI promotes this emphasis on quality of care and quality of life. Nursing homes have found that involving disciplines such as dietary, social work, physical therapy, occupational therapy, speech language pathology, pharmacy, and activities in the RAI process has fostered a more holistic approach to resident care and strengthened team communication. This interdisciplinary process also helps to support the spheres of influence on the resident's experience of care, including: workplace practices, the nursing home's cultural and physical environment, staff satisfaction, clinical and care practice delivery, shared leadership, family and community relationships, and Federal/State/local government regulations[1].

Persons generally enter a nursing home because of problems with functional status caused by physical deterioration, cognitive decline, the onset or exacerbation of an acute illness or condition, or other related factors. Sometimes, the individual's ability to manage independently has been limited to the extent that skilled nursing, medical treatment, and/or rehabilitation is needed for the resident to maintain and/or restore function or to live safely from day to day. While we recognize that there are often unavoidable declines, particularly in the last stages of life, all necessary resources and disciplines must be used to ensure that residents achieve the highest level of functioning possible (quality of care) and maintain their sense of individuality (quality of life). This is true for both long-term residents and residents in a rehabilitative program anticipating return to their previous environment or another environment of their choice.

1.2 Content of the RAI for Nursing Homes

The RAI consists of three basic components: The Minimum Data Set (MDS) Version 3.0, the Care Area Assessment (CAA) process and the RAI Utilization Guidelines. The utilization of the

---

[1] Healthcentric Advisors: The Holistic Approach to Transformational Change (HATCh™). CMS NH QIOSC Contract. Providence, RI. 2006. Available from http://healthcentricadvisors.org/images/stories/documents/inhc.pdf.

three components of the RAI yields information about a resident's functional status, strengths, weaknesses, and preferences, as well as offering guidance on further assessment once problems have been identified. Each component flows naturally into the next as follows:

- **Minimum Data Set.** A core set of screening, clinical, and functional status elements, including common definitions and coding categories, which forms the foundation of a comprehensive assessment for all residents of nursing homes certified to participate in Medicare or Medicaid. The items in the MDS standardize communication about resident problems and conditions within nursing homes, between nursing homes, and between nursing homes and outside agencies. The required subsets of data items for each MDS assessment and tracking document (e.g., admission, quarterly, annual, significant change, significant correction, discharge, entry tracking, PPS assessments, etc.) can be found in Appendix H.

- **Care Area Assessment (CAA) Process.** This process is designed to assist the assessor to systematically interpret the information recorded on the MDS. Once a care area has been triggered, nursing home providers use current, evidence-based clinical resources to conduct an assessment of the potential problem and determine whether or not to care plan for it. The CAA process helps the clinician to focus on key issues identified during the assessment process so that decisions as to whether and how to intervene can be explored with the resident. The CAA process is explained in detail in Chapter 4. Specific components of the CAA process include:

  — **Care Area Triggers (CATs)** are specific resident responses for one or a combination of MDS elements. The triggers identify residents who have or are at risk for developing specific functional problems and require further assessment.

  — **Care Area Assessment** is the further investigation of triggered areas, to determine if the care area triggers require interventions and care planning. The **CAA** resources are provided as a courtesy to facilities in Appendix C. These resources include a compilation of checklists and Web links that may be helpful in performing the assessment of a triggered care area. The use of these resources are not mandatory and represent neither an all-inclusive list nor government endorsement.

  — **CAA Summary (Section V of the MDS 3.0)** provides a location for documentation of the care area(s) that have triggered from the MDS and the decisions made during the CAA process regarding whether or not to proceed to care planning.

- **Utilization Guidelines.** The Utilization Guidelines provide instructions for when and how to use the RAI. These include instructions for completion of the RAI as well as structured frameworks for synthesizing MDS and other clinical information (available from http://cms.gov/manuals/Downloads/som107ap_pp_guidelines_ltcf.pdf).

1.3   Completion of the RAI

Over time, the various uses of the MDS have expanded. While its primary purpose is an assessment tool is used to identify resident care problems that are addressed in an individualized care plan, data collected from MDS assessments is also used for the SNF PPS Medicare reimbursement system, many State Medicaid reimbursement systems, and monitoring the quality of care provided to nursing home residents. The MDS instrument has also been adapted for use by non-critical access hospitals with a swing bed agreement. They are required to complete the MDS for reimbursement under the Skilled Nursing Facility Prospective Payment System (SNF PPS).

- **Medicare and Medicaid Payment Systems.** The MDS contains items that reflect the acuity level of the resident, including diagnoses, treatments, and an evaluation of the resident's functional status. The MDS is used as a data collection tool to classify Medicare residents into RUGs (Resource Utilization Groups). The RUG classification system is used in SNF PPS for skilled nursing facilities, non-critical access hospital swing bed programs, and in many State Medicaid case mix payment systems to group residents into similar resource usage categories for the purposes of reimbursement. More detailed information on the SNF PPS is provided in Chapters 2 and 6. Please refer to the Medicare Internet-Only Manuals, including the Medicare Benefit Policy Manual, located at www.cms.gov/Manuals/IOM/list.asp for comprehensive information on SNF PPS, including but not limited to SNF coverage, SNF policies, and claims processing.

- **Monitoring the Quality of Care.** MDS assessment data are also used to monitor the quality of care in the nation's nursing homes. MDS-based quality measures (QMs) were developed by researchers to assist: (1) State Survey and Certification staff in identifying potential care problems in a nursing home; (2) nursing home providers with quality improvement activities/efforts; (3) nursing home consumers in understanding the quality of care provided by a nursing home; and (4) CMS with long-term quality monitoring and program planning. CMS continuously evaluates the usefulness of the QMs, which may be modified in the future to enhance their effectiveness.

- **Consumer Access to Nursing Home Information**. Consumers are also able to access information about every Medicare- and/or Medicaid-certified nursing home in the country. The Nursing Home Compare tool (http://www.medicare.gov/NHCompare) provides public access to nursing home characteristics, staffing and quality of care measures for certified nursing homes.

The RAI process has multiple regulatory requirements. Federal regulations at 42 CFR 483.20 (b)(1)(xviii), (g), and (h) require that

(1) the assessment accurately reflects the resident's status

(2) a registered nurse conducts or coordinates each assessment with the appropriate participation of health professionals

(3) the assessment process includes direct observation, as well as communication with the resident and direct care staff on all shifts.

Nursing homes are left to determine

(1) who should participate in the assessment process

(2) how the assessment process is completed

(3) how the assessment information is documented while remaining in compliance with the requirements of the Federal regulations and the instructions contained within this manual.

Given the requirements of participation of appropriate health professionals and direct care staff, completion of the RAI is best accomplished by an interdisciplinary team (IDT) that includes nursing home staff with varied clinical backgrounds, including nursing staff and the resident's physician. Such a team brings their combined experience and knowledge to the table in providing an understanding of the strengths, needs and preferences of a resident to ensure the best possible quality of care and quality of life. It is important to note that even nursing homes that have been granted a RN waiver under 42 CFR 483.30 (c) or (d) must provide a RN to conduct or coordinate the assessment and sign off the assessment as complete.

In addition, an accurate assessment requires collecting information from multiple sources, some of which are mandated by regulations. Those sources must include the resident and direct care staff on all shifts, and should also include the resident's medical record, physician, and family, guardian, or significant other as appropriate or acceptable. It is important to note here that information obtained should cover the same observation period as specified by the MDS items on the assessment, and should be validated for accuracy (what the resident's actual status was during that observation period) by the IDT completing the assessment. As such, nursing homes are responsible for ensuring that all participants in the assessment process have the requisite knowledge to complete an accurate assessment.

While CMS does not impose specific documentation procedures on nursing homes in completing the RAI, documentation that contributes to identification and communication of a resident's problems, needs, and strengths, that monitors their condition on an on-going basis, and that records treatment and response to treatment, is a matter of good clinical practice and an expectation of trained and licensed health care professionals. Good clinical practice is an expectation of CMS. As such, it is important to note that completion of the MDS does not remove a nursing home's responsibility to document a more detailed assessment of particular issues relevant for a resident. In addition, documentation must substantiate a resident's need for Part A SNF-level services and the response to those services for the Medicare SNF PPS.

1.4 Problem Identification Using the RAI

Clinicians are generally taught a problem identification process as part of their professional education. For example, the nursing profession's problem identification model is called the nursing process, which consists of assessment, diagnosis, outcome identification, planning, implementation, and evaluation. All good problem identification models have similar steps to those of the nursing process.

The RAI simply provides a structured, standardized approach for applying a problem identification process in nursing homes. The RAI should not be, nor was it ever meant to be, an additional burden for nursing home staff.

The completion of the RAI can be conceptualized using the nursing process as follows:

a. **Assessment**—Taking stock of all observations, information, and knowledge about a resident from all available sources (e.g., medical records, the resident, resident's family, and/or guardian or other legally authorized representative).

b. **Decision Making**—Determining with the resident (resident's family and/or guardian or other legally authorized representative), the resident's physician and the interdisciplinary team, the severity, functional impact, and scope of a resident's clinical issues and needs. Decision making should be guided by a review of the assessment information, in-depth understanding of the resident's diagnoses and co-morbidities, and the careful consideration of the triggered areas in the CAA process. Understanding the causes and relationships between a resident's clinical issues and needs and discovering the "whats" and "whys" of the resident's clinical issues and needs; finding out who the resident is and consideration for incorporating his or her needs, interests, and lifestyle choices into the delivery of care, is key to this step of the process.

c. **Identification of Outcomes**—Determining the expected outcomes forms the basis for evaluating resident-specific goals and interventions that are designed to help residents achieve those goals. This also assists the interdisciplinary team in determining who needs to be involved to support the expected resident outcomes. Outcomes identification reinforces individualized care tenets by promoting residents' active participation in the process.

d. **Care Planning**—Establishing a course of action with input from the resident (resident's family and/or guardian or other legally authorized representative), resident's physician and interdisciplinary team that moves a resident toward resident-specific goals utilizing individual resident strengths and interdisciplinary expertise; crafting the "how" of resident care.

e. **Implementation**—Putting that course of action (specific interventions derived through interdisciplinary individualized care planning) into motion by staff knowledgeable about the resident's care goals and approaches; carrying out the "how" and "when" of resident care.

f. **Evaluation**—Critically reviewing individualized care plan goals, interventions and implementation in terms of achieved resident outcomes as identified and assessing the need to modify the care plan (i.e., change interventions) to adjust to changes in the resident's status, goals, or improvement or decline.

The following pathway illustrates a problem identification process flowing from MDS (and other assessments), to the CAA decision-making process, care plan development, care plan implementation, and finally to evaluation. This manual will refer to this process throughout several chapter discussions.

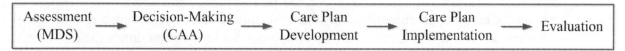

If you look at the RAI process as a solution oriented and dynamic process, it becomes a richly practical means of helping nursing home staff gather and analyze information in order to improve a resident's quality of care and quality of life. The RAI offers a clear path toward using all members of the interdisciplinary team in a proactive process. There is absolutely no reason to insert the RAI process as an added task or view it as another "layer" of labor.

The key to successfully using the RAI process is understanding that its structure is designed to enhance resident care, increase a resident's active participation in care, and promote the quality of a resident's life. This occurs not only because it follows an interdisciplinary problem-solving model, but also because staff (across all shifts), residents and families (and/or guardian or other legally authorized representative) and physicians (or other authorized healthcare professionals as allowable under state law) are all involved in its "hands on" approach. The result is a process that flows smoothly and allows for good communication and tracking of resident care. In short, it works.

Since the RAI has been implemented, nursing home staff who have applied the RAI process in the manner we have discussed have discovered that it works in the following ways:

- **Residents Respond to Individualized Care.** While we will discuss other positive responses to the RAI below, there is none more persuasive or powerful than good resident outcomes both in terms of a resident's quality of care and enhanced quality of life. Nursing home providers have found that when residents actively participate in their care, and care plans reflect appropriate resident-specific approaches to care based on careful consideration of individual problems and causes, linked with input from residents, residents' families (and/or guardian or other legally authorized representative), and the interdisciplinary team, residents have experienced goal achievement and either their level of functioning has improved or has deteriorated at a slower rate. Nursing home staff report that, as individualized attention increases, resident satisfaction with quality of life also increases.

- **Staff Communication Has Become More Effective.** When staff members are involved in a resident's ongoing assessment and have input into the determination and development of a resident's care plan, the commitment to and the understanding of that care plan is enhanced. All levels of staff, including nursing assistants, have a stake in the process. Knowledge gained from careful examination of possible causes and solutions of resident problems (i.e., from performing the CAAs) challenges staff to hone the professional skills of their discipline as well as focus on the individuality of the resident and holistically consider how that individuality is accommodated in the care plan.

- **Resident and Family Involvement in Care Has Increased.** There has been a dramatic increase in the frequency and nature of resident and family involvement in the care planning process. Input has been provided on individual resident goals, needs, interests, strengths, problems, preferences, and lifestyle choices. When considering all of this information, staff members have a much better picture of the resident, and residents and families have a better understanding of the goals and processes of care.

- **Increased Clarity of Documentation.** When the approaches to achieving a specific goal are understood and distinct, the need for voluminous documentation diminishes. Likewise, when staff members are communicating effectively among themselves with respect to resident care, repetitive documentation is not necessary and contradictory notes do not occur. In addition, new staff, consultants, or others who review records have found that the increased clarity of the information documented about a resident makes tracking care and outcomes easier to accomplish.

The purpose of this manual is to offer clear guidance, through instruction and example, for the effective use of the RAI, and thereby help nursing home staff achieve the benefits listed above.

In keeping with objectives set forth in the Institute of Medicine (IOM) study completed in 1986 (Committee on Nursing Home Regulation, IOM) that made recommendations to improve the quality of care in nursing homes, the RAI provides each resident with a standardized, comprehensive and reproducible assessment. This tool assesses a resident's ability to perform daily life functions, identifies significant impairments in a resident's functional capacity, and provides opportunities for direct resident interview. In essence, with an accurate RAI completed periodically, caregivers have a genuine and consistent recorded "look" at the resident and can attend to that resident's needs with realistic goals in hand.

Furthermore, with the consistent application of item definitions, the RAI ensures standardized communication both within the nursing home and between facilities (e.g., other long-term care facilities or hospitals). Basically, when everyone is speaking the same language, the opportunity for misunderstanding or error is diminished considerably.

1.5   MDS 3.0

In response to changes in nursing home care, resident characteristics, advances in resident assessment methods, and provider and consumer concerns about the performance of the MDS 2.0, the Centers for Medicare & Medicaid Services (CMS) contracted with the RAND Corporation and Harvard University to draft revisions and nationally test the MDS Version 3.0. Following is a synopsis of the goals and key findings as reported in the *Development & Validation of a Revised Nursing Home Assessment Tool: MDS 3.0* final report (Saliba and Buchanan, 2008).

Goals

The goals of the MDS 3.0 revision are to introduce advances in assessment measures, increase the clinical relevance of items, improve the accuracy and validity of the tool, increase user satisfaction, and increase the resident's voice by introducing more resident interview items. Providers, consumers, and other technical experts in nursing home care requested that MDS 3.0 revisions focus on improving the tool's clinical utility, clarity, and accuracy. CMS also wanted to increase the usability of the instrument while maintaining the ability to use MDS data for quality measure reporting and Medicare SNF PPS reimbursement (via resource utilization group [RUG] classification).

In addition to improving the content and structure of the MDS, the RAND/Harvard team also aimed to improve user satisfaction. User attitudes are key determinants of quality improvement implementation. Negative user attitudes toward the MDS are often cited as a reason that nursing homes have not fully implemented the information from the MDS into targeted care planning.

Methods

To address many of the issues and challenges previously identified and to provide an empirical foundation for examining revisions to the MDS before they were implemented, the RAND/Harvard team engaged in a careful iterative process that incorporated provider and consumer input, expert consultation, scientific advances in clinical knowledge about screening and assessment, CMS experience, and intensive item development and testing by a national Veterans Health Administration (VHA) consortium. This process allowed the final national testing of MDS 3.0 to include well-developed and tested items.

The national validation and evaluation of the MDS 3.0 included 71 community nursing homes (3,822 residents) and 19 VHA nursing homes (764 residents), regionally distributed throughout the United States. The evaluation was designed to test and analyze inter-rater agreement (reliability) between gold-standard (research) nurses and between nursing home and gold-standard nurses, validity of key sections, response rates for interview items, anonymous feedback on changes from participating nurses, and time to complete the MDS assessment. In addition, the national test design allowed comparison of item distributions between MDS 3.0 and MDS 2.0 and thus facilitated mapping into payment cells (Saliba and Buchanan, 2008).

Key Findings for MDS 3.0

- Improved Resident Input
- Improved Accuracy and Reliability
- Increased Efficiency
- Improved Staff Satisfaction and Perception of Clinical Utility

Improvements incorporated in MDS 3.0 produce a more efficient assessment instrument: better quality information was obtained in less time. Such gains should improve identification of resident needs and enhance resident-focused care planning. In addition, inclusion of items recognized in other care settings is likely to enhance communication among providers. These significant gains reflect the cumulative effect of changes across the tool, including:

- use of more valid items,
- direct inclusion of resident reports, and
- improved clarity of retained items.

1.6 Components of the MDS

The MDS is completed for all residents in Medicare- or Medicaid-certified nursing homes and non-critical access hospitals with Medicare swing bed agreements. The mandated assessment schedule is discussed in Chapter 2. States may also establish additional MDS requirements. For specific information on State requirements, please contact your State RAI Coordinator (see Appendix B).

1.7   Layout of the RAI Manual

The layout of the RAI manual is as follows:

- Chapter 1: Resident Assessment Instrument (RAI)
- Chapter 2: Assessments for the Resident Assessment Instrument (RAI)
- Chapter 3: Overview to the Item-by-Item Guide to the MDS 3.0
- Chapter 4: Care Area Assessment (CAA) Process and Care Planning
- Chapter 5: Submission and Correction of the MDS Assessments
- Chapter 6: Medicare Skilled Nursing Facility Prospective Payment System (SNF PPS)

APPENDICES

- Appendix A: Glossary and Common Acronyms
- Appendix B: State Agency and CMS Regional Office RAI/MDS Contacts
- Appendix C: Care Area Assessment (CAA) Resources
- Appendix D: Interviewing to Increase Resident Voice in MDS Assessments
- Appendix E: PHQ-9 Scoring Rules and Instruction for BIMS (When Administered In Writing)
- Appendix F: Item Matrix
- Appendix G: References
- Appendix H: MDS 3.0 Item Sets

Section	Title	Intent
A	Identification Information	Obtain key information to uniquely identify each resident, nursing home, type of record, and reasons for assessment.
B	Hearing, Speech, and Vision	Document the resident's ability to hear, understand, and communicate with others and whether the resident experiences visual, hearing or speech limitations and/or difficulties.
C	Cognitive Patterns	Determine the resident's attention, orientation, and ability to register and recall information.
D	Mood	Identify signs and symptoms of mood distress.
E	Behavior	Identify behavioral symptoms that may cause distress or are potentially harmful to the resident, or may be distressing or disruptive to facility residents, staff members or the environment.
F	Preferences for Customary Routine and Activities	Obtain information regarding the resident's preferences for his or her daily routine and activities.
G	Functional Status	Assess the need for assistance with activities of daily living (ADLs), altered gait and balance, and decreased range of motion.
H	Bladder and Bowel	Gather information on the use of bowel and bladder appliances, the use of and response to urinary toileting programs, urinary and bowel continence, bowel training programs, and bowel patterns.
I	Active Disease Diagnosis	Code diseases that have a relationship to the resident's current functional, cognitive, mood or behavior status, medical treatments, nursing monitoring, or risk of death.
J	Health Conditions	Document health conditions that impact the resident's functional status and quality of life.
K	Swallowing/Nutritional Status	Assess conditions that could affect the resident's ability to maintain adequate nutrition and hydration.
L	Oral/Dental Status	Record any oral or dental problems present.
M	Skin Conditions	Document the risk, presence, appearance, and change of pressure ulcers as well as other skin ulcers, wounds or lesions. Also includes treatment categories related to skin injury or avoiding injury.
N	Medications	Record the number of days that any type of injection, insulin, and/or select medications was received by the resident.
O	Special Treatments and Procedures	Identify any special treatments, procedures, and programs that the resident received during the specified time periods.
P	Restraints	Record the frequency that the resident was restrained by any of the listed devices at any time during the day or night.
Q	Participation in Assessment and Goal Setting	Record the participation of the resident, family and/or significant others in the assessment, and to understand the resident's overall goals.
V	Care Area Assessment (CAA) Summary	Document triggered care areas, whether or not a care plan has been developed for each triggered area, and the location of care area assessment documentation.
X	Correction Request	Request to modify or inactivate a record already present in the QIES ASAP database.
Z	Assessment Administration	Provide billing information and signatures of persons completing the assessment.

1.8   Protecting the Privacy of the MDS Data

MDS assessment data is personal information about nursing facility residents that facilities are required to collect and keep confidential in accordance with federal law. The 42 CFR Part 483.20 requires Medicare and Medicaid certified nursing facility providers to collect the resident assessment data that comprises the MDS. This data is considered part of the resident's medical record and is protected from improper disclosure by Medicare and Medicaid certified facilities by regulation at CFR 483.75(l)(2)(3) and 483.75(l)(2)(4)(i)(ii)(iii), release of information from the resident's clinical record is permissible only when required by:

1. transfer to another health care institution,

2. law (both State and Federal), and/or

3. the resident.

Otherwise, providers cannot release MDS data in individual level format or in the aggregate. Nursing facility providers are also required under CFR 483.20 to transmit MDS data to a Federal data repository. Any personal data maintained and retrieved by the Federal government is subject to the requirements of the Privacy Act of 1974. The Privacy Act specifically protects the confidentiality of personal identifiable information and safeguards against its misuse. Information regarding The Privacy Act can be found at https://www.cms.gov/Research-Statistics-Data-and-Systems/Computer-Data-and-Systems/Privacy/PrivacyActof1974.html.

The Privacy Act requires by regulation that all individuals whose data are collected and maintained in a federal database must receive notice. Therefore, residents in nursing facilities must be informed that the MDS data is being collected and submitted to the national system, Quality Improvement Evaluation System Assessment Submission and Processing System (QIES ASAP) and the State MDS database. The notice shown on page 1-14 of this section meets the requirements of the Privacy Act of 1974 for nursing facilities. The form is a notice and not a consent to release or use MDS data for health care information. Each resident or family member must be given the notice containing submission information at the time of admission. It is important to remember that resident consent is not required to complete and submit MDS assessments that are required under Omnibus Budget Reconciliation Act of 1987 (OBRA '87) or for Medicare payment purposes.

Contractual Agreements

Providers, who are part of a multi-facility corporation, may release data to their corporate office or parent company but not to other providers within the multi-facility corporation. The parent company is required to "act" in the same manner as the facility and is permitted to use data only to the extent the facility is permitted to do so (as described in the 42 CFR at 483.10(e)(3)).

In the case where a facility submits MDS data to CMS through a contractor or through its corporate office, the contractor or corporate office has the same rights and restrictions as the facility does under the Federal and State regulations with respect to maintaining resident data, keeping such data confidential, and making disclosures of such data. This means that a contractor may maintain a database, but must abide by the same rules and regulations as the facility. Moreover, the fact that there may have been a change of ownership of a facility that has been transferring data through a contractor should not alter the contractor's rights and responsibilities;

presumably, the new owner has assumed existing contractual rights and obligations, including those under the contract for submitting MDS information. All contractual agreements, regardless of their type, involving the MDS data should not violate the requirements of participation in the Medicare and/or Medicaid program, the Privacy Act of 1974 or any applicable State laws.

PRIVACY ACT STATEMENT – HEALTH CARE RECORDS (7/14/2005)

THIS FORM IS NOT A CONSENT FORM TO RELEASE OR USE HEALTH CARE INFORMATION PERTAINING TO YOU.

1. **AUTHORITY FOR COLLECTION OF INFORMATION INCLUDING SOCIAL SECURITY NUMBER (SSN)**
Sections 1819(f), 1919(f), 1819(b)(3)(A), 1919(b)(3)(A), and 1864 of the Social Security Act.

2. **PRINCIPAL PURPOSES FOR WHICH INFORMATION IS INTENDED TO BE USED**
This form provides you the advice required by The Privacy Act of 1974. The personal information will facilitate tracking of changes in your health and functional status over time for purposes of evaluating and assuring the quality of care provided by nursing homes that participate in Medicare or Medicaid.

3. **ROUTINE USES**
The primary use of this information is to aid in the administration of the survey and certification of Medicare/Medicaid long-term care facilities and to improve the effectiveness and quality of care given in those facilities. This system will also support regulatory, reimbursement, policy, and research functions. This system will collect the minimum amount of personal data needed to accomplish its stated purpose. The information collected will be entered into the Long-Term Care Minimum Data Set (LTC MDS) system of records, System No. 09-70-1517. Information from this system may be disclosed, under specific circumstances (routine uses), which include: To the Census Bureau and to: (1) Agency contractors, or consultants who have been engaged by the Agency to assist in accomplishment of a CMS function, (2) another Federal or State agency, agency of a State government, an agency established by State law, or its fiscal agent to administer a Federal health program or a Federal/State Medicaid program and to contribute to the accuracy of reimbursement made for such programs, (3) to Quality Improvement Organizations (QIOs) to perform Title XI or Title XVIII functions, (4) to insurance companies, underwriters, third party administrators (TPA), employers, self-insurers, group health plans, health maintenance organizations (HMO) and other groups providing protection against medical expenses to verify eligibility for coverage or to coordinate benefits with the Medicare program, (5) an individual or organization for a research, evaluation, or epidemiological project related to the prevention of disease of disability, or the restoration of health, or payment related projects, (6) to a member of Congress or congressional staff member in response to an inquiry from a constituent, (7) to the Department of Justice, (8) to a CMS contractor that assists in the administration of a CMS-administered health benefits program or to a grantee of a CMS-administered grant program, (9) to another Federal agency or to an instrumentality of any governmental jurisdiction that administers, or that has the authority to investigate potential fraud or abuse in a health benefits program funded in whole or in part by Federal funds to prevent, deter, and detect fraud and abuse in those programs, (10) to national accrediting organizations, but only for those facilities that these accredit and that participate in the Medicare program.

4. **WHETHER DISCLOSURE IS MANDATORY OR VOLUNTARY AND EFFECT ON INDIVIDUAL OF NOT PROVIDING INFORMATION**
For Nursing Home residents residing in a certified Medicare/Medicaid nursing facility the requested information is mandatory because of the need to assess the effectiveness and quality of care given in certified facilities and to assess the appropriateness of provided services. If the requested information is not furnished the determination of beneficiary services and resultant reimbursement may not be possible.

Your signature merely acknowledges that you have been advised of the foregoing. If requested, a copy of this form will be furnished to you.

_____	_____
Signature of Resident or Sponsor	Date

NOTE: Providers may request to have the Resident or his or her Representative sign a copy of this notice as a means to document that notice was provided. Signature is NOT required. If the

Resident or his or her Representative agrees to sign the form it merely acknowledges that they have been advised of the foregoing information. Residents or their Representative must be supplied with a copy of the notice. This notice may be included in the admission packet for all new nursing home admissions.

Legal Notice Regarding MDS 3.0 - Copyright 2011 United States of America and interRAI. This work may be freely used and distributed solely within the United States. Portions of the MDS 3.0 are under separate copyright protections; Pfizer Inc. holds the copyright for the PHQ-9 and the Annals of Internal Medicine holds the copyright for the CAM. Both Pfizer Inc. and the Annals of Internal Medicine have granted permission to freely use these instruments in association with the MDS 3.0.

CHAPTER 2:   ASSESSMENTS FOR THE RESIDENT ASSESSMENT INSTRUMENT (RAI)

This chapter presents the assessment types and instructions for the completion (including timing and scheduling) of the mandated OBRA and Medicare assessments in nursing homes and the mandated Medicare assessments in non-critical access hospitals with a swing bed agreement.

2.1   Introduction to the Requirements for the RAI

The statutory authority for the RAI is found in Section 1819(f)(6)(A-B) for Medicare, and 1919 (f)(6)(A-B) for Medicaid, of the Social Security Act (SSA), as amended by the Omnibus Budget Reconciliation Act of 1987 (OBRA 1987). These sections of the SSA require the Secretary of the Department of Health and Human Services (the Secretary) to specify a Minimum Data Set (MDS) of core elements for use in conducting assessments of nursing home residents. It furthermore requires the Secretary to designate one or more resident assessment instruments based on the MDS.

The OBRA regulations require nursing homes that are Medicare certified, Medicaid certified or both, to conduct initial and periodic assessments for all their residents. The Resident Assessment Instrument (RAI) process is the basis for the accurate assessment of each nursing home resident. The MDS 3.0 is part of that assessment process and is required by CMS. The OBRA required assessments will be described in detail in Section 2.6.

MDS assessments are also required for Medicare payment (Prospective Payment System [PPS]) purposes under Medicare Part A (described in detail in Section 2.9).

It is important to note that when the OBRA and Medicare PPS assessment time frames coincide, one assessment may be used to satisfy both requirements. In such cases, the most stringent requirement for MDS completion must be met. Therefore, it is imperative that nursing home staff fully understand the requirements for both types of assessments in order to avoid unnecessary duplication of effort and to remain in compliance with both OBRA and Medicare PPS requirements. (Refer to Sections 2.11 and 2.12 for combining OBRA and Medicare assessments).

2.2   State Designation of the RAI for Nursing Homes

Federal regulatory requirements at 42 CFR 483.20(b)(1) and 483.20(c) require facilities to use an RAI that has been specified by the State and approved by CMS. The Federal requirement also mandates facilities to encode and electronically transmit the MDS data. (Detailed submission requirements are located in Chapter 5.)

While states must use all Federally-required MDS 3.0 items, they have some flexibility in adding optional Section S items. As such, each State must have CMS approval of the State's Comprehensive and Quarterly assessments.

- CMS's approval of a State's RAI covers the core items included on the instrument, the wording and sequencing of those items, and all definitions and instructions for the RAI.

- CMS's approval of a State's RAI does not include characteristics related to formatting (e.g., print type, color coding, or changes such as printing triggers on the assessment form).

- All comprehensive RAIs authorized by States must include at least the CMS MDS Version 3.0 (with or without optional Section S) and use of the Care Area Assessment (CAA) process (including CATs and the CAA Summary (Section V)).

- If allowed by the State, facilities may have some flexibility in form design (e.g., print type, color, shading, integrating triggers) or use a computer generated printout of the RAI as long as the State can ensure that the facility's RAI in the resident's record accurately and completely represents the CMS-approved State's RAI in accordance with 42 CFR 483.20(b). This applies to either pre-printed forms or computer generated printouts.

- Facility assessment systems must always be based on the MDS (i.e., both item terminology and definitions). However, facilities may insert additional items within automated assessment programs, but must be able to "extract" and print the MDS in a manner that replicates the State's RAI (i.e., using the exact wording and sequencing of items as is found on the State RAI).

Additional information about State specification of the RAI, variations in format and CMS approval of a State's RAI can be found in Sections 4145.1 - 4145.7 of the CMS State Operations Manual (SOM). For more information about your State's assessment requirements, contact your State RAI coordinator (see Appendix B).

2.3 Responsibilities of Nursing Homes for Completing Assessments

The requirements for the RAI are found at 42 CFR 483.20 and are applicable to all residents in Medicare and/or Medicaid certified long-term care facilities. The requirements are applicable regardless of age, diagnosis, length of stay, payment source or payer source. Federal RAI requirements are not applicable to individuals residing in non-certified units of long-term care facilities or licensed-only facilities. This does not preclude a State from mandating the RAI for residents who live in these units. Please contact your State RAI Coordinator for State requirements. A list of RAI Coordinators can be found in Appendix B.

An RAI (MDS, CAA process, and Utilization Guidelines) must be completed for any resident residing in the facility, including:

- **All residents** of Medicare (Title 18) skilled nursing facilities (SNFs) or Medicaid (Title 19) nursing facilities (NFs). This includes certified SNFs or NFs in hospitals, regardless of payment source.

- **Hospice Residents:** When a SNF or NF is the hospice patient's residence for purposes of the hospice benefit, the facility must comply with the Medicare or Medicaid participation requirements, meaning the resident must be assessed using the RAI, have a care plan and be provided with the services required under the plan of care. This can be achieved through cooperation of both the hospice and long-term care facility staff (including participation in completing the RAI and care planning) with the consent of the resident.

- **Short-term or respite residents:** An RAI must be completed for any individual residing more than 14 days on a unit of a facility that is certified as a long-term care facility for participation in the Medicare or Medicaid programs. If the respite resident is in a certified bed, the OBRA assessment schedule and tracking document requirements must be followed. If the respite resident is in the facility for fewer than 14 days, an OBRA Admission assessment is not required; however, a Discharge assessment is required:
  - Given the nature of a short-term or respite resident, staff members may not have access to all information required to complete some MDS items prior to the resident's discharge. In that case, the "not assessed/no information" coding convention should be used ("-") (See Chapter 3 for more information).
  - Regardless of the resident's length of stay, the facility must still have a process in place to identify the resident's needs, and must initiate a plan of care to meet those needs upon admission.
  - If the resident is eligible for Medicare Part A benefits, a Medicare assessment will still be required to support payment under the SNF PPS.

- **Special population residents (e.g. pediatric or residents with a psychiatric diagnosis):** Certified facilities are required to complete an RAI for all residents who reside in the facility, regardless of age or diagnosis.

- **Swing bed facility residents:** Swing beds of non-critical access hospitals that provide Part A skilled nursing facility-level services were phased into the SNF PPS on July 1, 2002 (referred to as swing beds in this manual). Swing bed providers must assess the clinical condition of beneficiaries by completing the MDS assessment for each Medicare resident receiving Part A SNF level of care in order to be reimbursed under the SNF PPS. CMS collects MDS data for quality monitoring purposes of swing bed facilities effective October 1, 2010. Therefore, swing bed providers must also complete the Entry record, Discharge assessments, and Death in Facility record. Requirements for the Medicare-required PPS assessments, Entry record, Discharge assessments and Death in Facility record outlined in this manual also apply to swing bed facilities, including but not limited to, completion date, encoding requirements, submission time frame, and RN signature. There is no longer a separate swing bed MDS assessment manual.

The RAI process <u>must</u> be used with residents in facilities with different certification situations, including:

- **Newly Certified Nursing Homes:**
  - Nursing homes must admit residents and operate in compliance with certification requirements before a certification survey can be conducted.
  - Nursing homes must meet specific requirements, 42 Code of Federal Regulations, Part 483 (Requirements for States and Long Term Care Facilities, Subpart B), in order to participate in the Medicare and/or Medicaid programs.

— The OBRA assessments are a requirement for long-term care facilities; therefore resident assessments are conducted prior to certification as if the beds were already certified.

— Then, assuming a survey is completed where the nursing home has been determined to be in substantial compliance, the facility will be certified effective the last day of the survey.

— NOTE: Even in situations where the facility's certification date is delayed due to the need for a resurvey, the facility must continue performing OBRA assessments according to the original schedule.

— For OBRA assessments, the assessment schedule is determined from the resident's actual date of admission. If a facility completes an Admission assessment prior to the certification date, there is no need to do another Admission assessment. The facility simply continues the OBRA schedule using the actual admission date as Day 1.

— Medicare cannot be billed for any care provided prior to the certification date. Therefore, the facility must use the certification date as Day 1 of the covered Part A stay when establishing the Assessment Reference Date (ARD) for the Medicare PPS assessments.

- **Adding Certified Beds:**
  — If the nursing home is already certified and is just adding additional certified beds, the procedure for changing the number of certified beds is different from that of the initial certification.

  — Medicare and Medicaid residents should not be placed in a bed until the facility has been notified that the bed has been certified.

- **Change In Ownership:** There are two types of change in ownership transactions:
  — The more common situation requires the new owner to assume the assets and liabilities of the prior owner. In this case:
    o The assessment schedule for existing residents continues, and the facility continues to use the existing provider number.

    o **Example:** if the Admission assessment was done 10 days prior to the change in ownership, the next OBRA assessment would be due no later than 92 days after the ARD (A2300) of the Admission assessment, and would be submitted using the existing provider number. If the resident is in a Part A stay, and the 14-Day Medicare PPS assessment was combined with the OBRA Admission assessment, the next regularly scheduled Medicare assessment would be the 30-Day MDS, and would also be submitted under the existing provider number.

  — There are also situations where the new owner does not assume the assets and liabilities of the previous owner. In these cases:
    o The beds are no longer certified.

    o There are no links to the prior provider, including sanctions, deficiencies, resident assessments, Quality Measures, debts, provider number, etc.

o The previous owner would complete a Discharge assessment - return not anticipated, thus code A0310F=10, A2000=date of ownership change, and A2100=02 for those residents who will remain in the facility.

o The new owner would complete an Admission assessment and Entry tracking record for all residents, thus code A0310F=01, A1600=date of ownership change, A1700=1 (admission), and A1800=02.

o Compliance with OBRA regulations, including the MDS requirements, is expected at the time of survey for certification of the facility with a new owner. See information above regarding newly certified nursing homes.

- **Resident Transfers:**
  - When transferring a resident, the transferring facility must provide the new facility with necessary medical records, including appropriate MDS assessments, to support the continuity of resident care.
  - When admitting a resident from another nursing home, regardless of whether or not it is a transfer within the same chain, a new Admission assessment must be done within 14 days. The MDS schedule then starts with the new Admission assessment and, if applicable, a 5-day Medicare-required PPS assessment.
  - The admitting facility should look at the previous facility's assessment in the same way they would review other incoming documentation about the resident for the purpose of understanding the resident's history and promoting continuity of care. However, the admitting facility must perform a new Admission assessment for the purpose of planning care within that facility to which the resident has been transferred.
  - When there has been a transfer of residents as a result of a natural disaster(s) (e.g., flood, earthquake, fire) with an **anticipated return** to the facility, the evacuating facility should contact their Regional Office, State agency, and Medicare contractor for guidance.
  - When there has been a transfer as a result of a natural disaster(s) (e.g., flood, earthquake, fire) and it has been determined that the resident will not return to the evacuating facility, the evacuating provider will discharge the resident **return not anticipated** and the receiving facility will admit the resident, with the MDS cycle beginning as of the admission date to the receiving facility. For questions related to this type of situation, providers should contact their Regional Office, State agency, and Medicare contractor for guidance.

2.4 Responsibilities of Nursing Homes for Reproducing and Maintaining Assessments

The Federal regulatory requirement at 42 CFR 483.20(d) requires nursing homes to maintain all resident assessments completed within the previous 15 months in the resident's active clinical record. This requirement applies to all MDS assessment types regardless of the form of storage (i.e., electronic or hard copy).

- The 15-month period for maintaining assessment data may not restart with each readmission to the facility:
  — When a resident is **discharged return anticipated** and the resident **returns to the facility within 30 days**, the facility must copy the previous RAI and transfer that copy to the new record. The15-month requirement for maintenance of the RAI data must be adhered to.
  — When a resident is **discharged return anticipated and does not return within 30 days** or **discharged return not anticipated**, facilities may develop their own specific policies regarding how to handle return situations, whether or not to copy the previous RAI to the new record.
  — In cases where the resident returns to the facility after a long break in care (i.e., 15 months or longer), staff may want to review the older record and familiarize themselves with the resident history and care needs. However, the decision on retaining the prior stay record in the active clinical record is a matter of facility policy and is not a CMS requirement.
- After the 15-month period, RAI information may be thinned from the clinical record and stored in the medical records department, provided that it is easily retrievable if requested by clinical staff, State agency surveyors, CMS, or others as authorized by law. The **exception** is that demographic information (Items A0500-A1600) from the most recent Admission assessment must be maintained in the active clinical record until the resident is discharged return not anticipated.
- Nursing homes may use electronic signatures for clinical record documentation, including the MDS, when permitted to do so by State and local law and when authorized by the long-term care facility's policy. Use of electronic signatures for the MDS does not require that the entire clinical record be maintained electronically. Facilities must have written policies in place to ensure proper security measures to protect the use of an electronic signature by anyone other than the person to whom the electronic signature belongs.
- Nursing homes also have the option for a resident's clinical record to be maintained electronically rather than in hard copy. This also applies to portions of the clinical record such as the MDS. Maintenance of the MDS electronically does not require that the entire clinical record also be maintained electronically, nor does it require the use of electronic signatures.
- In cases where the MDS is maintained electronically without the use of electronic signatures, nursing homes must maintain, at a minimum, hard copies of signed and dated CAA(s) completion (Items V0200B-C), correction completion (Items X1100A-E), and assessment completion (Items Z0400-Z0500) data that is resident-identifiable in the resident's active clinical record.
- Nursing homes must ensure that proper security measures are implemented via facility policy to ensure the privacy and integrity of the record.
- Nursing homes must also ensure that clinical records, regardless of form, are maintained in a centralized location as deemed by facility policy and procedure (e.g., a facility with five units may maintain all records in one location or by unit or a facility may maintain the MDS assessments and care plans in a separate binder). Nursing homes must also

ensure that clinical records, regardless of form, are easily and readily accessible to staff (including consultants), State agencies (including surveyors), CMS, and others who are authorized by law and need to review the information in order to provide care to the resident.

- Nursing homes that are not capable of maintenance of the MDS electronically must adhere to the current requirement that either a hand written **or** a computer-generated copy be maintained in the clinical record. Either is equally acceptable. This includes all MDS (including Quarterly) assessments and CAA(s) summary data completed during the previous 15-month period.

- All State licensure and State practice regulations continue to apply to Medicare and/or Medicaid certified long-term care facilities. Where State law is more restrictive than Federal requirements, the provider needs to apply the State law standard.

- In the future, long-term care facilities may be required to conform to a CMS electronic signature standard should CMS adopt one.

2.5 Assessment Types and Definitions

In order to understand the requirements for conducting assessments of nursing home residents, it is first important to understand some of the concepts and definitions associated with MDS assessments. Concepts and definitions for assessments are only introduced in this section. Detailed instructions are provided throughout the rest of this chapter.

Admission refers to the date a person enters the facility and is admitted as a resident. A day begins at 12:00 a.m. and ends at 11:59 p.m. Regardless of whether admission occurs at 12:00 a.m. or 11:59 p.m., this date is considered the 1st day of admission. Completion of an OBRA Admission assessment must occur in any of the following admission situations:

- when the resident has never been admitted to this facility before; OR

- when the resident has been in this facility previously and was discharged prior to completion of the OBRA Admission assessment; OR

- when the resident has been in this facility previously and was discharged return not anticipated; OR

- when the resident has been in this facility previously and was discharged return anticipated and did not return within 30 days of discharge (see Discharge assessment below).

Assessment Combination refers to the use of one assessment to satisfy both OBRA and Medicare PPS assessment requirements when the time frames coincide for both required assessments. In such cases, the most stringent requirement of the two assessments for MDS completion must be met. Therefore, it is imperative that nursing home staff fully understand the requirements for both types of assessments in order to avoid unnecessary duplication of effort and to remain in compliance with both OBRA and Medicare PPS requirements. Sections 2.11 and 2.12 provide more detailed information on combining Medicare and OBRA assessments. In addition, when all requirements for both are met, one assessment may satisfy two OBRA assessment requirements, such as Admission and Discharge assessment, or two PPS assessments, such as a 30-day assessment and an End of Therapy OMRA.

Assessment Completion refers to the date that all information needed has been collected and recorded for a particular assessment type and staff have signed and dated that the assessment is complete.

- For OBRA-required Comprehensive assessments, assessment completion is defined as completion of the CAA process in addition to the MDS items, meaning that the RN assessment coordinator has signed and dated both the MDS (Item Z0500) and CAA(s) (Item V0200B) completion attestations. Since a Comprehensive assessment includes completion of both the MDS and the CAA process, the assessment timing requirements for a comprehensive assessment apply to both the completion of the MDS and the CAA process.

- For non-comprehensive and Discharge assessments, assessment completion is defined as completion of the MDS only, meaning that the RN assessment coordinator has signed and dated the MDS (Item Z0500) completion attestation.

Completion requirements are dependent on the assessment type and timing requirements. Completion specifics by assessment type are discussed in Section 2.6 for OBRA assessments and Section 2.9 for Medicare assessments.

Assessment Reference Date (ARD) refers to the last day of the observation (or "look back") period that the assessment covers for the resident. Since a day begins at 12:00 a.m. and ends at 11:59 p.m., the ARD must also cover this time period. The facility is required to set the ARD on the MDS Item Set or in the facility software within the required timeframe of the assessment type being completed. This concept of setting the ARD is used for all assessment types (OBRA and Medicare-required PPS) and varies by assessment type and facility determination.

Most of the MDS 3.0 items have a 7 day look back period. If a resident has an ARD of July 1, 2011 then all pertinent information starting at 12 AM on June 25th and ending on July 1st at 11:59PM should be included for MDS 3.0 coding.

Assessment Scheduling refers to the period of time during which assessments take place, setting the ARD, timing, completion, submission, and the observation periods required to complete the MDS items.

Assessment Submission refers to electronic MDS data being in record and file formats that conform to standard record layouts and data dictionaries, and passes standardized edits defined by CMS and the State. Chapter 5, CFR 483.20(f)(2), and the MDS 3.0 Data Submission Specifications on the CMS MDS 3.0 web site provide more detailed information.

Assessment Timing refers to when and how often assessments must be conducted, based upon the resident's length of stay and the length of time between ARDs. The table in Section 2.6 describes the assessment timing schedule for OBRA-required assessments, while information on the Medicare-required PPS assessment timing schedule is provided in Section 2.8.

- For OBRA-required assessments, regulatory requirements for each assessment type dictate assessment timing, the schedule for which is established with the Admission (comprehensive) assessment when the ARD is set by the RN assessment coordinator and the Interdisciplinary team (IDT).

- Assuming the resident did not experience a significant change in status, was not discharged, and did not have a Significant Correction to Prior Comprehensive assessment (SCPA) completed, assessment scheduling would then move through a cycle of three Quarterly assessments followed by an Annual (comprehensive) assessment.

- This cycle (Comprehensive assessment – Quarterly assessment – Quarterly assessment – Quarterly assessment – Comprehensive assessment) would repeat itself annually for the resident who: 1) the IDT determines the criteria for a Significant Change in Status Assessment (SCSA) has not occurred, 2) an uncorrected significant error in prior comprehensive or Quarterly assessment was not determined, and 3) was not discharged with return not anticipated.

- OBRA assessments may be scheduled early if a nursing home wants to stagger due dates for assessments. As a result, more than three OBRA Quarterly assessments may be completed on a particular resident in a given year, or the Annual may be completed early to ensure that regulatory time frames between assessments are met. However, States may have more stringent restrictions.

- When a resident does have a SCSA or SCPA completed, the assessment resets the assessment timing/scheduling. The next Quarterly assessment would be scheduled within 92 days after the ARD of the SCSA or SCPA, and the next comprehensive assessment would be scheduled within 366 days after the ARD of the SCSA or SCPA.

- Early Medicare-required assessments completed with an ARD prior to the beginning of the prescribed ARD window will have a payment penalty applied (see Section 2.13).

Assessment Transmission refers to the electronic transmission of submission files to the QIES Assessment Submission and Processing (ASAP) system using the Medicare Data Communication Network (MDCN). Chapter 5 and the CMS MDS 3.0 web site provide more detailed information.

Comprehensive MDS assessments include both the completion of the MDS as well as completion of the Care Area Assessment (CAA) process and care planning. Comprehensive MDSs include Admission, Annual, Significant Change in Status Assessment (SCSA), and Significant Correction to Prior Comprehensive Assessment (SCPA).

Death In Facility refers to when the resident dies in the facility or dies while on a leave of absence (LOA) (see LOA definition). The facility must complete a Death in Facility tracking record. A Discharge assessment is not required.

Discharge refers to the date a resident leaves the facility. A day begins at 12:00 a.m. and ends at 11:59 p.m. Regardless of whether discharge occurs at 12:00 a.m. or 11:59 p.m., this date is considered the actual date of discharge. There are two types of discharges – return anticipated and return not anticipated. A Discharge assessment is required with both types of discharges. Section 2.6 provides detailed instructions regarding both discharge types. Any of the following situations warrant a Discharge assessment, regardless of facility policies regarding opening and closing clinical records and bed holds:

- resident is discharged from the facility to a private residence (as opposed to going on an LOA);
- resident is admitted to a hospital or other care setting (regardless of whether the nursing home discharges or formally closes the record);
- resident has a hospital observation stay greater than 24 hours, regardless of whether the hospital admits the resident.

Discharge Assessment refers to an assessment required on resident discharge. This assessment includes clinical items for quality monitoring as well as discharge tracking information.

Entry is a term used for both an admission and a reentry, and requires completion of an Entry tracking record.

Entry and Discharge Reporting MDS assessments and tracking records that include a select number of items from the MDS used to track residents and gather important quality data at transition points, such as when they enter or leave a nursing home. Entry/Discharge reporting includes Entry tracking record, Discharge assessments, and Death in Facility tracking record.

Interdisciplinary Team (IDT[1]) is a group of clinicians from several medical fields that combines knowledge, skills, and resources to provide care to the resident.

Item Set refers to the MDS items that are active on a particular assessment type or tracking form. There are 10 different item subsets for nursing homes and 8 for swing bed providers as follows:

- **Nursing Home**
  - **Comprehensive (NC[2]) Item Set.** This is the set of items active on an OBRA Comprehensive assessment (Admission, Annual, Significant Change in Status, and Significant Correction of Prior Comprehensive Assessments). This item set is used whether the OBRA Comprehensive assessment is stand-alone or combined with any other assessment (PPS assessment and/or Discharge assessment).
  - **Quarterly (NQ) Item Set.** This is the set of items active on an OBRA Quarterly assessment (including Significant Correction of Prior Quarter Assessment). This item set is used for a stand-alone Quarterly assessment or a Quarterly assessment combined with any type of PPS assessment and/or Discharge assessment
  - **PPS (NP) Item Set.** This is the set of items active on a scheduled PPS assessment (5-day, 14-day, 30-day, 60-day, or 90-day). This item set is used for a standalone.

---

[1] 42 CFR 483.20(k)(2) A comprehensive care plan must be (ii) Prepared by an interdisciplinary team, that includes the attending physician, a registered nurse with responsibility for the resident, and other appropriate staff in disciplines as determined by the resident's needs, and, to the extent practicable, the participation of the resident, the resident's family or the resident's legal representative;"

[2] The codes in parentheses are the item set codes (ISCs) used in the data submission specifications.

scheduled PPS assessment or a scheduled PPS assessment combined with a PPS OMRA assessment and/or a Discharge assessment.

— **OMRA - Start of Therapy (NS) Item Set.** This is the set of items active on a standalone start of therapy OMRA assessment.

— **OMRA - Start of Therapy and Discharge (NSD) Item Set.** This is the set of items active on a PPS start of therapy OMRA assessment combined with a Discharge assessment (either return anticipated or not anticipated).

— **OMRA (NO) Item Set.** This is the set of items active on a standalone end of therapy OMRA and a change of therapy OMRA assessment. The code used is "NO" since this was the only type of OMRA when the code was initially assigned.

— **OMRA - Discharge (NOD) Item Subset.** This is the set of items active on a PPS end of therapy OMRA assessment combined with a Discharge assessment (either return anticipated or not anticipated).

— **Discharge (ND) Item Set.** This is the set of items active on a standalone Discharge assessment (either return anticipated or not anticipated).

— **Tracking (NT) Item Set.** This is the set of items active on an Entry Tracking Record or a Death in Facility Tracking Record.

— **Inactivation Request (XX) Item Set.** This is the set of items active on a request to inactivate a record in the national MDS QIES ASAP system.

- **Swing Beds**

— **PPS (SP) Item Set.** This is the set of items active on a scheduled PPS assessment (5-day, 14-day, 30-day, 60-day, or 90-day) or a Swing Bed Clinical Change assessment. This item set is used for a scheduled PPS assessment that is standalone or in any combination with other swing bed assessments (Swing Bed Clinical Change assessment, OMRA assessment, and/or Discharge assessment). This item set is also used for a Swing Bed Clinical Change assessment that is standalone or in any combination with other swing bed assessments (scheduled PPS assessment, OMRA assessment, and/or Discharge assessment).

— **OMRA – Start of Therapy (SS) Item Set.** This is the set of items active on a standalone start of therapy OMRA assessment.

— **OMRA – Start of Therapy and Discharge Assessment (SSD) Item Set.** This is the set of items active on a PPS start of therapy OMRA assessment combined with a Discharge assessment (either return anticipated or not anticipated).

— **OMRA (SO) Item Set.** This is the set of items active on a standalone end of therapy OMRA and change of therapy OMRA assessment.

— **OMRA - Discharge Assessment (SOD) Item Set.** This is the set of items active on a PPS end of therapy OMRA assessment combined with a Discharge assessment (either return anticipated or not anticipated).

— **Discharge (SD) Item Set.** This is the set of items active on a standalone Discharge assessment (either return anticipated or not anticipated).

— **Tracking (ST) Item Set.** This is the set of items active on an Entry Tracking Record or a Death in Facility Tracking Record.

— **Inactivation (XX) Item Set.** This is the set of items active on a request to inactivate a record in the national MDS QIES ASAP system.

Printed layouts for the item sets are available on the CMS website at: http://www.cms.gov/NursingHomeQualityInits/45_NHQIMDS30TrainingMaterials.asp#TopOfPage

The item set for a particular MDS record is completely determined by the reason for assessment Items (A0310A, A0310B, A0310C, A0310D, and A0310F). Item set determination is complicated and standard MDS software from CMS and private vendors will automatically make this determination. Section 2-15 of this chapter provides manual lookup tables for determining the item set, when automated software is unavailable.

Leave of Absence (LOA), which does not require completion of either a Discharge assessment or an Entry tracking record, occurs when a resident has a:

- Temporary home visit of at least one night; or
- Therapeutic leave of at least one night; or
- Hospital observation stay less than 24 hours and the hospital does not admit the patient.

Providers should refer to Chapter 6 and their State LOA policy for further information, if applicable.

Upon return, providers should make appropriate documentation in the medical record regarding any changes in the resident. If there are changes noted, they should be documented in the medical record.

MDS Assessment Codes are those values that correspond to the OBRA-required and Medicare- required PPS assessments represented in Items A0310A, A0310B, A0310C, and A0310F of the MDS 3.0. They will be used to reference assessment types throughout the rest of this chapter.

Medicare-Required PPS Assessments provide information about the clinical condition of beneficiaries receiving Part A SNF-level care in order to be reimbursed under the SNF PPS for both SNFs and Swing Bed providers. Medicare-required PPS MDSs can be scheduled or unscheduled. These assessments are coded on the MDS 3.0 in Items A0310B (PPS Assessment) and A0310C (PPS Other Medicare Required Assessment – OMRA). They include:

- 5-day
- 14-day
- 30-day
- 60-day
- 90-day
- Readmission/Return
- SCSA
- SCPA
- Swing Bed Clinical Change (CCA)

- Start of Therapy (SOT) Other Medicare Required (OMRA)
- End of Therapy (EOT) OMRA
- Both Start and End of Therapy OMRA
- Change of Therapy (COT) OMRA

Non-Comprehensive MDS assessments include a select number of items from the MDS used to track the resident's status between comprehensive assessments and to ensure monitoring of critical indicators of the gradual onset of significant changes in resident status. They do not include completion of the CAA process and care planning. Non-comprehensive assessments include Quarterly and Significant Correction to Prior Quarterly (SCQA) assessments.

Observation (Look Back) Period is the time period over which the resident's condition or status is captured by the MDS assessment. When the resident is first admitted to the nursing home, the RN assessment coordinator and the IDT will set the ARD. For subsequent assessments, the observation period for a particular assessment for a particular resident will be chosen based upon the regulatory requirements concerning timing and the ARDs of previous assessments. Most MDS items themselves require an observation period, such as 7 or 14 days, depending on the item. Since a day begins at 12:00 a.m. and ends at 11:59 p.m., the observation period must also cover this time period. When completing the MDS, only those occurrences during the look back period will be captured. In other words, if it did not occur during the look back period, it is not coded on the MDS.

OBRA-Required Tracking Records and Assessments are federally mandated, and therefore, must be performed for all residents of Medicare and/or Medicaid certified nursing homes. These assessments are coded on the MDS 3.0 in Items A0310A (Federal OBRA Reason for Assessment) and A0310F (Entry/discharge reporting). They include:

Tracking records

- Entry
- Death in facility

Assessments

- Admission (comprehensive)
- Quarterly
- Annual (comprehensive)
- SCSA (comprehensive)
- SCPA (comprehensive)
- SCQA
- Discharge (return not anticipated or return anticipated)

Reentry refers to the situation when a resident was previously in this nursing home **and** had an OBRA Admission assessment completed **and** was discharged return anticipated **and** returned within 30 days of discharge. Upon the resident's return to the facility, the facility is required to complete an Entry tracking record. In determining if the resident returned to facility within 30 days, the day of discharge from the facility is not counted in the 30 days. For example, a resident who is discharged return anticipated on December 1 would need to return to the facility by December 31 to meet the "within 30 day" requirement.

Respite refers to short-term, temporary care provided to a resident to allow family members to take a break from the daily routine of care giving. The nursing home is required to complete an Entry tracking record and a Discharge assessment for all respite residents. If the respite stay is 14 days or longer, the facility must have completed an OBRA Admission.

2.6   Required OBRA Assessments for the MDS

If the assessment is being used for OBRA requirements, the OBRA reason for assessment must be coded in Items A0310A and A0310F (Discharge Assessment). Medicare reasons for assessment are described later in this chapter (Section 2.9) while the OBRA reasons for assessment are described below.

The table provides a summary of the assessment types and requirements for the OBRA-required assessments, the details of which will be discussed throughout the remainder of this chapter.

RAI OBRA-required Assessment Summary

Assessment Type	MDS Assessment Code (A0310A or A0310F)	Assessment Reference Date (ARD) (Item A2300) No Later Than	7-day Observation Period (Look Back) Consists Of	14-day Observation Period (Look Back) Consists Of	MDS Completion Date (Item Z0500B) No Later Than	CAA(s) Completion Date (Item V0200B2) No Later Than	Care Plan Completion Date (Item V0200C2) No Later Than	Transmission Date No Later Than	Regulatory Requirement	Assessment Combination
Admission (Comprehensive)	A0310A = 01	14th calendar day of the resident's admission (admission date + 13 calendar days)	ARD + 6 previous calendar days	ARD +13 previous calendar days	14th calendar day of the resident's admission (admission date + 13 calendar days)	Same as MDS Completion Date	CAA(s) Completion Date + 7 calendar days	Care Plan Completion Date + 14 calendar days	42 CFR 483.20 (Initial) 42 CFR 483.20 (b)(2)(i) (by the 14th day)	May be combined with another assessment
Annual (Comprehensive)	A0310A = 03	ARD of previous OBRA comprehensive assessment + 366 calendar days AND ARD of previous OBRA Quarterly assessment + 92 calendar days	ARD + 6 previous calendar days	ARD +13 previous calendar days	ARD + 14 calendar days	Same as MDS Completion Date	CAA(s) Completion Date + 7 calendar days	Care Plan Completion Date + 14 calendar days	42 CFR 483.20 (b)(2)(iii) (every 12 months)	May be combined with another assessment
Significant Change in Status (SCSA) (Comprehensive)	A0310A = 04	14th calendar day after determination that significant change in resident's status occurred (determination date + 14 calendar days)	ARD + 6 previous calendar days	ARD + 13 previous calendar days	14th calendar day after determination that significant change in resident's status occurred (determination date + 14 calendar days)	Same as MDS Completion Date	CAA(s) Completion Date + 7 calendar days	Care Plan Completion Date + 14 calendar days	42 CFR 483.20 (b)(2)(ii) (within 14 days)	May be combined with another assessment
Significant Correction to Prior Comprehensive (SCPA) (Comprehensive)	A0310A = 05	14th calendar day after determination that significant error in prior comprehensive assessment occurred (determination date + 14 calendar days)	ARD + 6 previous calendar days	ARD + 13 previous calendar days	14th calendar day after determination that significant error in prior comprehensive assessment occurred (determination date + 14 calendar days)	Same as MDS Completion Date	CAA(s) Completion Date + 7 calendar days	Care Plan Completion Date + 14 calendar days	42 CFR 483.20(f)(3)(iv)	May be combined with another assessment

(continued)

RAI OBRA-required Assessment Summary (con't)

Assessment Type	MDS Assessment Code (A0310A or A0310F)	Assessment Reference Date (ARD) (Item A2300) No Later Than	7-day Observation Period (Look Back) Consists Of	14-day Observation Period (Look Back) Consists Of	MDS Completion Date (Item Z0500B) No Later Than	CAA(s) Completion Date (Item V0200B2) No Later Than	Care Plan Completion Date (Item V0200C2) No Later Than	Transmission Date No Later Than	Regulatory Requirement	Assessment Combination
Quarterly (Non-Comprehensive)	A0310A=02	ARD of previous OBRA assessment of any type + 92 calendar days	ARD + 6 previous calendar days	ARD + 13 previous calendar days	ARD + 14 calendar days	N/A	N/A	MDS Completion Date + 14 calendar days	42 CFR 483.20(c) (every 3 months)	May be combined with another assessment
Significant Correction to Prior Quarterly (SCQA) (Non-Comprehensive)	A0310A=06	14th day after determination that significant error in prior quarterly assessment occurred (determination date + 14 calendar days)	ARD + 6 previous calendar days	ARD + 13 previous calendar days	14th day after determination that significant error in prior quarterly assessment occurred (determination date + 14 calendar days)	N/A	N/A	MDS Completion Date + 14 calendar days	42 CFR 483.20(f) (3)(v)	May be combined with another assessment
Discharge Assessment – return not anticipated (Non-Comprehensive)	A0310F=10	N/A	N/A	N/A	Discharge Date + 14 calendar days	N/A	N/A	MDS Completion Date + 14 calendar days		May be combined with another assessment
Discharge Assessment – return anticipated (Non-Comprehensive)	A0310F=11	N/A	N/A	N/A	Discharge Date + 14 calendar days	N/A	N/A	MDS Completion Date + 14 calendar days		May be combined with another assessment
Entry tracking record	A0310F=01	N/A	N/A	N/A	Entry Date + 7 calendar days	N/A		Entry Date + 14 calendar days		May not be combined with another assessment
Death in facility tracking record	A0310F=12	N/A	N/A	N/A	Discharge (death) Date + 7 calendar days	N/A	N/A	Discharge (death) Date +14 calendar days		May not be combined with another assessment

Comprehensive Assessments

OBRA-required comprehensive assessments include the completion of both the MDS and the CAA process, as well as care planning. Comprehensive assessments are completed upon admission, annually, and when a significant change in a resident's status has occurred or a significant correction to a prior comprehensive assessment is required. They consist of:

- Admission Assessment
- Annual Assessment
- Significant Change in Status Assessment
- Significant Correction to Prior Comprehensive Assessment

Each of these assessment types will be discussed in detail in this section. They are **not** required for residents in swing bed facilities.

Assessment Management Requirements and Tips for Comprehensive Assessments:

- The ARD (Item A2300) is the last day of the observation/look back period, and day 1 for purposes of counting back to determine the beginning of observation/look back periods. For example, if the ARD is set for day 14 of a resident's admission, then the beginning of the observation period for MDS items requiring a 7-day observation period would be day 8 of admission (ARD + 6 previous calendar days), while the beginning of the observation period for MDS items requiring a 14-day observation period would be day 1 of admission (ARD + 13 previous calendar days).
- If a resident goes to the hospital **prior** to completion of the OBRA Admission assessment, when the resident returns, the nursing home must consider the resident as a new admission. The nursing home may not complete a Significant Change in Status Assessment until after an OBRA Admission assessment has been completed.
- If a resident had an OBRA Admission assessment completed and then goes to the hospital (discharge return anticipated and returns within 30 days) and returns during an assessment period and most of the assessment was completed prior to the hospitalization, then the nursing home may wish to continue with the original assessment, provided the resident does not meet the criteria for a SCSA. In this case, the ARD remains the same and the assessment must be completed by the completion dates required of the assessment type based on the timeframe in which the assessment was started. Otherwise, the assessment should be reinitiated with a new ARD and completed within 14 days after re-entry from the hospital. The portion of the resident's assessment that was previously completed should be stored on the resident's record with a notation that the assessment was reinitiated because the resident was hospitalized.
- If a resident is discharged prior to the completion deadline for the assessment, completion of the assessment is not required. Whatever portions of the RAI that have been completed

must be maintained in the resident's medical record.[3] In closing the record, the nursing home should note why the RAI was not completed.

- If a resident dies prior to the completion deadline for the assessment, completion of the assessment is not required. Whatever portions of the RAI that have been completed must be maintained in the resident's medical record.[4] In closing the record, the nursing home should note why the RAI was not completed.

- If a significant change in status is identified in the process of completing any assessment except Admission and SCSAs, code and complete the assessment as a comprehensive SCSA instead.

- The nursing home may combine a comprehensive assessment with a Discharge assessment.

- In the process of completing any assessment except an Admission and a SCPA, if it is identified that an uncorrected significant error occurred in a previous assessment that has already been submitted and accepted into the MDS system, and has not already been corrected in a subsequent comprehensive assessment, code and complete the assessment as a comprehensive SCPA instead. A correction request for the erroneous assessment should also be completed and submitted. See the section on SCPAs for detailed information on completing a SCPA, and chapter 5 for detailed information on processing corrections.

- In the process of completing any assessment except an Admission, if it is identified that a non-significant (minor) error occurred in a previous assessment, continue with completion of the assessment in progress and also submit a correction request for the erroneous assessment as per the instructions in Chapter 5.

- The MDS must be transmitted (submitted and accepted into the MDS database) electronically no later than 14 calendar days after the care plan completion date (V0200C2 + 14 calendar days).

- The ARD of an assessment drives the due date of the next assessment. The next comprehensive assessment is due within 366 days after the ARD of the most recent comprehensive assessment.

- May be combined with a Medicare-required PPS assessment (see Sections 2.11 and 2.12 for details).

OBRA-required comprehensive assessments include the following types, which are numbered according to their MDS 3.0 assessment code (Item A0310A).

01.   Admission Assessment (A0310A=01)

The Admission assessment is a comprehensive assessment for a new resident and, under some circumstances, a returning resident that must be completed by the end of day 14, counting the date of admission to the nursing home as day 1 if:

---

[3]   The RAI is considered part of the resident's clinical record and is treated as such by the RAI utilization guidelines, e.g., portions of the RAI that are "started" must be saved.

[4]   The RAI is considered part of the resident's clinical record and is treated as such by the RAI utilization guidelines, e.g., portions of the RAI that are "started" must be saved.

- this is the resident's first time in this facility, OR
- the resident had been in this facility previously and was discharged prior to completion of the OBRA Admission assessment, OR
- the resident has been admitted to this facility and was discharged return not anticipated, OR
- the resident has been admitted to this facility and was discharged return anticipated and did not return within 30 days of discharge.

Assessment Management Requirements and Tips for Admission Assessments:

- Since a day begins at 12:00 a.m. and ends at 11:59 p.m., the actual date of admission, regardless of whether admission occurs at 12:00 am or 11:59 pm, is considered day "1" of admission.
- The ARD (Item A2300) must be set no later than day 14, counting the date of admission as day 1. Since a day begins at 12:00 a.m. and ends at 11:59 p.m., the ARD must also cover this time period. For example, if a resident is admitted at 8:30 a.m. on Wednesday (day 1), a completed RAI is required by the end of the day Tuesday (day 14).
- Federal statute and regulations require that residents are assessed promptly upon admission (but no later than day 14) and the results are used in planning and providing appropriate care to attain or maintain the highest practicable well-being. This means it is imperative for nursing homes to assess a resident upon the individual's admission. The IDT may choose to start and complete the Admission comprehensive assessment at any time prior to the end of day 14. Nursing homes may find early completion of the MDS and CAA(s) beneficial to providing appropriate care, particularly for individuals with short lengths of stay when the assessment and care planning process is often accelerated.
- The MDS completion date (Item Z0500B) must be no later than day 14. This date may be earlier than or the same as the CAA(s) completion date, but not later than.
- The CAA(s) completion date (Item V0200B2) must be no later than day 14.
- The care plan completion date (Item V0200C2) must be no later than 7 calendar days after the CAA(s) completion date (Item V0200B2) (CAA(s) completion date + 7 calendar days).
- For a resident who goes in and out of the facility on a relatively frequent basis and return is expected within the next 30 days, the resident may be discharged with return anticipated. This status **requires** an Entry tracking record **each time** the resident returns to the facility and a Discharge assessment **each time** the resident is discharged. The nursing home may combine the Admission assessment with the Discharge assessment when applicable.

02. Annual Assessment (A0310A=03)

The Annual assessment is a comprehensive assessment for a resident that must be completed on an annual basis (at least every 366 days) unless a SCSA or a SCPA has been completed since the most recent comprehensive assessment was completed. Its completion dates (MDS/CAA(s)/care plan) depend on the most recent comprehensive and past assessments' ARDs and completion dates.

Assessment Management Requirements and Tips for Annual Assessments:

- The ARD (Item A2300) must be set within 366 days after the ARD of the previous OBRA comprehensive assessment (ARD of previous comprehensive assessment + 366 calendar days) AND within 92 days since the ARD of the previous OBRA Quarterly or Significant Correction to Prior Quarterly assessment (ARD of previous OBRA Quarterly assessment + 92 calendar days).

- The MDS completion date (Item Z0500B) must be no later than 14 days after the ARD (ARD + 14 calendar days). This date may be earlier than or the same as the CAA(s) completion date, but not later than.

- The CAA(s) completion date (Item V0200B2) must be no later than 14 days after the ARD (ARD + 14 calendar days). This date may be the same as the MDS completion date, but not earlier than.

- The care plan completion date (Item V0200C2) must be no later than 7 calendar days after the CAA(s) completion date (Item V0200B2) (CAA(s) completion date + 7 calendar days).

03. Significant Change In Status Assessment (SCSA) (A0310A=04)

The SCSA is a comprehensive assessment for a resident that must be completed when the IDT has determined that a resident meets the significant change guidelines for either improvement or decline. It can be performed at any time after the completion of an Admission assessment, and its completion dates (MDS/CAA(s)/care plan) depend on the date that the IDT's determination was made that the resident had a significant change.

A **"significant change"** is a decline or improvement in a resident's status that:

1. Will not normally resolve itself without intervention by staff or by implementing standard disease-related clinical interventions, is not "self-limiting" (for declines only);

2. Impacts more than one area of the resident's health status; and

3. Requires interdisciplinary review and/or revision of the care plan.

A significant change differs from a significant error because it reflects an actual significant change in the resident's health status and NOT incorrect coding of the MDS.
A significant change may require referral for a Preadmission Screening and Resident Review (PASRR) evaluation if a mental illness, intellectual disability (ID), or related condition is present or is suspected to be present.

Assessment Management Requirements and Tips for Significant Change in Status Assessments:

- When a resident's status changes and it is not clear whether the resident meets the SCSA guidelines, the nursing home may take up to 14 days to determine whether the criteria are met.

- After the IDT has determined that a resident meets the significant change guidelines, the nursing home should document the initial identification of a significant change in the resident's status in the progress notes.

- A SCSA is appropriate when:

  — There is a determination that a significant change (either improvement or decline) in a resident's condition from his/her baseline has occurred as indicated by comparison of the resident's current status to the most recent comprehensive assessment and any subsequent Quarterly assessments; and

  — The resident's condition is not expected to return to baseline within two weeks.

  — For a resident who goes in and out of the facility on a relatively frequent basis and reentry is expected within the next 30 days, the resident may be discharged with return anticipated. This status requires an Entry tracking record each time the resident returns to the facility and a Discharge assessment each time the resident is discharged. However, if the IDT determines that the resident would benefit from a Significant Change in Status Assessment during the intervening period, the staff must complete a SCSA. This is only allowed when the resident has had an OBRA Admission assessment completed and submitted prior to discharge return anticipated (and resident returns within 30 days) or when the OBRA Admission assessment is combined with the discharge return anticipated assessment (and resident returns within 30 days).

- A SCSA may **not** be completed prior to an OBRA Admission assessment.

- A SCSA is required to be performed when a terminally ill resident enrolls in a hospice program (Medicare Hospice or other structured hospice) and remains a resident at the nursing home. The ARD must be within 14 days from the effective date of the hospice election (which can be the same or later than the date of the hospice election statement, but not earlier than). A SCSA must be performed regardless of whether an assessment was recently conducted on the resident. This is to ensure a coordinated plan of care between the hospice and nursing home is in place. A Medicare-certified hospice must conduct an assessment at the initiation of its services. This is an appropriate time for the nursing home to evaluate the MDS information to determine if it reflects the current condition of the resident, since the nursing home remains responsible for providing necessary care and services to assist the resident in achieving his/her highest practicable well-being at whatever stage of the disease process the resident is experiencing.

- If a resident is admitted on the hospice benefit (i.e. the resident is coming into the facility having already elected hospice), the facility should complete the Admission assessment, checking the Hospice Care item, O0100K. Completing an Admission assessment followed by a SCSA is not required.

- A SCSA is required to be performed when a resident is receiving hospice services and then decides to discontinue those services (known as revoking of hospice care). The ARD must be within 14 days from one of the following: 1) the effective date of the hospice election revocation (which can be the same or later than the date of the hospice election revocation statement, but not earlier than); 2) the expiration date of the certification of terminal illness; or 3) the date of the physician's or medical director's order stating the resident is no longer terminally ill.

- The ARD must be within 14 days after the determination that the criteria are met for a SCSA (determination date + 14 calendar days) but no later than day 14 after the IDT's determination is made that the criteria for a SCSA are met.

- The MDS completion date (Item Z0500B) must be no later than 14 days from the ARD (ARD + 14 calendar days) and no later than 14 days after the determination that the criteria for a SCSA were met. This date may be earlier than or the same as the CAA(s) completion date, but not later than.

- When a SCSA is completed, the nursing home must review all triggered care areas compared to the resident's previous status. If the CAA process indicates no change in a care area, then the prior documentation for the particular care area may be carried forward, and the nursing home should specify where the supporting documentation can be located in the medical record.

- The CAA(s) completion date (Item V0200B2) must be no later than 14 days after the ARD (ARD + 14 calendar days) and no later than 14 days after the determination that the criteria for a SCSA were met. This date may be the same as the MDS completion date, but not earlier than MDS completion.

- The care plan completion date (Item V0200C2) must be no later than 7 calendar days after the CAA(s) completion date (Item V0200B2) (CAA(s) completion date + 7 calendar days).

Guidelines for Determining a Significant Change in a Resident's Status:
Note: this is not an exhaustive list

The final decision regarding what constitutes a significant change in status must be based upon the judgment of the IDT. MDS assessments are not required for minor or temporary variations in resident status - in these cases, the resident's condition is expected to return to baseline within 2 weeks. However, staff must note these transient changes in the resident's status in the resident's record and implement necessary assessment, care planning, and clinical interventions, even though an MDS assessment is not required.

Some Guidelines to Assist in Deciding if a Change is Significant or Not:

- A condition is defined as "self-limiting" when the condition will normally resolve itself without further intervention or by staff implementing standard disease-related clinical interventions. If the condition has not resolved within 2 weeks, staff should begin a SCSA. This timeframe may vary depending on clinical judgment and resident needs. For example, a 5% weight loss for a resident with the flu would not normally meet the requirements for a SCSA. In general, a 5% weight loss may be an expected outcome for a resident with the flu who experienced nausea and diarrhea for a week. In this situation, staff should monitor the resident's status and attempt various interventions to rectify the immediate weight loss. If the resident did not become dehydrated and started to regain weight after the symptoms subsided, a comprehensive assessment would not be required.

- A SCSA is appropriate if there are either two or more areas of decline or two or more areas of improvement. In this example, a resident with a 5% weight loss in 30 days would not generally require a SCSA unless a second area of decline accompanies it. Note that this assumes that the care plan has already been modified to actively treat the weight loss as opposed to continuing with the original problem, "potential for weight loss." This situation should be documented in the resident's clinical record along with the plan for subsequent monitoring and, if the problem persists or worsens, a SCSA may be warranted.

- **If there is only one change**, staff may still decide that the resident would benefit from a SCSA. It is important to remember that each resident's situation is unique and the IDT must make the decision as to whether or not the resident will benefit from a SCSA. Nursing homes must document a rationale, in the resident's medical record, for completing a SCSA that does not meet the criteria for completion.

- A SCSA is also appropriate if there is a consistent pattern of changes, with either two or more areas of decline or two or more areas of improvement. This may include two changes within a particular domain (e.g., two areas of ADL decline or improvement).

- A SCSA would not be appropriate in situations where the resident has stabilized but is expected to be discharged in the immediate future. The nursing home has engaged in discharge planning with the resident and family, and a comprehensive reassessment is not necessary to facilitate discharge planning;

- **Decline in two or more of the following:**
  - Resident's decision-making changes;
  - Presence of a resident mood item not previously reported by the resident or staff and/or an increase in the symptom frequency (PHQ-9$^©$), e.g., increase in the number of areas where behavioral symptoms are coded as being present and/or the frequency of a symptom increases for items in Section E (Behavior);
  - Any decline in an ADL physical functioning area where a resident is newly coded as Extensive assistance, Total dependence, or Activity did not occur since last assessment;
  - Resident's incontinence pattern changes or there was placement of an indwelling catheter;
  - Emergence of unplanned weight loss problem (5% change in 30 days or 10% change in 180 days);
  - Emergence of a new pressure ulcer at Stage II or higher or worsening in pressure ulcer status;
  - Resident begins to use trunk restraint or a chair that prevents rising when it was not used before; and/or
  - Overall deterioration of resident's condition.

Examples (SCSA):

1. Mr. T no longer responds to verbal requests to alter his screaming behavior. It now occurs daily and has neither lessened on its own nor responded to treatment. He is also starting to resist his daily care, pushing staff away from him as they attempt to assist with his ADLs. This is a significant change, and a SCSA is required, since there has been deterioration in the behavioral symptoms to the point where it is occurring daily and new approaches are needed to alter the behavior. Mr. T's behavioral symptoms could have many causes, and a SCSA

will provide an opportunity for staff to consider illness, medication reactions, environmental stress, and other possible sources of Mr. T's disruptive behavior.

2. Mrs. T required minimal assistance with ADLs. She fractured her hip and upon return to the facility requires extensive assistance with all ADLs. Rehab has started and staff is hopeful she will return to her prior level of function in 4-6 weeks.

    - **Improvement in two or more of the following:**
        - — Any improvement in an ADL physical functioning area where a resident is newly coded as Independent, Supervision, or Limited assistance since last assessment;
        - — Decrease in the number of areas where Behavioral symptoms are coded as being present and/or the frequency of a symptom decreases;
        - — Resident's decision making changes for the better;
        - — Resident's incontinence pattern changes for the better;
        - — Overall improvement of resident's condition.

3. Mrs. G has been in the nursing home for 5 weeks following an 8-week acute hospitalization. On admission she was very frail, had trouble thinking, was confused, and had many behavioral complications. The course of treatment led to steady improvement and she is now stable. She is no longer confused or exhibiting inappropriate behaviors. The resident, her family, and staff agree that she has made remarkable progress. A SCSA is required at this time. The resident is not the person she was at admission - her initial problems have resolved and she will be remaining in the facility. A SCSA will permit the interdisciplinary team to review her needs and plan a new course of care for the future.

Guidelines for When a Change in Resident Status in not Significant:
Note: this is not an exhaustive list

- Discrete and easily reversible cause(s) documented in the resident's record and for which the IDT can initiate corrective action (e.g., an anticipated side effect of introducing a psychoactive medication while attempting to establish a clinically effective dose level. Tapering and monitoring of dosage would not require a SCSA)

- Short-term acute illness, such as a mild fever secondary to a cold from which the IDT expects the resident to fully recover.

- Well-established, predictable cyclical patterns of clinical signs and symptoms associated with previously diagnosed conditions (e.g., depressive symptoms in a resident previously diagnosed with bipolar disease would not precipitate a Significant Change Assessment).

- Instances in which the resident continues to make steady progress under the current course of care. Reassessment is required only when the condition has stabilized.

- Instances in which the resident has stabilized but is expected to be discharged in the immediate future. The facility has engaged in discharge planning with the resident and family, and a comprehensive reassessment is not necessary to facilitate discharge planning.

Guidelines for Determining the Need for a SCSA for Residents with Terminal Conditions:
Note: this is not an exhaustive list

The key in determining if a SCSA is required for individuals with a terminal condition is whether or not the change in condition is an expected, well-defined part of the disease course and is consequently being addressed as part of the overall plan of care for the individual.

- If a terminally ill resident experiences a new onset of symptoms or a condition that is not part of the expected course of deterioration and the criteria are met for a SCSA, a SCSA assessment is required.

- If a resident elects the Medicare Hospice program, it is important that the two separate entities (nursing home and hospice program staff) coordinate their responsibilities and develop a care plan reflecting the interventions required by both entities. The nursing home and hospice plans of care should be reflective of the current status of the resident.

Examples (SCSA):

1. Mr. M has been in this nursing home for two and one-half years. He has been a favorite of staff and other residents, and his daughter has been an active volunteer on the unit. Mr. M is now in the end stage of his course of chronic dementia, diagnosed as probable Alzheimer's. He experiences recurrent pneumonias and swallowing difficulties, his prognosis is guarded, and family members are fully aware of his status. He is on a special dementia unit, staff has detailed palliative care protocols for all such end stage residents, and there has been active involvement of his daughter in the care planning process. As changes have occurred, staff has responded in a timely, appropriate manner. In this case, Mr. M's care is of a high quality, and as his physical state has declined, there is no need for staff to complete a new MDS assessment for this bedfast, highly dependent terminal resident.

2. Mrs. K came into the nursing home with identifiable problems and has steadily responded to treatment. Her condition has improved over time and has recently hit a plateau. She will be discharged within 5 days. The initial RAI helped to set goals and start her care. The course of care provided to Mrs. K was modified as necessary to ensure continued improvement. The IDT's treatment response reversed the causes of the resident's condition. An assessment need not be completed in view of the imminent discharge. Remember, facilities have 14 days to complete an assessment once the resident's condition has stabilized, and if Mrs. K is discharged within this period, a new assessment is not required. If the resident's discharge plans change, or if she is not discharged, an assessment is required by the end of the allotted 14-day period.

3. Mrs. P, too, has responded to care. Unlike Mrs. K, however, she continues to improve. Her discharge date has not been specified. She is benefiting from her care and full restoration of her functional abilities seems possible. In this case, treatment is focused appropriately, progress is being made, staff is on top of the situation, and there is nothing to be gained by requiring a SCSA at this time. However, if her condition was to stabilize and her discharge was not imminent, a SCSA would be in order.

Guidelines for Determining When A Significant Change Should Result in Referral for a Preadmission Screening and Resident Review (PASRR) Level II Evaluation:

- If a SCSA occurs for an individual *known* or *suspected* to have a mental illness, intellectual disability ("mental retardation" in the regulation), or related condition (as defined by 42 CFR 483.102), a referral to the state mental health or ID/DD authority (SMH/MR/DDA) for a possible Level II PASRR evaluation must promptly occur as required by Section 1919(e)(7)(B)(iii) of the Social Security Act[5].

- PASRR is not a requirement of the resident assessment process, but is an OBRA provision that is required to be coordinated with the resident assessment process. This guideline is intended to help facilities coordinate PASRR with the SCSA — the guideline does not require any actions to be taken in completing the SCSA itself.

- Facilities should look to their state PASRR program requirements for specific procedures. PASRR contact information for the state MH/MR/DD authorities and the state Medicaid agency is available at http://www.cms. gov/.

- The nursing facility must provide the SMH/MR/DDA authority with referrals as described below, independent of the findings of the SCSA. PASRR Level II is to function as an independent assessment process for this population with special needs, in parallel with the facility's assessment process. Nursing facilities should have a low threshold for referral to the SMH/MR/DDA, so that these authorities may exercise their expert judgment about when a Level II evaluation is needed.

- Referral should be made as soon as the criteria indicating such are evident — the facility should not wait until the SCSA is complete.

Referral for Level II Resident Review Evaluations are Required for Individuals Previously Identified by PASRR to Have Mental Illness, Intellectual Disability, or a Related Condition in the Following Circumstances:
Note: this is not an exhaustive list

- A resident who demonstrates increased behavioral, psychiatric, or mood-related symptoms.

- A resident with behavioral, psychiatric, or mood related symptoms that have not responded to ongoing treatment.

- A resident who experiences an improved medical condition—such that the resident's plan of care or placement recommendations may require modifications.

- A resident whose significant change is physical, but with behavioral, psychiatric, or mood-related symptoms, or cognitive abilities, that may influence adjustment to an altered pattern of daily living.

- A resident who indicates a preference (may be communicated verbally or through other forms of communication, including behavior) to leave the facility.

---

[5]   The statute may also be referenced as 42 U.S.C. 1396r(e)(7)(B)(iii). Note that as of this revision date the statute supersedes Federal regulations at 42 CFR 483.114(c), which still reads as requiring annual resident review. The regulation has not yet been updated to reflect the statutory change to resident review upon significant change in condition.

- A resident whose condition or treatment is or will be significantly different than described in the resident's most recent PASRR Level II evaluation and determination. (Note that a referral for a possible new Level II PASRR evaluation is required whenever such a disparity is discovered, whether or not associated with a SCSA.)

Examples (PASRR & SCSAs):

1. Mr. L has a diagnosis of serious mental illness, but his primary reason for admission was rehabilitation following a hip fracture. Once the hip fracture resolves and he becomes ambulatory, even if other conditions exist for which Mr. L receives medical care, he should be referred for a PASRR evaluation to determine whether a change in his placement or services is needed.

2. Ms. K has intellectual disability. She is normally cooperative, but after she had a fall and sustained a leg injury, she becomes agitated and combative with the physical therapist and with staff who try to assess her status. She does not understand why her normal routine has changed and why staff are touching a painful area of her body.

Referral for Level II Resident Review Evaluations are Also Required for Individuals Who May Not Have Previously Been Identified by PASRR to Have Mental Illness, Intellectual Disability, or a Related Condition in the Following Circumstances: Note: this is not an exhaustive list

- A resident who exhibits behavioral, psychiatric, or mood related symptoms suggesting the presence of a diagnosis of mental illness as defined under 42 CFR 483.100 (where dementia is not the primary diagnosis).

- A resident whose intellectual disability as defined under 42 CFR 483.100, or related condition as defined under 42 CFR 435.1010 was not previously identified and evaluated through PASRR.

- A resident transferred, admitted, or readmitted to a NF following an inpatient psychiatric stay or equally intensive treatment.

04. Significant Correction to Prior Comprehensive Assessment (SCPA) (A0310A=05)

The SCPA is a comprehensive assessment for an existing resident that must be completed when the IDT determines that a resident's prior comprehensive assessment contains a significant error. It can be performed at any time after the completion of an Admission assessment, and its ARD and completion dates (MDS/CAA(s)/care plan) depend on the date the determination was made that the significant error exists in a comprehensive assessment.

A **"significant error"** is an error in an assessment where:

1. The resident's overall clinical status is not accurately represented (i.e., miscoded) on the erroneous assessment; and

2. The error has not been corrected via submission of a more recent assessment.

A significant error differs from a significant change because it reflects incorrect coding of the MDS and NOT an actual significant change in the resident's health status.

Assessment Management Requirements and Tips for Significant Correction to Prior Comprehensive Assessments:

- Nursing homes should document the initial identification of a significant error in an assessment in the progress notes.
- A SCPA is appropriate when:
  — the erroneous comprehensive assessment has been completed and transmitted/submitted into the MDS system; and
  — there is not a more current assessment in progress or completed that includes a correction to the item(s) in error.
- The ARD must be within 14 days after the determination that a significant error in the prior comprehensive assessment occurred (determination date + 14 calendar days).
- The MDS completion date (Item Z0500B) must be no later than 14 days after the ARD (ARD + 14 calendar days) and no later than 14 days after the determination was made that a significant error occurred. This date may be earlier than or the same as the CAA(s) completion date, but not later than the CAA(s) completion date.
- The CAA(s) completion date (Item V0200B2) must be no later than 14 days after the ARD (ARD + 14 calendar days) and no more than 14 days after the determination was made that a significant error occurred. This date may be the same as the MDS completion date, but not earlier than the MDS completion date.
- The care plan completion date (Item V0200C2) must be no later than 7 calendar days after the CAA(s) completion date (Item V0200B2) (CAA(s) completion date + 7 calendar days).

Non-Comprehensive Assessments and Entry and Discharge Reporting

OBRA-required non-comprehensive MDS assessments include a select number of MDS items, but **not** completion of the CAA process and care planning. The OBRA non-comprehensive assessments include:

- Quarterly Assessment
- Significant Correction to Prior Quarterly Assessment
- Discharge Assessment – Return not Anticipated
- Discharge Assessment – Return Anticipated

The Quarterly and Significant Correction to Prior Quarterly assessments are **not** required for Swing Bed residents. However, Swing Bed providers are required to complete the Discharge assessments.

Tracking records include a select number of MDS items and are required for **all** residents in the nursing home and swing bed facility. They include:

- Entry Tracking Record
- Death in Facility Tracking Record

Assessment Management Requirements and Tips for Non-Comprehensive Assessments:

- The ARD is considered the last day of the observation/look back period, therefore it is day 1 for purposes of counting back to determine the beginning of observation/look back periods. For example, if the ARD is set for March 14, then the beginning of the observation period for MDS items requiring a 7-day observation period would be March 8 (ARD + 6 previous calendar days), while the beginning of the observation period for MDS items requiring a 14-day observation period would be March 1 (ARD + 13 previous calendar days).

  If a resident goes to the hospital (discharge return anticipated and returns within 30 days) and returns during the assessment period and most of the assessment was completed prior to the hospitalization, then the nursing home may wish to continue with the original assessment, provided the resident does not meet the criteria for a SCSA.

  For example:

  — Resident A has a Quarterly assessment with an ARD of March 20th. The facility staff finished most of the assessment. The resident is discharged (return anticipated) to the hospital on March 23rd and returns on March 25th. Review of the information from the discharging hospital reveals that there is not any significant change in status for the resident. Therefore, the facility staff continue with the assessment that was not fully completed before discharge and complete the assessment by April 3rd (which is day 14 after the ARD).

  — Resident B also has a Quarterly assessment with an ARD of March 20th. She goes to the hospital on March 20th and returns March 30th. While there is no significant change the facility decides to start a new assessment and sets the ARD for April 2nd and completes the assessment.

- If a resident is discharged during this assessment process, then whatever portions of the RAI that have been completed must be maintained in the resident's discharge record.[6] In closing the record, the nursing home should note why the RAI was not completed.

- If a resident dies during this assessment process, completion of the assessment is not required. Whatever portions of the RAI that have been completed must be maintained in the resident's medical record.[5] In closing the record, the nursing home should note why the RAI was not completed.

- If a significant change in status is identified in the process of completing any assessment except Admission and SCSAs, code and complete the assessment as a comprehensive SCSA instead.

---

[6] The RAI is considered part of the resident's clinical record and is treated as such by the RAI utilization guidelines, e.g., portions of the RAI that are "started" must be saved.

- In the process of completing any assessment except an Admission and a SCPA, if it is identified that a significant error occurred in a previous comprehensive assessment that has already been submitted and accepted into the MDS system and has not already been corrected in a subsequent comprehensive assessment, code and complete the assessment as a comprehensive SCPA instead. A correction request for the erroneous comprehensive assessment should also be completed and submitted. See the section on SCPAs for detailed information on completing a SCPA, and Chapter 5 for detailed information on processing corrections.

- In the process of completing any assessment except an Admission, if it is identified that a non-significant (minor) error occurred in a previous assessment, continue with completion of the assessment in progress and also submit a correction request for the erroneous assessment as per the instructions in Chapter 5.

- The ARD of an assessment drives the due date of the next assessment. The next non-comprehensive assessment is due within 92 days after the ARD of the most recent OBRA assessment (ARD of previous OBRA assessment - Admission, Annual, Significant Change in Status, or Significant Correction assessment - + 92 calendar days).

- While the CAA process is not required with a non-comprehensive assessment, nursing homes are still required to review the information from these assessments, determine if a revision to the resident's care plan is necessary, and make the applicable revision.

- The MDS must be transmitted (submitted and accepted into the MDS database) electronically no later than 14 calendar days after the MDS completion date (Z0500B + 14 calendar days).

- Non-comprehensive assessments may be combined with a Medicare-required PPS assessment (see Sections 2.11 and 2.12 for details).

05. Quarterly Assessment (A0310A=02)

The Quarterly assessment is an OBRA non-comprehensive assessment for a resident that must be completed at least every 92 days following the previous OBRA assessment of any type. It is used to track a resident's status between comprehensive assessments to ensure critical indicators of gradual change in a resident's status are monitored. As such, not all MDS items appear on the Quarterly assessment. The ARD (A2300) must be not more than 92 days after the ARD of the most recent OBRA assessment of any type.

Assessment Management Requirements and Tips:

- Federal requirements dictate that, at a minimum, three Quarterly assessments be completed in each 12-month period. Assuming the resident does not have a SCSA or SCPA completed and was not discharged from the nursing home, a typical 12-month OBRA schedule would look like this:

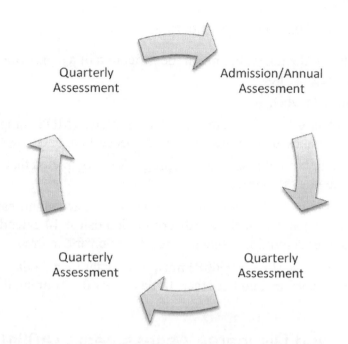

- OBRA assessments may be scheduled early if a nursing home wants to stagger due dates for assessments. As a result, more than three OBRA Quarterly assessments may be completed on a particular resident in a given year, or the Annual assessment may be completed early to ensure that the regulatory time frames are met. However, States may have more stringent restrictions.

- The ARD must be within 92 days after the ARD of the previous OBRA assessment (Quarterly, Admission, SCSA, SCPA, or Annual assessment + 92 calendar days).

- The MDS completion date (Item Z0500B) must be no later than 14 days after the ARD (ARD + 14 calendar days).

06. Significant Correction to Prior Quarterly Assessment (SCQA) (A0310A=06)

The SCQA is an OBRA non-comprehensive assessment that must be completed when the IDT determines that a resident's prior Quarterly assessment contains a significant error. It can be performed at any time after the completion of a Quarterly assessment, and the ARD (Item A2300) and completion dates (Item Z0500B) depend on the date the determination was made that there is a significant error in a previous Quarterly assessment.

A **"significant error"** is an error in an assessment where:

1. The resident's overall clinical status is not accurately represented (i.e., miscoded) on the erroneous assessment; and

2. The error has not been corrected via submission of a more recent assessment.

A significant error differs from a significant change because it reflects incorrect coding of the MDS and NOT an actual significant change in the resident's health status.

Assessment Management Requirements and Tips:

- Nursing homes should document the initial identification of a significant error in an assessment in the progress notes.
- A SCQA is appropriate when:
  — the erroneous Quarterly assessment has been completed (MDS completion date, Item Z0500B) and transmitted/submitted into the MDS system; and
  — there is not a more current assessment in progress or completed that includes a correction to the item(s) in error.
- The ARD must be within 14 days after the determination that a significant error in the prior Quarterly assessment has occurred (determination date + 14 calendar days) and no later than 14 days after determining that the significant error occurred.
- The MDS completion date (Item Z0500B) must be no later than 14 days after the ARD (ARD + 14 calendar days) and no later than 14 days after determining that the significant error occurred.

Tracking Records and Discharge Assessments (A0310F)

OBRA-required tracking records and assessments consist of the Entry tracking record, the Discharge assessments, and the Death in Facility tracking record. These include the completion of a select number of MDS items in order to track residents when they enter or leave a facility. They do not include completion of the CAA process and care planning. The Discharge assessments include items for quality monitoring. Entry and discharge reporting **is** required for Swing Bed residents and respite residents.

If the resident has one or more admissions to the hospital before the Admission assessment is completed, the nursing home should continue to submit Discharge assessments and Entry records every time until the resident is in the nursing home long enough to complete the comprehensive Admission assessment.

OBRA-required Tracking Records and Discharge Assessments include the following types (Item A0310F):

07. Entry Tracking Record (Item A0310F=01)

There are two types of entries – admission and reentry.

Admission (Item A1700=1)

- Entry tracking record is coded an Admission every time a resident:
  — is admitted for the first time to this facility; or
  — is readmitted after a discharge prior to completion of the OBRA Admission assessment; or
  — is readmitted after a discharge return not anticipated; or

— is readmitted after a discharge return anticipated when return was not within 30 days of discharge.

- For swing bed facilities, the Entry tracking record will always be coded 1, Admission, since these providers do not complete an OBRA Admission assessment.

Example (Admission):

1. Mr. S. was admitted to the nursing home on February 5, 2011 following a stroke. He regained most of his function and returned to his home on March 29, 2011. He was discharged return not anticipated. Five months later, Mr. S. underwent surgery for a total knee replacement. He returned to the nursing home for rehabilitation therapy on August 27, 2011. Code the Entry tracking record for the August 27, 2011 return as follows:

    A0310F = 01
    A1600 = 08-27-2011
    A1700 = 1

Reentry (Item A1700=2)

- Entry tracking record is coded Reentry every time a person is readmitted to a nursing home when the resident was previously admitted to this nursing home (i.e., an OBRA Admission was completed), **and** was discharged return anticipated from this nursing home, **and** returned within 30 days of discharge. See Section 2.5, Reentry, for greater detail.

Example (Reentry):

1. Mr. W. was admitted to the nursing home on April 11, 2011. Four weeks later he became very short of breath during lunch. The nurse assessed him and noted his lung sounds were not clear. His breathing became very labored. He was discharged return anticipated and admitted to the hospital. On May 18, 2011, Mr. W. returned to the facility. Code the Entry tracking record for the May 18, 2011 return, as follows:

    A0310F = 01
    A1600 = 05-18-2011
    A1700 = 2

Assessment Management Requirements and Tips for Entry Tracking Records:

- The Entry tracking record is the first item set completed for all residents.
- Must be completed every time a resident is admitted (admission) or readmitted (reentry) into a nursing home (or swing bed facility).
- Must be completed for a respite resident every time the resident enters the facility.
- Must be completed within 7 days after the admission/reentry.
- Must be submitted no later than the 14th calendar day after the entry (entry date (A1600) + 14 calendar days).

- Required in addition to the initial Admission assessment or other OBRA or PPS assessments that might be required.
- Contains administrative and demographic information.
- Is a stand-alone tracking record.
- May **not** be combined with an assessment.

08. Death in Facility Tracking Record (A0310F=12)

- Must be completed when the resident dies in the facility or when on LOA
- Must be completed within 7 days after the resident's death, which is recorded in item A2000, Discharge Date (A2000 + 7 calendar days).
- Must be submitted within 14 days after the resident's death, which is recorded in item A2000, Discharge Date (A2000 + 14 calendar days).
- Consists of demographic and administrative items.
- May not be combined with any type of assessment.

Example (Death in Facility):

1. Mr. W. was admitted to the nursing home for hospice care due to a terminal illness on September 9, 2011. He passed away on November 13, 2011. Code the November 13, 2011 Death in Facility tracking record as follows:

   A0310F = 12
   A2000 = 11-13-2011
   A2100 = 08

Discharge Assessments (A0310F)

Discharge assessments consist of discharge return anticipated and discharge return not anticipated. These are OBRA required assessments.

09. Discharge Assessment–Return Not Anticipated (A0310F=10)

- Must be completed when the resident is discharged from the facility and the resident is not expected to return to the facility within 30 days.
- Must be completed (Item Z0500B) within 14 days after the discharge date (A2000 + 14 calendar days).
- Must be submitted within 14 days after the MDS completion date (Z0500B + 14 calendar days).
- Consists of demographic, administrative, and clinical items.
- If the resident returns, the Entry tracking record will be coded A1700=1, Admission. The OBRA schedule for assessments will start with a new Admission assessment. If the resident's stay will be covered by Medicare Part A, the PPS schedule starts with a

Medicare-required 5-day scheduled assessment or combination of the Admission and 5-day PPS assessment.

Example (Discharge-return not anticipated):

1. Mr. S. was admitted to the nursing home on February 5, 2011 following a stroke. He regained most of his function and was discharged return not anticipated to his home on March 29, 2011. Code the March 29, 2011 Discharge assessment as follows:

> A0310F = 10
> A2000 = 03-29-2011
> A2100 = 01

10. Discharge Assessment–Return Anticipated (A0310F=11)

- Must be completed when the resident is discharged from the facility and the resident is expected to return to the facility within 30 days.

- For a resident discharged to a hospital or other setting (such as a respite resident) who comes in and out of the facility on a relatively frequent basis and reentry can be expected, the resident is discharged return anticipated unless it is known on discharge that he or she will not return within 30 days. This status requires an Entry tracking record each time the resident returns to the facility and a Discharge assessment each time the resident is discharged.

- Must be completed (Item Z0500B) within 14 days after the discharge date (Item A2000) (i.e., discharge date (A2000) + 14 calendar days).

- Must be submitted within 14 days after the MDS completion date (Item Z0500B) (i.e., MDS completion date (Z0500B) + 14 calendar days).

- Consists of demographic, administrative, and clinical items.

- When the resident returns to the nursing home, the IDT must determine if criteria are met for a SCSA (only when the OBRA Admission assessment was completed prior to discharge).

  — If criteria are met, complete a Significant Change in Status assessment.

  — If criteria are not met, continue with the OBRA schedule as established prior to the resident's discharge.

- If a SCSA is not indicated and an OBRA assessment was due while the resident was in the hospital, the facility has 13 days after reentry to complete the assessment (this does not apply to Admission assessment).

- When a resident had a prior Discharge assessment completed indicating that the resident was expected to return (A0310E=11) to the facility, but later learned that the resident will not be returning to the facility, there is no Federal requirement to inactivate the resident's record nor to complete another Discharge assessment. Please contact your State RAI Coordinator for specific State requirements.

Example (Discharge-return anticipated):

1. Ms. C. was admitted to the nursing home on May 22, 2011. She tripped while at a restaurant with her daughter. She was discharged return anticipated and admitted to the hospital on May 31, 2011. Code the May 31, 2011 Discharge assessment as follows:

   A0310F = 11
   A2000 = 05-31-2011
   A2100 = 03

Assessment Management Requirements and Tips for Discharge Assessments:

- Must be completed when the resident is discharged from the facility (see definition of Discharge on page 2-10).
- Must be completed when the resident is admitted to an acute care hospital.
- Must be completed when the resident has a hospital observation stay greater than 24 hours.
- Must be completed on a respite resident every time the resident is discharged from the facility.
- May be combined with another OBRA required assessment when requirements for all assessments are met.
- May be combined with a PPS Medicare required assessment when requirements for all assessments are met.
- Discharge date (Item A2000) must be the ARD (Item A2300) of the Discharge assessment.
- For **unplanned discharges**, the facility should complete the Discharge assessment to the best of its abilities. The use of the dash, "-", is appropriate when the staff are unable to determine the response to an item, including the interview items. In some cases, the facility may have already completed some items of the assessment and should record those responses or may be in the process of completing an assessment. The facility may combine the Discharge assessment with another assessment(s) when requirements for all assessments are met.
  - An unplanned discharge includes, for example:
    o Acute-care transfer of the resident to a hospital or an emergency department in order to either stabilize a condition or determine if an acute-care admission is required based on emergency department evaluation; or
    o Resident unexpectedly leaving the facility against medical advice; or
    o Resident unexpectedly deciding to go home or to another setting (e.g., due to the resident deciding to complete treatment in an alternate setting).
- Nursing home bed hold status and opening and closing of the medical record have no effect on these requirements.

The following chart details the sequencing and coding of Tracking records and Discharge assessments.

Entry, Discharge, and Reentry Algorithms

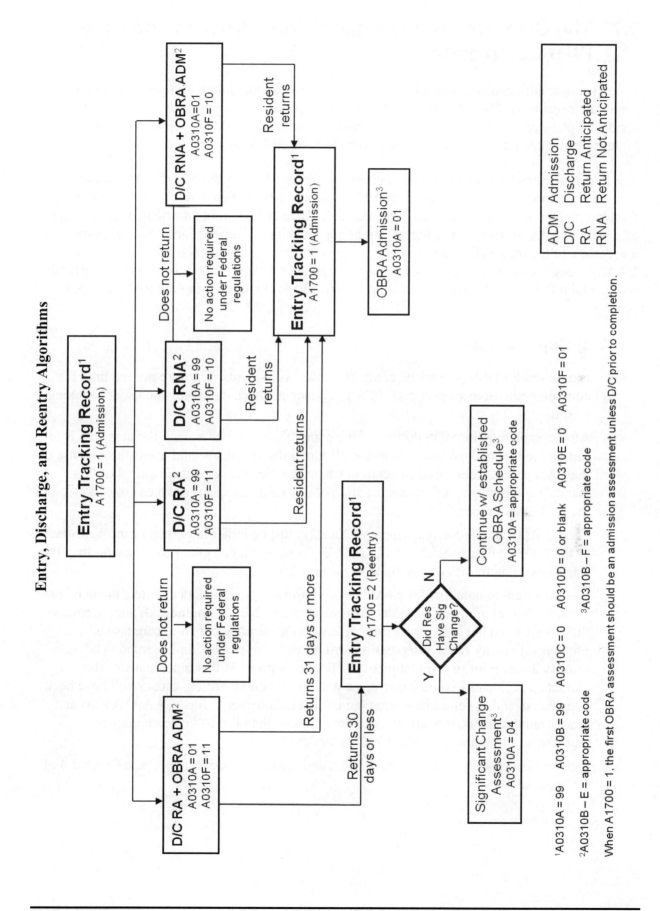

Entry Tracking Record[1]
A1700 = 1 (Admission)

D/C RA + OBRA ADM[2]
A0310A = 01
A0310F = 11

D/C RA[2]
A0310A = 99
A0310F = 11

Does not return

No action required under Federal regulations

Returns 31 days or more

Returns 30 days or less

Entry Tracking Record[1]
A1700 = 2 (Reentry)

Did Res Have Sig Change?

Y

Significant Change Assessment[3]
A0310A = 04

N

Continue w/ established OBRA Schedule[3]
A0310A = appropriate code

D/C RNA + OBRA ADM[2]
A0310A = 01
A0310F = 10

D/C RNA[2]
A0310A = 99
A0310F = 10

Does not return

No action required under Federal regulations

Resident returns

Resident returns

Resident returns

Entry Tracking Record[1]
A1700 = 1 (Admission)

OBRA Admission[3]
A0310A = 01

ADM   Admission
D/C   Discharge
RA   Return Anticipated
RNA   Return Not Anticipated

[1]A0310A = 99   A0310B = 99   A0310C = 0   A0310D = 0 or blank   A0310E = 0   A0310F = 01

[2]A0310B – E = appropriate code   [3]A0310B – F = appropriate code

When A1700 = 1, the first OBRA assessment should be an admission assessment unless D/C prior to completion.

2.7 The Care Area Assessment (CAA) Process and Care Plan Completion

Federal statute and regulations require nursing homes to conduct initial and periodic assessments for all their residents. The assessment information is used to develop, review, and revise the resident's plans of care that will be used to provide services to attain or maintain the resident's highest practicable physical, mental, and psychosocial well-being.

The RAI process, which includes the Federally-mandated MDS, is the basis for an accurate assessment of nursing home residents. The MDS information and the CAA process provide the foundation upon which the care plan is formulated. There are 20 problem-oriented CAAs, each of which includes MDS-based "trigger" conditions that signal the need for additional assessment and review of the triggered care area. Detailed information regarding each care area and the CAA process, including definitions and triggers, appear in Chapter 4 of this manual. Chapter 4 also contains detailed information on care planning development utilizing the RAI and CAA process.

CAA(s) Completion

- Is required for OBRA-required comprehensive assessments. They are not required for non-comprehensive assessments, PPS assessments, Discharge assessments, or Tracking records.

- After completing the MDS portion of the comprehensive assessment, the next step is to further identify and evaluate the resident's strengths, problems, and needs through use of the CAA process (described in detail in Chapter 3, Section V, and Chapter 4 of this manual) and through further investigation of any resident-specific issues not addressed in the RAI/CAA process.

- The CAA(s) completion date (Item V0200B2) must be either later than or the same date as the MDS completion date (Item Z0500B). In no event can either date be later than the established timeframes as described in Section 2.6.

- It is important to note that for an Admission assessment, the resident enters the nursing home with a set of physician-based treatment orders. Nursing home staff should review these orders and begin to assess the resident and to identify potential care issues/problems. In many cases, interventions will already have been implemented to address priority issues prior to completion of the final care plan. At this time, many of the resident's problems in the 20 care areas will have been identified, causes will have been considered, and a preliminary care plan initiated. However, a final CAA(s) review and associated documentation are still required no later than the 14th calendar day of admission (admission date plus 13 calendar days).

- Detailed information regarding each CAA and the CAA process appears in Chapter 4 of this manual.

Care Plan Completion

- Care plan completion based on the CAA process is required for OBRA-required comprehensive assessments. It is not required for non-comprehensive assessments, PPS assessments, Discharge assessments, or Tracking records.

- After completing the MDS and CAA portions of the comprehensive assessment, the next step is to evaluate the information gained through both assessment processes in order to identify problems, causes, contributing factors, and risk factors related to the problems. Subsequently, the IDT must evaluate the information gained to develop a care plan that addresses those findings in the context of the resident's strengths, problems, and needs (described in detail in Chapter 4 of this manual).

- The care plan completion date (Item V0200C2) must be either later than or the same date as the CAA completion date (Item V0200B2), but no later than 7 calendar days after the CAA completion date. The MDS completion date (Item Z0500B) must be earlier than or the same date as the care plan completion date. In no event can either date be later than the established timeframes as described in Section 2.6.

- For Annual assessments, SCSAs, and SCPAs, the process is basically the same as that described with an Admission assessment. In these cases, however, the care plan will already be in place. Review of the CAA(s) when the MDS is complete for these assessment types should raise questions about the need to modify or continue services and result in either the continuance or revision of the existing care plan. A new care plan does not need to be developed after each Annual assessment, SCSA, or SCPA.

- Nursing homes should also evaluate the appropriateness of the care plan after each Quarterly assessment and modify the care plan on an ongoing basis, if appropriate.

- Detailed information regarding the care planning process appears in Chapter 4 of this manual.

2.8 The Skilled Nursing Facility Medicare Prospective Payment System Assessment Schedule

Skilled nursing facilities (SNFs) must assess the clinical condition of beneficiaries by completing the MDS assessment for each Medicare resident receiving Part A SNF-level care for reimbursement under the SNF PPS. In addition to the Medicare-required assessments, the SNF must also complete the OBRA assessments. All requirements for the OBRA assessments apply to the Medicare-required assessments, such as completion and submission time frames.

Assessment Window

Each of the Medicare-required scheduled assessments has defined days within which the Assessment Reference Date (ARD) must be set. The facility is required to set the ARD on the MDS form itself or in the facility software within the appropriate timeframe of the assessment type being completed. For example, the ARD for the Medicare-required 5-day scheduled assessment must be set on days 1 through 8. Timeliness of the PPS assessment is defined by selecting an ARD within the prescribed ARD window. See Scheduled Medicare PPS

Assessments chart below for the allowed ARDs for each of the Medicare-required assessments and other assessment information.

When coding a standalone Change of Therapy OMRA (COT), a standalone End of Therapy OMRA (EOT), or a standalone Start of Therapy OMRA (SOT), facilities must set the ARD for the assessment for a day within the allowable ARD window for that assessment type, but may do so no more than two days after the window has passed.

The first day of Medicare Part A coverage for the current stay is considered day 1 for PPS assessment scheduling purposes. In most cases, the first day of Medicare Part A coverage is the date of admission or reentry. However, there are situations in which the Medicare beneficiary may qualify for Part A services at a later date. See Chapter 6, Section 6.7, for more detailed information.

Grace Days

There may be situations when an assessment might be delayed (e.g., illness of RN assessor, a high volume of assessments due at approximately the same time) or additional days are needed to more fully capture therapy or other treatments. Therefore, CMS has allowed for these situations by defining a number of grace days for each Medicare assessment. For example, the Medicare-required 5-Day ARD can be extended 1 to 3 grace days (i.e., days 6 to 8). The use of grace days allows clinical flexibility in setting ARDs. See chart below for the allowed grace days for each of the scheduled Medicare-required assessments. Grace days are not applied to unscheduled Medicare PPS Assessments.

Scheduled Medicare PPS Assessments

The Medicare-required standard assessment schedule includes 5-day, 14-day, 30-day, 60-day, and 90-day scheduled assessments, each with a predetermined time period for setting the ARD for that assessment. The Readmission/Return assessment is also a scheduled assessment.

The SNF provider must complete the Medicare-required assessments according to the following schedule to assure compliance with the SNF PPS requirements.

Medicare MDS Scheduled Assessment Type	Reason for Assessment (A0310B code)	Assessment Reference Date	Assessment Reference Date Grace Days+	Applicable Standard Medicare Payment Days^
5-day Readmission/Return	01 06	Days 1-5	6-8	1 through 14
14-day	02	Days 13-14	15-18	15 through 30
30-day	03	Days 27-29	30-33	31 through 60
60-day	04	Days 57-59	60-63	61 through 90
90-day	05	Days 87-89	90-93	91 through 100

+Grace Days: a specific number of days that can be added to the ARD window without penalty.

^Applicable Standard Medicare Payment Days may vary when assessment types are combined. For example, when a provider combines an unscheduled assessment, such as a Significant Change in Status Assessment (SCSA), with a scheduled assessment, such as a 30-day Medicare-required assessment, the new resource utilization group (RUG) would take effect on the ARD of the assessment. If the ARD of this assessment was day 28, the new RUG would take effect on day 28 of the stay. The exception would be if the ARD fell within the grace days. In that case, the new RUG would be effective on the first day of the regular payment period. For example, if the ARD of an unscheduled assessment combined with the 60-day assessment, was day 62, the new RUG would take effect on day 61.

Unscheduled Medicare PPS Assessments

There are situations when a SNF provider must complete an assessment outside of the standard scheduled Medicare-required assessments. These assessments are known as unscheduled assessments. When indicated, a provider must complete the following unscheduled assessments:

1. *Significant Change in Status Assessment* (for swing bed providers this unscheduled assessment is called the *Swing Bed Clinical Change Assessment*): Complete when the SNF interdisciplinary team has determined that a resident meets the significant change guidelines for either improvement or decline (see section 2.6).
2. *Significant Correction to Prior Comprehensive Assessment*: Complete because a significant error was made in the prior comprehensive assessment (see section 2.6).
3. *Start of Therapy Other Medicare Required Assessment (SOT-OMRA):* Complete to classify a resident into a RUG-IV Rehabilitation Plus Extensive Services or Rehabilitation group. This is an optional assessment (see section 2.9).
4. *End of Therapy Other Medicare Required Assessment* (EOT- OMRA): Complete in two circumstances: (a) When the beneficiary who was receiving rehabilitation services (occupational therapy [OT], and/or physical therapy [PT], and/or speech-language pathology services [SLP]), was classified in a RUG-IV Rehabilitation Plus Extensive Services or Rehabilitation group, all therapies have ended and the beneficiary continues to receive skilled services. (b) When the beneficiary who was receiving rehabilitation services (occupational therapy [OT], and/or physical therapy [PT], and/or speech-language pathology services [SLP]), was classified in a RUG-IV Rehabilitation Plus Extensive Services or Rehabilitation group and did not receive any therapy services for three or more consecutive calendar days. The EOT would be completed to classify the beneficiary into a non-therapy RUG group beginning on the day after the last day of therapy provided.
5. *Change of Therapy Other Medicare Required Assessment (COT-OMRA):* Complete when the intensity of therapy, which includes the total reimbursable therapy minutes (RTM), and other therapy qualifiers such as number of therapy days and disciplines providing therapy, changes to such a degree that the beneficiary would classify into a different RUG-IV category than the RUG-IV category for which the resident is currently being billed for the 7-day COT observation period following the ARD of the most recent assessment used for Medicare payment(see section 2.9). The requirement to complete a change of therapy is reevaluated with additional 7-day COT observation periods ending on the 14th, 21st, and 28th days after the most recent Medicare payment assessment ARD and a COT OMRA is to be completed if the RUG-IV category changes. If a new assessment used for Medicare payment has occurred, the COT observation period will restart beginning on the day following the ARD of the most recent assessment used for Medicare payment.

A Medicare unscheduled assessment in a scheduled assessment window cannot be followed by the scheduled assessment later in that window—the two assessments must be combined with an ARD appropriate to the unscheduled assessment. If a scheduled assessment has been completed and an unscheduled assessment falls in that assessment window, the unscheduled assessment may supersede the scheduled assessment and the payment may be modified until the next unscheduled or scheduled assessment. See Chapter 6 (Section 6.4) for complete details.

Tracking Records and Discharge Assessments Reporting

Tracking records and discharge assessments reporting are required on **all** residents in the SNF and swing bed facilities. Tracking records and standalone Discharge assessments do not impact payment.

The following chart summarizes the Medicare-required scheduled and unscheduled assessments, tracking records, and discharge assessments:

Medicare Scheduled and Unscheduled MDS Assessment, Tracking Records, and Discharge Assessment Reporting Schedule for SNFs and Swing Bed Facilities

Codes for Assessments Required for Medicare	Assessment Reference Date (ARD) Can be Set on Any of Following Days	Grace Days ARD Can Also be Set on These Days	Allowed ARD Window	Billing Cycle Used by the Business Office	Special Comment
5-day A0310B = 01 and Readmission/return A0310B = 06	Days 1-5	6-8	Days 1-8	Sets payment rate for days 1-14	• See Section 2.12 for instructions involving beneficiaries who transfer or expire day 8 or earlier. • CAAs must be completed only if the Medicare 5-day scheduled assessment is dually coded as an OBRA Admission or Annual assessment, SCSA or SCPA.
14-day A0310B = 02	Days 13-14	15-18	Days 13-18	Sets payment rate for days 15-30	• CAAs must be completed only if the 14-day assessment is dually coded as an OBRA Admission or Annual assessment, SCSA or SCPA. • Grace days do not apply when the 14-day scheduled assessment is dually coded as an OBRA Admission.
30-day A0310B = 03	Days 27-29	30-33	Days 27-33	Sets payment rate for days 31-60	
60-day A0310B = 04	Days 57-59	60-63	Days 57-63	Sets payment rate for days 61-90	
90-day A0310B = 05	Days 87-89	90-93	Days 87-93	Sets payment rate for days 91-100	• If combined with the OBRA Quarterly assessment the completion date requirements for the OBRA Quarterly assessment must also be met.

Medicare Scheduled and Unscheduled MDS Assessment Schedule for SNFs (cont.)

Codes for Assessments Required for Medicare	Assessment Reference Date (ARD) Can be Set on Any of Following Days	Grace Days ARD Can Also be Set on These Days	Allowed ARD Window	Billing Cycle Used by the Business Office	Special Comment
Start of Therapy Other Medicare-required Assessment (OMRA) A0310B = 01 - 07 and A0310C = 1 or 3	• 5-7 days after the start of therapy • The day of the first therapy evaluation counts as day 1	N/A	N/A	Modifies payment rate starting on the date of the first therapy evaluation	• Voluntary assessment used to establish a Rehabilitation Plus Extensive Services or Rehabilitation RUG.
End of Therapy OMRA A0310B = 01-07 and A0310C = 2 or 3	• 1-3 days after all therapy (PT, OT, SLP) services are discontinued. • The first non-therapy day counts as day 1.	N/A	N/A	Modifies payment rate starting on the day after the latest therapy end date	• Not required if the resident has been determined to no longer meet Medicare skilled level of care. • Establishes a new non-therapy RUG Classification. • Only required for patients who are classified into Rehabilitation Plus Extensive Services or Rehabilitation RUG on most recent PPS assessment. • For circumstances when an End of Therapy with Resumption option would be used, See Section 2.9.
Change of Therapy OMRA A0310B = 01-07 And A0310C = 4	• Day 7 of the COT observation period	N/A	N/A	Modifies payment rate starting on Day 1 of that COT observation period and continues for the remainder of the current payment period, unless the payment is modified by a subsequent COT OMRA or other scheduled or unscheduled PPS assessment	• Required only if the intensity of therapy during the 7-day look back period would change the RUG category classification of the most recent PPS Assessment • Establishes a new RUG classification

(continued)

Medicare Scheduled and Unscheduled MDS Assessment Schedule for SNFs (cont.)

Codes for Assessments Required for Medicare	Assessment Reference Date (ARD) Can be Set on Any of Following Days	Grace Days ARD Can Also be Set on These Days	Allowed ARD Window	Billing Cycle Used by the Business Office	Special Comment
Significant Change in Status Assessment (SCSA) A0310A = 04	Completed by the end of the 14th calendar day after determination that a significant change has occurred.	N/A	N/A	Modifies payment rate effective with the ARD when not combined with another assessment*	May establish a new RUG Classification.
Swing Bed Clinical Change Assessment (CCA) A0310B = 01-07 and A0310D = 1	Completed by the end of the 14th calendar day after determination that a clinical change has occurred.	N/A	N/A	Modifies payment rate effective with the ARD when not combined with another assessment*	May establish a new RUG Classification.
Significant Correction to Prior Comprehensive Assessment (SCPA) A0310A = 05	Completed by the end of the 14th calendar day after identification of a significant, uncorrected error in prior comprehensive assessment.	N/A	N/A	Modifies payment rate effective with the ARD when not combined with another assessment*	May establish a new RUG Classification.
Entry tracking record A0310F = 01	N/A	N/A	N/A	N/A	May not be combined with another assessment
Discharge Assessment A0310F = 10 or 11	Must be set for the day of discharge	N/A	N/A	N/A	May be combined with another assessment when the date of discharge is the ARD of the Medicare-required assessment
Death in facility tracking record A0310F = 12	N/A	N/A	N/A	N/A	May not be combined with another assessment

*NOTE: When SCSA, SCPA, and CCA are combined with another assessment, payment rate may not be effective on the ARD. For example, a provider combines the 30-day Medicare-required assessment with a Significant Change in Status assessment with an ARD of day 33, a grace day, payment rate would become effective on day 31, not day 33. See Chapter 6, Section 6.4.

2.9 MDS Medicare Assessments for SNFs

The MDS has been constructed to identify the OBRA Reasons for Assessment and the SNF PPS Reasons for Assessment in Items A0310A and A0310B respectively. If the assessment is being used for Medicare reimbursement, the Medicare Reason for Assessment must be coded in Item A0310B. The OBRA Reason for Assessment is described earlier in this section while the Medicare PPS assessments are described below. A SNF provider may combine assessments to meet both OBRA and Medicare requirements. When combining assessments, all completion deadlines and other requirements for both types of assessments must be met. If all requirements cannot be met, the assessments must be completed separately. The relationship between OBRA and Medicare assessments are discussed below and in more detail in Sections 2.11 and 2.12.

PPS Scheduled Assessments for a Medicare Part A Stay

01. Medicare-required 5-Day Scheduled Assessment

- ARD (Item A2300) must be set on days 1 through 5 of the Part A SNF covered stay.
- ARD may be extended up to day 8 if using the designated grace days.
- Must be completed (Item Z0500B) within 14 days after the ARD (ARD + 14 days).
- Authorizes payment from days 1 through 14 of the stay, as long as the resident meets all criteria for Part A SNF-level services.
- Must be submitted electronically and accepted into the QIES Assessment Submission and Processing (ASAP) system within 14 days after completion (Item Z0500B) (completion + 14 days).
- If combined with the OBRA Admission assessment, the assessment must be completed by the end of day 14 of admission (admission date plus 13 calendar days).
- Is the first Medicare-required assessment to be completed when the resident is first admitted for SNF Part A stay.
- Is the first Medicare-required assessment to be completed when the Part A resident is re-admitted to the facility following a discharge assessment – return not anticipated or if the resident returns more than 30 days after a discharge assessment-return anticipated.
- If a resident goes from Medicare Advantage to Medicare Part A, the Medicare PPS schedule must start over with a 5-day PPS assessment as the resident is now beginning a Medicare Part A stay.

02. Medicare-required 14-Day Scheduled Assessment

- ARD (Item A2300) must be set on days 13 through 14 of the Part A SNF covered stay.
- ARD may be extended up to day 18 if using the designated grace days.
- Must be completed (Item Z0500B) within 14 days after the ARD (ARD + 14 days).
- Authorizes payment from days 15 through 30 of the stay, as long as all the coverage criteria for Part A SNF-level services continue to be met.
- Must be submitted electronically and accepted into the QIES ASAP system within 14 days after completion (Item Z0500B) (completion + 14 days).
- If combined with the OBRA Admission assessment, the assessment must be completed by the end of day 14 of admission and grace days may not be used when setting the ARD.

03. Medicare-required 30-Day Scheduled Assessment

- ARD (Item A2300) must be set on days 27 through 29 of the Part A SNF covered stay.
- ARD may be extended up to day 33 if using the designated grace days.
- Must be completed (Item Z0500B) within 14 days after the ARD (ARD + 14 days).
- Authorizes payment from days 31 through 60 of the stay, as long as all the coverage criteria for Part A SNF-level services continue to be met.
- Must be submitted electronically and accepted into the QIES ASAP system within 14 days after completion (Item Z0500B) (completion + 14 days).

04. Medicare-required 60-Day Scheduled Assessment

- ARD (Item A2300) must be set on days 57 through 59 of the Part A SNF covered stay.
- ARD may be extended up to day 63 if using the designated grace days.
- Must be completed (Item Z0500B) within 14 days after the ARD (ARD + 14 days).
- Authorizes payment from days 61 through 90 of the stay, as long as all the coverage criteria for Part A SNF-level services continue to be met.
- Must be submitted electronically and accepted into the QIES ASAP system within 14 days after completion (Item Z0500B) (completion + 14 days).

05. Medicare-required 90-Day Scheduled Assessment

- ARD (Item A2300) must be set on days 87 through 89 of the Part A SNF covered stay.
- ARD may be extended up to day 93 if using the designated grace days.
- Must be completed (Item Z0500B) within 14 days after the ARD (ARD + 14 days).
- Authorizes payment from days 91 through 100 of the stay, as long as all the coverage criteria for Part A SNF-level services continue to be met.
- Must be submitted electronically and accepted into the QIES ASAP system within 14 days after completion (Item Z0500B) (completion + 14 days).

06. Medicare-required Readmission/Return Assessment

- Completed when a resident whose SNF stay was being reimbursed by Medicare Part A is hospitalized, discharged return anticipated, and then returns to the SNF from the hospital within 30 days and continues to require and receive Part A SNF-level care services. Under these conditions, the entry tracking record completed upon return to the SNF will be coded as a reentry with Item A1700 = 2.
- ARD (Item A2300) must be set on days 1 through 5 of the Part A SNF covered stay.
- ARD may be extended up to day 8 if using the designated grace days.
- Must be completed (Item Z0500B) within 14 days after the ARD (ARD + 14 days).
- Authorizes payment from days 1 through 14 of the stay, as long as all the coverage criteria for Part A SNF-level services continue to be met.
- Must be submitted electronically and accepted into the QIES ASAP system within 14 days after completion (Item Z0500B) (completion + 14 days).
- If combined with the OBRA Admission assessment, the assessment must be completed by the Day 14 counting the date of admission as Day 1 (admission date plus 13 calendar days).

PPS Unscheduled Assessments for a Medicare Part A Stay

07. Unscheduled Assessments Used for PPS

There are several unscheduled assessment types that may be required to be completed during a resident's Part A SNF covered stay.

Start of Therapy (SOT) OMRA

- Optional.

- Completed only to classify a resident into a RUG-IV Rehabilitation Plus Extensive Services or Rehabilitation group. If the RUG-IV classification is not a Rehabilitation Plus Extensive Services or a Rehabilitation (therapy) group, the assessment will not be accepted by CMS and cannot be used for Medicare billing.

- Completed only if the resident is not already classified into a RUG-IV Rehabilitation Plus Extensive Services or Rehabilitation group.

- ARD (Item A2300) must be set on days 5-7 after the start of therapy (Item O0400A5 or O0400B5 or O0400C5, whichever is the earliest date) with the exception of the Short Stay Assessment (see Chapter 6, Section 6.4). The date of the earliest therapy evaluation is counted as day 1 when determining the ARD for the Start of Therapy OMRA, regardless if treatment is provided or not on that day.

- May be combined with scheduled PPS assessments.

- An SOT OMRA is not necessary if rehabilitation services start within the ARD window (including grace days) of the 5-day assessment, since the therapy rate will be paid starting Day 1 of the SNF stay.

- The ARD may not precede the ARD of first scheduled PPS assessment of the Medicare stay (5-day or readmission/return assessment).

  — For example if the 5-day assessment is performed on Day 8 and an SOT is performed in that window, the ARD for the SOT would be Day 8 as well.

- Must be completed (Item Z0500B) within 14 days after the ARD (ARD + 14 days).

- Establishes a RUG-IV classification and Medicare payment (see Chapter 6, Section 6.4 for policies on determining RUG-IV payment), which begins on the day therapy started.

- Must be submitted electronically and accepted into the QIES ASAP system within 14 days after completion (Item Z0500B) (completion + 14 days).

End of Therapy (EOT) OMRA

- Required when the resident was classified in a RUG-IV Rehabilitation Plus Extensive Services or Rehabilitation group and continues to need Part A SNF-level services after the planned or unplanned discontinuation of all rehabilitation therapies for three or more consecutive days.

- ARD (Item A2300) must be set on day 1, 2, or 3 after all rehabilitation therapies have been discontinued for any reason (Item O0400A6 or O0400B6 or O0400C6, whichever is the latest). The last day on which therapy treatment was furnished is considered day 0 when determining the ARD for the End of Therapy OMRA. Day 1 is the first day after the last therapy treatment was provided whether therapy was scheduled or not scheduled for that day. For example:

  — If the resident was discharged from all therapy services on Tuesday, day 1 is Wednesday.

  — If the resident was discharged from all therapy services on Friday, Day 1 would be Saturday.

— If the resident received therapy Friday, was not scheduled for therapy on Saturday or Sunday and refused therapy for Monday, Day 1 would be Saturday.

- May be combined with any scheduled PPS assessment. In such cases, the item set for the scheduled assessment should be used.

- The ARD for the End of Therapy OMRA may not precede the ARD of the first scheduled PPS assessment of the Medicare stay (5-day or readmission/return assessment).

— For example: if the 5-day assessment is completed on day 8 and an EOT is completed in that window, the ARD for the EOT should be Day 8 as well.

- Must be completed (Item Z0500B) within 14 days after the ARD (ARD + 14 days).

- Establishes a new non-therapy RUG classification and Medicare payment rate (Item Z0150A), which begins the day after the last day of therapy treatment regardless of day selected for ARD.

- Must be submitted electronically to the QIES ASAP system and accepted into the QIES ASAP system within 14 days after completion (Item Z0500B) (completion + 14 days).

- In cases where a resident is classified into a Rehabilitation or Rehabilitation plus Extensive Services RUG category and experiences a planned or unplanned discontinuation of therapy services for three or more consecutive calendar days and the resident is discharged from the facility *on* the third day of missed therapy services, then no EOT OMRA is required. If the facility chooses to complete an EOT OMRA in this situation, it may be combined with the discharge assessment.

- In cases where a resident is discharged from the SNF *on or prior to* the third consecutive day of missed therapy services, then no EOT is required. More precisely, in cases where the date coded for Item A2000 is on or prior to the third consecutive day of missed therapy services, then no EOT OMRA is required. If a SNF chooses to complete the EOT OMRA in this situation, they may combine the EOT OMRA with the discharge assessment.

- If the EOT OMRA is performed because three or more consecutive days of therapy were missed, and it is determined that therapy will resume, there are three options for completion:

1. Complete only the EOT OMRA and keep the resident in a non-Rehabilitation RUG category until the next scheduled PPS assessment is completed. For example:

   - Mr. K. was discharged from all therapy services on Day 22 of his SNF stay. The EOT OMRA was performed on Day 24 of his SNF stay and classified into HD1. Payment continued at HD1 until the 30- day assessment was completed. At that point, therapy resumed (with a new therapy evaluation) and the resident was classified into RVB.

2. In cases where therapy resumes after an EOT OMRA is performed and more than 5 consecutive calendar days have passed since the last day of therapy provided, or therapy services will not resume at the same RUG-IV therapy classification level that had been in effect prior to the EOT OMRA, an SOT OMRA is required to classify the resident back into a RUG-IV therapy group and a new therapy evaluation is required as well. For example:

- Mr. G. who had been classified into RVX did not receive therapy on Saturday and Sunday. He also missed therapy on Monday because his family came to visit, on Tuesday he missed therapy due to a doctor's appointment and refused therapy on Wednesday. An EOT OMRA was performed on Monday classifying him into the ES2 non-therapy RUG. He missed 5 consecutive calendar days of therapy. A new therapy evaluation was completed and he resumed therapy services on Thursday. An SOT OMRA was then completed and Mr. G. was placed back into the RVX therapy RUG category.

- Mrs. B., who had been classified into RHC did not receive therapy on Monday, Tuesday, and Wednesday because of an infection, and it was determined that she would be able to start therapy again on Thursday. An EOT OMRA was completed to pay for the three days she did not have therapy with a non-therapy RUG classification of HC2. It was determined that Mrs. B. would not be able to resume therapy at the same RUG-IV therapy classification, and an SOT OMRA was completed to place her into the RMB RUG-IV therapy category. A new therapy evaluation was required.

3. In cases where therapy resumes after the EOT OMRA is performed and the resumption of therapy date is no more than 5 consecutive calendar days after the last day of therapy provided, and the therapy services have resumed at the same RUG-IV classification level, and with the same therapy plan of care that had been in effect prior to the EOT OMRA, an End of Therapy OMRA with Resumption (EOT-R) may be completed. For Example:

- Mrs. A. who was in RVL did not receive therapy on Saturday and Sunday because the facility did not provide weekend services and she missed therapy on Monday because of a doctor's appointment, but resumed therapy Tuesday. The IDT determined that her RUG-IV therapy classification level did not change as she had not had any significant clinical changes during the lapsed therapy days. An EOT-R was completed and Mrs. A was placed into ES3 for the three days she did not receive therapy. On Tuesday, Mrs. A. was placed back into RVL, which was the same therapy RUG group she was in prior to the discontinuation of therapy. A new therapy evaluation was not required.

NOTE: If the EOT OMRA has not been accepted in the QIES ASAP when therapy resumes, code the EOT-R items (O0450A and O0450B) on the assessment and submit the record. If the EOT OMRA without the EOT-R items has been accepted into the QIES ASAP system, then submit a modification request for that EOT OMRA with the only changes being the completion of the EOT-R items and check X0900E to indicate that the reason for modification is the addition of the Resumption of Therapy date.

NOTE: When an EOT-R is completed, the Therapy Start Date (O0400A5, O0400B5, and O0400C5) on the next PPS assessment is the same as the Therapy Start Date on the EOT-R. If therapy is ongoing, the Therapy End Date (O0400A6, O0400B6, and O0400C6) would be filled out with dashes.

4. In cases when the therapy end date is in one payment period and the resumption date is in the next payment period, the facility should bill the non-therapy RUG given on the EOT OMRA beginning the day after the last day of therapy treatment and begin billing the therapy RUG that was in effect prior to the EOT OMRA beginning on the day that

therapy resumed (O0450B). If the resumption of therapy occurs after the next billing period has started, then this therapy RUG should be used until modified by a future scheduled or unscheduled assessment.

For example, a resident misses therapy on Days 11, 12, and 13 and resumes therapy on Day 15. In this case the facility should bill the non-therapy RUG for Days 11, 12, 13, and 14 and on Day 15 the facility should bill the RUG that was in effect prior to the EOT.

Change of Therapy (COT) OMRA

- Required when the resident was receiving any amount of skilled therapy services and when the intensity of therapy (as indicated by the total reimbursable therapy minutes (RTM) delivered, and other therapy qualifiers such as number of therapy days and disciplines providing therapy) changes to such a degree that it would no longer reflect the RUG-IV classification and payment assigned for a given SNF resident based on the most recent assessment used for Medicare payment.

- ARD is set for Day 7 of a COT observation period. The COT observation periods are successive 7-day windows with the first observation period beginning on the day following the ARD set for the most recent scheduled or unscheduled PPS assessment, except for an EOT-R assessment (see below). For example:
  — If the ARD for a patient's 30-day assessment is set for day 30, and there are no intervening assessments, then the COT observation period ends on Day 37.
  — If the ARD for the patient's most recent COT (whether the COT was completed or not) was day Day 37, the next COT observation period would end on Day 44.

- In cases where the last PPS Assessment was an EOT-R, the end of the first COT observation period is Day 7 after the Resumption of Therapy date (O0450B) on the EOT-R, rather than the ARD. The resumption of therapy date is counted as day 1 when determining Day 7 of the COT observation period. For example:
  — If the ARD for an EOT-R is set for day 35 and the resumption date is the equivalent of day 37, then the COT observation period ends on day 43.

- An evaluation of the necessity for a COT OMRA (that is, an evaluation of the therapy intensity, as described above) must be completed after the COT observation period is over.

- The COT would be completed if the patient's therapy intensity, as described above, has changed to classify the resident into a higher or lower RUG category. For example:
  — If a facility sets the ARD for its 14-day assessment to day 14, Day 1 for purposes of the COT period would be Day 15 of the SNF stay, and the facility would be required to review the therapy services provided to the patient for the week consisting of Day 15 through 21. The ARD for the COT OMRA would then be set for Day 21, if the facility were to determine that, for example, the total RTM has changed such that the resident's RUG classification would change from that found on the 14-day assessment (assuming no intervening assessments). If the total RTM would not result in a RUG classification change, and all other therapy category qualifiers have

remained consistent with the patient's current RUG classification, then the COT OMRA would not be completed.

- If Day 7 of the COT observation period falls within the ARD window of a scheduled PPS Assessment, the SNF may choose to complete the PPS Assessment alone by setting the ARD of the scheduled PPS assessment for an allowable day that is *on or before* Day 7 of the COT observation period. This effectively resets the COT observation period to the 7 days following that scheduled PPS Assessment ARD. Alternatively, the SNF may choose to combine the COT OMRA and scheduled assessment following the instructions discussed in Section 2.10.

- In cases where a resident is discharged <u>from the SNF</u> *on or before* Day 7 of the COT observation period, then no COT OMRA is required. More precisely, in cases where the date coded for Item A2000 is on or before Day 7 of the COT observation period, then no COT OMRA is required. If a SNF chooses to complete the COT OMRA in this situation, they may combine the COT OMRA with the discharge assessment.

- The COT ARD may not precede the ARD of the first scheduled or unscheduled PPS assessment of the Medicare stay used to establish the patient's current RUG-IV therapy classification.

- Must be completed (Item Z0500B) within 14 days after the ARD (ARD + 14 days)

- Establishes a new RUG-IV category. Payment begins on Day 1 of that COT observation period and continues for the remainder of the current payment period, unless the payment is modified by a subsequent COT OMRA or other PPS assessment.

- Must be submitted electronically and accepted into the QIES ASAP system within 14 days after completion (Item Z0500B) (completion + 14 days).

Significant Change in Status Assessment (SCSA)

- Is an OBRA required assessment. See Section 2.6 of this chapter for definition, guidelines in completion, and scheduling.

- May establish a new RUG-IV classification.

- When a SCSA for a SNF PPS resident is not combined with a PPS assessment (A0310A = 04 and A0310B = 99), the RUG-IV classification and associated payment rate begin on the ARD. For example, a SCSA is completed with an ARD of day 20 then the RUG-IV classification begins on day 20.

- When the SCSA is completed with a scheduled Medicare-required assessment and grace days are not used when setting the ARD, the RUG-IV classification begins on the ARD. For example, the SCSA is combined with the Medicare-required 14-day scheduled assessment and the ARD is set on day 13, the RUG-IV classification begins on day 13.

- When the SCSA is completed with a scheduled Medicare-required assessment and the ARD is set within the grace days, the RUG-IV classification begins on the first day of the payment period of the scheduled Medicare-required assessment standard payment period. For example, the SCSA is combined with the Medicare-required 30-day scheduled assessment, which pays for days 31 to 60, and the ARD is set at day 33, the RUG-IV classification begins day 31.

Swing Bed Clinical Change Assessment

- Is a required assessment for swing bed providers. Staff is responsible for determining whether a change (either an improvement or decline) in a patient's condition constitutes a "clinical change" in the patient's status.

- Is similar to the OBRA Significant Change in Status Assessment with the exceptions of the CAA process and the timing related to the OBRA Admission assessment. See Section 2.6 of this chapter.

- May establish a new RUG-IV classification. See previous Significant Change in Status subsection for ARD implications on the payment schedule.

Significant Correction to Prior Comprehensive Assessment

- Is an OBRA required assessment. See Section 2.6 of this chapter for definition, guidelines in completion, and scheduling.

- May establish a new RUG-IV classification. See previous Significant Change in Status subsection for ARD implications on the payment schedule.

Coding Tips and Special Populations

- When coding a standalone Change of Therapy OMRA (COT), a standalone End of Therapy OMRA (EOT), or a standalone Start of Therapy OMRA (SOT), the interview items may be coded using the responses provided by the resident on a previous assessment **only** if the DATE of the interview responses from the previous assessment (as documented in item Z0400) were obtained no more than 14 days before the DATE of completion for the interview items on the unscheduled assessment (as documented in item Z0400) for which those responses will be used.

- When coding a standalone Change of Therapy OMRA (COT), a standalone End of Therapy OMRA (EOT), or a standalone Start of Therapy OMRA (SOT), facilities must set the ARD for the assessment for a day within the allowable ARD window for that assessment type, but may only do so no more than two days after the window has passed. For example, if Day 7 of the COT observation period is May 23rd and the COT is required, then the ARD for this COT must be set for May 23rd and this must be done by May 25th. Facilities may still exercise the use of this flexibility period in cases where the resident discharges from the facility during that period.

2.10 Combining Medicare Scheduled and Unscheduled Assessments

There may be instances when more than one Medicare-required assessment is due in the same time period. To reduce provider burden, CMS allows the combining of assessments. Two Medicare-required Scheduled Assessments may **never** be combined since these assessments have specific ARD windows that do not occur at the same time. However, it is possible that a Medicare-required Scheduled Assessment and a Medicare Unscheduled Assessment may be combined or that two Medicare Unscheduled assessments may be combined.

When combining assessments, the more stringent requirements must be met. For example, when a nursing home Start of Therapy OMRA is combined with a 14-Day Medicare-required Assessment, the PPS item set must be used. The PPS item set contains all the required items for the 14-Day Medicare-required assessment, whereas the Start of Therapy OMRA item set consists of fewer items, thus the provider would need to complete the PPS item set. The ARD window (including grace days) for the 14-day assessment is days 13-18, therefore, the ARD must be set no later than day 18 to ensure that all required time frames are met. For a swing bed provider, the swing bed PPS item set would need to be completed.

If an unscheduled PPS assessment (OMRA, SCSA, SCPA, or Swing Bed CCA) is required in the assessment window (including grace days) of a scheduled PPS assessment that has not yet been performed, then facilities must combine the scheduled and unscheduled assessments by setting the ARD of the scheduled assessment for the same day that the unscheduled assessment is required. In such cases, facilities should provide the proper response to the A0310 items to indicate which assessments are being combined, as completion of the combined assessment will be taken to fulfill the requirements for both the scheduled and unscheduled assessments. A scheduled PPS assessment cannot occur after an unscheduled assessment in the assessment window—the scheduled assessment must be combined with the unscheduled assessment using the appropriate ARD for the unscheduled assessment. The purpose of this policy is to minimize the number of assessments required for SNF PPS payment purposes and to ensure that the assessments used for payment provide the most accurate picture of the resident's clinical condition and service needs. More details about combining PPS assessments are provided in this chapter and in Chapter 6, Section 30.3 of the Medicare Claims Processing Manual (CMS Pub. 100-04) available on the CMS web site. Listed below are some of the possible assessment combinations allowed. A provider may choose to combine more than two assessment types when all requirements are met. When entered directly into the software the coding of Item A0310 will provide the item set that the facility is required to complete. For SNFs that use a paper format to collect MDS data, the provider must ensure that the item set selected meets the requirements of all assessments coded in Item A0310 (see Section 2.15).

In cases when a facility fails to combine a scheduled and unscheduled PPS assessment as required by the combined assessment policy, the payment is controlled by the unscheduled assessment. For example: if the ARD of an EOT OMRA is set for Day 14 and the ARD of a 14-day assessment is set for Day 15, this would violate the combined assessment policy. Consequently, the EOT OMRA would control the payment. The EOT would begin payment on Day 12, and continue paying into the 14-day payment window until the next scheduled or unscheduled assessment used for payment.

> **DEFINITIONS**
>
> **USED FOR PAYMENT**
> An assessment is considered to be "used for payment" in that it either controls the payment for a given period or, with scheduled assessments may set the basis for payment for a given period.

PPS Scheduled Assessment and Start of Therapy OMRA

- ARD (Item A2300) must be set within the ARD window for the Medicare-required scheduled assessment **and** 5-7 days after the start of therapy (Item O0400A5 or O0400B5 or O0400C5, whichever is the earliest date). If both ARD requirements are not met, the assessments may not be combined.

- An SOT OMRA is not necessary if rehabilitation services start within the ARD window (including grace days) of the 5-day assessment, since the therapy rate will be paid starting Day 1 of the SNF stay.
- If the ARD for the SOT OMRA falls within the ARD window (including grace days) of a PPS scheduled assessment that has not been performed yet, the assessments MUST be combined.
- Complete the PPS item set.
- Code the Item A0310 of the MDS 3.0 as follows:

  A0310A = 99
  A0310B = 01, 02, 03, 04, 05, or 06 as appropriate
  A0310C = 1
  A0310D = 0 (Swing Beds only)

PPS Scheduled Assessment and End of Therapy OMRA

- ARD (Item A2300) must be set within the window for the Medicare scheduled assessment **and** 1-3 days after the last day therapy was furnished (Item O0400A6 or O0400B6 or O0400C6, whichever is the latest date). If both ARD requirements are not met, the assessments may not be combined.
- If the ARD for the EOT OMRA falls within the ARD window (including grace days) of a PPS scheduled assessment that has not been performed yet, the assessments MUST be combined.
- Must complete the PPS item set.
- Code the Item A0310 of the MDS 3.0 as follows:

  A0310A = 99
  A0310B = 01, 02, 03, 04, 05, or 06 as appropriate
  A0310C = 2
  A0310D = 0 (Swing Beds only)

PPS Scheduled Assessment and Start and End of Therapy OMRA

- ARD (Item A2300) must be set within the window for the Medicare-required scheduled assessment **and** 5-7 days after the start of therapy (Item O0400A5 or O0400B5 or O0400C5, whichever is earliest) **and** 1-3 days after the last day therapy was furnished (Item O0400A6 or O0400B6 or O0400C6, whichever is latest). If all three ARD requirements are not met, the assessments may not be combined.
- If the ARD for the EOT and SOT OMRA falls within the ARD window (including grace days) of a PPS scheduled assessment that has not been performed yet, the assessments MUST be combined.
- Must complete the PPS item set.
- Code the Item A0310 of the MDS 3.0 as follows:

  A0310A = 99
  A0310B = 01, 02, 03, 04, 05, or 06 as appropriate
  A0310C = 3
  A0310D = 0 (Swing Beds only)

PPS Scheduled Assessment and Change of Therapy OMRA

- If Day 7 of the COT observation period falls within the ARD window (including grace days) of a scheduled PPS Assessment, then a SNF must elect to either combine the COT OMRA with the scheduled PPS assessment or may choose to complete the scheduled PPS assessment alone, as described in Section 2.9. If the scheduled PPS assessment is to be completed alone, then the ARD for the scheduled PPS assessment must be set for on or before Day 7 of the COT observation period. If the SNF chooses to combine the scheduled PPS assessment with the COT OMRA, then the ARD of the combined assessment must be set for Day 7 of the COT observation period.

- Must complete the scheduled PPS assessment item set.

- Since the scheduled assessment is combined with the COT OMRA, the combined assessment will set payment at the new RUG-IV level beginning on Day 1 of the COT observation period and that payment will continue through the remainder of the current standard payment period and the next payment period appropriate to the given scheduled assessment, assuming no intervening assessments. For example:

  — Based on her 14-day assessment, Mrs. T is currently classified into group RVB. Based on the ARD set for the 14-day assessment, a change of therapy evaluation for Mrs. T is necessary on Day 28. The change of therapy evaluation reveals that the therapy services Mrs. T received during that COT observation period were only sufficient to qualify Mrs. T for RHB. Therefore, a COT OMRA is required. Since the facility has not yet completed a 30-day assessment for Mrs. T, the facility must combine the 30-day assessment with the required COT OMRA. The combined assessment confirms Mrs. T's appropriate classification into RHB. The payment for the revised RUG classification will begin on Day 22 and, assuming no intervening assessments, will continue until Day 60.

PPS Scheduled Assessment and Swing Bed Clinical Change Assessment

- ARD (Item A2300) must be set within the window for the Medicare-required scheduled assessment **and** within 14 days after the interdisciplinary team (IDT) determination that a change in the patient's condition constitutes a clinical change **and** the assessment must be completed (Item Z0500B) within 14 days after the IDT determines that a change in the patient's condition constitutes a clinical change. If all requirements are not met, the assessments may not be combined.

- If the ARD for the Swing Bed Clinical Change Assessment falls within the ARD (including grace days) of a PPS scheduled assessment that has not been completed yet, the assessments MUST be combined.

- Must complete the Swing Bed PPS item set.

- Code the Item A0310 of the MDS 3.0 as follows:

  A0310A = 99 (only value allowed for Swing Beds)
  A0310B = 01, 02, 03, 04, 05, or 06, as appropriate
  A0310C = 0
  A0310D = 1

Swing Bed Clinical Change Assessment and Start of Therapy OMRA

- ARD (Item A2300) must be set within 14 days after the IDT determination that a change in the patient's condition constitutes a clinical change **and** 5-7 days after the start of therapy (Item O0400A5 or O0400B5 or O0400C5, whichever is earliest) **and** the assessment must be completed (Item Z0500B) within 14 days after the IDT determination that a change in the patient's condition constitutes a clinical change. If all requirements are not met, the assessments may not be combined.

- Must complete the Swing Bed PPS item set.

- Code the Item A0310 of the MDS 3.0 as follows:

   A0310A = 99
   A0310B = 07
   A0310C = 1
   A0310D = 1

Swing Bed Clinical Change Assessment and End of Therapy OMRA

- ARD (Item A2300) must be set within 14 days after the IDT determination that a change in the patient's condition constitutes a clinical change **and** 1-3 days after the last day therapy was furnished (Item O0400A6 or O0400B6 or O0400C6, whichever is the latest) **and** the assessment must be completed (Item Z0500B) within 14 days after the IDT determination that a change in the patient's condition constitutes a clinical change. If all requirements are not met, the assessments may not be combined.

- Must complete the Swing Bed PPS item set.

- Code the Item A0310 of the MDS 3.0 as follows:

   A0310A = 99
   A0310B = 07
   A0310C = 2
   A0310D = 1

Swing Bed Clinical Change Assessment and Start and End of Therapy OMRA

- ARD (Item A2300) must be set within 14 days after the IDT determination that a change in the patient's condition constitutes a clinical change **and** 5-7 days after the start of therapy (Item O0400A5 or O0400B5 or O0400C5, whichever is the earliest) **and** 1-3 days after the last day therapy was furnished (Item O0400A6 or O0400B6 or O0400C6, whichever is the latest) **and** the assessment must be completed (Item Z0500B) within 14 days after the IDT determination that a change in the patient's condition constitutes a clinical change. If all requirements are not met, the assessments may not be combined.

- Must complete the Swing Bed PPS item set.

- Code the Item A0310 of the MDS 3.0 as follows:

   A0310A = 99
   A0310B = 07
   A0310C = 3
   A0310D = 1

2.11 Combining Medicare Assessments and OBRA Assessments[7]

SNF providers are required to meet two assessment standards in a Medicare certified nursing facility:

- The OBRA standards are designated by the reason selected in Item A0310A, **Federal OBRA Reason for Assessment**, and Item A0130F, **Entry/Discharge Reporting** and are required for all residents.

- The Medicare standards are designated by the reason selected in Item A0310B, **PPS Assessment**, and Item A0310C, **PPS Other Medicare Required Assessment - OMRA** and are required for resident's whose stay is covered by Medicare Part A.

- When the OBRA and Medicare assessment time frames coincide, one assessment may be used to satisfy both requirements. PPS and OBRA assessments may be combined when the ARD windows overlap allowing for a common assessment reference date. When combining the OBRA and Medicare assessments, the most stringent requirements for ARD, item set, and CAA completion requirements must be met. For example, the skilled nursing facility staff must be very careful in selecting the ARD for an OBRA Admission assessment combined with a 14-day Medicare assessment. For the OBRA Admission standard, the ARD must be set between days 1 and 14 counting the date of admission as day 1. For Medicare, the ARD must be set for days 13 or 14, but the regulation allows grace days up to day 18. However, when combining a 14-day Medicare assessment with the Admission assessment, the use of grace days for the PPS assessment would result in a late OBRA Admission assessment. To assure the assessment meets both standards, an ARD of day 13 or 14 would have to be chosen in this situation. In addition, the completion standards must be met. While a PPS assessment can be completed within 14 days after the ARD when it is not combined with an OBRA assessment, the CAA completion date for the OBRA Admission assessment (Item V0200B2) must be day 14 or earlier. With the combined OBRA Admission/Medicare 14-day assessment, completion by day 14 would be required. Finally, when combining a Medicare assessment with an OBRA assessment, the SNF staff must ensure that all required items are completed. For example, when combining the Medicare-required 30-day assessment with a Significant Change in Status Assessment, the provider would need to complete a comprehensive item set, including CAAs.

Some states require providers to complete additional state-specific items (Section S) for selected assessments. States may also add comprehensive items to the Quarterly and/or PPS item sets. Providers must ensure that they follow their state requirements in addition to any OBRA and/or Medicare requirements.

The following tables provide the item set for each type of assessment or tracking record. When two or more assessments are combined then the appropriate item set contains all items that would be necessary if each of the combined assessments were being completed individually.

---

[7] OBRA-required comprehensive and Quarterly assessments do not apply to Swing Bed Providers. However, Swing Bed Providers are required to complete the Entry Record, Discharge Assessments, and Death in Facility Record.

Minimum Required Item Set By Assessment Type for Skilled Nursing Facilities

	Comprehensive Item Set	Quarterly/ PPS* Item Sets	Other Required Assessments/Tracking Item Sets for Skilled Nursing Facilities
Stand-alone Assessment Types	• OBRA Admission • Annual • Significant Change in Status (SCSA) • Significant Correction to Prior Comprehensive (SCPA)	• Quarterly • Significant Correction to Prior Quarterly • PPS 5-Day (5-Day) • PPS 14-Day (14-Day) • PPS 30-Day (30-Day) • PPS 60-Day (60-Day) • PPS 90-Day (90-Day) • PPS Readmission/Return	• Entry Tracking Record • Discharge assessments • Death in Facility Tracking Record • Start of Therapy OMRA • Start of Therapy OMRA and Discharge • Change of Therapy OMRA • OMRA • OMRA and Discharge
Combined Assessment Types	• OBRA Admission and 5-Day • OBRA Admission and 14-Day • OBRA Admission and any OMRA • Annual and any Medicare-required • Annual and any OMRA • SCSA and any Medicare-required • SCSA and any OMRA • SCPA and any Medicare-required • SCPA and any OMRA • Any OBRA comprehensive and any Discharge	• Quarterly and any Medicare-scheduled • Quarterly and any OMRA • Significant Correction to Prior Quarterly and any Medicare-required • Significant Correction to Prior Quarterly and any OMRA • Any Discharge and any Medicare-required • Quarterly and any Discharge • Significant Correction to Prior Quarterly and any Discharge • Any Medicare-required and any Discharge	N/A

*Provider must check with State Agency to determine if the state requires additional items to be completed for the required OBRA Quarterly and PPS assessments.

Minimum Required Item Set By Assessment Type for Swing Bed Providers

	Swing Bed PPS	Other Required Assessments/Tracking Item Sets for Swing Bed Providers
Assessment Type	• PPS 5-Day (5-Day) • PPS 14-Day (14-Day) • PPS 30-Day (30-Day) • PPS 60-Day (60-Day) • PPS 90-Day (90-Day) • PPS Readmission/Return • Clinical Change Assessment	• Entry Record • Discharge assessments • Death in Facility record • Start of Therapy OMRA • Start of Therapy OMRA and Discharge • Change of Therapy OMRA • OMRA • OMRA and Discharge
Assessment Type Combinations	• Clinical Change and any Medicare-required • Any Medicare-required and any Discharge	N/A

Tracking records (Entry and Death in Facility) are never combined with other assessments.

The OMRA item sets are all unique item sets and are never completed when combining with other assessments, which require completion of additional items. For example, a **Start of Therapy OMRA** item set is completed only when an assessment is conducted to capture the start of therapy **and** assign a RUG-IV therapy group. In addition, a **Start of Therapy OMRA and Discharge** item set is only completed when the facility staff choose to complete an assessment to reflect the start of therapy and discharge from facility. If those assessments are completed in combination with another assessment type, an item set that contains all items required for both assessments must be selected.

2.12 Medicare and OBRA Assessment Combinations

Below are some of the possible assessment combinations allowed. A provider may choose to combine more than two assessment types when all requirements are met. The coding of Item A0310 will provide the item set that the facility is required to complete. For SNFs that use a paper format to collect MDS data, the provider must ensure that the item set selected meets the requirements of all assessments coded in Item A0310 (see Section 2.15).

Medicare-required 5-Day and OBRA Admission Assessment

- Comprehensive item set.
- ARD (Item A2300) must be set on days 1 through 5 of the Part A SNF stay.
- ARD may be extended up to day 8 using the designated grace days.
- Must be completed (Item Z0500B) by the end of day 14 of the stay (admission date plus 13 calendar days).
- See Section 2.7 for requirements for CAA process and care plan completion.

Medicare-required 14-Day and OBRA Admission Assessment

- Comprehensive item set.
- ARD (Item A2300) must be set on days 13 or 14 of the Part A SNF stay.
- ARD may not be extended from day 15 to day 18 (i.e., grace days may not be used).
- Must be completed (Item Z0500B) by the end of day 14 of the stay (admission date plus 13 calendar days).
- See Section 2.7 for requirements for CAA process and care plan completion.

Medicare-required Scheduled Assessment and OBRA Quarterly Assessment

- Quarterly item set as required by the State.
- ARD (Item A2300) must be set on a day that meets the requirements described earlier for each Medicare-required scheduled assessment in Section 2.9 and for the OBRA Quarterly assessment in Section 2.6.
- ARD may be extended to grace days as long as the requirement for the Quarterly ARD is met.

- See Section 2.6 for OBRA Quarterly assessment completion requirements.

Medicare-required Scheduled Assessment and Annual Assessment

- Comprehensive item set.
- ARD (Item A2300) must be set on a day that meets the requirements described earlier for each Medicare-required scheduled assessment in Section 2.9 and for the OBRA Annual assessment in Section 2.6.
- ARD may be extended to grace days as long as the requirement for the Annual ARD is met.
- See Section 2.6 for OBRA Annual assessment completion requirements.
- See Section 2.7 for requirements for CAA process and care plan completion.

Medicare-required Scheduled Assessment and Significant Change in Status Assessment

- Comprehensive item set.
- ARD (Item A2300) must be set within the window for the Medicare-required scheduled assessment and within 14 days after determination that criteria are met for a Significant Change in Status assessment.
- Must be completed (Item Z0500B) within 14 days after the determination that the criteria are met for a Significant Change in Status assessment.
- See Section 2.7 for requirements for CAA process and care plan completion.

Medicare-required Scheduled Assessment and Significant Correction to Prior Comprehensive Assessment

- Comprehensive item set.
- ARD (Item A2300) must be set within the window for the Medicare-required scheduled assessment **and** within 14 days after the determination that an uncorrected significant error in the prior comprehensive assessment has occurred.
- Must be completed (Item Z0500B) within 14 days after the determination that an uncorrected significant error in the prior comprehensive assessment has occurred.
- See Section 2.7 for requirements for CAA process and care plan completion.

Medicare-required Scheduled Assessment and Significant Correction to Prior Quarterly Assessment

- See Medicare-required Scheduled Assessment and OBRA Quarterly Assessment.

Medicare-required Scheduled Assessment and Discharge Assessment

- PPS item set.

- ARD (Item A2300) must be set for the day of discharge (Item A2000) **and** the date of discharge must fall within the allowed window of the Medicare scheduled assessment as described earlier in Section 2.9.
- Must be completed (Item Z0500B) within 14 days after the ARD.

Start of Therapy OMRA and OBRA Admission Assessment

- Comprehensive item set.
- ARD (Item A2300) must be set on day 14 or earlier of the stay and 5-7 days after the start of therapy (Item O0400A5 or O0400B5 or O0400C5, whichever is the earliest date).
- Completed to classify a resident into a RUG-IV Rehabilitation Plus Extensive Services or Rehabilitation group. If the RUG-IV classification is not a therapy group, the assessment will not be accepted by CMS and cannot be used for Medicare billing.
- Must be completed (Item Z0500B) by day 14 of the stay (admission date plus 13 calendar days).
- See Section 2.7 for requirements for CAA process and care plan completion

Start of Therapy OMRA and OBRA Quarterly Assessment

- Quarterly item set as required by the State.
- ARD (Item A2300) must be set 5-7 days after the start of therapy (Item O0400A5 or O0400B5 or O0400C5, whichever is the earliest date) and meet the requirements for an OBRA Quarterly assessment as described in Section 2.6.
- Completed to classify a resident into a RUG-IV Rehabilitation Plus Extensive Services or Rehabilitation group. If the RUG-IV classification is not a therapy group, the assessment will not be accepted by CMS and cannot be used for Medicare billing.
- See Section 2.6 for OBRA Quarterly assessment completion requirements.

Start of Therapy OMRA and Annual Assessment

- Comprehensive item set
- ARD (Item A2300) must be set 5-7 days after the start of therapy (Item O0400A5 or O0400B5 or O0400C5) **and** meet the requirements for an OBRA Annual assessment as described in Section 2.6.
- Completed to classify a resident into a RUG-IV Rehabilitation Plus Extensive Services or Rehabilitation group. If the RUG-IV classification is not a therapy group, the assessment will not be accepted by CMS and cannot be used for Medicare billing.
- See Section 2.7 for requirements for CAA process and care plan completion.

Start of Therapy OMRA and Significant Change in Status Assessment

- Comprehensive item set.
- ARD (Item A2300) must be set within 14 days after the determination that criteria are met for a Significant Change in Status assessment **and** 5-7 days after the start of therapy (Item O0400A5 or O0400B5 or O0400C5, whichever is the earliest date).

- Must be completed (Item Z0500B) within 14 days after the ARD and within 14 days after the determination that the criteria are met for a Significant Change in Status assessment.
- Completed to classify a resident into a RUG-IV Rehabilitation Plus Extensive Services or Rehabilitation group. If the RUG-IV classification is not a therapy group, the assessment will **not** be accepted by CMS and cannot be used for Medicare billing.
- See Section 2.7 for requirements for CAA process and care plan completion.

Start of Therapy OMRA and Significant Correction to Prior Comprehensive Assessment

- Comprehensive item set.
- ARD (Item A2300) must be set within 14 days after determination that an uncorrected significant error in a comprehensive assessment has occurred **and** 5-7 days after the start of therapy (Item O0400A5 or O0400B5 or O0400C5, whichever is the earliest date).
- Must be completed (Item Z0500B) within 14 days after the ARD and within 14 days after the determination that an uncorrected significant error in a comprehensive assessment has occurred.
- Completed to classify a resident into a RUG-IV Rehabilitation Plus Extensive Services or Rehabilitation group. If the RUG-IV classification is not a therapy group, the assessment will **not** be accepted by CMS and cannot be used for Medicare billing.
- See Section 2.7 for requirements for CAA process and care plan completion.

Start of Therapy OMRA and Significant Correction to Prior Quarterly Assessment

- See SOT OMRA and OBRA Quarterly Assessment

Start of Therapy OMRA and Discharge Assessment

- Start of Therapy OMRA and Discharge item set.
- ARD (Item A2300) must be set for the day of discharge (Item A2000) **and** the date of discharge must fall within 5-7 days after the start of therapy (Item O0400A5 or O0400B5 or O0400C5, whichever is the earliest date). The ARD must be set by no more than two days after the date of discharge. (See Section 2.8 for further clarification.)
- Completed to classify a resident into a RUG-IV Rehabilitation Plus Extensive Services or Rehabilitation group. If the RUG-IV classification is not a therapy group, the assessment will **not** be accepted by CMS and cannot be used for Medicare billing.
- Must be completed (Item Z0500B) within 14 days after the ARD.

End of Therapy OMRA and OBRA Admission Assessment

- Comprehensive item set.
- ARD (Item A2300) must be set on day 14 or earlier of the stay **and** 1-3 days after the last day therapy was furnished (difference is 3 or less for Item A2300 minus Item O0400A6 or O0400B6 or O0400C6, whichever is the latest).

- Must be completed (Item Z0500B) by day 14 of the stay (admission date plus 13 calendar days).

- Completed only when the resident was classified in a RUG-IV Rehabilitation Plus Extensive Services or Rehabilitation group and continues to need Part A SNF-level services after the discontinuation of all therapies.

- Establishes a new non-therapy RUG classification and Medicare payment rate (Item Z0150A), which begins the day after the last day of therapy treatment.

- See Section 2.7 for requirements for CAA process and care plan completion.

End of Therapy OMRA and OBRA Quarterly Assessment

- Quarterly item set as required by the State.

- ARD (Item A2300) must be 1-3 days after the last day therapy was furnished (Item O0400A6 or O0400B6 or O0400C6, whichever is the latest) **and** meet the requirements for an OBRA Quarterly assessment as described in Section 2.6.

- Completed only when the resident was classified in a RUG-IV Rehabilitation Plus Extensive Services or Rehabilitation group and continues to need Part A SNF-level services after the discontinuation of all therapies.

- Establishes a new non-therapy RUG classification and Medicare payment rate (Item Z0150A), which begins the day after the last day of therapy treatment.

- See Section 2.6 for OBRA Quarterly assessment completion requirements.

End of Therapy OMRA and Annual Assessment

- Comprehensive item set.

- ARD (Item A2300) must be set 1-3 days after the last day therapy was furnished (Item O0400A6 or O0400B6 or O0400C6, whichever is the latest) **and** meet the requirements for an OBRA Annual assessment as described in Section 2.6.

- Completed only when the resident was classified in a RUG-IV Rehabilitation Plus Extensive Services or Rehabilitation group and continues to need Part A SNF-level services after the discontinuation of all therapies.

- Establishes a new non-therapy RUG classification and Medicare payment rate (Item Z0150A), which begins the day after the last day of therapy treatment.

- See Section 2.6 for OBRA Annual assessment completion requirements.

- See Section 2.7 for requirements for CAA process and care plan completion.

End of Therapy OMRA and Significant Change in Status Assessment

- Comprehensive item set.

- ARD (Item A2300) must be set within 14 days after the determination that the criteria are met for a Significant Change in Status assessment **and** 1-3 days after the end of therapy (O0400A6 or O0400B6 or O0400C6, whichever is the latest date).

- Must be completed (Item Z0500B) within 14 days after the ARD and within 14 days after the determination that the criteria are met for a Significant Change in Status assessment.

- Completed only when the resident was classified in a RUG-IV Rehabilitation Plus Extensive Services or Rehabilitation group and continues to need Part A SNF-level services after the discontinuation of all therapies.

- Establishes a new non-therapy RUG classification and Medicare payment rate (Item Z0150A), which begins the day after the last day of therapy treatment.

- See Section 2.7 for requirements for CAA process and care plan completion.

End of Therapy OMRA and Significant Correction to Prior Comprehensive Assessment

- Comprehensive item set.

- ARD (Item A2300) must be set within 14 days after the determination that an uncorrected significant error in the prior comprehensive assessment has occurred **and** 1-3 days after the end of therapy (Item O0400A6 or O0400B6 or O0400C6, whichever is the latest date).

- Must be completed (Item Z0500B) within 14 days after the ARD and within 14 days after the determination that an uncorrected significant error in prior comprehensive assessment has occurred.

- Completed only when the resident was classified in a RUG-IV Rehabilitation Plus Extensive Services or Rehabilitation group and continues to need Part A SNF-level services after the discontinuation of all therapies.

- Establishes a new non-therapy RUG classification and Medicare payment rate (Item Z0150A), which begins the day after the last day of therapy treatment.

- See Section 2.7 for requirements for CAA process and care plan completion.

End of Therapy OMRA and Significant Correction to Prior Quarterly Assessment

- See EOT OMRA and OBRA Quarterly Assessment.

End of Therapy OMRA and Discharge Assessment

- OMRA and Discharge item set.

- ARD (Item A2300) must be set for the day of discharge (Item A2000) **and** the date of discharge must fall within 1-3 days after the last day therapy was furnished (Item O0400A6 or O0400B6 or O0400C6, whichever is the latest). The ARD must be set by no more than two days after the date of discharge. (See Section 2.8 for further clarification).

- Completed only when the resident was classified in a RUG-IV Rehabilitation Plus Extensive Services or Rehabilitation group and continues to need Part A SNF-level services after the discontinuation of all therapies.

- Establishes a new non-therapy RUG classification and Medicare payment rate (Item Z0150A), which begins the day after the last day of therapy treatment.

- Must be completed (Item Z0500B) within 14 days after the ARD.

Start and End of Therapy OMRA and OBRA Admission Assessment

- Comprehensive item set.

- ARD (Item A2300) must be set on day 14 or earlier of the stay **and** 5-7 days after the start of therapy (Item O0400A5 or O0400B5 or O0400C5, whichever is earliest) **and** 1-3 days after the last day therapy was furnished (Item O0400A6 or O0400B6 or O0400C6, whichever is the latest).

- Must be completed (Item Z0500B) by day 14 of the stay (admission date plus 13 calendar days).

- Completed to classify a resident into a RUG-IV Rehabilitation Plus Extensive Services or Rehabilitation group (Item Z0100A) **and** into a non-therapy group (Item Z0150A) when the resident continues to need Part A SNF-level services after the discontinuation of all therapies. If the RUG-IV classification (Item Z0100) is not a therapy group, the assessment will **not** be accepted by CMS and cannot be used for Medicare billing.

- Establishes a new non-therapy RUG classification and Medicare payment rate (Item Z0150A), which begins the day after the last day of therapy treatment.

- See Section 2.7 for requirements for CAA process and care plan completion.

Start and End of Therapy OMRA and OBRA Quarterly Assessment

- Quarterly item set.

- ARD (Item A2300) must be 5-7 days after the start of therapy (Item O0400A5 or O0400B5 or O0400C5, whichever is earliest) **and** 1-3 days after the last day therapy was furnished (Item O0400A6 or O0400B6 or O0400C6, whichever is the latest) **and** meet the requirements for OBRA Quarterly assessment as described in Section 2.6.

- Completed to classify a resident into a RUG-IV Rehabilitation Plus Extensive Services or Rehabilitation group (Item Z0100A) **and** into a non-therapy group (Item Z0150A) when the resident continues to need Part A SNF-level services after the discontinuation of all therapies. If the RUG-IV classification (Item Z0100A) is not a therapy group, the assessment will **not** be accepted by CMS and cannot be used for Medicare billing.

- Establishes a new non-therapy RUG classification and Medicare payment rate (Item Z0150A), which begins the day after the last day of therapy treatment.

- See Section 2.6 for OBRA Quarterly assessment completion requirements.

Start and End of Therapy OMRA and Annual Assessment

- Comprehensive item set.

- ARD (Item A2300) must be set 5-7 days after the start of therapy (Item O0400A5 or O0400B5 or O0400C5, whichever is the earliest) **and** 1-3 days after the last day therapy was furnished (Item O0400A6 or O0400B6 or O0400C6, whichever is the latest) **and** meet the requirements for OBRA Annual assessment requirements as described in Section 2.6.

- Completed to classify a resident into a RUG-IV Rehabilitation Plus Extensive Services or Rehabilitation group (Item Z0100A) **and** into a non-therapy group (Item Z0150A) when the resident continues to need Part A SNF-level services after the discontinuation of all therapies. If the RUG-IV classification (Item Z0100A) is not a therapy group, the assessment will **not** be accepted by CMS and cannot be used for Medicare billing.

- Establishes a new non-therapy RUG classification and Medicare payment rate (Item Z0150A), which begins the day after the last day of therapy treatment.
- See Section 2.6 for OBRA Annual assessment completion requirements.
- See Section 2.7 for requirements for CAA process and care plan completion.

Start and End of Therapy OMRA and Significant Change in Status Assessment

- Comprehensive item set.
- ARD (A2300) must be set within 14 days after the determination that the criteria are met for a Significant Change in Status assessment **and** 5-7 days after the start of therapy (Item O0400A5 or O0400B5 or O0400C5, whichever is earliest) **and** 1-3 days after the end of therapy (O0400A6 or O0400B6 or O0400C6, whichever is the latest date).
- Must be completed (Z0500B) within 14 days after the ARD and within 14 days after the determination that criteria are met for a Significant Change in Status assessment.
- Completed to classify a resident into a RUG-IV Rehabilitation Plus Extensive Services or Rehabilitation group (Item Z0100A) **and** into a non-therapy group (Item Z0150A) when the resident continues to need Part A SNF-level services after the discontinuation of all therapies. If the RUG-IV classification (Item Z0100A) is not a therapy group, the assessment will **not** be accepted by CMS and cannot be used for Medicare billing.
- Establishes a new non-therapy RUG classification and Medicare payment rate (Item Z0150A), which begins the day after the last day of therapy treatment.
- See Section 2.7 for requirements for CAA process and care plan completion.

Start and End of Therapy OMRA and Significant Correction to Prior Comprehensive Assessment

- Comprehensive item set.
- ARD (Item A2300) must be set within 14 days after the determination that an uncorrected significant error in the prior comprehensive assessment has occurred **and** 5-7 days after the start of therapy (Item O0400A5 or O0400B5 or O0400C5, whichever is earliest) **and** 1-3 days after the end of therapy (Item O0400A6 or O0400B6 or O0400C6, whichever is the latest date).
- Must be completed (Item Z0500B) within 14 days after the ARD and within 14 days after the determination that an uncorrected significant error in prior comprehensive assessment has occurred.
- Completed to classify a resident into a RUG-IV Rehabilitation Plus Extensive Services or Rehabilitation group (Item Z0100A) **and** into a non-therapy group (Item Z0150A) when the resident continues to need Part A SNF-level services after the discontinuation of all therapies. If the RUG-IV classification (Item Z0100A) is not a therapy group, the assessment will **not** be accepted by CMS and cannot be used for Medicare billing.
- Establishes a new non-therapy RUG classification and Medicare payment rate (Item Z0150A), which begins the day after the last day of therapy treatment.
- See Section 2.7 for requirements for CAA process and care plan completion.

Start and End of Therapy OMRA and Significant Correction to Prior Quarterly Assessment

- See Start and End of Therapy OMRA and OBRA Quarterly Assessment.

Start and End of Therapy OMRA and Discharge Assessment

- OMRA-Start of Therapy and Discharge item set.

- ARD (Item A2300) must be set for the day of discharge (Item A2000) and the date of discharge must fall within 5-7 days after the start of therapy (Item O0400A5 or O0400B5 or O0400C5, whichever is earliest) and 1-3 days after the last day therapy was furnished (Item O0400A6 or O0400B6 or O0400C6). The ARD must be set by no more than two days after the date of discharge. (See Section 2.8 for further clarification).

- Completed to classify a resident into a RUG-IV Rehabilitation Plus Extensive Services or Rehabilitation group (Item Z0100A) **and** into a non-therapy group (Item Z0150A) when the resident continues to need Part A SNF-level services after the discontinuation of all therapies. If the RUG-IV classification (Item Z0100A) is not a therapy group, the assessment will **not** be accepted by CMS and cannot be used for Medicare billing..

- Establishes a new non-therapy RUG classification and Medicare payment rate (Item Z0150A), which begins the day after the last day of therapy treatment.

- Must be completed (Item Z0500B) within 14 days after the ARD.

Change of Therapy OMRA and OBRA Admission Assessment

- Comprehensive item set.

- ARD (Item A2300) must be set on day 14 or earlier after admission **and** be on the last day of a COT 7-day observation period. Must be completed (Item Z0500B) by day 14 after admission (admission date plus 13 calendar days).

- Completed when the patient received skilled therapy services and a change of therapy evaluation determines that a COT OMRA is necessary, based on a determination that the intensity of therapy (as indicated by the total reimbursable therapy minutes (RTM) delivered and other therapy qualifiers such as number of therapy days and disciplines providing therapy), in the COT observation window differed from the therapy intensity on the last PPS assessment to such an extent that the RUG IV category would change).

- Establishes a new RUG-IV classification and Medicare payment rate (Item Z0100A), which begins on Day 1 of that COT observation period and continues for the remainder of the current payment period, unless the payment is modified by a subsequent COT OMRA or other unscheduled PPS assessment.

- See Section 2.7 for requirements for CAA process and care plan completion.

Change of Therapy OMRA and OBRA Quarterly Assessment

- Quarterly item set as required by the State.

- ARD (Item A2300) must meet the requirements for an OBRA Quarterly assessment as described in Section 2.6 **and** be on the last day of a COT 7-day observation period.

- Completed when the patient received skilled therapy services and a change of therapy evaluation determines that a COT OMRA is necessary, based on a determination that the intensity of therapy (as indicated by the total reimbursable therapy minutes (RTM) and other therapy qualifiers such as number of therapy days and disciplines providing therapy), in the COT observation window differed from the therapy intensity on the last PPS assessment to such an extent that the RUG IV category would change.

- Establishes a new RUG-IV classification and Medicare payment rate (Item Z0100A), which begins on Day 1 of that COT observation period and continues for the remainder of the current payment period, unless the payment is modified by a subsequent COT OMRA or other unscheduled PPS assessment.

- See Section 2.6 for OBRA Quarterly assessment completion requirements.

Change of Therapy OMRA and Annual Assessment

- Comprehensive item set.

- ARD (Item A2300) must meet the requirements for an OBRA Annual assessment as described in Section 2.6 **and** be on the last day of a COT 7-day observation period.

- Completed when the patient received skilled therapy services and a change of therapy evaluation determines that a COT OMRA is necessary, based on a determination that the intensity of therapy (as indicated by the total reimbursable therapy minutes (RTM) and other therapy qualifiers such as the number of therapy days and disciplines providing therapy), in the COT observation window differed from the therapy intensity on the last PPS assessment to such an extent that the RUG IV category would change.

- Establishes a new RUG-IV classification and Medicare payment rate (Item Z0150A), which begins on Day 1 of that COT observation period and continues for the remainder of the current payment period, unless the payment is modified by a subsequent COT OMRA or other unscheduled PPS assessment.

- See Section 2.6 for OBRA Annual assessment completion requirements.

- See Section 2.7 for requirements for CAA process and care plan completion.

Change of Therapy OMRA and Significant Change in Status Assessment

- Comprehensive item set.

- ARD (Item A2300) must be set within 14 days after the determination that the criteria are met for a Significant Change in Status assessment **and** be on the last day of a COT 7-day observation period.

- Must be completed (Item Z0500B) within 14 days after the ARD and within 14 days after the determination that the criteria are met for a Significant Change in Status assessment.

- Completed when the patient received skilled therapy services and a change of therapy evaluation determines that a COT OMRA is necessary, based on a determination that the intensity of therapy (as indicated by the total reimbursable therapy minutes (RTM) delivered and other therapy qualifiers such as the number of therapy days and disciplines providing therapy), in the COT observation window differed from the therapy intensity on the last PPS assessment to such an extent that the RUG IV category would change.

- Establishes a new RUG-IV classification and Medicare payment rate (Item Z0150A), which begins on Day 1 of that COT observation period and continues for the remainder of the current payment period, unless the payment is modified by a subsequent COT OMRA or other unscheduled PPS assessment.
- See Section 2.7 for requirements for CAA process and care plan completion.

Change of *Therapy* OMRA and Significant Correction to Prior Comprehensive Assessment

- Comprehensive item set.
- ARD (Item A2300) must be set within 14 days after the determination that an uncorrected error in the prior comprehensive assessment has occurred **and** be on the last day of a COT 7-day observation period.
- Must be completed (Item Z0500B) within 14 days after the ARD and within 14 days after the determination that the criteria are met for a Significant Correction assessment.
- Completed when the patient received skilled therapy services and a change of therapy evaluation determines that a COT OMRA is necessary, based on a determination that the intensity of therapy (as indicated by the total reimbursable therapy minutes (RTM) and other therapy qualifiers such as the number of therapy days and disciplines providing therapy), in the COT observation window differed from the therapy intensity on the last PPS assessment to such an extent that the RUG IV category would change.
- Establishes a new RUG-IV classification and Medicare payment rate (Item Z0150A), which begins on Day 1 of that COT observation period and continues for the remainder of the current payment period, unless the payment is modified by a subsequent COT OMRA or other unscheduled PPS assessment.
- See Section 2.7 for requirements for CAA process and care plan completion.

Change of Therapy OMRA and Significant Correction to Prior Quarterly Assessment

- See COT OMRA and OBRA Quarterly Assessment.

Change of Therapy OMRA and Discharge Assessment

- COT OMRA and Discharge item set.
- ARD (Item A2300) must be set for the day of discharge (Item A2000) **and** be on the last day of a COT 7-day observation period. The ARD must be set by no more than two days after the date of discharge. (See Section 2.8 for further clarification.)
- Completed when the patient received skilled therapy services and a change of therapy evaluation determines that a COT OMRA is necessary, based on a determination that the intensity of therapy (as indicated by the total reimbursable therapy minutes (RTM) and other therapy qualifiers such as the number of therapy days and disciplines providing therapy), in the COT observation window differed from the therapy intensity on the last PPS assessment to such an extent that the RUG IV category would change.

- Establishes a new RUG-IV classification and Medicare payment rate (Item Z0150A), which begins on Day 1 of that COT observation period and continues for the remainder of the current payment period, unless the payment is modified by a subsequent COT OMRA or other unscheduled PPS assessment.

- Must be completed (Item Z0500B) within 14 days after the ARD.

2.13 Factors Impacting the SNF Medicare Assessment Schedule[8]

Resident Expires Before or On the Eighth Day of SNF Stay

If the beneficiary dies in the SNF or while on a leave of absence before or on the eighth day of the covered SNF stay, the provider should prepare a Medicare-required assessment as completely as possible and submit the assessment as required. If there is not a PPS MDS in the QIES ASAP system, the provider must bill the default rate for any Medicare days. The Medicare Short Stay Policy may apply (see Chapter 6, Section 6.4 for greater detail). The provider must also complete a Death in Facility Tracking Record (see Section 2.6 for greater detail).

Resident Transfers or Discharged Before or On the Eighth Day of SNF Stay

If the beneficiary is discharged from the SNF or transferred to another payer source before or on the eighth day of the covered SNF stay, the provider should prepare a Medicare-required assessment as completely as possible and submit the assessment as required. If there is not a PPS MDS in the QIES ASAP system, the provider must bill the default rate for any Medicare days. The Medicare Short Stay Policy may apply (see Chapter 6, Section 6.4 for greater detail). When the beneficiary is discharged from the SNF, the provider must also complete a Discharge assessment (see Sections 2.11 and 2.12 for details on combining a Medicare-required assessment with a discharge assessment).

Short Stay

If the beneficiary dies, is discharged from the SNF, or discharged from Part A level of care on or before the eighth day of covered SNF stay, the resident may be a candidate for the short stay policy. The short stay policy allows the assignment into a Rehabilitation Plus Extensive Services or Rehabilitation category when a resident received rehabilitation therapy and was not able to have received 5 days of therapy due to discharge from Medicare Part A. See Chapter 6, Section 6.4 for greater detail.

Resident is Admitted to an Acute Care Facility and Returns

If a Medicare Part A resident is admitted to an acute care facility and later returns to the SNF (even if the acute stay facility is less than 24 hours and/or not over midnight) to resume Part A coverage, the Medicare assessment schedule is restarted. The type of entry on the Entry Tracking record (as described in Section 2.6) completed by the provider determines whether a Medicare-required 5-day or a Medicare Readmission/Return assessment should be completed.

---

[8] These requirements/policies also apply to swing bed providers.

When the Medicare resident returns to the SNF and the entry type on the Entry Tracking record is a Reentry (Item A1700=2), the first required Medicare assessment is the Medicare Readmission/ Return assessment (Item A0310B = 06) as long as the resident is eligible for Medicare Part A services, requires and receives skilled services and has days remaining in the benefit period.

When the Medicare resident returns to the SNF and the entry type on the Entry Tracking record is an Admission (Item A1700=1), the first required Medicare assessment is the Medicare-required 5-Day assessment (Item A0310B = 01) as long as the resident is eligible for Medicare Part A services, requires and receives skilled services and has days remaining in the benefit period.

For Swing bed providers, the first required Medicare assessment is always the Medicare-required 5-Day assessment (Item A0310B = 01) as long as the resident is eligible for Medicare Part A services, requires and receives skilled services and has days remaining in the benefit period.

Resident Is Sent to Acute Care Facility, Not in SNF over Midnight, and Is Not Admitted to Acute Care Facility

If a resident is out of the facility over a midnight, but for less than 24 hours, and is not admitted to an acute care facility, the Medicare assessment schedule is not restarted. However, there are payment implications: the day preceding the midnight on which the resident was absent from the nursing home is not a covered Part A day. This is known as the "midnight rule." The Medicare assessment schedule must then be adjusted. The day preceding the midnight is not a covered Part A day and therefore, the Medicare assessment clock is adjusted by skipping that day in calculating when the next Medicare assessment is due. For example, if the resident goes to the emergency room at 10 p.m. Wednesday, day 22 of his Part A stay, and returns at 3 a.m. the next day, Wednesday is not billable to Part A. As a result, the day of his return to the SNF, Thursday, becomes day 22 of his Part A stay.

Resident Takes a Leave of Absence from the SNF

If a resident is out of the facility for a Leave of Absence (LOA) as defined on page 2-12 in this chapter, the Medicare assessment schedule may be adjusted for certain assessments. For **scheduled PPS assessments**, the Medicare assessment schedule is adjusted to exclude the LOA when determining the appropriate ARD for a given assessment. For example, if a resident leaves a SNF at 6:00pm on Wednesday, which is Day 27 of the resident's stay and returns to the SNF on Thursday at 9:00am, then Wednesday becomes a non-billable day and Thursday becomes Day 27 of the resident's stay. Therefore, a facility that would choose Day 27 for the ARD of their 30-day assessment would select Thursday as the ARD date rather than Wednesday, as Wednesday is no longer a billable Medicare Part A day.

In the case of **unscheduled PPS assessments**, the ARD of the relevant assessment is not affected by the LOA because the ARDs for unscheduled assessments are not tied directly to the Medicare assessment calendar or to a particular day of the resident's stay. For instance, Day 7 of the COT observation period occurs 7 days following the ARD of the most recent PPS assessment used for payment, regardless if a LOA occurs at any point during the COT observation period. For example, if the ARD for a resident's 30-day assessment were set for November 7 and the resident went to the emergency room at 11:00pm on November 9, returning on November 10, Day 7 of the COT observation period would remain November 14.

Resident Leaves the Facility and Returns During an Observation Period

The ARD is not altered if the beneficiary is out of the facility for a temporary leave of absence during part of the observation period. In this case, the facility may include services furnished during the beneficiary's temporary absence (when permitted under MDS coding guidelines; see Chapter 3) but may not extend the observation period.

Resident Discharged from Part A Skilled Services and Returns to SNF Part A Skilled Level Services

In the situation when a beneficiary is discharged from Medicare Part A services but remains in the facility in a Medicare and/or Medicaid certified bed with another pay source, the OBRA schedule will be continued. Since the beneficiary remained in a certified bed after the Medicare benefits were discontinued, the facility must continue with the OBRA schedule from the beneficiary's original date of admission. There is no reason to change the OBRA schedule when Part A benefits resume. If and when the Medicare Part A benefits resume, the Medicare schedule starts again with a 5-Day Medicare-required assessment, MDS Item A0310B = 01. See Chapter 6, Section 6.7 for greater detail to determine whether or not the resident is eligible for Part A SNF coverage.

The original date of entry (Item A1600) is retained. The beneficiary should be assessed to determine if there was a significant change in status. A SCSA could be completed with either the Medicare-required 5-day or 14-day assessment or separately.

Delay in Requiring and Receiving Skilled Services

There are instances when the beneficiary does not require SNF level of care services when initially admitted to the SNF. See Chapter 6, Section 6.7.

Non-Compliance with the PPS Assessment Schedule

According to Part 42 Code of Federal Regulation (CFR) Section 413.343, an assessment that does not have its ARD within the prescribed ARD window will be paid at the default rate for the number of days the ARD is out of compliance. Frequent early or late assessment scheduling practices may result in a review. The default rate takes the place of the otherwise applicable Federal rate. It is equal to the rate paid for the RUG group reflecting the lowest acuity level, and would generally be lower than the Medicare rate payable if the SNF had submitted an assessment in accordance with the prescribed assessment schedule.

Early PPS Assessment

An assessment should be completed according to the Medicare-required assessment schedule. **If an assessment is performed earlier than the schedule indicates (the ARD is not in the defined window), the provider will be paid at the default rate for the number of days the assessment was out of compliance.** For example, a Medicare-required 14-Day assessment with an ARD of day 12 (1 day early) would be paid at the default rate for the first day of the payment period that begins on day 15.

In the case of an early COT OMRA, the early COT would reset the COT calendar such that the next COT OMRA, if deemed necessary, would have an ARD set for 7 days from the early COT ARD. For example, a facility completes a 30-day assessment with an ARD of November 1 which classifies a resident into a therapy RUG. On November 8, which is Day 7 of the COT observation period, it is determined that a COT is required. A COT OMRA is completed for this resident with an ARD set for November 6, which is Day 5 of the COT observation period as opposed to November 8 which is Day 7 of the COT observation period. This COT OMRA would be considered an early assessment and, based on the ARD set for this early assessment would be paid at the default rate for the two days this assessment was out of compliance. The next seven day COT observation period would begin on November 7, and end on November 13.

Late PPS Assessment

If the SNF fails to set the ARD within the defined ARD window for a Medicare-required assessment, including the grace days, and the resident is still on Part A, the SNF must complete a late assessment. The ARD can be no earlier than the day the error was identified.

If the ARD on the late assessment is set for **prior to the end of the period during which the late assessment would have controlled the payment,** had the ARD been set timely, and/or **no intervening assessments have occurred, the SNF will bill the default rate for the number of days that the assessment is out of compliance.** This is equal to the number of days between the day following the last day of the available ARD window (including grace days when appropriate) and the late ARD (including the late ARD). **The SNF would then bill the Health Insurance Prospective Payment System (HIPPS) code established by the late assessment for the remaining period of time that the assessment would have controlled payment.** For example, a Medicare-required 30-day assessment with an ARD of Day 41 is out of compliance for 8 days and therefore would be paid at the default rate for 8 days and the HIPPS code from the late 30-day assessment until the next scheduled or unscheduled assessment that controls payment. In this example, if there are no other assessments until the 60-day assessment, the remaining 22 days are billed according to the HIPPS code on the late assessment.

DEFINITIONS
INTERVENING ASSESSMENT
Refers to an assessment with an ARD set for a day in the interim period between the last day of the appropriate ARD window for a late assessment (including grace days, when appropriate) and the actual ARD of the late assessment.
DAYS OUT OF COMPLIANCE
Refers to the number of days between the day following the last day of the available ARD window, including grace days when appropriate, and the late ARD (including the late ARD) of an assessment.

A second example, involving a late unscheduled assessment would be if a COT OMRA was completed with an ARD of Day 39, while Day 7 of the COT observation period was Day 37. In this case, the COT OMRA would be considered 2 days late and the facility would bill the default rate for 2 days and then bill the HIPPS code from the late COT OMRA until the next scheduled or unscheduled assessment controls payment, in this case, for at least 5 days. NOTE: In such cases where a late assessment is completed and no intervening assessments occur, the late assessment is used to establish the COT calendar.

If the ARD of the late assessment is set **after the end of the period during which the late assessment would have controlled payment,** had the assessment been completed timely, or in cases where **an intervening assessment** has occurred and the resident is still on Part A, the provider must still complete the assessment. The ARD can be no earlier than the day the error was identified. **The SNF must bill all covered days during which the late assessment would have controlled payment had the ARD been set timely at the default rate regardless of the HIPPS code calculated from the late assessment.** For example, a Medicare-required 14-day assessment with an ARD of Day 32 would be paid at the default rate for Days 15 through 30. A late assessment cannot be used to replace a different Medicare-required assessment. In the example above, the SNF would also need to complete the 30-day Medicare-required assessment within Days 27-33, which includes grace days. The 30-day assessment would cover Days 31 through 60 as long as the beneficiary has SNF days remaining and is eligible for SNF Part A services. In this example, the late 14-day assessment would not be considered an assessment used for payment and would not impact the COT calendar, as only an assessment used for payment can affect the COT calendar (see section 2.8).

A second example involving an unscheduled assessment would be the following. A 30-day assessment is completed with an ARD of Day 30. Day 7 of the COT observation period is Day 37. An EOT OMRA is performed timely for this resident with an ARD set for Day 42 and the resident's last day of therapy was Day 39. Upon further review of the resident's record on Day 52, the facility determines that a COT should have been completed with an ARD of Day 37 but was not. The ARD for the COT OMRA is set for day 52. The late COT OMRA should have controlled payment from Day 31 until the next assessment used for payment. Because there was an intervening assessment (in this case the EOT OMRA) prior to the ARD of the late COT OMRA, the facility would bill the default rate for 9 days (the period during which the COT OMRA would have controlled payment). The facility would bill the RUG from the EOT OMRA as per normal beginning the first non-therapy day, in this case Day 40, until the next scheduled or unscheduled assessment used for payment.

Missed PPS Assessment

If the SNF fails to set the ARD of a scheduled PPS assessment prior to the end of the last day of the ARD window, including grace days, and the resident was already discharged from Medicare Part A when this error is discovered, the provider cannot complete an assessment for SNF PPS purposes and the days cannot be billed to Part A. An existing OBRA assessment (except a stand-alone discharge assessment) in the QIES ASAP system may be used to bill for some Part A days when specific circumstances are met. See Chapter 6, Section 6.8 for greater detail.

In the case of an unscheduled PPS assessment, if the SNF fails to set the ARD for an unscheduled PPS assessment within the defined ARD window for that assessment, and the resident has been discharged from Part A, the assessment is missed and cannot be completed. All days that would have been paid by the missed assessment (had it been completed timely) are considered provider-liable. However, as with the late unscheduled assessment policy, the provider-liable period only lasts until the point when an intervening assessment controls the payment.

Errors on a + Medicare Assessment

To correct an error on an MDS that has been submitted to the QIES ASAP system, the nursing facility must follow the normal MDS correction procedures (see Chapter 5).

*These requirements/policies also apply to swing bed providers.

2.14 Expected Order of MDS Records

The MDS records for a nursing home resident are expected to occur in a specific order. For example, the first record for a resident is expected to be an Entry record with entry type (Item A1700) indicating admission, and the next record is expected to be an admission assessment, a 5 day PPS assessment, a discharge, or death in facility. The QIES ASAP system will issue a warning when an unexpected record is submitted. Examples include, an assessment record after a discharge (an entry is expected) or any record after a death in facility record.

The target date, rather than the submission date, is used to determine the order of records. The target date is the assessment reference date (Item A2300) for assessment records, the entry date (Item A1600) for entry records, and the discharge date (Item A2000) for discharge or death in facility records. In the following table, the prior record is represented in the columns and the next (subsequent) record is represented in the rows. A "no" has been placed in a cell when the next record is not expected to follow the prior record; the QIES ASAP system will issue a record order warning for record combinations that contain a "no". A blank cell indicates that the next record is expected to follow the prior record; a record order warning will *not* be issued for these combinations.

For the first MDS 3.0 record with event date on or after October 1, 2010, the last MDS 2.0 record (if available) should be used to determine if the record order is expected. The QIES ASAP system will find the last MDS 2.0 record and issue a warning if the order of these two records is unexpected.

Note that there are not any QIES ASAP record order warnings produced for Swing Bed MDS records.

Expected Order of MDS Records

Next Record	Prior Record												
	Entry	OBRA Admission	OBRA annual	OBRA quarterly	PPS 5-day or readmission/ return	PPS 14-day	PPS 30-day	PPS 60-day	PPS 90-day	PPS unscheduled	Discharge	Death in facility	No prior record
Entry	no	no	no	no	no	no	no	no	no	no		no	
OBRA Admission		no	no	no	no	no	no	no	no	no	no	no	no
OBRA Annual	no										no	no	no
OBRA Quarterly, sign. change, sign correction	no										no	no	no
PPS 5-day or readmission/return					no	no	no	no	no			no	no
PPS 14-day	no	no	no	no			no	no	no		no	no	no
PPS 30-day	no	no	no	no	no			no	no		no	no	no
PPS 60-day	no	no	no	no	no	no			no		no	no	no
PPS 90-day	no	no	no	no	no	no	no				no	no	no
PPS unscheduled	no											no	no
Discharge											no	no	no
Death in facility											no	no	no

Note: "no" indicates that the record sequence is not expected; record order warnings will be issued for these combinations. Blank cells indicate expected record sequences; no record order warning will be issued for these combinations.

2.15 Determining the Item Set for an MDS Record

The item set for a particular MDS record is completely determined by the reason for assessment Items (A0310A, A0310B, A0310C, A0310D, and A0310 F). Item set determination is complicated and standard MDS software from CMS and private vendors will automatically make this determination. This section provides manual lookup tables for determining the item set, when automated software is unavailable.

The first lookup table is for nursing home records. The first 4 columns are entries for the reason for assessment (RFA) Items A0310A, A0310B, A0310C, and A0310F. Item A0310D (swing bed clinical change assessment) has been omitted because it will always be skipped on a nursing home record. To determine the item set for a record, locate the row that includes the values of Items A0310A, A0310B, A0310C, and A0310F for that record. When the row is located, then the item set is identified in the ISC and Description columns for that row. If the combination of Items A0310A, A0310B, A0310C, and A0310F values for the record cannot be located in any row, then that combination of RFAs is not allowed and any record with that combination will be rejected by the QIES ASAP system.

Nursing Home Item Set Code (ISC) Reference Table

OBRA RFA (A0310A)	PPS RFA (A0310B)	OMRA (A0310C)	Entry/ Discharge (A0310F)	ISC	Description
01	01,02,06,99	0	10,11,99	NC	Comprehensive
01	01,02,06,07	1,2,3	10,11,99	NC	Comprehensive
01	02,07	4	10,11,99	NC	Comprehensive
03	01 thru 06,99	0	10,11,99	NC	Comprehensive
03,04,05	01 thru 07	1,2,3	10,11,99	NC	Comprehensive
03,04,05	02 thru 05,07	4	10,11,99	NC	Comprehensive
04,05	01 thru 07,99	0	10,11,99	NC	Comprehensive
02,06	01 thru 06,99	0	10,11,99	NQ	Quarterly
02,06	01 thru 07	1,2,3	10,11,99	NQ	Quarterly
02,06	02 thru 05,07	4	10,11,99	NQ	Quarterly
99	01 thru 06	0,1,2,3	10,11,99	NP	PPS
99	02 thru 05	4	10,11,99	NP	PPS
99	07	1	99	NS	SOT OMRA
99	07	1	10,11	NSD	SOT OMRA and Discharge
99	07	2,3,4	99	NO	EOT, EOT-R or COT OMRA
99	07	2,3,4	10,11	NOD	EOT, EOT-R or COT OMRA and Discharge
99	99	0	10,11	ND	Discharge
99	99	0	01,12	NT	Tracking

Consider examples of the use of this table. If Items A0310A = 01, A0310B = 99, A0310C= 0 and Item A0310F = 99 (a standalone admission assessment), then these values are matched in row 1 and the item set is an OBRA comprehensive assessment (NC). The same row would be selected if Item A0310F is changed to 10 (admission assessment combined with a return not anticipated discharge assessment). The item set is again an OBRA comprehensive assessment (NC). If Items A0310A = 99, A0310B = 99, A0310C= 0 and Item A0310F = 12 (a death in facility tracking record), then these values are matched in the last row and the item set is a tracking record (NT). Finally, if Items A0310A = 99, A0310B = 99, A0310C= 0 and A0310F = 99, then no row matches these entries, and the record is invalid and would be rejected.

There is one additional item set for inactivation request records. This is the set of items active on a request to inactivate a record in the national MDS QIES ASAP system. An inactivation request is indicated by A0050 = 3. The item set for this type of record is "Inactivation" with an ISC code of XX.

The next lookup table is for swing bed records. The first 5 columns are entries for the reason for assessment (RFA) Items A0310A, A0310B, A0310C, A0310D, and A0310F. To determine the item set for a record, locate the row that includes the values of Items A0310A, A0310B, A0310C, A0310D, and A0310F for that record. When the row is located, then the item set is identified in the ISC and Description columns for that row. If the combination of A0310A, A0310B, A0310C, A0310D, and A0310F values for the record cannot be located in any row, then that combination of RFAs is not allowed and any record with that combination will be rejected by the QIES ASAP system.

Swing Bed Item Set Code (ISC) Reference Table

OBRA RFA (A0310A)	PPS RFA (A0310B)	OMRA (A0310C)	SB Clinical Change (A0310D)	Entry/ Discharge (A0310F)	ISC	Description
99	01 thru 06	0,1,2,3	0	10,11,99	SP	PPS
99	01 thru 07	0,1,2,3	1	10,11,99	SP	PPS
99	02 thru 05	4	0	10,11,99	SP	PPS
99	02 thru 05,07	4	1	10,11,99	SP	PPS
99	07	1	0	99	SS	SOT OMRA
99	07	1	0	10,11	SSD	SOT OMRA and Discharge
99	07	2,3,4	0	99	SO	EOT , EOT-R or COT OMRA
99	07	2,3,4	0	10,11	SOD	EOT , EOT-R or COT OMRA and Discharge
99	99	0	0	10,11	SD	Discharge
99	99	0	0	01,12	ST	Tracking

The "Inactivation" (XX) item set is also used for swing beds when Item A0050 = 3.

CHAPTER 3:   OVERVIEW TO THE ITEM-BY-ITEM GUIDE TO THE MDS 3.0

This chapter provides item-by-item coding instructions for all required sections and items in the comprehensive MDS Version 3.0 item set. The goal of this chapter is to facilitate the accurate coding of the MDS resident assessment and to provide assessors with the rationale and resources to optimize resident care and outcomes.

3.1   Using this Chapter

Throughout this chapter, MDS assessment sections are presented using a standard format for ease of review and instruction. In addition, screenshots of each section are available for illustration purposes. Note: There are images imbedded in this manual and if you are using a screen reader to access the content contained in the manual you should refer to the MDS 3.0 item set to review the referenced information. The order of the sections is as follows:

- **Intent.** The reason(s) for including this set of assessment items in the MDS.

- **Item Display.** To facilitate accurate resident assessment using the MDS, each assessment section is accompanied by screen shots, which display the item from the MDS 3.0 item set.

- **Item Rationale.** The purpose of assessing this aspect of a resident's clinical or functional status.

- **Health-related Quality of Life.** How the condition, impairment, improvement, or decline being assessed can affect a resident's quality of life, along with the importance of staff understanding the relationship of the clinical or functional issue related to quality of life.

- **Planning for Care.** How assessment of the condition, impairment, improvement, or decline being assessed can contribute to appropriate care planning.

- **Steps for Assessment.** Sources of information and methods for determining the correct response for coding each MDS item.

- **Coding Instructions.** The proper method of recording each response, with explanations of individual response categories.

- **Coding Tips and Special Populations.** Clarifications, issues of note, and conditions to be considered when coding individual MDS items.

- **Examples.** Case examples of appropriate coding for most, if not all, MDS sections/items.

Additional layout issues to note include (1) the ◖))◗ symbol is displayed in all MDS 3.0 sections/items that require a resident interview, and (2) important definitions are highlighted in the columns, and these and other definitions of interest may be found in the glossary.

3.2 Becoming Familiar with the MDS-recommended Approach

1. **First, reading the Manual is essential.**
   - **The CMS Long-Term Care Facility Resident Assessment Instrument User's Manual is the <u>primary</u> source of information for completing an MDS assessment.**
   - Notice how the manual is organized.
   - Using it correctly will increase the accuracy of your assessments.
   - While it is important to understand and apply the information in Chapter 3, facilities should also become familiar with Chapters 1, 2, 4, 5 and 6. These Chapters provide the framework and supporting information for data collected on the item set as well as the process for further assessment and care planning.
   - It is important to understand the entire process of the RAI in conjunction with the intent and rationale for coding items on the MDS 3.0 item set.
   - Check the MDS 3.0 Web site regularly for updates at: http://www.cms.gov/NursingHomeQualityInits/45_NHQIMDS30TrainingMaterials.asp
   - If you <u>require</u> further assistance, submit your question to your State RAI Coordinator listed in **Appendix B: State Agency and CMS Regional Office RAI/MDS Contacts** available on CMS' website: http://www.cms.gov/NursingHomeQualityInits/45_NHQIMDS30TrainingMaterials.asp

2. **Second, review the MDS item sets.**
   - Notice how sections are organized and where information should be recorded.
   - Work through one section at a time.
   - Examine item definitions and response categories as <u>provided</u> on the item sets, realizing that more detailed definitions and coding information is found in each Section of Chapter 3.
   - There are <u>several</u> item sets, and depending on which item set you are completing, the skip patterns and items active for each item set may be different.

3. **Complete a thorough review of Chapter 3.**
   - Review procedural instructions, time frames, and general coding conventions.
   - Become familiar with the intent of each item, rationale and steps for assessment.
   - Become familiar with the item itself with its coding choices and responses, keeping in mind the clarifications, issues of note, and other pertinent information needed to understand how to code the item.
   - Do the definitions and instructions differ from current practice at your facility?
   - Does your facility processes require updating to comply with MDS requirements?
   - Complete a test MDS assessment for a resident at your facility. Enter the appropriate codes on the MDS.

- Make a note where your review could benefit from additional information, training, and using the varying skill sets of the interdisciplinary team. Be certain to explore resources available to you.

- As you are completing this test case, read through the instructions that apply to each section as you are completing the MDS. Work through the Manual and item set one section at a time until you are comfortable coding items. Make sure you understand this information before going on to another section.

- Review the test case you completed. Would you still code it the same way? Are you surprised by any definitions, instructions, or case examples? For example, do you understand how to code ADLs?

- As you review the coding choices in your test case against the manual, make notations corresponding to the section(s) of this Manual where you need further clarification, or where questions arose. Note sections of the manual that help to clarify these coding and procedural questions.

- Would you now complete your initial case differently?

- It will take time to go through all this material. Do it slowly and carefully without rushing. Discuss any clarifications, questions or issues with your State RAI Coordinator (see **Appendix B: State Agency and CMS Regional Office RAI/MDS Contacts** available on CMS' website: http://www.cms.gov/NursingHomeQualityInits/45_NHQIMDS30TrainingMaterials.asp)

4. **Use of information in this chapter:**
   - Keep this chapter with you during the assessment process.
   - Where clarification is needed, review the intent, rationale and specific coding instructions for each item in question.

3.3 Coding Conventions

There are several standard conventions to be used when completing the MDS assessment, as follows.

- Unlike the MDS 2.0, the standard look-back period for the MDS 3.0 is **7 days**, unless otherwise stated.

- **With the exception of certain items (e.g., some items in Sections K and O), the look-back period generally <u>does not</u> include hospital stay.**

- There are a few instances in which scoring on one item will govern how scoring is completed for one or more additional items. This is called a skip pattern. The instructions direct the assessor to "skip" over the next item (or several items) and go on to another. When you encounter a skip pattern, leave the item blank and move on to the next item as directed (e.g., item B0100, **Comatose**, directs the assessor to skip to item G0110, **Activities of Daily Living Assistance**, if B0100 is answered **code 1, yes.** The intervening items from B0200-F0800 would not be coded (i.e. left blank). If B0100 was recorded as **code 0, no,** then the assessor would continue to code the MDS at the next item, B0200).

- Use a check mark for boxes with where the instructions state to "check all that apply," if specified condition is met; otherwise these boxes remain blank (e.g., F0800, **Staff Assessment of Daily and Activity Preferences**, boxes A-Z).

- Use a numeric response (a number or pre-assigned value) for blank boxes (e.g., D0350, **Safety Notification**).

- When completing hard copy forms to be used for data entry, capital letters may be easiest to read. Print legibly.

- When recording month, day, and year for dates, enter two digits for the month and the day and four digits for the year. For example, the third day of January in the year 2011 is recorded as:

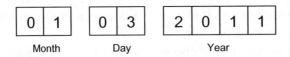

| 0 | 1 | | 0 | 3 | | 2 | 0 | 1 | 1 |
| Month | | | Day | | | Year | | | |

- Almost all MDS 3.0 items allow a dash (-) value to be entered and submitted to the MDS QIES ASAP system.

  — A dash value indicates that an item was not assessed. This most often occurs when a resident is discharged before the item could be assessed.

  — Dash values allow a partial assessment to be submitted when an assessment is required for payment purposes.

  — There are four date items (A2400C, O0400A6, O0400B6, and O0400C6) that use a dash-filled value to indicate that the event has not yet occurred. For example, if there is an ongoing Medicare stay, then the end date for that Medicare stay (A2400C) has not occurred, therefore, this item would be dash-filled.

  — The few items that do not allow dash values include identification items in Section A [e.g., Legal Name of Resident (Item A0500), Assessment Reference Date (Item A2300), Type of Assessment (Item A0310), and Gender (Item A0800)] and ICD-9 diagnosis codes (Item I8000). All items for which a dash is not an acceptable value can be found on the CMS MDS 3.0 Technical Information web page at the following link: http://www.cms.gov/Medicare/Quality-Initiatives-Patient-Assessment-Instruments/NursingHomeQualityInits/NHQIMDS30TechnicalInformation.html

- When the term "physician" is used in this manual, it should be interpreted as including nurse practitioners, physician assistants, or clinical nurse specialists, if allowable under state licensure laws and Medicare.

- Residents should be the primary source of information for resident assessment items. Should the resident not be able to participate in the assessment, the resident's family, significant other, and guardian or legally authorized representative should be consulted.

- Several times throughout the manual the word "significant" is used. The term may have different connotations depending on the circumstance in which it is used. For the MDS 3.0 , the term "significant" when discussing clinical, medical, or laboratory findings refers to measures of supporting evidence that are considered when developing or assigning a diagnosis, and therefore reflects clinical judgment. When the term "significant" is used in discussing relationships between people, as in "significant other," it means a person, who may be a family member or a close friend that is important or influential in the life of the resident.

- When completing the MDS 3.0, there are some items that require a count or measurement, however, there are instances where the actual results of the count or measurement are greater than the number of available boxes. For example, number of pressure ulcers, or weight. When the result of a count or measurement is greater than the number of available boxes, facilities are instructed to maximize the count/measurement by placing a "9" in each box (e.g. k0200B if the weight was 1010 lbs you would enter 999 in the available boxes). Even though the number is not exact, the facility should document the correct number in the resident's medical record and ensure that an appropriate plan of care is completed that addresses the additional counts/measurements.

Section	Title	Intent
A	Identification Information	Obtain key information to uniquely identify each resident, nursing home, type of record, and reasons for assessment.
B	Hearing, Speech, and Vision	Document the resident's ability to hear, understand, and communicate with others and whether the resident experiences visual, hearing or speech limitations and/or difficulties.
C	Cognitive Patterns	Determine the resident's attention, orientation, and ability to register and recall information.
D	Mood	Identify signs and symptoms of mood distress.
E	Behavior	Identify behavioral symptoms that may cause distress or are potentially harmful to the resident, or may be distressing or disruptive to facility residents, staff members or the environment.
F	Preferences for Customary Routine and Activities	Obtain information regarding the resident's preferences for his or her daily routine and activities.
G	Functional Status	Assess the need for assistance with activities of daily living (ADLs), altered gait and balance, and decreased range of motion.
H	Bladder and Bowel	Gather information on the use of bowel and bladder appliances, the use of and response to urinary toileting programs, urinary and bowel continence, bowel training programs, and bowel patterns.
I	Active Disease Diagnosis	Code diseases that have a relationship to the resident's current functional, cognitive, mood or behavior status, medical treatments, nursing monitoring, or risk of death.
J	Health Conditions	Document health conditions that impact the resident's functional status and quality of life.
K	Swallowing/Nutritional Status	Assess conditions that could affect the resident's ability to maintain adequate nutrition and hydration.
L	Oral/Dental Status	Record any oral or dental problems present.
M	Skin Conditions	Document the risk, presence, appearance, and change of pressure ulcers as well as other skin ulcers, wounds or lesions. Also includes treatment categories related to skin injury or avoiding injury.
N	Medications	Record the number of days that any type of injection, insulin, and/or select medications was received by the resident.
O	Special Treatments and Procedures	Identify any special treatments, procedures, and programs that the resident received during the specified time periods.
P	Restraints	Record the frequency that the resident was restrained by any of the listed devices at any time during the day or night.
Q	Participation in Assessment and Goal Setting	Record the participation of the resident, family and/or significant others in the assessment, and to understand the resident's overall goals.
V	Care Area Assessment (CAA) Summary	Document triggered care areas, whether or not a care plan has been developed for each triggered area, and the location of care area assessment documentation.
X	Correction Request	Request to modify or inactivate a record already present in the QIES ASAP database.
Z	Assessment Administration	Provide billing information and signatures of persons completing the assessment.

SECTION A: IDENTIFICATION INFORMATION

Intent: The intent of this section is to obtain key information to uniquely identify each resident, the home in which he or she resides, and the reasons for assessment.

A0050: Type of Record

A0050. Type of Record	
Enter Code ☐	1. **Add new record** → Continue to A0100, Facility Provider Numbers 2. **Modify existing record** → Continue to A0100, Facility Provider Numbers 3. **Inactivate existing record** → Skip to X0150, Type of Provider

Coding Instructions for A0050, Type of Record

- **Code 1, Add new record:** if this is a **new record** that has not been previously submitted and accepted in the QIES ASAP system. If this item is **coded as 1**, continue to A0100 Facility Provider Numbers.

  If there is an existing database record for the same resident, the same facility, the same reasons for assessment/tracking, and the same date (assessment reference date, entry date, or discharge date), then the current record is a duplicate and not a new record. In this case, the submitted record will be rejected and not accepted in the QIES ASAP system and a "fatal" error will be reported to the facility on the Final Validation Report.

- **Code 2, Modify existing record:** if this is a **request to modify** the MDS items for a record that already has been submitted and accepted in the QIES ASAP system.

  If this item is **coded as 2**, continue to A0100, Facility Provider Numbers.

  When a modification request is submitted, the QIES ASAP System will take the following steps:

  1. The system will attempt to locate the existing record in the QIES ASAP database for this facility with the resident, reasons for assessment/tracking, and date (assessment reference date, entry date, or discharge date) indicated in subsequent Section X items.

  2. If the existing record is not found, the submitted modification record will be rejected and not accepted in the QIES ASAP system. A "fatal" error will be reported to the facility on the Final Validation Report.

  3. If the existing record is found, then the items in all sections of the submitted modification record will be edited. If there are any fatal errors, the modification record will be rejected and not accepted in the QIES ASAP system. The "fatal" error(s) will be reported to the facility on the Final Validation Report.

  4. If the modification record passes all the edits, it will replace the prior record being modified in the QIES ASAP database. The prior record will be moved to a history file in the QIES ASAP database.

A0050: Type of Record (cont.)

- **Code 3, Inactivate existing record:** if this is a **request to inactivate** a record that already has been submitted and accepted in the QIES ASAP system.

  If this item is **coded as 3**, skip to X0150, Type of Provider.

  When an inactivation request is submitted, the QIES ASAP system will take the following steps:

  1. The system will attempt to locate the existing record in the QIES ASAP system for this facility with the resident, reasons for assessment/tracking, and date (assessment reference date, entry date, or discharge date) indicated in subsequent Section X items.

  2. If the existing record is not found in the QIES ASAP database, the submitted inactivation request will be rejected and a "fatal" error will be reported to the facility on the Final Validation Report.

  3. All items in Section X of the submitted record will be edited. If there are any fatal errors, the current inactivation request will be rejected and no record will be inactivated in the QIES ASAP system.

  4. If the existing record is found, it will be removed from the active records in the QIES ASAP database and moved to a history file.

Identification of Record to be Modified/Inactivated

The Section X items from X0200 through X0700 identify the existing QIES ASAP database assessment or tracking record that is in error. In this section, reproduce the information **EXACTLY** as it appeared on the existing erroneous record, even if the information is incorrect. This information is necessary to locate the existing record in the database.

> **Example:** A MDS assessment for Joan L. Smith is submitted and accepted by the QIES ASAP system. A data entry error is then identified on the previously submitted and accepted record: The encoder mistakenly entered "John" instead of "Joan" when entering a prior assessment for Joan L. Smith. To correct this data entry error, the facility will modify the erroneous record and complete the items in Section X including items under Identification of Record to be Modified/Inactivated. When completing X0200A, the Resident First Name, "John" will be entered in this item. This will permit the MDS system to locate the previously submitted assessment that is being corrected. If the correct name "Joan" were entered, the QIES ASAP system would not locate the prior assessment.

The correction to the name from "John" to "Joan" will be made by recording "Joan" in the "normal" A0500A, Resident First Name in the modification record. The modification record must include all items appropriate for that assessment, not just the corrected name. This modification record will then be submitted and accepted into the QIES ASAP system which causes the desired correction to be made.

A0100: Facility Provider Numbers

A0100. Facility Provider Numbers

A. National Provider Identifier (NPI):

B. CMS Certification Number (CCN):

C. State Provider Number:

Item Rationale

- Allows the identification of the nursing home submitting assessment.

Coding Instructions

- Nursing homes must have a National Provider Number (NPI) and a CMS Certified Number (CCN).
- Enter the nursing home provider numbers:
  - A. National Provider Identifier (NPI)
  - B. CMS Certified Number (CCN)
  - C. State Provider Number (optional) This number is assigned by the Regional Office and provided to the intermediary/carrier and the State survey agency. When known enter the State Provider Number in A0100C. Completion of this is not required; however, your State may require the completion of this item.

DEFINITIONS

NATIONAL PROVIDER IDENTIFIER (NPI) A unique Federal number that identifies providers of health care services. The NPI applies to the nursing home for all of its residents.

CMS CERTIFICATION NUMBER (CCN) Replaces the term "Medicare/Medicaid Provider Number" in survey, certification, and assessment-related activities.

STATE PROVIDER NUMBER Medicaid Provider Number established by a state.

A0200: Type of Provider

A0200. Type of Provider

Enter Code

Type of provider
1. Nursing home (SNF/NF)
2. Swing Bed

Item Rationale

- Allows designation of type of provider.

Coding Instructions

- **Code 1, nursing home (SNF/NF):** if a Medicare skilled nursing facility (SNF) or Medicaid nursing facility (NF).
- **Code 2, swing bed:** if a hospital with swing bed approval.

DEFINITION

SWING BED

A rural hospital with less than 100 beds that participates in the Medicare program that has CMS approval to provide post-hospital SNF care. The hospital may use its beds, as needed, to provide either acute or SNF care.

A0310 Type of Assessment

For Comprehensive, Quarterly, and PPS Assessments, Entry and Discharge Records.

A0310. Type of Assessment	
Enter Code	**A. Federal OBRA Reason for Assessment** 01. **Admission** assessment (required by day 14) 02. **Quarterly** review assessment 03. **Annual** assessment 04. **Significant change in status** assessment 05. **Significant correction** to **prior comprehensive** assessment 06. **Significant correction** to **prior quarterly** assessment 99. **None of the above**
Enter Code	**B. PPS Assessment** <u>PPS Scheduled Assessments for a Medicare Part A Stay</u> 01. **5-day** scheduled assessment 02. **14-day** scheduled assessment 03. **30-day** scheduled assessment 04. **60-day** scheduled assessment 05. **90-day** scheduled assessment 06. **Readmission/return** assessment <u>PPS Unscheduled Assessments for a Medicare Part A Stay</u> 07. **Unscheduled assessment used for PPS** (OMRA, significant or clinical change, or significant correction assessment) <u>Not PPS Assessment</u> 99. **None of the above**
Enter Code	**C. PPS Other Medicare Required Assessment - OMRA** 0. **No** 1. **Start of therapy** assessment 2. **End of therapy** assessment 3. **Both Start and End of therapy** assessment 4. **Change of therapy** assessment
Enter Code	**D. Is this a Swing Bed clinical change assessment?** Complete only if A0200 = 2 0. **No** 1. **Yes**
Enter Code	**E. Is this assessment the first assessment** (OBRA, Scheduled PPS, or Discharge) **since the most recent admission/entry or reentry?** 0. **No** 1. **Yes**
Enter Code	**F. Entry/discharge reporting** 01. **Entry** tracking record 10. **Discharge** assessment-**return not anticipated** 11. **Discharge** assessment-**return anticipated** 12. **Death in facility** tracking record 99. **None of the above**
Enter Code	**G. Type of discharge** - Complete only if A0310F = 10 or 11 1. **Planned** 2. **Unplanned**

Item Rationale

- Allows identification of needed assessment content.

Coding Instructions for A0310, Type of Assessment

Enter the code corresponding to the reason or reasons for completing this assessment.

If the assessment is being completed for both Omnibus Budget Reconciliation Act (OBRA)–required clinical reasons (A0310A) and Prospective Payment System (PPS) reasons (A0310B and A0310C) all requirements for both types of assessments must be met. See Chapter 2 on assessment schedules for details of these requirements.

A0310: Type of Assessment (cont.)

Coding Instructions for A0310A, Federal OBRA Reason for Assessment

- Document the reason for completing the assessment, using the categories of assessment types. For detailed information on the requirements for scheduling and timing of the assessments, see Chapter 2 on assessment schedules.

- Enter the number corresponding to the OBRA reason for assessment. This item contains 2 digits. For codes 01-06, enter "0" in the first box and place the correct number in the second box. If the assessment is not coded 01-06, enter code "99".
  - **01.** Admission assessment (required by day 14)
  - **02.** Quarterly review assessment
  - **03.** Annual assessment
  - **04.** Significant change in status assessment
  - **05.** Significant correction to prior comprehensive assessment
  - **06.** Significant correction to prior quarterly assessment
  - **99.** None of the above

Coding Tips and Special Populations

- If a nursing home resident elects the hospice benefit, the nursing home is required to complete an MDS significant change in status assessment (SCSA). The nursing home is required to complete a SCSA when they come off the hospice benefit (revoke). See Chapter 2 for details on this requirement.

- It is a CMS requirement to have a SCSA completed EVERY time the hospice benefit has been elected, even if a recent MDS was done and the only change is the election of the hospice benefit.

Coding Instructions for A0310B, PPS Assessment

- Enter the number corresponding to the PPS reason for completing this assessment. This item contains 2 digits. For codes 01-07, enter "0" in the first box and place the correct number in the second box. If the assessment is not coded as 01-07, enter code "99".

- See Chapter 2 on assessment schedules for detailed information on the scheduling and timing of the assessments.

PPS Scheduled Assessments for a Medicare Part A Stay
  - **01.** 5-day scheduled assessment
  - **02.** 14-day scheduled assessment
  - **03.** 30-day scheduled assessment
  - **04.** 60-day scheduled assessment
  - **05.** 90-day scheduled assessment
  - **06.** Readmission/return assessment

> **DEFINITION**
>
> **PROSPECTIVE PAYMENT SYSTEM (PPS)**
> Method of reimbursement in which Medicare payment is made based on the classification system of that service (e.g., resource utilization groups, RUGs, for skilled nursing facilities).

A0310: Type of Assessment (cont.)

PPS Unscheduled Assessments for Medicare Part A Stay

07. Unscheduled assessment used for PPS (OMRA, significant change, or significant correction assessment)

99. None of the above

Coding Instructions for A0310C, PPS Other Medicare Required Assessment—OMRA

- **Code 0, no:** if this assessment is not an OMRA.

- **Code 1, Start of therapy assessment (OPTIONAL):** with an assessment reference date (ARD) that is 5 to 7 days after the first day therapy services are provided (except when the assessment is used as a Short Stay assessment, see Chapter 6). No need to combine with the 5-day assessment except for short stay. Only complete if therapy RUG (index maximized), otherwise the assessment will be rejected.

- **Code 2, End of therapy assessment:** with an ARD that is 1 to 3 days after the last day therapy services were provided.

- **Code 3, both the Start and End of therapy assessment:** with an ARD that is <u>both</u> 5 to 7 days after the first day therapy services were provided <u>and</u> that is 1 to 3 days after the last day therapy services were provided (except when the assessment is used as a Short Stay assessment, see Chapter 6).

- **Code 4, Change of therapy assessment:** with an ARD that is Day 7 of the COT observation period.

Coding Instructions for A0310D, Is This a Swing Bed Clinical Change Assessment?

- **Code 0, no:** if this assessment is not a Swing Bed Clinical Change assessment.

- **Code 1, yes:** if this assessment is a swing bed clinical change assessment.

Coding Instructions for A0310E, Is This Assessment the First Assessment (OBRA, PPS, or Discharge) since the Most Recent Admission/Entry or Reentry?

- **Code 0, no:** if this assessment is not the first assessment since the most recent admission/entry or reentry.

- **Code 1, yes:** if this assessment is the first assessment since the most recent admission/entry or reentry.

Coding Tips and Special Populations

- A0310E = 0 for any tracking record (Entry or Death in Facility) because tracking records are not considered assessments.

A0310: Type of Assessment (cont.)

Coding Instructions for A0310F, Federal OBRA & PPS Entry/Discharge Reporting

- Enter the number corresponding to the reason for completing this assessment or tracking record. This item contains 2 digits. For code 01, enter "0" in the first box and place "1" in the second box. If the assessment is not coded as "01" or "10 or "11" or "12," enter "99":

    01. Entry tracking record

    10. Discharge assessment-return not anticipated

    11. Discharge assessment-return anticipated

    12. Death in facility tracking record

    99. None of the above

Coding Instructions for A0310G, Type of Discharge

- **Code 1:** if type of discharge is a planned discharge.

- **Code 2:** if type of discharge is an unplanned discharge.

A0410: Submission Requirement

A0410. Submission Requirement	
Enter Code ☐	1. **Neither federal nor state required submission** 2. **State but not federal required submission** (FOR NURSING HOMES ONLY) 3. **Federal required submission**

Item Rationale

- There must be a federal and/or state authority to submit MDS assessment data to the MDS National Repository.

- Nursing homes must be certain they are submitting MDS assessments under the appropriate authority. With this item, the nursing home indicates the submission authority.

Steps for Assessment

1. Ask the nursing home administrator or representative which units in the nursing home are Medicare certified, if any, and which units are Medicaid certified, if any.
2. Identify all units in the nursing home that are not certified, if any.

    - If some or all of the units in the nursing home are neither Medicare nor Medicaid certified, ask the nursing home administrator or representative whether the State has authority to collect MDS information for residents on units that are neither Medicare nor Medicaid certified.

A0410: Submission Requirement (cont.)

Coding Instructions

- **Code 1, neither federal nor state required submission:** if the MDS record is for a resident on a unit that is neither Medicare nor Medicaid certified, and the state does not have authority to collect MDS information for residents on this unit. If the record is submitted, it will be rejected and all information from that record will be purged.

- **Code 2, State but not federal required submission:** if the MDS record is for a resident on a unit that is neither Medicare nor Medicaid certified, but the state has authority, under state licensure or other requirements, to collect MDS information for these residents.

- **Code 3, Federal required submission:** if the MDS record is for a resident on a Medicare and/or Medicaid certified unit. There is CMS authority to collect MDS information for residents on this unit.

A0500: Legal Name of Resident

A0500. Legal Name of Resident	
A. First name:	B. Middle initial:
C. Last name:	D. Suffix:

Item Rationale

- Allows identification of resident
- Also used for matching each of the resident's records

> **DEFINITION**
> **LEGAL NAME**
> Resident's name as it appears on the Medicare card. If the resident is not enrolled in the Medicare program, use the resident's name as it appears on a Medicaid card or other government-issued document.

Steps for Assessment

1. Ask resident, family, significant other, guardian, or legally authorized representative.
2. Check the resident's name on his or her Medicare card, or if not in the program, check a Medicaid card or other government-issued document.

Coding Instructions

Use printed letters. Enter in the following order:

- A. First Name
- B. Middle Initial (if the resident has no middle initial, leave Item A0500B blank; if the resident has two or more middle names, use the initial of the first middle name)
- C. Last Name
- D. Suffix (e.g., Jr./Sr.)

A0600: Social Security and Medicare Numbers

A0600. Social Security and Medicare Numbers
A. Social Security Number:
☐☐☐ – ☐☐ – ☐☐☐☐
B. Medicare number (or comparable railroad insurance number):
☐☐☐☐☐☐☐☐☐☐☐☐

Item Rationale

- Allows identification of the resident.
- Allows records for resident to be matched in system.

Coding Instructions

- Enter the Social Security Number (SSN) in A0600A, one number per space starting with the leftmost space. If no social security number is available for the resident (e.g., if the resident is a recent immigrant or a child) the item may be left blank.

- Enter Medicare number in A0600B exactly as it appears on the resident's documents.

- If the resident does not have a Medicare number, a Railroad Retirement Board (RRB) number may be substituted. These RRB numbers contain both letters and numbers. To enter the RRB number, enter the first letter of the code in the leftmost space followed by one letter/digit per space. If no Medicare number or RRB number is known or available, the item may be left blank.

- For PPS assessments (A0310B = 01, 02, 03, 04, 05, 06, and 07), either the SSN (A0600A) or Medicare number/RRB number (A0600B) must be present and both may not be blank.

- A0600B can only be a Medicare (HIC) number or a Railroad Retirement Board number.

> **DEFINITIONS**
>
> **SOCIAL SECURITY NUMBER**
> A tracking number assigned to an individual by the U.S. Federal government for taxation, benefits, and identification purposes.
>
> **MEDICARE NUMBER (OR COMPARABLE RAILROAD INSURANCE NUMBER)**
> An identifier assigned to an individual for participation in national health insurance program. The Medicare Health Insurance identifier may be different from the resident's social security number (SSN), and may contain both letters and numbers. For example, many residents may receive Medicare benefits based on a spouse's Medicare eligibility.

A0700: Medicaid Number

A0700. Medicaid Number - Enter "+" if pending, "N" if not a Medicaid recipient
☐☐☐☐☐☐☐☐☐☐☐☐☐☐☐☐☐

Item Rationale

- Assists in correct resident identification.

A0700: Medicaid Number (cont.)

Coding Instructions

- Record this number if the resident is a Medicaid recipient.
- Enter one number per box beginning in the leftmost box.
- Recheck the number to make sure you have entered the digits correctly.
- Enter a "+" in the leftmost box if the number is pending. If you are notified later that the resident does have a Medicaid number, just include it on the next assessment.
- If not applicable because the resident is not a Medicaid recipient, enter "N" in the leftmost box.

Coding Tips and Special Populations

- To obtain the Medicaid number, check the resident's Medicaid card, admission or transfer records, or medical record.
- Confirm that the resident's name on the MDS matches the resident's name on the Medicaid card.
- It is not necessary to process an MDS correction to add the Medicaid number on a prior assessment. However, a correction may be a State-specific requirement.

A0800: Gender

A0800. Gender	
Enter Code	1. Male 2. Female

Item Rationale

- Assists in correct identification.
- Provides demographic gender specific health trend information.

Coding Instructions

- **Code 1:** if resident is male.
- **Code 2:** if resident is female.

Coding Tips and Special Populations

- Resident gender on the MDS should match what is in the Social Security system.

A0900: Birth Date

A0900. Birth Date
□□ - □□ - □□□□ Month   Day   Year

A0900: Birth Date (cont.)

Item Rationale

- Assists in correct identification.
- Allows determination of age.

Coding Instructions

- Fill in the boxes with the appropriate birth date. If the complete birth date is known, do not leave any boxes blank. If the month or day contains only a single digit, fill the first box in with a "0." For example: January 2, 1918, should be entered as 01-02-1918.
- Sometimes, only the birth year or the birth year and birth month will be known. These situations are handled as follows:
  — If only the birth year is known (e.g., 1918), then enter the year in the "year" portion of A0900, and leave the "month" and "day" portions blank. If the birth year and birth month are known, but the day of the month is not known, then enter the year in the "year" portion of A0900, enter the month in the "month" portion of A0900, and leave the "day" portion blank.

A1000: Race/Ethnicity

A1000. Race/Ethnicity	
↓ Check all that apply	
☐	A. American Indian or Alaska Native
☐	B. Asian
☐	C. Black or African American
☐	D. Hispanic or Latino
☐	E. Native Hawaiian or Other Pacific Islander
☐	F. White

Item Rationale

- This item uses the common uniform language approved by the Office of Management and Budget (OMB) to report racial and ethnic categories. The categories in this classification are social-political constructs and should not be interpreted as being scientific or anthropological in nature.
- Provides demographic race/ethnicity specific health trend information.
- These categories are NOT used to determine eligibility for participation in any Federal program.

A1000: Race/Ethnicity (cont.)

Steps for Assessment: Interview Instructions

1. Ask the resident to select the category or categories that most closely correspond to his or her race/ethnicity from the list in A1000.

    • Individuals may be more comfortable if this and the preceding question are introduced by saying, "We want to make sure that all our residents get the best care possible, regardless of their race or ethnic background. We would like you to tell us your ethnic and racial background so that we can review the treatment that all residents receive and make sure that everyone gets the highest quality of care" (Baker et al., 2005).

2. If the resident is unable to respond, ask a family member or significant other.

3. Category definitions are provided to resident or family only if requested by them in order to answer the item.

4. Respondents should be offered the option of selecting one or more racial designations.

5. Only if the resident is unable to respond and no family member or significant other is available, observer identification or medical record documentation may be used.

Coding Instructions

Check all that apply.

    • Enter the race or ethnic category or categories the resident, family or significant other uses to identify him or her.

DEFINITIONS

RACE/ETHNICITY

AMERICAN INDIAN OR ALASKA NATIVE

A person having origins in any of the original peoples of North and South America (including Central America), and who maintains tribal affiliation or community attachment.

ASIAN

A person having origins in any of the original peoples of the Far East, Southeast Asia, or the Indian subcontinent including, for example, Cambodia, China, India, Japan, Korea, Malaysia, Pakistan, the Philippine Islands, Thailand, Vietnam.

BLACK OR AFRICAN AMERICAN

A person having origins in any of the black racial groups of Africa. Terms such as "Haitian" or "Negro" can be used in addition to "Black" or "African American."

HISPANIC OR LATINO

A person of Cuban, Mexican, Puerto Rican, South or Central American or other Spanish culture or origin regardless of race. The term "Spanish Origin" can be used in addition to "Hispanic" or "Latino."

NATIVE HAWAIIAN OR OTHER PACIFIC ISLANDER

A person having origins in any of the original peoples of Hawaii, Guam, Samoa, or other Pacific Islands.

WHITE

A person having origins in any of the original peoples of Europe, the Middle East, or North Africa.

A1100: Language

A1100. Language	
Enter Code ☐	**A. Does the resident need or want an interpreter to communicate with a doctor or health care staff?** 0. **No** 1. **Yes** → Specify in A1100B, Preferred language 9. **Unable to determine** **B. Preferred language:** ☐☐☐☐☐☐☐☐☐☐☐☐☐☐☐☐

Item Rationale

Health-related Quality of Life

- Inability to make needs known and to engage in social interaction because of a language barrier can be very frustrating and can result in isolation, depression, and unmet needs.
- Language barriers can interfere with accurate assessment.

Planning for Care

- When a resident needs or wants an interpreter, the nursing home should ensure that an interpreter is available.
- An alternate method of communication also should be made available to help to ensure that basic needs can be expressed at all times, such as a communication board with pictures on it for the resident to point to (if able).
- Identifies residents who need interpreter services in order to answer interview items or participate in consent process.

Steps for Assessment

1. Ask the resident if he or she needs or wants an interpreter to communicate with a doctor or health care staff.
2. If the resident is unable to respond, a family member or significant other should be asked.
3. If neither source is available, review record for evidence of a need for an interpreter.
4. If an interpreter is wanted or needed, ask for preferred language.
5. It is acceptable for a family member or significant other to be the interpreter if the resident is comfortable with it and if the family member or significant other will translate exactly what the resident says without providing his or her interpretation.

Coding Instructions for A1100A

- **Code 0, no:** if the resident (or family or medical record if resident unable to communicate) indicates that the resident does not want or need an interpreter to communicate with a doctor or health care staff.
- **Code 1, yes:** if the resident (or family or medical record if resident unable to communicate) indicates that he or she needs or wants an interpreter to communicate with a doctor or health care staff. Specify preferred language. Proceed to 1100B and enter the resident's preferred language.
- **Code 9, unable to determine:** if no source can identify whether the resident wants or needs an interpreter.

A1100: Language (cont.)

Coding Instructions for A1100B

- Enter the preferred language the resident primarily speaks or understands after interviewing the resident and family, observing the resident and listening, and reviewing the medical record.

Coding Tips and Special Populations

- An organized system of signing such as American Sign Language (ASL) can be reported as the preferred language if the resident needs or wants to communicate in this manner.

A1200: Marital Status

A1200. Marital Status	
Enter Code	1. **Never married** 2. **Married** 3. **Widowed** 4. **Separated** 5. **Divorced**

Item Rationale

- Allows understanding of the formal relationship the resident has and can be important for care and discharge planning.
- Demographic information.

Steps for Assessment

1. Ask the resident about his or her marital status.
2. If the resident is unable to respond, ask a family member or other significant other.
3. If neither source can report, review the medical record for information.

Coding Instructions

- Choose the answer that best describes the current marital status of the resident and enter the corresponding number in the code box:

    1. Never Married

    2. Married

    3. Widowed

    4. Separated

    5. Divorced

A1300: Optional Resident Items

A1300. Optional Resident Items
A. Medical record number:
[ ][ ][ ][ ][ ][ ][ ][ ][ ][ ][ ][ ]
B. Room number:
[ ][ ][ ][ ][ ][ ][ ][ ][ ][ ]
C. Name by which resident prefers to be addressed:
[ ]
D. Lifetime occupation(s) - put "/" between two occupations:
[ ]

Item Rationale

- Some facilities prefer to include the nursing home medical record number on the MDS to facilitate tracking.
- Some facilities conduct unit reviews of MDS items in addition to resident and nursing home level reviews. The unit may be indicated by the room number.
- Preferred name and lifetime occupation help nursing home staff members personalize their interactions with the resident.
- Many people are called by a nickname or middle name throughout their life. It is important to call residents by the name they prefer in order to establish comfort and respect between staff and resident. Also, some cognitively impaired or hearing impaired residents might have difficulty responding when called by their legal name, if it is not the name most familiar to them.
- Others may prefer a more formal and less familiar address. For example, a physician might appreciate being referred to as "Doctor."
- Knowing a person's lifetime occupation is also helpful for care planning and conversation purposes. For example, a carpenter might enjoy pursuing hobby shop activities.
- These are optional items because they are not needed for CMS program function.

Coding Instructions for A1300A, Medical Record Number

- Enter the resident's medical record number (from the nursing home medical record, admission office or Health Information Management Department) if the nursing home chooses to exercise this option.

Coding Instructions for A1300B, Room Number

- Enter the resident's room number if the nursing home chooses to exercise this option.

Coding Instructions for A1300C, Name by Which Resident Prefers to Be Addressed

- Enter the resident's preferred name. This field captures a preferred nickname, middle name, or title that the resident prefers staff use.
- Obtained from resident self-report or family or significant other if resident is unable to respond.

A1300: Optional Resident Items (cont.)

Coding Instructions for A1300D, Lifetime Occupation(s)

- Enter the job title or profession that describes the resident's main occupation(s) before retiring or entering the nursing home. When two occupations are identified, place a slash (/) between each occupation.

- The lifetime occupation of a person whose primary work was in the home should be recorded as "homemaker." For a resident who is a child or an intellectually disabled/developmentally disabled adult resident who has never had an occupation, record as "none."

A1500: Preadmission Screening and Resident Review (PASRR)

A1500. Preadmission Screening and Resident Review (PASRR)
Complete only if A0310A = 01, 03, 04, or 05
Enter Code [ ] **Is the resident currently considered by the state level II PASRR process to have serious mental illness and/or intellectual disability ("mental retardation" in federal regulation) or a related condition?** 0. **No** → Skip to A1550, Conditions Related to ID/DD Status 1. **Yes** → Continue to A1510, Level II Preadmission Screening and Resident Review (PASRR) Conditions 9. **Not a Medicaid-certified unit** → Skip to A1550, Conditions Related to ID/DD Status

Item Rationale

Health-related Quality of Life

- All individuals who are admitted to a Medicaid certified nursing facility must have a Level I PASRR completed to screen for possible mental illness (MI), intellectual disability (ID), ("mental retardation" (MR) in federal regulation)/developmental disability (DD), or related conditions regardless of the resident's method of payment (please contact your local State Medicaid Agency for details regarding PASRR requirements and exemptions).

- Individuals who have or are suspected to have MI or ID/DD or related conditions may not be admitted to a Medicaid-certified nursing facility unless approved through Level II PASRR determination. Those residents covered by Level II PASRR process may require certain care and services provided by the nursing home, and/or specialized services provided by the State.

- A resident with MI or ID/DD must have a Resident Review (RR) conducted when there is a significant change in the resident's physical or mental condition. Therefore, when a significant change in status MDS assessment is completed for a resident with MI or ID/DD, the nursing home is required to notify the State mental health authority, intellectual disability or developmental disability authority (depending on which operates in their State) in order to notify them of the resident's change in status. Section 1919(e)(7)(B)(iii) of the Social Security Act requires the notification or referral for a significant change.[1]

---

[1] The statute may also be referenced as 42 USC 1396r(e)(7)(B)(iii). Note that as of this revision date the statute supersedes Federal regulations at 42 CFR 483.114(c), which still reads as requiring annual resident review. The regulation has not yet been updated to reflect the statutory change to resident review upon significant change in condition.

A1500: Preadmission Screening and Resident Review (PASRR) (cont.)

- Each State Medicaid agency might have specific processes and guidelines for referral, and which types of significant changes should be referred. Therefore, facilities should become acquainted with their own State requirements.
- Please see https://www.cms.gov/PASRR/01_Overview.asp for CMS information on PASRR.

Planning for Care

- The Level II PASRR determination and the evaluation report specify services to be provided by the nursing home and/or specialized services defined by the State.
- The State is responsible for providing specialized services to individuals with MI or ID/DD. In some States specialized services are provided to residents in Medicaid-certified facilities (in other States specialized services are only provided in other facility types such as a psychiatric hospital). The nursing home is required to provide all other care and services appropriate to the resident's condition.
- The services to be provided by the nursing home and/or specialized services provided by the State that are specified in the Level II PASRR determination and the evaluation report should be addressed in the plan of care.
- Identifies individuals who are subject to Resident Review upon change in condition.

Steps for Assessment

1. Complete if A0310A = 01, 03, 04 or 05 (Admission assessment, Annual assessment, Significant Change in Status Assessment, Significant Correction to Prior Comprehensive Assessment).
2. Review the Level I PASRR form to determine whether a Level II PASRR was required.
3. Review the PASRR report provided by the State if Level II screening was required.

Coding Instructions

- **Code 0, no:** and skip to A1550, Conditions Related to ID/DD Status, if any of the following apply:
  - PASRR Level I screening did not result in a referral for Level II screening, or
  - Level II screening determined that the resident does not have a serious mental illness and/or intellectual/developmental disability or related condition, or
  - PASRR screening is not required because the resident was admitted from a hospital after requiring acute inpatient care, is receiving services for the condition for which he or she received care in the hospital, and the attending physician has certified before admission that the resident is likely to require less than 30 days of nursing home care.

A1500: Preadmission Screening and Resident Review (PASRR) (cont.)

- **Code 1, yes:** if PASRR Level II screening determined that the resident has a serious mental illness and/or ID/DD or related condition, and continue to A1510, Level II Preadmission Screening and Resident Review (PASRR) Conditions.

- **Code 9, not a Medicaid-certified unit:** if bed is not in a Medicaid-certified nursing home. Skip to A1550, Conditions Related to ID/DD Status. The PASRR process does not apply to nursing home units that are not certified by Medicaid (unless a State requires otherwise) and therefore the question is not applicable.

  — Note that the requirement is based on the certification of the part of the nursing home the resident will occupy. In a nursing home in which some parts are Medicaid certified and some are not, this question applies when a resident is admitted, or transferred to, a Medicaid certified part of the building.

A1510: Level II Preadmission Screening and Resident Review (PASRR) Conditions

A1510. Level II Preadmission Screening and Resident Review (PASRR) Conditions
Complete only if A0310A = 01, 03, 04, or 05
↓ Check all that apply
☐   A. Serious mental illness
☐   B. Intellectual Disability ("mental retardation" in federal regulation)
☐   C. Other related conditions

Steps for Assessment

1. Complete if A0310A = 01, 03, 04 or 05 (admission assessment, annual assessment, significant change in status assessment, significant correction to prior comprehensive assessment).

2. Check all that apply.

Coding Instructions

- **Code A, Serious mental illness:** if resident has been diagnosed with a serious mental illness.

- **Code B, Intellectual Disability ("mental retardation" in federal regulation)/Developmental Disability:** if resident has been diagnosed with intellectual disability/developmental disability.

- **Code C, Other related conditions:** if resident has been diagnosed with other related conditions.

A1550: Conditions Related to Intellectual Disability/Developmental Disability (ID/DD) Status

A1550. Conditions Related to ID/DD Status

If the resident is 22 years of age or older, complete only if A0310A = 01

If the resident is 21 years of age or younger, complete only if A0310A = 01, 03, 04, or 05

↓ **Check all conditions that are related to ID/DD status** that were manifested before age 22, and are likely to continue indefinitely

	ID/DD With Organic Condition
☐	A. Down syndrome
☐	B. Autism
☐	C. Epilepsy
☐	D. Other organic condition related to ID/DD
	ID/DD Without Organic Condition
☐	E. ID/DD with no organic condition
	No ID/DD
☐	Z. None of the above

Item Rationale

- To document conditions associated with intellectual or developmental disabilities.

Steps for Assessment

1. If resident is 22 years of age or older on the assessment reference date, complete only if A0310A = 01 (Admission assessment).

2. If resident is 21 years of age or younger on the assessment reference date, complete if A0310A = 01, 03, 04, or 05 (Admission assessment, Annual assessment, Significant Change in Status Assessment, Significant Correction to Prior Comprehensive Assessment).

Coding Instructions

- Check all conditions related to ID/DD status that were present before age 22.
- When age of onset is not specified, assume that the condition meets this criterion AND is likely to continue indefinitely.
- **Code A:** if Down syndrome is present.
- **Code B:** if autism is present.
- **Code C:** if epilepsy is present.
- **Code D:** if other organic condition related to ID/DD is present.

DEFINITIONS

DOWN SYNDROME

A common genetic disorder in which a child is born with 47 rather than 46 chromosomes, resulting in developmental delays, intellectual disability, low muscle tone, and other possible effects.

AUTISM

A developmental disorder that is characterized by impaired social interaction, problems with verbal and nonverbal communication, and unusual, repetitive, or severely limited activities and interests.

EPILEPSY

A common chronic neurological disorder that is characterized by recurrent unprovoked seizures.

A1550: Conditions Related to Intellectual Disability/Developmental Disability (ID/DD) Status (cont.)

- **Code E:** if an ID/DD condition is present but the resident does not have any of the specific conditions listed.
- **Code Z:** if ID/DD condition is not present.

> **DEFINITION**
>
> **OTHER ORGANIC CONDITION RELATED TO ID/DD**
>
> Examples of diagnostic conditions include congenital syphilis, maternal intoxication, mechanical injury at birth, prenatal hypoxia, neuronal lipid storage diseases, phenylketonuria (PKU), neurofibromatosis, microcephalus, macroencephaly, meningomyelocele, congenital hydrocephalus, etc.

A1600: Entry Date (date of this admission/entry or reentry into the facility)

A1600. Entry Date (date of this admission/entry or reentry into the facility)
☐☐ - ☐☐ - ☐☐☐☐   Month   Day   Year

Item Rationale

- To document the date of admission/entry or reentry into the nursing home.

Coding Instructions

- Enter the most recent date of admission/entry or reentry to this nursing home. Use the format: Month-Day-Year: XX-XX-XXXX. For example, October 12, 2010, would be entered as 10-12-2010.

> **DEFINITION**
>
> **ENTRY DATE**
>
> The initial date of admission to the nursing facility, or the date the resident most recently returned to your nursing facility after being discharged.

A1700: Type of Entry

A1700. Type of Entry	
Enter Code ☐	1. Admission 2. Reentry

Item Rationale

- Captures whether date in A1600 is an admission/entry or reentry date.

Coding Instructions

- **Code 1, admission/entry:** when one of the following occurs:

A1700: Type of Entry (cont.)

1. resident has never been admitted to this facility before; OR
2. resident has been in this facility previously and was discharged prior to completion of the OBRA Admission assessment; OR
3. resident has been in this facility previously and was discharged return not anticipated; OR
4. resident has been in this facility previously and was discharged return anticipated and did not return within 30 days of discharge.

- **Code 2, reentry:** when all 3 of the following occurred prior to the this entry, the resident was:
  1. admitted to this nursing home (i.e., OBRA Admission assessment was completed), AND
  2. discharged return anticipated, AND
  3. returned to facility within 30 days of discharge.

Coding Tips and Special Populations

- Swing bed facilities will always code the resident's entry as an admission, '1', since an OBRA Admission assessment must have been completed to code as a reentry. OBRA Admission assessments are not completed for swing bed residents.
- In determining if a resident returns to the facility within 30 days, the day of discharge from the facility is not counted in the 30 days. For example, a resident is discharged return anticipated on December 1 would need to return to the facility by December 31 to meet the "within 30 day" requirement.

A1800: Entered From

Enter Code	A1800. Entered From
	01. **Community** (private home/apt., board/care, assisted living, group home)
	02. **Another nursing home or swing bed**
	03. **Acute hospital**
	04. **Psychiatric hospital**
	05. **Inpatient rehabilitation facility**
	06. **ID/DD facility**
	07. **Hospice**
	09. **Long Term Care Hospital** (LTCH)
	99. **Other**

Item Rationale

- Understanding the setting that the individual was in immediately prior to nursing home admission informs care planning and may also inform discharge planning and discussions.
- Demographic information.

Steps for Assessment

1. Review transfer and admission records.
2. Ask the resident and/or family or significant others.

A1800: Entered From (cont.)

Coding Instructions

Enter the 2-digit code that corresponds to the location or program the resident was admitted from for this admission.

- **Code 01, community (private home/apt, board/care, assisted living, group home):** if the resident was admitted from a private home, apartment, board and care, assisted living facility or group home.

- **Code 02, another nursing home or swing bed:** if the resident was admitted from an institution (or a distinct part of an institution) that is primarily engaged in providing skilled nursing care and related services for residents who require medical or nursing care or rehabilitation services for injured, disabled, or sick persons. Includes swing beds.

- **Code 03, acute hospital:** if the resident was admitted from an institution that is engaged in providing, by or under the supervision of physicians for inpatients, diagnostic services, therapeutic services for medical diagnosis, and the treatment and care of injured, disabled, or sick persons.

- **Code 04, psychiatric hospital:** if the resident was admitted from an institution that is engaged in providing, by or under the supervision of a physician, psychiatric services for the diagnosis and treatment of mentally ill residents.

- **Code 05, inpatient rehabilitation facility (IRF):** if the resident was admitted from an institution that is engaged in providing, under the supervision of physicians, services for the rehabilitation of injured, disabled, or sick persons. Includes IRFs that are units within acute care hospitals.

- **Code 06, ID/DD facility:** if the resident was admitted from an institution that is engaged in providing, under the supervision of a physician, any health and rehabilitative services for individuals who have intellectual or developmental disabilities.

- **Code 07, hospice:** if the resident was admitted from a program for terminally ill persons where an array of services is necessary for the palliation and management of terminal illness and related conditions. The hospice must be licensed by the State as a hospice provider and/or certified under the Medicare program as a hospice provider. Includes community-based or inpatient hospice programs.

- **Code 09, long term care hospital (LTCH):** if the resident was admitted from a hospital that is certified under Medicare as a short-term, acute-care hospital which has been excluded from the Inpatient Acute Care Hospital Prospective Payment System (IPPS) under §1886(d)((1)(B)(iv) of the Social Security Act. For the purpose of Medicare payment, LTCHs are defined as having an average inpatient length of stay (as determined by the Secretary) of greater than 25 days.

DEFINITIONS

PRIVATE HOME OR APARTMENT

Any house, condominium, or apartment in the community whether owned by the resident or another person. Also included in this category are retirement communities and independent housing for the elderly.

BOARD AND CARE/ ASSISTED LIVING/ GROUP HOME

A non-institutional community residential setting that includes services of the following types: home health services, homemaker/personal care services, or meal services.

A1800: Entered From (cont.)

- **Code 99, other:** if the resident was admitted from none of the above.

Coding Tips and Special Populations

- If an individual was enrolled in a home-based hospice program enter **07, Hospice**, instead of **01, Community**.

A2000: Discharge Date

A2000. Discharge Date
Complete only if A0310F = 10, 11, or 12
[ ][ ] – [ ][ ] – [ ][ ][ ][ ] Month   Day   Year

Item Rationale

- Closes case in system.

Coding Instructions

- Enter the date the resident was discharged (whether or not return is anticipated). This is the date the resident leaves the facility.
- For discharge assessments, the discharge date (A2000) and ARD (A2300) must be the same date.
- Do not include leave of absence or hospital observational stays less than 24 hours unless admitted to the hospital.
- Obtain data from the medical, admissions or transfer records.

Coding Tips and Special Populations

- If a resident was receiving services under SNF Part A PPS, the discharge date may be later than the end of Medicare stay date (A2400C).

A2100: Discharge Status

A2100. Discharge Status		
Complete only if A0310F = 10, 11, or 12		
Enter Code [ ][ ]	01. **Community** (private home/apt., board/care, assisted living, group home) 02. **Another nursing home or swing bed** 03. **Acute hospital** 04. **Psychiatric hospital** 05. **Inpatient rehabilitation facility** 06. **ID/DD facility** 07. **Hospice** 08. **Deceased** 09. **Long Term Care Hospital** (LTCH) 99. **Other**	

A2100: Discharge Status (cont.)

Item Rationale

- Demographic and outcome information.

Steps for Assessment

1. Review the medical record including the discharge plan and discharge orders for documentation of discharge location.

Coding Instructions

Select the 2-digit code that corresponds to the resident's discharge status.

- **Code 01, community (private home/apt., board/care, assisted living, group home):** if discharge location is a private home, apartment, board and care, assisted living facility, or group home.

- **Code 02, another nursing home or swing bed:** if discharge location is an institution (or a distinct part of an institution) that is primarily engaged in providing skilled nursing care and related services for residents who require medical or nursing care or rehabilitation services for injured, disabled, or sick persons. Includes swing beds.

- **Code 03, acute hospital:** if discharge location is an institution that is engaged in providing, by or under the supervision of physicians for inpatients, diagnostic services, therapeutic services for medical diagnosis, and the treatment and care of injured, disabled, or sick persons.

- **Code 04, psychiatric hospital:** if discharge location is an institution that is engaged in providing, by or under the supervision of a physician, psychiatric services for the diagnosis and treatment of mentally ill residents.

- **Code 05, inpatient rehabilitation facility:** if discharge location is an institution that is engaged in providing, under the supervision of physicians, rehabilitation services for the rehabilitation of injured, disabled or sick persons. Includes IRFs that are units within acute care hospitals.

- **Code 06, ID/DD facility:** if discharge location is an institution that is engaged in providing, under the supervision of a physician, any health and rehabilitative services for individuals who have intellectual or developmental disabilities.

- **Code 07, hospice:** if discharge location is a program for terminally ill persons where an array of services is necessary for the palliation and management of terminal illness and related conditions. The hospice must be licensed by the State as a hospice provider and/or certified under the Medicare program as a hospice provider. Includes community-based (e.g., home) or inpatient hospice programs.

- **Code 08, deceased:** if resident is deceased.

- **Code 09, long term care hospital (LTCH):** if discharge location is an institution that is certified under Medicare as a short-term, acute-care hospital which has

A2100: Discharge Status (cont.)

been excluded from the Inpatient Acute Care Hospital Prospective Payment System (IPPS) under §1886(d)((1)(B)(iv) of the Social Security Act. For the purpose of Medicare payment, LTCHs are defined as having an average inpatient length of stay (as determined by the Secretary) of greater than 25 days.

- **Code 99, other:** if discharge location is none of the above.

A2200: Previous Assessment Reference Date for Significant Correction

A2200. Previous Assessment Reference Date for Significant Correction
Complete only if A0310A = 05 or 06
☐☐ - ☐☐ - ☐☐☐☐
Month   Day   Year

Item Rationale

- To identify the ARD of a previous comprehensive or Quarterly assessment (A0310A = 05 or 06) in which a significant error is discovered.

Coding Instructions

- Complete only if A0310A = 05 (Significant Correction to Prior Comprehensive Assessment) or A0310A = 06 (Significant Correction to Prior Quarterly Assessment).
- Enter the ARD of the prior comprehensive or Quarterly assessment in which a significant error has been identified and a correction is required.

A2300: Assessment Reference Date

A2300. Assessment Reference Date
Observation end date:
☐☐ - ☐☐ - ☐☐☐☐
Month   Day   Year

Item Rationale

- Designates the end of the look-back period so that all assessment items refer to the resident's status during the same period of time.

  As the last day of the look-back period, the ARD serves as the reference point for determining the care and services captured on the MDS assessment. Anything that happens after the ARD will not be captured on that MDS. For example, for a MDS item with a 7-day look-back period, assessment information is collected for a 7-day period ending on and including the ARD which is the 7th day of this look-back period. For an item with a 14-day look-back period, the information is collected for a 14-day period ending on and including the ARD. The look-back period includes observations and events through the end of the day (midnight) of the ARD.

A2300: Assessment Reference Date (cont.)

Steps for Assessment

1. Interdisciplinary team members should select the ARD based on the reason for the assessment and compliance with all timing and scheduling requirements outlined in Chapter 2.

Coding Instructions

- Enter the appropriate date on the lines provided. Do not leave any spaces blank. If the month or day contains only a single digit, enter a "0" in the first space. Use four digits for the year. For example, October 2, 2010, should be entered as: 10-02-2010.

- For detailed information on the timing of the assessments, see Chapter 2 on assessment schedules.

- For discharge assessments, the discharge date item (A2000) and the ARD item (A2300) must contain the same date.

> **DEFINITION**
>
> **ASSESSMENT REFERENCE DATE (ARD)**
> The specific end-point for the look-back periods in the MDS assessment process. Almost all MDS items refer to the resident's status over a designated time period referring back in time from the Assessment Reference Date (ARD). Most frequently, this look-back period, also called the observation or assessment period, is a 7-day period ending on the ARD. Look-back periods may cover the 7 days ending on this date, 14 days ending on this date, etc.

Coding Tips and Special Populations

- When the resident dies or is discharged prior to the end of the look-back period for a required assessment, the ARD must be adjusted to equal the discharge date.

- The look-back period may not be extended simply because a resident was out of the nursing home during part of the look-back period (e.g., a home visit, therapeutic leave, or hospital observation stay less than 24 hours when resident is not admitted). For example, if the ARD is set at day 13 and there is a 2-day temporary leave during the look-back period, the 2 leave days are still considered part of the look-back period.

- When collecting assessment information, data from the time period of the leave of absence is captured as long as the particular MDS item permits. For example, if the family takes the resident to the physician during the leave, the visit would be counted in Item O0600, **Physician Examination** (if criteria are otherwise met).

    This requirement applies to all assessments, regardless of whether they are being completed for clinical or payment purposes.

A2400: Medicare Stay

A2400. Medicare Stay	
Enter Code ☐	**A. Has the resident had a Medicare-covered stay since the most recent entry?** 0. **No** → Skip to B0100, Comatose 1. **Yes** → Continue to A2400B, Start date of most recent Medicare stay
	B. Start date of most recent Medicare stay: ☐☐ – ☐☐ – ☐☐☐☐ Month Day Year
	C. End date of most recent Medicare stay - Enter dashes if stay is ongoing: ☐☐ – ☐☐ – ☐☐☐☐ Month Day Year

A2400: Medicare Stay (cont.)

Item Rationale

- Identifies when a resident is receiving services under the scheduled PPS.
- Identifies when a resident's Medicare Part A stay begins and ends.
- The end date is used to determine if the resident's stay qualifies for the short stay assessment.

Coding Instructions for A2400A, Has the Resident Had a Medicare-covered Stay since the Most Recent Entry?

- **Code 0, no:** if the resident has not had a covered Medicare Part A covered stay since the most recent admission/entry or reentry. Skip to B0100, Comatose.
- **Code 1, yes:** if the resident has had a Medicare Part A covered stay since the most recent admission/entry or reentry. Continue to A2400B.

Coding Instructions for A2400B, Start of Most Recent Medicare Stay

- **Code the date of day 1** of this Medicare stay if A2400A is **coded 1, yes**.

Coding Instructions for A2400C, End Date of Most Recent Medicare Stay

- **Code the date of last day** of this Medicare stay if A2400A is **coded 1, yes**.
- If the Medicare Part A stay is ongoing there will be no end date to report. Enter dashes to indicate that the stay is ongoing.
- The end of Medicare date is coded as follows, whichever occurs first:
  — Date SNF benefit exhausts (i.e., the 100th day of the benefit); or
  — Date of last day covered as recorded on the effective date from the Generic Notice; or
  — The last paid day of Medicare A when payer source changes to another payer (regardless if the resident was moved to another bed or not); or
  — Date the resident was discharged from the facility (see Item A2000, Discharge Date).

> **DEFINITIONS**
>
> **MOST RECENT MEDICARE STAY**
> This is a Medicare Part A covered stay that has started on or after the most recent admission/entry or reentry to the nursing facility.
>
> **MEDICARE-COVERED STAY**
> Skilled Nursing Facility stays billable to Medicare Part A. Does not include stays billable to Medicare Advantage HMO plans.
>
> **CURRENT MEDICARE STAY**
> NEW ADMISSION:
> Day 1 of Medicare Part A stay.
>
> READMISSION:
> Day 1 of Medicare Part A coverage after readmission following a discharge.

Medicare Stay End Date Algorithm
A2400C

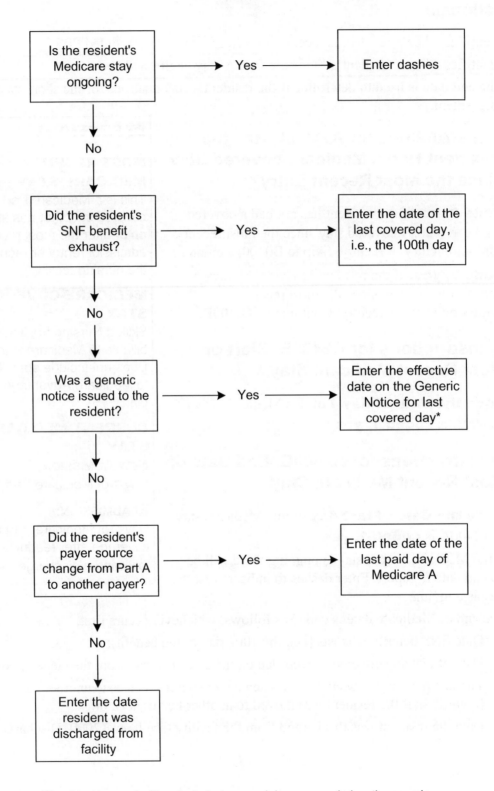

*if resident leaves facility prior to last covered day as recorded on the generic notice, enter date resident left facility.

A2400: Medicare Stay (cont.)

Coding Tips and Special Populations

- When a resident on Medicare Part A returns following a therapeutic leave of absence or a hospital observation stay of less than 24 hours (without hospital admission), this is a continuation of the Medicare Part A stay, not a new Medicare Part A stay.
- The end date of the Medicare stay may be earlier than actual discharge date from the facility (Item A2000).

Examples

1. Mrs. G. began receiving services under Medicare Part A on October 14, 2010. Due to her stable condition and ability to manage her medications and dressing changes, the facility determined that she no longer qualified for Part A SNF coverage and issued an Advanced Beneficiary Notice (ABN) and a Generic Notice with the last day of coverage as November 23, 2010. Mrs. G. was discharged from the facility on November 24, 2010. Code the following on her Discharge assessment:

   - A2000 = 11-24-2010
   - A2400A = 1
   - A2400B = 10-14-2010
   - A2400C = 11-23-2010

2. Mr. N began receiving services under Medicare Part A on December 11, 2010. He was sent to the ER on December 19, 2010 at 8:30pm and was not admitted to the hospital. He returned to the facility on December 20, 2010, at 11:00 am. The facility completed his 14-day PPS assessment with an ARD of December 23, 2010. Code the following on his 14-day PPS assessment:

   - A2400A = 1
   - A2400B = 12-11-2010
   - A2400C = ----------

3. Mr. R. began receiving services under Medicare Part A on October 15, 2010. He was discharged return anticipated on October 20, 2010, to the hospital. Code the following on his Discharge assessment:

   - A2000 = 10-20-2010
   - A2400A = 1
   - A2400B = 10-15-2010
   - A2400C = 10-20-2010

SECTION B: HEARING, SPEECH, AND VISION

Intent: The intent of items in this section is to document the resident's ability to hear (with assistive hearing devices, if they are used), understand, and communicate with others and whether the resident experiences visual limitations or difficulties related to diseases common in aged persons.

B0100: Comatose

B0100. Comatose	
Enter Code [ ]	**Persistent vegetative state/no discernible consciousness** 0. **No** → Continue to B0200, Hearing 1. **Yes** → Skip to G0110, Activities of Daily Living (ADL) Assistance

Item Rationale

Health-related Quality of Life

- Residents who are in a coma or persistent vegetative state are at risk for the complications of immobility, including skin breakdown and joint contractures.

Planning for Care

- Care planning should center on eliminating or minimizing complications and providing care consistent with the resident's health care goals.

> **DEFINITIONS**
>
> **COMATOSE (coma)**
> A pathological state in which neither arousal (wakefulness, alertness) nor awareness exists. The person is unresponsive and cannot be aroused; he/she does not open his/her eyes, does not speak and does not move his/her extremities on command or in response to noxious stimuli (e.g., pain).

Steps for Assessment

1. Review the medical record to determine if a neurological diagnosis of comatose or persistent vegetative state has been documented by a physician, or nurse practitioner, physician assistant, or clinical nurse specialist if allowable under state licensure laws.

Coding Instructions

- **Code 0, no:** if a diagnosis of coma or persistent vegetative state is not present during the 7-day look-back period. Continue to B0200 **Hearing**.

- **Code 1, yes:** if the record indicates that a physician, nurse practitioner or clinical nurse specialist has documented a diagnosis of coma or persistent vegetative state that is applicable during the 7-day look-back period. Skip to Section G0110, **Activities of Daily Living (ADL) Assistance**.

B0100: Comatose (cont.)

Coding Tips

- Only code if a diagnosis of coma or persistent vegetative state has been assigned. For example, some residents in advanced stages of progressive neurologic disorders such as Alzheimer's disease may have severe cognitive impairment, be non-communicative and sleep a great deal of time; however, they are usually not comatose or in a persistent vegetative state, as defined here.

> **DEFINITIONS**
>
> **PERSISTENT VEGETATIVE STATE**
> Sometimes residents who were comatose after an anoxic-ischemic injury (i.e., not enough oxygen to the brain) from a cardiac arrest, head trauma, or massive stroke, regain wakefulness but do not evidence any purposeful behavior or cognition. Their eyes are open, and they may grunt, yawn, pick with their fingers, and have random body movements. Neurological exam shows extensive damage to both cerebral hemispheres.

B0200: Hearing

B0200. Hearing	
Enter Code ☐	**Ability to hear** (with hearing aid or hearing appliances if normally used) 0. **Adequate** - no difficulty in normal conversation, social interaction, listening to TV 1. **Minimal difficulty** - difficulty in some environments (e.g., when person speaks softly or setting is noisy) 2. **Moderate difficulty** - speaker has to increase volume and speak distinctly 3. **Highly impaired** - absence of useful hearing

Item Rationale

Health-related Quality of Life

- Problems with hearing can contribute to sensory deprivation, social isolation, and mood and behavior disorders.
- Unaddressed communication problems related to hearing impairment can be mistaken for confusion or cognitive impairment.

Planning for Care

- Address reversible causes of hearing difficulty (such as cerumen impaction).
- Evaluate potential benefit from hearing assistance devices.
- Offer assistance to residents with hearing difficulties to avoid social isolation.

B0200: Hearing (cont.)

- Consider other communication strategies for persons with hearing loss that is not reversible or is not completely corrected with hearing devices.

- Adjust environment by reducing background noise by lowering the sound volume on televisions or radios, because a noisy environment can inhibit opportunities for effective communication.

Steps for Assessment

1. Ensure that the resident is using his or her normal hearing appliance if they have one. Hearing devices may not be as conventional as a hearing aid. Some residents by choice may use hearing amplifiers or a microphone and headphones as an alternative to hearing aids. Ensure the hearing appliance is operational.

2. Interview the resident and ask about hearing function in different situations (e.g. hearing staff members, talking to visitors, using telephone, watching TV, attending activities).

3. Observe the resident during your verbal interactions and when he or she interacts with others throughout the day.

4. Think through how you can best communicate with the resident. For example, you may need to speak more clearly, use a louder tone, speak more slowly or use gestures. The resident may need to see your face to understand what you are saying, or you may need to take the resident to a quieter area for them to hear you. All of these are cues that there is a hearing problem.

5. Review the medical record.

6. Consult the resident's family, direct care staff, activities personnel, and speech or hearing specialists.

Coding Instructions

- **Code 0, adequate:** No difficulty in normal conversation, social interaction, or listening to TV. The resident hears all normal conversational speech and telephone conversation and announcements in group activities.

- **Code 1, minimal difficulty:** Difficulty in some environments (e.g., when a person speaks softly or the setting is noisy). The resident hears speech at conversational levels but has difficulty hearing when not in quiet listening conditions or when not in one-on-one situations. The resident's hearing is adequate after environmental adjustments are made, such as reducing background noise by moving to a quiet room or by lowering the volume on television or radio.

- **Code 2, moderate difficulty:** Speaker has to increase volume and speak distinctly. Although hearing-deficient, the resident compensates when the speaker adjusts tonal quality and speaks distinctly; or the resident can hear only when the speaker's face is clearly visible.

B0200: Hearing (cont.)

- **Code 3, highly impaired:** Absence of useful hearing. The resident hears only some sounds and frequently fails to respond even when the speaker adjusts tonal quality, speaks distinctly, or is positioned face-to-face. There is no comprehension of conversational speech, even when the speaker makes maximum adjustments.

Coding Tips for Special Populations

- Residents who are unable to respond to a standard hearing assessment due to cognitive impairment will require alternate assessment methods. The resident can be observed in their normal environment. Does he or she respond (e.g., turn his or her head) when a noise is made at a normal level? Does the resident seem to respond only to specific noise in a quiet environment? Assess whether the resident responds only to loud noise or do they not respond at all.

B0300: Hearing Aid

B0300. Hearing Aid	
Enter Code	**Hearing aid or other hearing appliance used** in completing B0200, Hearing 0. No 1. Yes

Item Rationale

Health-related Quality of Life

- Problems with hearing can contribute to social isolation and mood and behavior disorders.

- Many residents with impaired hearing could benefit from hearing aids or other hearing appliances.

- Many residents who own hearing aids do not have the hearing aids with them or have nonfunctioning hearing aids upon arrival.

Planning for Care

- Knowing if a hearing aid was used when determining hearing ability allows better identification of evaluation and management needs.

- For residents with hearing aids, use and maintenance should be included in care planning.

- Residents who do not have adequate hearing without a hearing aid should be asked about history of hearing aid use.

- Residents who do not have adequate hearing despite wearing a hearing aid might benefit from a re-evaluation of the device or assessment for new causes of hearing impairment.

Steps for Assessment

1. Prior to beginning the hearing assessment, ask the resident if he or she owns a hearing aid or other hearing appliance and, if so, whether it is at the nursing home.

2. If the resident cannot respond, write the question down and allow the resident to read it.

B0300: Hearing Aid (cont.)

3. If the resident is still unable, check with family and care staff about hearing aid or other hearing appliances.

4. Check the medical record for evidence that the resident had a hearing appliance in place when hearing ability was recorded.

5. Ask staff and significant others whether the resident was using a hearing appliance when they observed hearing ability (above).

Coding Instructions

*   **Code 0, no:** if the resident did not use a hearing aid (or other hearing appliance) for the 7-day hearing assessment coded in **B0200, Hearing.**

*   **Code 1, yes:** if the resident did use a hearing aid (or other hearing appliance) for the hearing assessment coded in **B0200, Hearing.**

B0600: Speech Clarity

B0600. Speech Clarity	
Enter Code	**Select best description of speech pattern** 0. **Clear speech** - distinct intelligible words 1. **Unclear speech** - slurred or mumbled words 2. **No speech** - absence of spoken words

Item Rationale

Health-related Quality of Life

*   Unclear speech or absent speech can hinder communication and be very frustrating to an individual.

*   Unclear speech or absent speech can result in physical and psychosocial needs not being met and can contribute to depression and social isolation.

Planning for Care

*   If speech is absent or is not clear enough for the resident to make needs known, other methods of communication should be explored.

*   Lack of speech clarity or ability to speak should not be mistaken for cognitive impairment.

> **DEFINITIONS**
>
> **SPEECH**
> The verbal expression of articulate words.

Steps for Assessment

1. Listen to the resident.

2. Ask primary assigned caregivers about the resident's speech pattern.

3. Review the medical record.

B0600: Speech Clarity (cont.)

4. Determine the quality of the resident's speech, not the content or appropriateness—just words spoken.

Coding Instructions

- **Code 0, clear speech:** if the resident usually utters distinct, intelligible words.

- **Code 1, unclear speech:** if the resident usually utters slurred or mumbled words.

- **Code 2, no speech:** if there is an absence of spoken words.

B0700: Makes Self Understood

B0700. Makes Self Understood	
Enter Code ☐	**Ability to express ideas and wants,** consider both verbal and non-verbal expression 0. **Understood** 1. **Usually understood** - difficulty communicating some words or finishing thoughts **but** is able if prompted or given time 2. **Sometimes understood** - ability is limited to making concrete requests 3. **Rarely/never understood**

Item Rationale

Health-related Quality of Life

- Problems making self understood can be very frustrating for the resident and can contribute to social isolation and mood and behavior disorders.

- Unaddressed communication problems can be inappropriately mistaken for confusion or cognitive impairment.

Planning for Care

- Ability to make self understood can be optimized by not rushing the resident, breaking longer questions into parts and waiting for reply, and maintaining eye contact (if appropriate).

- If a resident has difficulty making self understood:

  — Identify the underlying cause or causes.

  — Identify the best methods to facilitate communication for that resident.

DEFINITIONS

MAKES SELF UNDERSTOOD
Able to express or communicate requests, needs, opinions, and to conduct social conversation in his or her primary language, whether in speech, writing, sign language, gestures, or a combination of these. Deficits in the ability to make one's self understood (expressive communication deficits) can include reduced voice volume and difficulty in producing sounds, or difficulty in finding the right word, making sentences, writing, and/or gesturing.

B0700: Makes Self Understood (cont.)

Steps for Assessment

1. Assess using the resident's preferred language.

2. Interact with the resident. Be sure he or she can hear you or have access to his or her preferred method for communication. If the resident seems unable to communicate, offer alternatives such as writing, pointing or using cue cards.

3. Observe his or her interactions with others in different settings and circumstances.

4. Consult with the primary nurse assistant (over all shifts), if available, the resident's family, and speech-language pathologist.

Coding Instructions

- **Code 0, understood:** if the resident expresses requests and ideas clearly.

- **Code 1, usually understood:** if the resident has difficulty communicating some words or finishing thoughts **but** is able if prompted or given time. He or she may have delayed responses or may require some prompting to make self understood.

- **Code 2, sometimes understood:** if the resident has limited ability but is able to express concrete requests regarding at least basic needs (e.g., food, drink, sleep, toilet).

- **Code 3, rarely or never understood:** if, at best, the resident's understanding is limited to staff interpretation of highly individual, resident-specific sounds or body language (e.g., indicated presence of pain or need to toilet).

B0800: Ability to Understand Others

B0800. Ability To Understand Others	
Enter Code	**Understanding verbal content, however able** (with hearing aid or device if used) 0. **Understands** - clear comprehension 1. **Usually understands** - misses some part/intent of message **but** comprehends most conversation 2. **Sometimes understands** - responds adequately to simple, direct communication only 3. **Rarely/never understands**

Item Rationale

Health-related Quality of Life

- Inability to understand direct person-to-person communication

  — Can severely limit association with others.

  — Can inhibit the individual's ability to follow instructions that can affect health and safety.

B0800: Ability to Understand Others (cont.)

Planning for Care

- Thorough assessment to determine underlying cause or causes is critical in order to develop a care plan to address the individual's specific deficits and needs.

- Every effort should be made by the facility to provide information to the resident in a consistent manner that he or she understands based on an individualized assessment.

Steps for Assessment

1. Assess in the resident's preferred language.

2. If the resident uses a hearing aid, hearing device or other communications enhancement device, the resident should use that device during the evaluation of the resident's understanding of person-to-person communication.

3. Interact with the resident and observe his or her understanding of other's communication.

4. Consult with direct care staff over all shifts, if possible, the resident's family, and speech-language pathologist (if involved in care).

5. Review the medical record for indications of how well the resident understands others.

> **DEFINITIONS**
>
> **ABILITY TO UNDERSTAND OTHERS**
> Comprehension of direct person-to-person communication whether spoken, written, or in sign language or Braille. Includes the resident's ability to process and understand language. Deficits in one's ability to understand (receptive communication deficits) can involve declines in hearing, comprehension (spoken or written) or recognition of facial expressions.

Coding Instructions

- **Code 0, understands:** if the resident clearly comprehends the message(s) and demonstrates comprehension by words or actions/behaviors.

- **Code 1, usually understands:** if the resident misses some part or intent of the message **but** comprehends most of it. The resident may have periodic difficulties integrating information but generally demonstrates comprehension by responding in words or actions.

- **Code 2, sometimes understands:** if the resident demonstrates frequent difficulties integrating information, and responds adequately only to simple and direct questions or instructions. When staff rephrase or simplify the message(s) and/or use gestures, the resident's comprehension is enhanced.

- **Code 3, rarely/never understands:** if the resident demonstrates very limited ability to understand communication. Or, if staff have difficulty determining whether or not the resident comprehends messages, based on verbal and nonverbal responses. Or, the resident can hear sounds but does not understand messages.

B1000: Vision

B1000. Vision	
Enter Code [ ]	**Ability to see in adequate light** (with glasses or other visual appliances) 0. **Adequate** - sees fine detail, including regular print in newspapers/books 1. **Impaired** - sees large print, but not regular print in newspapers/books 2. **Moderately impaired** - limited vision; not able to see newspaper headlines but can identify objects 3. **Highly impaired** - object identification in question, but eyes appear to follow objects 4. **Severely impaired** - no vision or sees only light, colors or shapes; eyes do not appear to follow objects

Item Rationale

Health-related Quality of Life

- A person's reading vision often diminishes over time.

- If uncorrected, vision impairment can limit the enjoyment of everyday activities such as reading newspapers, books or correspondence, and maintaining and enjoying hobbies and other activities. It also limits the ability to manage personal business, such as reading and signing consent forms.

- Moderate, high or severe impairment can contribute to sensory deprivation, social isolation, and depressed mood.

> **DEFINITIONS**
>
> **ADEQUATE LIGHT**
> Lighting that is sufficient or comfortable for a person with normal vision to see fine detail.

Planning for Care

- Reversible causes of vision impairment should be sought.

- Consider whether simple environmental changes such as better lighting or magnifiers would improve ability to see.

- Consider large print reading materials for persons with impaired vision.

- For residents with moderate, high, or severe impairment, consider alternative ways of providing access to content of desired reading materials or hobbies.

Steps for Assessment

1. Ask direct care staff over all shifts if possible about the resident's usual vision patterns during the 7-day look-back period (e.g., is the resident able to see newsprint, menus, greeting cards?).

2. Then ask the resident about his or her visual abilities.

3. Test the accuracy of your findings:

   - Ensure that the resident's customary visual appliance for close vision is in place (e.g., eyeglasses, magnifying glass).

   - Ensure adequate lighting.

B1000: Vision (cont.)

- Ask the resident to look at regular-size print in a book or newspaper. Then ask the resident to read aloud, starting with larger headlines and ending with the finest, smallest print. If the resident is unable to read a newspaper, provide material with larger print, such as a flyer or large textbook.

- When the resident is unable to read out loud (e.g. due to aphasia, illiteracy), you should test this by another means such as, but not limited to:

  — Substituting numbers or pictures for words that are displayed in the appropriate print size (regular-size print in a book or newspaper)

Coding Instructions

- **Code 0, adequate:** if the resident sees fine detail, including regular print in newspapers/books.

- **Code 1, impaired:** if the resident sees large print, but not regular print in newspapers/books.

- **Code 2, moderately impaired:** if the resident has limited vision and is not able to see newspaper headlines but can identify objects in his or her environment.

- **Code 3, highly impaired:** if the resident's ability to identify objects in his or her environment is in question, but the resident's eye movements appear to be following objects (especially people walking by).

- **Code 4, severely impaired:** if the resident has no vision, sees only light, colors or shapes, or does not appear to follow objects with eyes.

Coding Tips and Special Populations

- Some residents have never learned to read or are unable to read English. In such cases, ask the resident to read numbers, such as dates or page numbers, or to name items in small pictures. Be sure to display this information in two sizes (equivalent to regular and large print).

- If the resident is unable to communicate or follow your directions for testing vision, observe the resident's eye movements to see if his or her eyes seem to follow movement of objects or people. These gross measures of visual acuity may assist you in assessing whether or not the resident has any visual ability. For residents who appear to do this, **code 3, highly impaired.**

B1200: Corrective Lenses

B1200. Corrective Lenses	
Enter Code ☐	**Corrective lenses (contacts, glasses, or magnifying glass) used** in completing B1000, Vision 0. **No** 1. **Yes**

B1200: Corrective Lenses (cont.)

Item Rationale

Health-related Quality of Life

- Decreased ability to see can limit the enjoyment of everyday activities and can contribute to social isolation and mood and behavior disorders.

- Many residents who do not have corrective lenses could benefit from them, and others have corrective lenses that are not sufficient.

- Many persons who benefit from and own visual aids do not have them on arrival at the nursing home.

Planning for Care

- Knowing if corrective lenses were used when determining ability to see allows better identification of evaluation and management needs.

- Residents with eyeglasses or other visual appliances should be assisted in accessing them. Use and maintenance should be included in care planning.

- Residents who do not have adequate vision without eyeglasses or other visual appliances should be asked about history of corrective lens use.

- Residents who do not have adequate vision, despite using a visual appliance, might benefit from a re-evaluation of the appliance or assessment for new causes of vision impairment.

Steps for Assessment

1. Prior to beginning the assessment, ask the resident whether he or she uses eyeglasses or other vision aids and whether the eyeglasses or vision aids are at the nursing home. Visual aids do not include surgical lens implants.

2. If the resident cannot respond, check with family and care staff about the resident's use of vision aids during the 7-day look-back period.

3. Observe whether the resident used eyeglasses or other vision aids during reading vision test (B1000).

4. Check the medical record for evidence that the resident used corrective lenses when ability to see was recorded.

5. Ask staff and significant others whether the resident was using corrective lenses when they observed the resident's ability to see.

B1200: Corrective Lenses (cont.)

Coding Instructions

- **Code 0, no:** if the resident did not use eyeglasses or other vision aid during the **B1000, Vision** assessment.

- **Code 1, yes:** if corrective lenses or other visual aids were used when visual ability was assessed in completing **B1000, Vision.**

SECTION C: COGNITIVE PATTERNS

Intent: The items in this section are intended to determine the resident's attention, orientation and ability to register and recall new information. These items are crucial factors in many care-planning decisions.

C0100: Should Brief Interview for Mental Status Be Conducted?

C0100. Should Brief Interview for Mental Status (C0200-C0500) be Conducted?
Attempt to conduct interview with all residents

Enter Code
[ ]

  0. **No** (resident is rarely/never understood) → Skip to and complete C0700-C1000, Staff Assessment for Mental Status
  1. **Yes** → Continue to C0200, Repetition of Three Words

Item Rationale

Health-related Quality of Life

- This information identifies if the interview will be attempted.
- Most residents are able to attempt the Brief Interview for Mental Status (BIMS).
- A structured cognitive test is more accurate and reliable than observation alone for observing cognitive performance.
  — Without an attempted structured cognitive interview, a resident might be mislabeled based on his or her appearance or assumed diagnosis.
  — Structured interviews will efficiently provide insight into the resident's current condition that will enhance good care.

Planning for Care

- Structured cognitive interviews assist in identifying needed supports.
- The structured cognitive interview is helpful for identifying possible delirium behaviors (C1300).

Steps for Assessment

1. Determine if the resident is rarely/never understood verbally or in writing. If rarely/never understood, skip to C0700 – C1000, Staff Assessment of Mental Status.
2. Review **Language** item (A1100), to determine if the resident needs or wants an interpreter.
   - If the resident needs or wants an interpreter, complete the interview with an interpreter.

Coding Instructions

Record whether the cognitive interview should be attempted with the resident.

- **Code 0, no:** if the interview should not be attempted because the resident is rarely/never understood, cannot respond verbally or in writing, or an interpreter is needed but not available. Skip to C0700, **Staff Assessment of Mental Status**.

- **Code 1, yes:** if the interview should be attempted because the resident is at least sometimes understood verbally or in writing, and if an interpreter is needed, one is available. Proceed to C0200, **Repetition of Three Words**.

C0100: Should Brief Interview for Mental Status Be Conducted? (cont.)

Coding Tips

- If the resident needs an interpreter, every effort should be made to have an interpreter present for the BIMS. If it is not possible for a needed interpreter to participate on the day of the interview, code C0100 = 0 to indicate interview not attempted and complete C0700-C1000, **Staff Assessment of Mental Status**, instead of C0200-C0500, **Brief Interview for Mental Status**.
- Includes residents who use American Sign Language (ASL).

C0200-C0500: Brief Interview for Mental Status (BIMS)

Brief Interview for Mental Status (BIMS)	
C0200. Repetition of Three Words	
Enter Code ☐	Ask resident: *"I am going to say three words for you to remember. Please repeat the words after I have said all three. The words are: **sock, blue, and bed.** Now tell me the three words."* **Number of words repeated after first attempt** 0. None 1. One 2. Two 3. Three After the resident's first attempt, repeat the words using cues ("sock, something to wear; blue, a color; bed, a piece of furniture"). You may repeat the words up to two more times.
C0300. Temporal Orientation (orientation to year, month, and day)	
Enter Code ☐	Ask resident: *"Please tell me what year it is right now."* **A. Able to report correct year** 0. Missed by > 5 years or no answer 1. Missed by 2-5 years 2. Missed by 1 year 3. Correct
Enter Code ☐	Ask resident: *"What month are we in right now?"* **B. Able to report correct month** 0. Missed by > 1 month or no answer 1. Missed by 6 days to 1 month 2. Accurate within 5 days
Enter Code ☐	Ask resident: *"What day of the week is today?"* **C. Able to report correct day of the week** 0. Incorrect or no answer 1. Correct
C0400. Recall	
Enter Code ☐	Ask resident: *"Let's go back to an earlier question. What were those three words that I asked you to repeat?"* If unable to remember a word, give cue (something to wear; a color; a piece of furniture) for that word. **A. Able to recall "sock"** 0. No - could not recall 1. Yes, after cueing ("something to wear") 2. Yes, no cue required
Enter Code ☐	**B. Able to recall "blue"** 0. No - could not recall 1. Yes, after cueing ("a color") 2. Yes, no cue required
Enter Code ☐	**C. Able to recall "bed"** 0. No - could not recall 1. Yes, after cueing ("a piece of furniture") 2. Yes, no cue required
C0500. Summary Score	
Enter Score ☐☐	Add scores for questions C0200-C0400 and fill in total score (00-15) Enter 99 if unable to complete one or more questions of the interview

C0200-C0500: Brief Interview for Mental Status (BIMS) (cont.)

Item Rationale

Health-related Quality of Life

- Direct or performance-based testing of cognitive function decreases the chance of incorrect labeling of cognitive ability and improves detection of delirium.
- Cognitively intact residents may appear to be cognitively impaired because of extreme frailty, hearing impairment or lack of interaction.
- Some residents may appear to be more cognitively intact than they actually are.
- When cognitive impairment is incorrectly diagnosed or missed, appropriate communication, worthwhile activities and therapies may not be offered.
- A resident's performance on cognitive tests can be compared over time.
  - If performance worsens, then an assessment for delirium and or depression should be considered.
- The BIMS is an opportunity to observe residents for signs and symptoms of delirium (C1300).

Planning for Care

- Assessment of a resident's mental state provides a direct understanding of resident function that may:
  - enhance future communication and assistance and
  - direct nursing interventions to facilitate greater independence such as posting or providing reminders for self-care activities.
- A resident's performance on cognitive tests can be compared over time.
  - An abrupt change in cognitive status may indicate delirium and may be the only indication of a potentially life threatening illness.
  - A decline in mental status may also be associated with a mood disorder.
- Awareness of possible impairment may be important for maintaining a safe environment and providing safe discharge planning.

Steps for Assessment: Basic Interview Instructions for BIMS (C0200-C0500)

1. Refer to Appendix D for a review of basic approaches to effective interviewing techniques.
2. Interview any resident not screened out by **Should Brief Interview for Mental Status Be Conducted?** (Item C0100).
3. Conduct the interview in a private setting.
4. Be sure the resident can hear you.

- Residents with hearing impairment should be tested using their usual communication devices/techniques, as applicable.

C0200-C0500: Brief Interview for Mental Status (BIMS) (cont.)

- Try an external assistive device (headphones or hearing amplifier) if you have any doubt about hearing ability.
- Minimize background noise.

5. Sit so that the resident can see your face. Minimize glare by directing light sources away from the resident's face.
6. Give an introduction before starting the interview.

   Suggested language: "I would like to ask you some questions. We ask everyone these same questions. This will help us provide you with better care. Some of the questions may seem very easy, while others may be more difficult."

7. If the resident expresses concern that you are testing his or her memory, he or she may be more comfortable if you reply: "We ask these questions of everyone so we can make sure that our care will meet your needs."
8. Directly ask the resident each item in C0200 through C0400 at one sitting and in the order provided.
9. If the resident chooses not to answer a particular item, accept his or her refusal and move on to the next questions. For C0200 through C0400, code refusals as incorrect.

Coding Instructions

See coding instructions for individual items.

Coding Tips

- On occasion, the interviewer may not be able to state the items clearly because of an accent or slurred speech. If the interviewer is unable to pronounce any cognitive items clearly, have a different staff member complete the BIMS.
- Nonsensical responses should be coded as zero.
- Rules for stopping the interview before it is complete:
  — Stop the interview after completing (C0300C) "Day of the Week" if:
    1. all responses have been nonsensical (i.e., any response that is unrelated, incomprehensible, or incoherent; not informative with respect to the item being rated), OR
    2. there has been no verbal or written response to any of the questions up to this point, OR
    3. there has been no verbal or written response to some questions up to this point and for all others, the resident has given a nonsensical response.
- If the interview is stopped, do the following:
  1. Code **-, dash** in C0400A, C0400B, and C0400C.
  2. Code **99** in the summary score in C0500.
  3. Code **1, yes** in **C0600 Should the Staff Assessment for Mental Status (C0700-C1000) be Conducted?**
  4. Complete the **Staff Assessment for Mental Status**.

C0200-C0500: Brief Interview for Mental Status (BIMS) (cont.)

- When staff identify that the resident's primary method of communication is in written format, the BIMS can be administered in writing. **The administration of the BIMS in writing should be limited to this circumstance.**
- See Appendix E for details regarding how to administer the BIMS in writing.

> **DEFINITIONS**
>
> **NONSENSICAL RESPONSE** Any response that is unrelated, incomprehensible, or incoherent; it is not informative with respect to the item being rated.

Examples of Incorrect and Nonsensical Responses

1. Interviewer asks resident to state the year. The resident replies that it is 1935. This answer is incorrect but related to the question.

   Coding: This answer is **coded 0, incorrect** but would NOT be considered a nonsensical response.

   Rationale: The answer is wrong, but it is logical and relates to the question.

2. Interviewer asks resident to state the year. The resident says, "Oh what difference does the year make when you're as old as I am?" The interviewer asks the resident to try to name the year, and the resident shrugs.

   Coding: This answer is **coded 0, incorrect** but would NOT be considered a nonsensical response.

   Rationale: The answer is wrong because refusal is considered a wrong answer, but the resident's comment is logical and clearly relates to the question.

3. Interviewer asks the resident to name the day of the week. Resident answers, "Sylvia, she's my daughter."

   Coding: The answer is **coded 0, incorrect**; the response is illogical and nonsensical.

   Rationale: The answer is wrong, and the resident's comment clearly does not relate to the question; it is nonsensical.

C0200: Repetition of Three Words

Brief Interview for Mental Status (BIMS)	
C0200. Repetition of Three Words	
Enter Code	Ask resident: *"I am going to say three words for you to remember. Please repeat the words after I have said all three. The words are: sock, blue, and bed. Now tell me the three words."* **Number of words repeated after first attempt** 0. **None** 1. **One** 2. **Two** 3. **Three** After the resident's first attempt, repeat the words using cues (*"sock, something to wear; blue, a color; bed, a piece of furniture"*). You may repeat the words up to two more times.

C0200: Repetition of Three Words (cont.)

Item Rationale

Health-related Quality of Life

- Inability to repeat three words on first attempt may indicate:
  — a hearing impairment,
  — a language barrier, or
  — inattention that may be a sign of delirium.

Planning for Care

- A cue can assist learning.
- Cues may help residents with memory impairment who can store new information in their memory but who have trouble retrieving something that was stored (e.g., not able to remember someone's name but can recall if given part of the first name).
- Staff can use cues when assisting residents with learning and recall in therapy, and in daily and restorative activities.

Steps for Assessment

Basic BIMS interview instructions are shown on page C-5. In addition, for repetition of three words:

1. Say to the resident: "I am going to say three words for you to remember. Please repeat the words after I have said all three. The words are: sock, blue, and bed." Interviewers need to use the words and related category cues as indicated. If the interview is being conducted with an interpreter present, the interpreter should use the equivalent words and similar, relevant prompts for category cues.
2. Immediately after presenting the three words, say to the resident: "Now please tell me the three words."
3. After the resident's first attempt to repeat the items:

> **DEFINITIONS**
>
> **CATEGORY CUE**
> Phrase that puts a word in context to help with learning and to serve as a hint that helps prompt the resident. The category cue for sock is "something to wear." The category cue for blue is "a color." For bed, the category cue is "a piece of furniture."

- If the resident correctly stated all three words, say, "That's right, the words are sock, something to wear; blue, a color; and bed, a piece of furniture" [category cues].
- Category cues serve as a hint that helps prompt residents' recall ability. Putting words in context stimulates learning and fosters memory of the words that residents will be asked to recall in item C0400, even among residents able to repeat the words immediately.
- If the resident recalled two or fewer words, say to the resident: "Let me say the three words again. They are sock, something to wear; blue, a color; and bed, a piece of furniture. Now tell me the three words." If the resident still does not recall all three words correctly, you may repeat the words and category cues one more time.

C0200: Repetition of Three Words (cont.)

- If the resident does not repeat all three words after three attempts, re-assess ability to hear. If the resident can hear, move on to the next question. If he or she is unable to hear, attempt to maximize hearing (alter environment, use hearing amplifier) before proceeding.

Coding Instructions

*Record the maximum number of words that the resident correctly repeated on the **first** attempt. This will be any number between 0 and 3.*

- The words may be recalled in any order and in any context. For example, if the words are repeated back in a sentence, they would be counted as repeating the words.
- Do not score the number of repeated words on the second or third attempt. These attempts help with learning the item, but only the number correct on the first attempt go into the total score. Do not record the number of attempts that the resident needed to complete.
- **Code 0, none:** if the resident did not repeat any of the 3 words on the first attempt.
- **Code 1, one:** if the resident repeated only 1 of the 3 words on the first attempt.
- **Code 2, two:** if the resident repeated only 2 of the 3 words on the first attempt.
- **Code 3, three:** if the resident repeated all 3 words on the first attempt.

Coding Tips

- On occasion, the interviewer may not be able to state the words clearly because of an accent or slurred speech. If the interviewer is unable to pronounce any of the 3 words clearly, have a different staff member conduct the interview.

Examples

1. The interviewer says, "The words are sock, blue, and bed. Now please tell me the three words." The resident replies, "Bed, sock, and blue." The interviewer repeats the three words with category cues, by saying, "That's right, the words are sock, something to wear; blue, a color; and bed, a piece of furniture."

   Coding: C0200 would be **coded 3, three** words correct.
   Rationale: The resident repeated all three items on the first attempt. The order of repetition does not affect the score.

2. The interviewer says, "The words are sock, blue, and bed. Now please tell me the three words." The resident replies, "Sock, bed, black." The interviewer repeats the three words plus the category cues, saying, "Let me say the three words again. They are sock, something to wear; blue, a color; and bed, a piece of furniture. Now tell me the three words." The resident says, "Oh yes, that's right, sock, blue, bed."

   Coding: C0200 would be **coded 2, two** of three words correct.
   Rationale: The resident repeated two of the three items on the first attempt. Residents are scored based on the first attempt.

C0200: Repetition of Three Words (cont.)

3. The interviewer says, "The words are sock, blue, and bed. Now please tell me the three words." The resident says, "Blue socks belong in the dresser." The interviewer repeats the three words plus the category cues.

> **Coding:** C0200 would be **coded 2, two** of the three words correct.
>
> **Rationale:** The resident repeated two of the three items—blue and sock. The resident put the words into a sentence, resulting in the resident repeating two of the three words.

4. The interviewer says, "The words are sock, blue, and bed. Now please tell me the three words." The resident replies, "What were those three words?" The interviewer repeats the three words plus the category cues.

> **Coding:** C0200 would be **coded 0, none** of the words correct.
>
> **Rationale:** The resident did not repeat any of the three words after the first time the interviewer said them.

C0300: Temporal Orientation (Orientation to Year, Month, and Day)

C0300. Temporal Orientation (orientation to year, month, and day)	

Enter Code ☐	Ask resident: *"Please tell me what year it is right now."*
	A. Able to report correct year
	  0. **Missed by > 5 years** or no answer
	  1. **Missed by 2-5 years**
	  2. **Missed by 1 year**
	  3. **Correct**

Enter Code ☐	Ask resident: *"What month are we in right now?"*
	B. Able to report correct month
	  0. **Missed by > 1 month** or no answer
	  1. **Missed by 6 days to 1 month**
	  2. **Accurate within 5 days**

Enter Code ☐	Ask resident: *"What day of the week is today?"*
	C. Able to report correct day of the week
	  0. **Incorrect** or no answer
	  1. **Correct**

Item Rationale

Health-related Quality of Life

- A lack of temporal orientation may lead to decreased communication or participation in activities.
- Not being oriented may be frustrating or frightening.

Planning for Care

- If staff know that a resident has a problem with orientation, they can provide reorientation aids and verbal reminders that may reduce anxiety.

> **DEFINITIONS**
>
> **TEMPORAL ORIENTATION**
> In general, the ability to place oneself in correct time. For the BIMS, it is the ability to indicate the correct date in current surroundings.

C0300: Temporal Orientation (Orientation to Year, Month, and Day) (cont.)

- Reorienting those who are disoriented or at risk of disorientation may be useful in treating symptoms of delirium.
- Residents who are not oriented may need further assessment for delirium, especially if this fluctuates or is recent in onset.

Steps for Assessment

Basic BIMS interview instructions are shown on page C-5.

1. Ask the resident each of the 3 questions in Item C0300 separately.
2. Allow the resident up to 30 seconds for each answer and do not provide clues.
3. If the resident specifically asks for clues (e.g., "is it bingo day?") respond by saying, "I need to know if you can answer this question without any help from me."

Coding Instructions for C0300A, Able to Report Correct Year

- **Code 0, missed by >5 years or no answer:** if the resident's answer is incorrect and is greater than 5 years from the current year or the resident chooses not to answer the item.
- **Code 1, missed by 2-5 years:** if the resident's answer is incorrect and is within 2 to 5 years from the current year.
- **Code 2, missed by 1 year:** if the resident's answer is incorrect and is within one year from the current year.
- **Code 3, correct:** if the resident states the correct year.

Examples

1. The date of interview is May 5, 2011. The resident, responding to the statement, "Please tell me what year it is right now," states that it is 2011.

    Coding: C0300A would be **coded 3, correct.**
    Rationale: 2011 is the current year.

2. The date of interview is June 16, 2011. The resident, responding to the statement, "Please tell me what year it is right now," states that it is 2007.

    Coding: C0300A would be **coded 1, missed by 2-5 years.**
    Rationale: 2007 is within 2 to 5 years of 2011.

3. The date of interview is January 10, 2011. The resident, responding to the statement, "Please tell me what year it is right now," states that it is 1911.

    Coding: C0300A would be **coded 0, missed by more than 5 years.**
    Rationale: Even though the '11 part of the year would be correct, 1911 is more than 5 years from 2011.

C0300: Temporal Orientation (Orientation to Year, Month, and Day) (cont.)

4. The date of interview is April 1, 2011. The resident, responding to the statement, "Please tell me what year it is right now," states that it is "'11". The interviewer asks, "Can you tell me the full year?" The resident still responds "'11," and the interviewer asks again, "Can you tell me the full year, for example, nineteen-eighty-two." The resident states, "2011."

    Coding: C0300A would be **coded 3, correct.**

    Rationale: Even though '11 is partially correct, the only correct answer is the exact year. The resident must state "2011," not "'11" or "1811" or "1911."

Coding Instructions for C0300B, Able to Report Correct Month

Count the current day as day 1 when determining whether the response was accurate within 5 days or missed by 6 days to 1 month.

- **Code 0, missed by >1 month or no answer:** if the resident's answer is incorrect by more than 1 month or if the resident chooses not to answer the item.

- **Code 1, missed by 6 days to 1 month:** if the resident's answer is accurate within 6 days to 1 month.

- **Code 2, accurate within 5 days:** if the resident's answer is accurate within 5 days, count current date as day 1.

Coding Tips

- In most instances, it will be immediately obvious which code to select. In some cases, you may need to write the resident's response in the margin and go back later to count days if you are unsure whether the date given is within 5 days.

Examples

1. The date of interview is June 25, 2011. The resident, responding to the question, "What month are we in right now?" states that it is June.

    Coding: C0300B would be **coded 2, accurate within 5 days.**

    Rationale: The resident correctly stated the month.

2. The date of interview is June 28, 2011. The resident, responding to the question, "What month are we in right now?" states that it is July.

    Coding: C0300B would be **coded 2, accurate within 5 days.**

    Rationale: The resident correctly stated the month within 5 days, even though the correct month is June. June 28th (day 1) + 4 more days is July 2nd, so July is within 5 days of the interview.

C0300: Temporal Orientation (Orientation to Year, Month, and Day) (cont.)

3. The date of interview is June 25, 2011. The resident, responding to the question, "What month are we in right now?" states that it is July.

> **Coding:** C0300B would be **coded 1, missed by 6 days to 1 month**.
>
> **Rationale:** The resident missed the correct month by six days. June 25th (day 1) + 5 more days = June 30th. Therefore, the resident's answer is incorrect within 6 days to 1 month.

4. The date of interview is June 30, 2011. The resident, responding to the question, "What month are we in right now?" states that it is August.

> **Coding:** C0300B would be **coded 0, missed by more than 1 month**.
>
> **Rationale:** The resident missed the month by more than 1 month.

5. The date of interview is June 2, 2011. The resident, responding to the question, "What month are we in right now?" states that it is May.

> **Coding:** C0300B would be **coded 2, accurate within 5 days.**
>
> **Rationale:** June 2 minus 5 days = May 29th. The resident correctly stated the month within 5 days even though the current month is June.

Coding Instructions for C0300C. Able to Report Correct Day of the Week

- **Code 0, incorrect, or no answer:** if the answer is incorrect or the resident chooses not to answer the item.
- **Code 1, correct:** if the answer is correct.

Examples

1. The day of interview is Monday, June 25, 2011. The interviewer asks: "What day of the week is it today?" The resident responds, "It's Monday."

> **Coding:** C0300C would be **coded 1, correct**.
>
> **Rationale:** The resident correctly stated the day of the week.

2. The day of interview is Monday, June 25, 2011. The resident, responding to the question, "What day of the week is it today?" states, "Tuesday."

> **Coding:** C0300C would be **coded 0, incorrect**.
>
> **Rationale:** The resident incorrectly stated the day of the week.

3. The day of interview is Monday, June 25, 2011. The resident, responding to the question, "What day of the week is it today?" states, "Today is a good day."

> **Coding:** C0300C would be **coded 0, incorrect**.
>
> **Rationale:** The resident did not answer the question correctly.

C0400: Recall

C0400. Recall	
	Ask resident: *"Let's go back to an earlier question. What were those three words that I asked you to repeat?"* If unable to remember a word, give cue (something to wear; a color; a piece of furniture) for that word.

Enter Code ☐	**A. Able to recall "sock"**
	   0. **No** - could not recall
	   1. **Yes, after cueing** ("something to wear")
	   2. **Yes, no cue required**

Enter Code ☐	**B. Able to recall "blue"**
	   0. **No** - could not recall
	   1. **Yes, after cueing** ("a color")
	   2. **Yes, no cue required**

Enter Code ☐	**C. Able to recall "bed"**
	   0. **No** - could not recall
	   1. **Yes, after cueing** ("a piece of furniture")
	   2. **Yes, no cue required**

Item Rationale

Health-related Quality of Life

- Many persons with cognitive impairment can be helped to recall if provided cues.
- Providing memory cues can help maximize individual function and decrease frustration for those residents who respond.

Planning for Care

- Care plans should maximize use of cueing for resident who respond to recall cues. This will enhance independence.

Steps for Assessment

Basic BIMS interview instructions are shown on page C-5.

1. Ask the resident the following: "Let's go back to an earlier question. What were those three words that I asked you to repeat?"
2. Allow up to 5 seconds for spontaneous recall of each word.
3. For any word that is not correctly recalled after 5 seconds, provide a category cue (refer to "Steps for Assessment," pages C-7–C-8 for the definition of category cue). Category cues should be used only after the resident is unable to recall one or more of the three words.
4. Allow up to 5 seconds after category cueing for each missed word to be recalled.

Coding Instructions

*For **each** of the three words the resident is asked to remember:*

- **Code 0, no—could not recall:** if the resident cannot recall the word even after being given the category cue or if the resident responds with a nonsensical answer or chooses not to answer the item.
- **Code 1, yes, after cueing:** if the resident requires the category cue to remember the word.
- **Code 2, yes, no cue required:** if the resident correctly remembers the word spontaneously without cueing.

C0400: Recall (cont.)

Coding Tips

- If on the first try (without cueing), the resident names multiple items in a category, one of which is correct, they should be coded as correct for that item.
- If, however, the interviewer gives the resident the cue and the resident then names multiple items in that category, the item is coded as could not recall, even if the correct item was in the list.

Examples

1. The resident is asked to recall the three words that were initially presented. The resident chooses not to answer the question and states, "I'm tired, and I don't want to do this anymore."

   Coding: C0400A-C0400C would be **coded 0, no—could not recall**, could not recall for each of the three words.

   Rationale: Choosing not to answer a question often indicates an inability to answer the question, so refusals are **coded 0, no—could not recall**. This is the most accurate way to score cognitive function, even though, on occasion, residents might choose not to answer for other reasons.

2. The resident is asked to recall the three words. The resident replies, "Socks, shoes, and bed." The examiner then cues, "One word was a color." The resident says, "Oh, the shoes were blue."

   Coding: C0400A, sock, would be **coded 2, yes, no cue required.**

   Rationale: The resident's initial response to the question included "sock." He is given credit for this response, even though he also listed another item in that category (shoes), because he was answering the initial question, without cueing.

   Coding: C0400B, blue, would be **coded 1, yes, after cueing.**

   Rationale: The resident did not recall spontaneously, but did recall after the category cue was given. Responses that include the word in a sentence are acceptable.

   Coding: C0400C, bed, would be **coded 2, yes, no cue required.**

   Rationale: The resident independently recalled the item on the first attempt.

3. The resident is asked to recall the three words. The resident answers, "I don't remember." The assessor then says, "One word was something to wear." The resident says, "Clothes." The assessor then says, "OK, one word was a color." The resident says, "Blue." The assessor then says, "OK, the last word was a piece of furniture." The resident says, "Couch."

   Coding: C0400A, sock, would be **coded 0, no—could not recall.**

   Rationale: The resident did not recall the item, even with a cue.

   Coding: C0400B, blue, would be **coded 1, yes, after cueing.**

   Rationale: The resident did recall after being given the cue.

   Coding: C0400C, bed, would be **coded 0, no—could not recall.**

   Rationale: The resident did not recall the item, even with a cue.

C0400: Recall (cont.)

4. The resident is asked to recall the three words. The resident says, "I don't remember." The assessor then says, "One word was something to wear." The resident says, "Hat, shirt, pants, socks, shoe, belt."

> **Coding:** C0400A, sock, would be **coded 0, no—could not recall.**
>
> **Rationale:** After getting the category cue, the resident named more than one item (i.e., a laundry list of items) in the category. The resident's response is coded as incorrect, even though one of the items was correct, because the resident did not demonstrate recall and likely named the item by chance.

C0500: Summary Score

C0500. Summary Score	
Enter Score	Add **scores** for questions C0200-C0400 and fill in total score (00-15) Enter 99 if unable to complete one or more questions of the interview

Item Rationale

Health-related Quality of Life

- The total score:
  - — Allows comparison with future and past performance.
  - — Decreases the chance of incorrect labeling of cognitive ability and improves detection of delirium.
  - — Provides staff with a more reliable estimate of resident function and allows staff interactions with residents that are based on more accurate impressions about resident ability.

Planning for Care

- The BIMS is a brief screener that aids in detecting cognitive impairment. It does not assess all possible aspects of cognitive impairment. A diagnosis of dementia should only be made after a careful assessment for other reasons for impaired cognitive performance. The final determination of the level of impairment should be made by the resident's physician or mental health care specialist; however, these practitioners can be provided specific BIMS results and the following guidance:

  The BIMS total score is highly correlated with Mini-Mental State Exam (MMSE; Folstein, Folstein, & McHugh, 1975) scores. Scores from a carefully conducted BIMS assessment where residents can hear all questions and the resident is not delirious suggest the following distributions:

  13-15: cognitively intact

  8-12: moderately impaired

  0-7: severe impairment

C0500: Summary Score (cont.)

- Abrupt changes in cognitive status (as indicative of a delirium) often signal an underlying potentially life threatening illness and a change in cognition may be the only indication of an underlying problem.

- Care plans can be more individualized based upon reliable knowledge of resident function.

Steps for Assessment

After completing C0200-C0400:

1. Add up the values for all questions from C0200 through C0400.
2. Do not add up the score while you are interviewing the resident. Instead, focus your full attention on the interview.

Coding Instructions

Enter the total score as a two-digit number. The total possible BIMS score ranges from 00 to 15.

- If the resident chooses not to answer a specific question(s), that question is coded as incorrect and the item(s) counts in the total score. If, however, the resident chooses not to answer four or more items, then the interview is coded as incomplete and a staff assessment is completed.

- To be considered a completed interview, the resident had to attempt and provide relevant answers to at least four of the questions included in C0200-C0400. To be relevant, a response only has to be related to the question (logical); it does not have to be correct. See general coding tips on page C-6 for residents who choose not to participate at all.

- **Code 99, unable to complete interview:** if (a) the resident chooses not to participate in the BIMS, (b) if four or more items were coded 0 because the resident chose not to answer or gave a nonsensical response, *or* (c) if any of the BIMS items is coded with a dash.

    — Note: a zero score does not mean the BIMS was incomplete. To be incomplete, a resident had to choose not to answer or give completely unrelated, nonsensical responses to four or more items.

Coding Tips

- Occasionally, a resident can communicate but chooses not to participate in the BIMS and therefore does not attempt any of the items in the section. This would be considered an incomplete interview; enter 99 for C0500, **Summary Score**, and complete the staff assessment of mental status.

C0500: Summary Score (cont.)

Example

1. The resident's scores on items C0200-C0400 were as follows:

C0200 (repetition)	3
C0300A (year)	2
C0300B (month)	2
C0300C (day)	1
C0400A (recall "sock")	2
C0400B (recall "blue")	2
C0400C (recall "bed")	0

   Coding: C0500 would be **coded 12**.

C0600: Should the Staff Assessment for Mental Status (C0700-C1000) Be Conducted?

C0600. Should the Staff Assessment for Mental Status (C0700 - C1000) be Conducted?
Enter Code	0. **No** (resident was able to complete interview) → Skip to C1300, Signs and Symptoms of Delirium 1. **Yes** (resident was unable to complete interview) → Continue to C0700, Short-term Memory OK

Item Rationale

Health-related Quality of Life

- Direct or performance-based testing of cognitive function using the BIMS is preferred as it decreases the chance of incorrect labeling of cognitive ability and improves detection of delirium. However, a minority of residents are unable or unwilling to participate in the BIMS.
- Mental status can vary among persons unable to communicate or who do not complete the interview.
  - Therefore, report of observed behavior is needed for persons unable to complete the BIMS interview.
  - When cognitive impairment is incorrectly diagnosed or missed, appropriate communication, activities, and therapies may not be offered.

Planning for Care

- Abrupt changes in cognitive status (as indicative of delirium) often signal an underlying potentially life-threatening illness and a change in cognition may be the only indication of an underlying problem.
  - This remains true for persons who are unable to communicate or to complete the BIMS.
- Specific aspects of cognitive impairment, when identified, can direct nursing interventions to facilitate greater independence and function.

C0600: Should the Staff Assessment for Mental Status (C0700-C1000) Be Conducted? (cont.)

Steps for Assessment

1. Review whether **Summary Score** item (C0500), is **coded 99**, unable to complete interview.

Coding Instructions

- **Code 0, no:** if the BIMS was completed and scored between 00 and 15. Skip to C1300.

- **Code 1, yes:** if the resident chooses not to participate in the BIMS or if four or more items were **coded 0** because the resident chose not to answer or gave a nonsensical response. Continue to C0700-C1000 and perform the Staff Assessment for Mental Status. Note: C0500 should be **coded 99**.

Coding Tips

- If a resident is scored 00 on C0500, C0700-C1000, Staff Assessment, should not be completed. **00** is a legitimate value for C0500 and indicates that the interview was complete. To have an incomplete interview, a resident had to choose not to answer or had to give completely unrelated, nonsensical responses to four or more BIMS items.

C0700-C1000: Staff Assessment of Mental Status Item

Staff Assessment for Mental Status
Do not conduct if Brief Interview for Mental Status (C0200-C0500) was completed
C0700. Short-term Memory OK

Enter Code ☐ — Seems or appears to recall after 5 minutes
   0. Memory OK
   1. Memory problem

C0800. Long-term Memory OK

Enter Code ☐ — Seems or appears to recall long past
   0. Memory OK
   1. Memory problem

C0900. Memory/Recall Ability
↓ Check all that the resident was normally able to recall
☐ A. Current season
☐ B. Location of own room
☐ C. Staff names and faces
☐ D. That he or she is in a nursing home
☐ Z. None of the above were recalled
C1000. Cognitive Skills for Daily Decision Making

Enter Code ☐ — Made decisions regarding tasks of daily life
   0. Independent - decisions consistent/reasonable
   1. Modified independence - some difficulty in new situations only
   2. Moderately impaired - decisions poor; cues/supervision required
   3. Severely impaired - never/rarely made decisions

C0700-C1000: Staff Assessment of Mental Status Item (cont.)

Item Rationale

Health-related Quality of Life

- Cognitive impairment is prevalent among some groups of residents, but not all residents are cognitively impaired.
- Many persons with memory problems can function successfully in a structured, routine environment.
- Residents may appear to be cognitively impaired because of communication challenges or lack of interaction but may be cognitively intact.
- When cognitive impairment is incorrectly diagnosed or missed, appropriate communication, worthwhile activities, and therapies may not be offered.

Planning for Care

- Abrupt changes in cognitive status (as indicative of a delirium) often signal an underlying potentially life-threatening illness and a change in cognition may be the only indication of an underlying problem.
- The level and specific areas of impairment affect daily function and care needs. By identifying specific aspects of cognitive impairment, nursing interventions can be directed toward facilitating greater function.
- Probing beyond first, perhaps mistaken, impressions is critical to accurate assessment and appropriate care planning.

C0700: Short-term Memory OK

C0700. Short-term Memory OK	
Enter Code ☐	Seems or appears to recall after 5 minutes 0. Memory OK 1. Memory problem

Item Rationale

Health-related Quality of Life

- To assess the mental state of residents who cannot be interviewed, an intact 5-minute recall ("short-term memory OK") indicates greater likelihood of normal cognition.
- An observed "memory problem" should be taken into consideration in Planning for Care.

Planning for Care

- Identified memory problems typically indicate the need for:

C0700: Short-term Memory OK (cont.)

— Assessment and treatment of an underlying related medical problem (particularly if this is a new observation) or adverse medication effect, or

— possible evaluation for other problems with thinking

— additional nursing support

— at times frequent prompting during daily activities

— additional support during recreational activities.

Steps for Assessment

1. Determine the resident's short-term memory status by asking him or her:

   • to describe an event 5 minutes after it occurred if you can validate the resident's response, or

   • to follow through on a direction given 5 minutes earlier.

2. Observe how often the resident has to be re-oriented to an activity or instructions.
3. Staff members also should observe the resident's cognitive function in varied daily activities.
4. Observations should be made by staff across all shifts and departments and others with close contact with the resident.
5. Ask direct care staff across all shifts and family or significant others about the resident's short-term memory status.
6. Review the medical record for clues to the resident's short-term memory during the look-back period.

Coding Instructions

Based on all information collected regarding the resident's short-term memory during the 7-day look-back period, identify and code according to the most representative level of function.

   • **Code 0, memory OK:** if the resident recalled information after 5 minutes.

   • **Code 1, memory problem:** if the most representative level of function shows the absence of recall after 5 minutes.

Coding Tips

   • If the test cannot be conducted (resident will not cooperate, is non-responsive, etc.) and staff members were unable to make a determination based on observing the resident, use the standard "no information" code (a dash, "-") to indicate that the information is not available because it could not be assessed.

C0700: Short-term Memory OK (cont.)

Example

1. A resident has just returned from the activities room where she and other residents were playing bingo. You ask her if she enjoyed herself playing bingo, but she returns a blank stare. When you ask her if she was just playing bingo, she says, "no." **Code 1, memory problem.**

> **Coding:** C0700, would be **coded 1, memory problem.**
>
> **Rationale:** The resident could not recall an event that took place within the past 5 minutes.

C0800: Long-term Memory OK

C0800. Long-term Memory OK	
Enter Code ☐	Seems or appears to recall long past 0. Memory OK 1. Memory problem

Item Rationale

Health-related Quality of Life

- An observed "long-term memory problem" may indicate the need for emotional support, reminders, and reassurance. It may also indicate delirium if this represents a change from the resident's baseline.
- An observed "long-term memory problem" should be taken into consideration in Planning for Care.

Planning for Care

- Long-term memory problems indicate the need for:
  — Exclusion of an underlying related medical problem (particularly if this is a new observation) or adverse medication effect, or
  — possible evaluation for other problems with thinking
  — additional nursing support
  — at times frequent prompting during daily activities
  — additional support during recreational activities.

Steps for Assessment

1. Determine resident's long-term memory status by engaging in conversation, reviewing memorabilia (photographs, memory books, keepsakes, videos, or other recordings that are meaningful to the resident) with the resident or observing response to family who visit.
2. Ask questions for which you can validate the answers from review of the medical record, general knowledge, the resident's family, etc.

   - Ask the resident, "Are you married?" "What is your spouse's name?" "Do you have any children?" "How many?" "When is your birthday?"

C0800: Long-term Memory OK (cont.)

3. Observe if the resident responds to memorabilia or family members who visit.
4. Observations should be made by staff across all shifts and departments and others with close contact with the resident.
5. Ask direct care staff across all shifts and family or significant others about the resident's memory status.
6. Review the medical record for clues to the resident's long-term memory during the look-back period.

Coding Instructions

- **Code 0, memory OK:** if the resident accurately recalled long past information.
- **Code 1, memory problem:** if the resident did not recall long past information or did not recall it correctly.

Coding Tips

- If the test cannot be conducted (resident will not cooperate, is non-responsive, etc.) and staff were unable to make a determination based on observation of the resident, use the standard "no information" code (a dash, "-"), to indicate that the information is not available because it could not be assessed.

C0900: Memory/Recall Ability

C0900. Memory/Recall Ability	
↓ Check all that the resident was normally able to recall	
☐	A. Current season
☐	B. Location of own room
☐	C. Staff names and faces
☐	D. That he or she is in a nursing home
☐	Z. None of the above were recalled

Item Rationale

Health-related Quality of Life

- An observed "memory/recall problem" with these items may indicate:
  — cognitive impairment and the need for additional support with reminders to support increased independence; or
  — delirium, if this represents a change from the resident's baseline.

Planning for Care

- An observed "memory/recall problem" with these items may indicate the need for:
  — Exclusion of an underlying related medical problem (particularly if this is a new observation) or adverse medication effect; or
  — possible evaluation for other problems with thinking;
  — additional signs, directions, pictures, verbal reminders to support the resident's independence;

C0900: Memory/Recall Ability (cont.)

— an evaluation for acute delirium if this represents a change over the past few days to weeks;

— an evaluation for chronic delirium if this represents a change over the past several weeks to months; or

— additional nursing support;

— the need for emotional support, reminders and reassurance to reduce anxiety and agitation.

Steps for Assessment

1. Ask the resident about each item. For example, "What is the current season? Is it fall, winter, spring, or summer?" "What is the name of this place?" If the resident is not in his or her room, ask, "Will you show me to your room?" Observe the resident's ability to find the way.

2. For residents with limited communication skills, in order to determine the most representative level of function, ask direct care staff across all shifts and family or significant other about recall ability.

   • Ask whether the resident gave indications of recalling these subjects or recognizing them during the look-back period.

3. Observations should be made by staff across all shifts and departments and others with close contact with the resident.

4. Review the medical record for indications of the resident's recall of these subjects during the look-back period.

Coding Instructions

For each item that the resident recalls, check the corresponding answer box. If the resident recalls none, check none of above.

• **Check C0900A, current season:** if resident is able to identify the current season (e.g., correctly refers to weather for the time of year, legal holidays, religious celebrations, etc.).

• **Check C0900B, location of own room:** if resident is able to locate and recognize own room. It is not necessary for the resident to know the room number, but he or she should be able to find the way to the room.

• **Check C0900C, staff names and faces:** if resident is able to distinguish staff members from family members, strangers, visitors, and other residents. It is not necessary for the resident to know the staff member's name, but he or she should recognize that the person is a staff member and not the resident's son or daughter, etc.

• **Check C0900D, that he or she is in a nursing home:** if resident is able to determine that he or she is currently living in a nursing home. To check this item, it is not necessary that the resident be able to state the name of the nursing home, but he or she should be able to refer to the nursing home by a term such as a "home for older people," a "hospital for the elderly," "a place where people who need extra help live," etc.

• **Check C0900Z, none of above was recalled.**

C1000: Cognitive Skills for Daily Decision Making

C1000. Cognitive Skills for Daily Decision Making	
Enter Code ☐	**Made decisions regarding tasks of daily life** 0. **Independent** - decisions consistent/reasonable 1. **Modified independence** - some difficulty in new situations only 2. **Moderately impaired** - decisions poor; cues/supervision required 3. **Severely impaired** - never/rarely made decisions

Item Rationale

Health-related Quality of Life

- An observed "difficulty with daily decision making" may indicate:
  — underlying cognitive impairment and the need for additional coaching and support or
  — possible anxiety or depression.

Planning for Care

- An observed "difficulty with daily decision making" may indicate the need for:
  — a more structured plan for daily activities and support in decisions about daily activities,
  — encouragement to participate in structured activities, or
  — an assessment for underlying delirium and medical evaluation.

Steps for Assessment

1. Review the medical record. Consult family and direct care staff across all shifts. Observe the resident.
2. Observations should be made by staff across all shifts and departments and others with close contact with the resident.
3. The intent of this item is to record what the resident is doing (performance). Focus on whether or not the resident is actively making these decisions and not whether staff believes the resident might be capable of doing so.
4. Focus on the resident's actual performance. Where a staff member takes decision-making responsibility away from the resident regarding tasks of everyday living, or the resident does not participate in decision making, whatever his or her level of capability may be, the resident should be coded as impaired performance in decision making.

> **DEFINITIONS**
>
> **DAILY DECISION MAKING**
> Includes: choosing clothing; knowing when to go to meals; using environmental cues to organize and plan (e.g., clocks, calendars, posted event notices); in the absence of environmental cues, seeking information appropriately (i.e. not repetitively) from others in order to plan the day; using awareness of one's own strengths and limitations to regulate the day's events (e.g., asks for help when necessary); acknowledging need to use appropriate assistive equipment such as a walker.

C1000: Cognitive Skills for Daily Decision Making (cont.)

Coding Instructions

Record the resident's actual performance in making everyday decisions about tasks or activities of daily living. Enter one number that corresponds to the most correct response.

- **Code 0, independent:** if the resident's decisions in organizing daily routine and making decisions were consistent, reasonable and organized reflecting lifestyle, culture, values.
- **Code 1, modified independence:** if the resident organized daily routine and made safe decisions in familiar situations, but experienced some difficulty in decision making when faced with new tasks or situations.
- **Code 2, moderately impaired:** if the resident's decisions were poor; the resident required reminders, cues, and supervision in planning, organizing, and correcting daily routines.
- **Code 3, severely impaired:** if the resident's decision making was severely impaired; the resident never (or rarely) made decisions.

Coding Tips

- If the resident "rarely or never" made decisions, despite being provided with opportunities and appropriate cues, Item C1000 would be **coded 3, severely impaired**. If the resident makes decisions, although poorly, **code 2, moderately impaired**.
- A resident's considered decision to exercise his or her right to decline treatment or recommendations by interdisciplinary team members should **not** be captured as impaired decision making in Item C1000, **Cognitive Skills for Daily Decision Making**.

Examples

1. Mr. B. seems to have severe cognitive impairment and is non-verbal. He usually clamps his mouth shut when offered a bite of food.
2. Mrs. C. does not generally make conversation or make her needs known, but replies "yes" when asked if she would like to take a nap.

> **Coding:** For the examples listed in 1A and 1B, Item C1000 would be **coded 3, severe impairment.**
>
> **Rationale:** In both examples, the residents are primarily non-verbal and do not make their needs known, but they do give basic verbal or non-verbal responses to simple gestures or questions regarding care routines. More information about how the residents function in the environment is needed to definitively answer the questions. From the limited information provided it appears that their communication of choices is limited to very particular circumstances, which would be regarded as "rarely/never" in the relative number of decisions a person could make during the course of a week on the MDS. If such decisions are more frequent or involved more activities, the resident may be only moderately impaired or better.

C1000: Cognitive Skills for Daily Decision Making (cont.)

3. A resident makes her own decisions throughout the day and is consistent and reasonable in her decision-making except that she constantly walks away from the walker she has been using for nearly 2 years. Asked why she doesn't use her walker, she replies, "I don't like it. It gets in my way, and I don't want to use it even though I know all of you think I should."

   Coding: C1000 would be **coded 0, independent.**

   Rationale: This resident is making and expressing understanding of her own decisions, and her decision is to decline the recommended course of action – using the walker. Other decisions she made throughout the look-back period were consistent and reasonable.

4. A resident routinely participates in coffee hour on Wednesday mornings, and often does not need a reminder. Due to renovations, however, the meeting place was moved to another location in the facility. The resident was informed of this change and was accompanied to the new location by the activities director. Staff noticed that the resident was uncharacteristically agitated and unwilling to engage with other residents or the staff. She eventually left and was found sitting in the original coffee hour room. Asked why she came back to this location, she responded, "the aide brought me to the wrong room, I'll wait here until they serve the coffee."

   Coding: C1000 would be **coded 1, modified independent.**

   Rationale: The resident is independent under routine circumstances. However, when the situation was new or different, she had difficulty adjusting.

5. Mr. G. enjoys congregate meals in the dining and is friendly with the other residents at his table. Recently, he has started to lose weight. He appears to have little appetite, rarely eats without reminders and willingly gives his food to other residents at the table. Mr. G. requires frequent cueing from staff to eat and supervision to prevent him from sharing his food.

   Coding: C1000 would be **coded 2, moderately impaired.**

   Rationale: The resident is making poor decisions by giving his food away. He requires cueing to eat and supervision to be sure that he is eating the food on his plate.

C1300: Signs and Symptoms of Delirium

Delirium		
C1300. Signs and Symptoms of Delirium (from CAM©)		
Code **after completing** Brief Interview for Mental Status or Staff Assessment, and reviewing medical record		
Coding: 0. **Behavior not present** 1. **Behavior continuously present, does not fluctuate** 2. **Behavior present, fluctuates** (comes and goes, changes in severity)	↓ Enter Codes in Boxes	
	☐	**A. Inattention** - Did the resident have difficulty focusing attention (easily distracted, out of touch or difficulty following what was said)?
	☐	**B. Disorganized thinking** - Was the resident's thinking disorganized or incoherent (rambling or irrelevant conversation, unclear or illogical flow of ideas, or unpredictable switching from subject to subject)?
	☐	**C. Altered level of consciousness** - Did the resident have altered level of consciousness (e.g., **vigilant** - startled easily to any sound or touch; **lethargic** - repeatedly dozed off when being asked questions, but responded to voice or touch; **stuporous** - very difficult to arouse and keep aroused for the interview; **comatose** - could not be aroused)?
	☐	**D. Psychomotor retardation** - Did the resident have an unusually decreased level of activity such as sluggishness, staring into space, staying in one position, moving very slowly?

*Item C1300 is adapted from the Confusion Assessment Method (CAM; Inouye et al., 1990) that has copyright protection and cannot be modified.

Item Rationale

Health-related Quality of Life

- Delirium is associated with:
  - increased mortality,
  - functional decline,
  - development or worsening of incontinence,
  - behavior problems,
  - withdrawal from activities
  - rehospitalizations and increased length of nursing home stay.
- Delirium can be misdiagnosed as dementia.
- A recent deterioration in cognitive function may indicate delirium, which may be reversible if detected and treated in a timely fashion.

Planning for Care

- Delirium may be a symptom of an acute, treatable illness such as infection or reaction to medications.
- Prompt detection is essential in order to identify and treat or eliminate the cause.

C1300: Signs and Symptoms of Delirium (cont.)

Steps for Assessment

1. Observe resident behavior during the **BIMS** items (C0200-C0400) for the signs and symptoms of delirium. Some experts suggest that increasing the frequency of assessment (as often as daily for new admissions) will improve the level of detection.
2. If the **Staff Assessment for Mental Status** items (C0700-C1000) was completed instead of the BIMS, ask staff members who conducted the interview about their observations of signs and symptoms of delirium.
3. Review medical record documentation during the 7-day look-back period to determine the resident's baseline status, fluctuations in behavior, and behaviors that might have occurred during the 7-day look-back period that were not observed during the BIMS.
4. Interview staff, family members and others in a position to observe the resident's behavior during the 7-day look-back period.

For additional guidance on the signs and symptoms of delirium can be found in Appendix C.

> **DEFINITIONS**
>
> **DELIRIUM**
> A mental disturbance characterized by new or acutely worsening confusion, disordered expression of thoughts, change in level of consciousness or hallucinations.

Steps for Assessment for C1300A, Inattention

Basic delirium assessment instructions are on page C-33. In addition, for C1300 (Inattention):

1. Assess attention separately from level of consciousness. Evidence of inattention may be found during the resident interview, in the medical record, or from family or staff reports of inattention during the 7-day look-back period.
2. An additional step to identify difficulty with attention is to ask the resident to count backwards from 20.

Coding Instructions for C1300A, Inattention

- **Code 0, behavior not present:** if the resident remains focused during the interview and all other sources agree that the resident was attentive during other activities.

- **Code 1, behavior continuously present, did not fluctuate:** if the resident had difficulty focusing attention, was easily distracted, or had difficulty keeping track of what was said AND the inattention did not vary during the look-back period. All sources must agree that inattention was consistently present to select this code.

> **DEFINITIONS**
>
> **INATTENTION**
> Reduced ability to maintain attention to external stimuli and to appropriately shift attention to new external stimuli. Resident seems unaware or out of touch with environment (e.g., dazed, fixated or darting attention).
>
> **FLUCTUATION** The behavior tends to come and go and/or increase or decrease in severity. The behavior may fluctuate over the course of the interview or during the 7-day look-back period. Fluctuating behavior may be noted by the interviewer, reported by staff or family or documented in the medical record.

C1300: Signs and Symptoms of Delirium (cont.)

- **Code 2, behavior present, fluctuates:** if inattention is noted during the interview or any source reports that the resident had difficulty focusing attention, was easily distracted, or had difficulty keeping track of what was said AND the inattention varied during interview or during the look-back period or if information sources disagree in assessing level of attention.

Examples

1. The resident tries to answer all questions during the BIMS. Although she answers several items incorrectly and responds "I don't know" to others, she pays attention to the interviewer. Medical record and staff indicate that this is her consistent behavior.

   Coding: Item C1300A would be **coded 0, behavior not present.**

   Rationale: The resident remained focused throughout the interview and this was constant during the look-back period.

2. Questions during the BIMS must be frequently repeated because resident's attention wanders. This behavior occurs throughout the interview and medical records and staff agree that this behavior is consistently present. The resident has a diagnosis of dementia.

   Coding: Item C1300A would be **coded 1, behavior continuously present, does not fluctuate.**

   Rationale: The resident's attention consistently wandered throughout the 7-day look-back period. The resident's dementia diagnosis does not affect the coding.

3. During the BIMS interview, the resident was not able to focus on all questions asked and his gaze wandered. However, several notes in the resident's medical record indicate that the resident was attentive when staff communicated with him.

   Coding: Item C1300A would be **coded 2, behavior present, fluctuates.**

   Rationale: Evidence of inattention was found during the BIMS but was noted to be absent in the medical record. This disagreement shows possible fluctuation in the behavior. If any information source reports the symptom as present, C1300A **cannot be coded as 0, Behavior not present.**

4. Resident is dazedly staring at the television for the first several questions. When you ask a question, she looks at you momentarily but does not answer. Midway through questioning, she seems to pay more attention and tries to answer.

   Coding: Item C1300A would be **coded 2, behavior present, fluctuates.**

   Rationale: Resident's attention fluctuated during the interview. If as few as one source notes fluctuation, then the behavior should be **coded 2.**

C1300: Signs and Symptoms of Delirium (cont.)

Coding Instructions for C1300B, Disorganized Thinking

- **Code 0, behavior not present:** if all sources agree that the resident's thinking was organized and coherent, even if answers were inaccurate or wrong.

- **Code 1, behavior continuously present, did not fluctuate:** if, during the interview and according to other sources, the resident's responses were consistently disorganized or incoherent, conversation was rambling or irrelevant, ideas were unclear or flowed illogically, or the resident unpredictably switched from subject to subject.

- **Code 2, behavior present, fluctuates:** if, during the interview or according to other data sources, the resident's responses fluctuated between disorganized/incoherent and organized/clear. Also code as fluctuating if information sources disagree.

> **DEFINITIONS**
>
> **DISORGANIZED THINKING** Evidenced by rambling, irrelevant, or incoherent speech.

Examples

1. The interviewer asks the resident, who is often confused, to give the date, and the response is: "Let's go get the sailor suits!" The resident continues to provide irrelevant or nonsensical responses throughout the interview, and medical record and staff indicate this is constant.

   Coding: C1300B would be **coded 1, behavior continuously present, does not fluctuate.**

   Rationale: All sources agree that the disorganized thinking is constant.

2. The resident responds that the year is 1837 when asked to give the date. The medical record and staff indicate that the resident is never oriented to time but has coherent conversations. For example, staff reports he often discusses his passion for baseball.

   Coding: C1300B would be **coded 0, behavior not present.**

   Rationale: The resident's answer was related to the question, even though it was incorrect. No other sources report disorganized thinking.

3. The resident was able to tell the interviewer her name, the year and where she was. She was able to talk about the activity she just attended and the residents and staff that also attended. Then the resident suddenly asked the interviewer, "Who are you? What are you doing in my daughter's home?"

   Coding: C1300B would be **coded 2, behavior present, fluctuates.**

   Rationale: The resident's thinking fluctuated between coherent and incoherent at least once. If as few as one source notes fluctuation, then the behavior should be **coded 2.**

C1300: Signs and Symptoms of Delirium (cont.)

Coding Instructions for C1300C, Altered Level of Consciousness

- **Code 0, behavior not present:** if all sources agree that the resident was alert and maintained wakefulness during conversation, interview(s), and activities.

- **Code 1, behavior continuously present, did not fluctuate:** if, during the interview and according to other sources, the resident was consistently lethargic (difficult to keep awake), stuporous (very difficult to arouse and keep aroused), vigilant (startles easily to any sound or touch), or comatose.

- **Code 2, behavior present, fluctuates:** if, during the interview or according to other sources, the resident varied in levels of consciousness. For example, was at times alert and responsive, while at other times resident was lethargic, stuporous, or vigilant. Also code as fluctuating if information sources disagree.

> **DEFINITIONS**
>
> **ALTERED LEVEL OF CONSCIOUSNESS**
>
> **VIGILANT** – startles easily to any sound or touch;
>
> **LETHARGIC** – repeatedly dozes off when you are asking questinos, but responds to voice or touch;
>
> **STUPOR** – very difficult to arouse and keep aroused for the interview;
>
> **COMATOSE** – cannot be aroused despite shaking and shouting.

Coding Tips

- A diagnosis of coma or stupor does not have to be present for staff to note the behavior in this section.

Examples

1. Resident is alert and conversational and answers all questions during the BIMS interview, although not all answers are correct. Medical record documentation and staff report during the 7-day look-back period consistently noted that the resident was alert.

   Coding: C1300C would be **coded 0, behavior not present.**

   Rationale: All evidence indicates that the resident is alert during conversation, interview(s) and activities.

2. The resident is lying in bed. He arouses to soft touch but is only able to converse for a short time before his eyes close, and he appears to be sleeping. Again, he arouses to voice or touch but only for short periods during the interview. Information from other sources indicates that this was his condition throughout the look-back period.

   Coding: C1300C would be **coded 1, behavior continuously present, does not fluctuate.**

   Rationale: The resident's lethargy was consistent throughout the interview, and there is consistent documentation of lethargy in the medical record during the look-back period.

C1300: Signs and Symptoms of Delirium (cont.)

3. Resident is usually alert, oriented to time, place, and person. Today, at the time of the BIMS interview, resident is conversant at the beginning of the interview but becomes lethargic and difficult to arouse.

> **Coding:** C1300C would be **coded 2, behavior present, fluctuates.**
>
> **Rationale:** The level of consciousness fluctuated during the interview. If as few as one source notes fluctuation, then the behavior should be **coded 2, fluctuating**.

Coding Instructions for C1300D, Psychomotor Retardation

- **Code 0, behavior not present:** if the resident's movements and responses were noted to be appropriate during BIMS and across all information sources.

- **Code 1, behavior continuously present, did not fluctuate:** if, during the interview and according to other sources, the resident consistently had an unusually decreased level of activity such as being sluggish, staring into space, staying in one position, or moving or speaking very slowly.

- **Code 2, behavior present, fluctuates:** if, during the BIMS interview or according to other sources, the resident showed slowness or decreased movement and activity which varied during the interview(s) or during the look-back period.

> **DEFINITIONS**
>
> **PSYCHOMOTOR RETARDATION**
>
> Greatly reduced or slowed level of activity or mental processing. Psychomotor retardation differs from altered level of consciousness. Resident need not be lethargic (altered level of consciousness) to have slowness of response. Psychomotor retardation may be present with normal level of consciousness; also residents with lethargy or stupor do not necessarily have psychomotor retardation.

Examples

1. Resident answers questions promptly during interview and staff and medical record note similar behavior.

> **Coding:** Item C1300D would be **coded 0, behavior not present.**
>
> **Rationale:** There is no evidence of psychomotor retardation from any source.

2. The resident is alert, but has a prolonged delay before answering the interviewer's question. Staff reports that the resident has always been very slow in answering questions.

> **Coding:** C1300D would be **coded 1, behavior continuously present, does not fluctuate.**
>
> **Rationale:** The psychomotor retardation was continuously present according to sources that described the resident's response speed to questions.

3. Resident moves body very slowly (i.e., to pick up a glass). Staff reports that they have not noticed any slowness.

> **Coding:** C1300D would be **coded 2, behavior present, fluctuates.**
>
> **Rationale:** There is evidence that psychomotor retardation comes and goes.

C1600: Acute Onset of Mental Status Change

C1600. Acute Onset Mental Status Change	
Enter Code [ ]	**Is there evidence of an acute change in mental status** from the resident's baseline? 0. **No** 1. **Yes**

Item Rationale

Health-related Quality of Life

- Acute onset mental status change may indicate delirium or other serious medical complications, which may be reversible if detected and treated in a timely fashion.

Planning for Care

- Prompt detection of acute mental status change is essential in order to identify and treat or eliminate the cause.

Coding Instructions

- **Code 0, no:** if there is no evidence of acute mental status change from the resident's baseline.
- **Code 1, yes:** if resident has an alteration in mental status observed in the past 7 days or in the BIMS that represents a change from baseline.

Coding Tips

- Interview resident's family or significant others.
- Review medical record prior to 7-day look-back.

Examples

1. Resident was admitted to the nursing home 4 days ago. Her family reports that she was alert and oriented prior to admission. During the BIMS interview, she is lethargic and incoherent.

   Coding: Item C1600 would be **coded 1, yes.**

   Rationale: There is an acute change of the resident's behavior from alert and oriented (family report) to lethargic and incoherent during interview.

2. Nurse reports that a resident with poor short-term memory and disorientation to time suddenly becomes agitated, calling out to her dead husband, tearing off her clothes, and being completely disoriented to time, person, and place.

   Coding: Item C1600 would be **coded 1, yes.**

   Rationale: The new behaviors represent an acute change in mental status.

C1600: Acute Onset of Mental Status Change (cont.)

Other Examples of Acute Mental Status Changes

- A resident who is usually noisy or belligerent becomes quiet, lethargic, or inattentive.
- A resident who is normally quiet and content suddenly becomes restless or noisy.
- A resident who is usually able to find his or her way around the unit begins to get lost.

SECTION D: MOOD

Intent: The items in this section address mood distress, a serious condition that is underdiagnosed and undertreated in the nursing home and is associated with significant morbidity. It is particularly important to identify signs and symptoms of mood distress among nursing home residents because these signs and symptoms can be treatable.

It is important to note that coding the presence of indicators in Section D does not automatically mean that the resident has a diagnosis of depression or other mood disorder. Assessors do not make or assign a diagnosis in Section D, they simply record the presence or absence of specific clinical mood indicators. Facility staff should recognize these indicators and consider them when developing the resident's individualized care plan.

- Depression can be associated with:
  — psychological and physical distress (e.g., poor adjustment to the nursing home, loss of independence, chronic illness, increased sensitivity to pain),
  — decreased participation in therapy and activities (e.g., caused by isolation),
  — decreased functional status (e.g., resistance to daily care, decreased desire to participate in activities of daily living [ADLs]), and
  — poorer outcomes (e.g., decreased appetite, decreased cognitive status).
- Findings suggesting mood distress should lead to:
  — identifying causes and contributing factors for symptoms,
  — identifying interventions (treatment, personal support, or environmental modifications) that could address symptoms, and
  — ensuring resident safety.

D0100: Should Resident Mood Interview Be Conducted?

D0100. Should Resident Mood Interview be Conducted? - Attempt to conduct interview with all residents
Enter Code	0. **No** (resident is rarely/never understood) → Skip to and complete D0500-D0600, Staff Assessment of Resident Mood (PHQ-9-OV) 1. **Yes** → Continue to D0200, Resident Mood Interview (PHQ-9©)

Item Rationale

This item helps to determine whether or not a resident or staff mood interview should be conducted.

Health-related Quality of Life

- Most residents who are capable of communicating can answer questions about how they feel.
- Obtaining information about mood directly from the resident, sometimes called "hearing the resident's voice," is more reliable and accurate than observation alone for identifying a mood disorder.

D0100: Should Resident Mood Interview Be Conducted? (cont.)

Planning for Care

- Symptom-specific information from direct resident interviews will allow for the incorporation of the resident's voice in the individualized care plan.

- If a resident cannot communicate, then **Staff Mood Interview** (D0500 A-J) should be conducted.

Steps for Assessment

1. Determine if the resident is rarely/never understood. If rarely/never understood, skip to D0500, Staff Assessment of Resident Mood (PHQ-9-OV©).

2. Review **Language** item (A1100) to determine if the resident needs or wants an interpreter to communicate with doctors or health care staff (A1100 = 1).

    - If the resident needs or wants an interpreter, complete the interview with an interpreter.

Coding Instructions

- **Code 0, no:** if the interview should not be conducted. This option should be selected for residents who are rarely/never understood, or who need an interpreter (A1100 = 1) but one was not available. Skip to item D0500, Staff Assessment of Resident Mood (PHQ-9-OV©).

- **Code 1, yes:** if the resident interview should be conducted. This option should be selected for residents who are able to be understood, and for whom an interpreter is not needed or is present. Continue to item D0200, Resident Mood Interview (PHQ-9©).

Coding Tips and Special Populations

- If the resident needs an interpreter, every effort should be made to have an interpreter present for the PHQ-9© interview. If it is absolutely not possible for a needed interpreter to be present on the day of the interview, code D0100 = 0 to indicate that an interview was not attempted and complete items D0500-D0650.

D0200: Resident Mood Interview (PHQ-9©)

D0200. Resident Mood Interview (PHQ-9©)		
Say to resident: *"Over the last 2 weeks, have you been bothered by any of the following problems?"*		
If symptom is present, enter 1 (yes) in column 1, Symptom Presence. If yes in column 1, then ask the resident: *"About **how often** have you been bothered by this?"* Read and show the resident a card with the symptom frequency choices. Indicate response in column 2, Symptom Frequency.		

1. **Symptom Presence**
  0. **No** (enter 0 in column 2)
  1. **Yes** (enter 0-3 in column 2)
  9. **No response** (leave column 2 blank)
	2. **Symptom Frequency**
	  0. **Never or 1 day**
	  1. **2-6 days** (several days)
	  2. **7-11 days** (half or more of the days)
	  3. **12-14 days** (nearly every day)
		1.
		Symptom
		Presence
			2.
			Symptom
			Frequency

		↓ Enter Scores in Boxes ↓	
A. *Little interest or pleasure in doing things*		☐	☐
B. *Feeling down, depressed, or hopeless*		☐	☐
C. *Trouble falling or staying asleep, or sleeping too much*		☐	☐
D. *Feeling tired or having little energy*		☐	☐
E. *Poor appetite or overeating*		☐	☐
F. *Feeling bad about yourself - or that you are a failure or have let yourself or your family down*		☐	☐
G. *Trouble concentrating on things, such as reading the newspaper or watching television*		☐	☐
H. *Moving or speaking so slowly that other people could have noticed. Or the opposite - being so fidgety or restless that you have been moving around a lot more than usual*		☐	☐
I. *Thoughts that you would be better off dead, or of hurting yourself in some way*		☐	☐

Item Rationale

Health-related Quality of Life

- Depression can be associated with:
  — psychological and physical distress,
  — decreased participation in therapy and activities,
  — decreased functional status, and
  — poorer outcomes.
- Mood disorders are common in nursing homes and are often underdiagnosed and undertreated.

Planning for Care

- Findings suggesting mood distress could lead to:
  — identifying causes and contributing factors for symptoms and
  — identifying interventions (treatment, personal support, or environmental modifications) that could address symptoms.

> **DEFINITIONS**
>
> **9-ITEM PATIENT HEALTH QUESTIONNAIRE (PHQ-9©)**
> A validated interview that screens for symptoms of depression. It provides a standardized severity score and a rating for evidence of a depressive disorder.

D0200: Resident Mood Interview (PHQ-9©) (cont.)

Steps for Assessment

Look-back period for this item is 14 days.

1. Conduct the interview preferably the day before or day of the ARD.
2. Interview any resident when D0100 = 1.
3. Conduct the interview in a private setting.
4. If an interpreter is used during resident interviews, the interpreter should not attempt to determine the intent behind what is being translated, the outcome of the interview, or the meaning or significance of the resident's responses. Interpreters are people who translate oral or written language from one language to another.
5. Sit so that the resident can see your face. Minimize glare by directing light sources away from the resident's face.
6. Be sure the resident can hear you.
   - Residents with a hearing impairment should be tested using their usual communication devices/techniques, as applicable.
   - Try an external assistive device (headphones or hearing amplifier) if you have any doubt about hearing ability.
   - Minimize background noise.
7. If you are administering the PHQ-9© in paper form, be sure that the resident can see the print. Provide large print or assistive device (e.g., page magnifier) if necessary.
8. Explain the reason for the interview before beginning.
   Suggested language: "I am going to ask you some questions about your mood and feelings over the past 2 weeks. I will also ask about some common problems that are known to go along with feeling down. Some of the questions might seem personal, but everyone is asked to answer them. This will help us provide you with better care."
9. Explain and /or show the interview response choices. A cue card with the response choices clearly written in large print might help the resident comprehend the response choices.
   Suggested language: "I am going to ask you how often you have been bothered by a particular problem over the last 2 weeks. I will give you the choices that you see on this card." (Say while pointing to cue card): "0-1 days—never or 1 day, 2-6 days—several days, 7-11 days—half or more of the days, or 12-14 days—nearly every day."
10. Interview the resident.
    Suggested language: "Over the last 2 weeks, have you been bothered by any of the following problems?"
    Then, for each question in **Resident Mood Interview** (D0200):
    - Read the item as it is written.
    - Do not provide definitions because the meaning **must be** based on the resident's interpretation. For example, the resident defines for himself what "tired" means; the item should be scored based on the resident's interpretation.
    - Each question **must be** asked in sequence to assess presence (column 1) and frequency (column 2) before proceeding to the next question.
    - Enter code 9 for any response that is unrelated, incomprehensible, or incoherent or if the resident's response is not informative with respect to the item being rated; this is considered a **nonsensical** response (e.g., when asked the question about "poor appetite or overeating," the resident answers, "I always win at poker.").

D0200: Resident Mood Interview (PHQ-9©) (cont.)

- For a **yes** response, ask the resident to tell you how often he or she was bothered by the symptom over the last 14 days. Use the response choices in D0200 Column 2, **Symptom Frequency**. Start by asking the resident the number of days that he or she was bothered by the symptom and read and show cue card with frequency categories/descriptions (0-1 days—never or 1 day, 2-6 days—several days, 7-11 days—half or more of the days, or 12-14 days—nearly every day).

Coding Instructions for Column 1. Symptom Presence

- **Code 0, no:** if resident indicates symptoms listed are not present enter 0. Enter 0 in Column 2 as well.

- **Code 1, yes:** if resident indicates symptoms listed are present enter 1. Enter 0, 1, 2, or 3 in Column 2, Symptom Frequency.

- **Code 9, no response:** if the resident was unable or chose not to complete the assessment, responded nonsensically and/or the facility was unable to complete the assessment. Leave Column 2, Symptom Frequency, blank.

Coding Instructions for Column 2. Symptom Frequency

Record the resident's responses as they are stated, regardless of whether the resident or the assessor attributes the symptom to something other than mood. Further evaluation of the clinical relevance of reported symptoms should be explored by the responsible clinician.

- **Code 0, never or 1 day:** if the resident indicates that he or she has never or has only experienced the symptom on 1 day.

- **Code 1, 2-6 days (several days):** if the resident indicates that he or she has experienced the symptom for 2-6 days.

- **Code 2, 7-11 days (half or more of the days):** if the resident indicates that he or she has experienced the symptom for 7-11 days.

- **Code 3, 12-14 days (nearly every day):** if the resident indicates that he or she has experienced the symptom for 12-14 days.

Coding Tips and Special Populations

- For question D0200I, **Thoughts That You Would Be Better Off Dead or of Hurting Yourself in Some Way:**
  — The checkbox in item D0350 reminds the assessor to notify a responsible clinician (psychologist, physician, etc). Follow facility protocol for evaluating possible self- harm.
  — Beginning interviewers may feel uncomfortable asking this item because they may fear upsetting the resident or may feel that the question is too personal. Others may worry that it will give the resident inappropriate ideas. However,
    o Experienced interviewers have found that most residents who are having this feeling appreciate the opportunity to express it.

D0200: Resident Mood Interview (PHQ-9©) (cont.)

o Asking about thoughts of self-harm does not give the person the idea. It does let the provider better understand what the resident is already feeling.

o The best interviewing approach is to ask the question openly and without hesitation.

- If the resident uses his or her own words to describe a symptom, this should be briefly explored. If you determine that the resident is reporting the intended symptom but using his or her own words, ask him to tell you how often he or she was bothered by that symptom.

- Select only one frequency response per item.

- If the resident has difficulty selecting between two frequency responses, code for the higher frequency.

- Some items (e.g., item F) contain more than one phrase. If a resident gives different frequencies for the different parts of a single item, select the highest frequency as the score for that item.

- Residents may respond to questions:
  — verbally,
  — by pointing to their answers on the cue card, OR
  — by writing out their answers.

Interviewing Tips and Techniques

- Repeat a question if you think that it has been misunderstood or misinterpreted.

- Some residents may be eager to talk with you and will stray from the topic at hand. When a person strays, you should gently guide the conversation back to the topic.
  — **Example:** Say, "That's interesting, now I need to know…"; "Let's get back to…"; "I understand, can you tell me about…."

- Validate your understanding of what the resident is saying by asking for clarification.
  — **Example:** Say, "I think I hear you saying that…"; "Let's see if I understood you correctly."; "You said…. Is that right?"

- If the resident has difficulty selecting a frequency response, start by offering a single frequency response and follow with a sequence of more specific questions. This is known as unfolding.
  — **Example:** Say, "Would you say [name symptom] bothered you more than half the days in the past 2 weeks?"
    o If the resident says "yes," show the cue card and ask whether it bothered him or her nearly every day (12-14 days) or on half or more of the days (7-11 days).
    o If the resident says "no," show the cue card and ask whether it bothered him or her several days (2-6 days) or never or 1 day (0-1 day).

D0200: Resident Mood Interview (PHQ-9©) (cont.)

- Noncommittal responses such as "not really" should be explored. Residents may be reluctant to report symptoms and should be gently encouraged to tell you if the symptom bothered him or her, even if it was only some of the time. This is known as probing. Probe by asking neutral or nondirective questions such as:
  — "What do you mean?"
  — "Tell me what you have in mind."
  — "Tell me more about that."
  — "Please be more specific."
  — "Give me an example."

- Sometimes respondents give a long answer to interview items. To narrow the answer to the response choices available, it can be useful to summarize their longer answer and then ask them which response option best applies. This is known as echoing.
  — **Example:** Item D0200E, **Poor Appetite or Overeating**. The resident responds "the food is always cold and it just doesn't taste like it does at home. The doctor won't let me have any salt."
    o Possible interviewer response: "You're telling me the food isn't what you eat at home and you can't add salt. How often would you say that you were bothered by poor appetite or over-eating during the last 2 weeks?"
  — **Example:** Item D0200A, **Little Interest or Pleasure in Doing Things**. The resident, when asked how often he or she has been bothered by little interest or pleasure in doing things, responds, "There's nothing to do here, all you do is eat, bathe, and sleep. They don't do anything I like to do."
    o Possible interview response: "You're saying there isn't much to do here and I want to come back later to talk about some things you like to do. Thinking about how you've been feeling over the past 2 weeks, how often have you been bothered by little interest or pleasure in doing things."
  — **Example:** Item D0200B, **Feeling Down, Depressed, or Hopeless**. The resident, when asked how often he or she has been bothered by feeling down, depressed, or hopeless, responds: "How would you feel if you were here?"
    o Possible interview response: "You asked how I would feel, but it is important that I understand **your** feelings right now. How often would you say that you have been bothered by feeling down, depressed, or hopeless during the last 2 weeks?"

- If the resident has difficulty with longer items, separate the item into shorter parts, and provide a chance to respond after each part. This method, known as disentangling, is helpful if a resident has moderate cognitive impairment but can respond to simple, direct questions.
  — **Example**: Item D0200E, **Poor Appetite or Overeating**.
    o You can simplify this item by asking: "In the last 2 weeks, how often have you been bothered by poor appetite?" (pause for a response) "Or overeating?"

D0200: Resident Mood Interview (PHQ-9©) (cont.)

— **Example:** Item D0200C, **Trouble Falling or Staying Asleep, or Sleeping Too Much**.

   o You can break the item down as follows: "How often are you having problems falling asleep?" (pause for response) "How often are you having problems staying asleep?" (pause for response) "How often do you feel you are sleeping too much?"

— **Example:** Item D0200H, **Moving or Speaking So Slowly That Other People Could Have Noticed. Or the Opposite—Being So Fidgety or Restless That You Have Been Moving Around a Lot More than Usual**.

   o You can simplify this item by asking: "How often are you having problems with moving or speaking so slowly that other people could have noticed?" (pause for response) "How often have you felt so fidgety or restless that you move around a lot more than usual?"

D0300: Total Severity Score

D0300. Total Severity Score	
☐☐ Enter Score	Add scores for all frequency responses in Column 2, Symptom Frequency. Total score must be between 00 and 27. Enter 99 if unable to complete interview (i.e., Symptom Frequency is blank for 3 or more items).

Item Rationale

Health-related Quality of Life

- The score does not diagnose a mood disorder or depression but provides a standard score which can be communicated to the resident's physician, other clinicians and mental health specialists for appropriate follow up.

- The **Total Severity Score** is a summary of the frequency scores on the PHQ-9© that indicates the extent of potential depression symptoms and can be useful for knowing when to request additional assessment by providers or mental health specialists.

> **DEFINITIONS**
>
> **TOTAL SEVERITY SCORE**
> A summary of the frequency scores that indicates the extent of potential depression symptoms. The score does not diagnose a mood disorder, but provides a standard of communication with clinicians and mental health specialists.

Planning for Care

- The PHQ-9© **Total Severity Score** also provides a way for health care providers and clinicians to easily identify and track symptoms and how they are changing over time.

D0300: Total Severity Score (cont.)

Steps for Assessment

After completing D0200 A-I:

1. Add the numeric scores across all frequency items in **Resident Mood Interview** (D0200) Column 2.
2. Do not add up the score while you are interviewing the resident. Instead, focus your full attention on the interview.
3. The maximum resident score is 27 (3 x 9).

Coding Instructions

- The interview is successfully completed if the resident answered the frequency responses of at least 7 of the 9 items on the PHQ-9$^{©}$.
- If symptom frequency is blank for 3 or more items, the interview is deemed **NOT** complete. **Total Severity Score** should be coded as "99" and the **Staff Assessment of Mood** should be conducted.
- Enter the total score as a two-digit number. The **Total Severity Score** will be between **00** and **27** (or "**99**" if symptom frequency is blank for 3 or more items).
- The software will calculate the Total Severity Score. For detailed instructions on manual calculations and examples, see Appendix E: PHQ-9$^{©}$ Total Severity Score Scoring Rules.

Coding Tips and Special Populations

- Responses to PHQ-9$^{©}$ can indicate possible depression. Responses can be interpreted as follows:
  — Major Depressive Syndrome is suggested if—of the 9 items—5 or more items are identified at a frequency of half or more of the days (7-11 days) during the look-back period and at least one of these, (1) little interest or pleasure in doing things, or (2) feeling down, depressed, or hopeless is identified at a frequency of half or more of the days (7-11 days) during the look-back period.
  — Minor Depressive Syndrome is suggested if, of the 9 items, (1) feeling down, depressed or hopeless, (2) trouble falling or staying asleep, or sleeping too much, or (3) feeling tired or having little energy are identified at a frequency of half or more of the days (7-11 days) during the look-back period and at least one of these, (1) little interest or pleasure in doing things, or (2) feeling down, depressed, or hopeless is identified at a frequency of half or more of the days (7-11 days).
  — In addition, PHQ-9$^{©}$ **Total Severity Score** can be used to track changes in severity over time. **Total Severity Score** can be interpreted as follows:
    - 1-4: minimal depression
    - 5-9: mild depression
    - 10-14: moderate depression
    - 15-19: moderately severe depression
    - 20-27: severe depression

D0350: Follow-up to D0200I

D0350. Safety Notification - Complete only if D0200I1 = 1 indicating possibility of resident self harm	
Enter Code [ ]	**Was responsible staff or provider informed that there is a potential for resident self harm?** 0. No 1. Yes

Item Rationale

Health-related Quality of Life

- This item documents if appropriate clinical staff and/or mental health provider were informed that the resident expressed that he or she had thoughts of being better off dead, or hurting him or herself in some way.

- It is well-known that untreated depression can cause significant distress and increased mortality in the geriatric population beyond the effects of other risk factors.

- Although rates of suicide have historically been lower in nursing homes than for comparable individuals living in the community, indirect self-harm and life threatening behaviors, including poor nutrition and treatment refusal are common.

- Recognition and treatment of depression in the nursing home can be lifesaving, reducing the risk of mortality within the nursing home and also for those discharged to the community (available at http://www.agingcare.com/Featured-Stories/125788/Suicide- and-the-Elderly.htm).

Planning for Care

- Recognition and treatment of depression in the nursing home can be lifesaving, reducing the risk of mortality within the nursing home and also for those discharged to the community.

Steps for Assessment

- Complete item D0350 **only** if item D0200I1 **Thoughts That You Would Be Better Off Dead, or of Hurting Yourself in Some Way** = 1 indicating the possibility of resident self-harm.

Coding Instructions

- **Code 0, no:** if responsible staff or provider was not informed that there is a potential for resident self-harm.

- **Code 1, yes:** if responsible staff or provider was informed that there is a potential for resident self-harm.

D0500: Staff Assessment of Resident Mood (PHQ-9-OV©)

D0500. Staff Assessment of Resident Mood (PHQ-9-OV*)
Do not conduct if Resident Mood Interview (D0200-D0300) was completed

Over the last 2 weeks, did the resident have any of the following problems or behaviors?

If symptom is present, enter 1 (yes) in column 1, Symptom Presence.
Then move to column 2, Symptom Frequency, and indicate symptom frequency.

1. Symptom Presence
  0. **No** (enter 0 in column 2)
  1. **Yes** (enter 0-3 in column 2)

2. Symptom Frequency
  0. **Never or 1 day**
  1. **2-6 days** (several days)
  2. **7-11 days** (half or more of the days)
  3. **12-14 days** (nearly every day)

	1. Symptom Presence	2. Symptom Frequency
	↓ Enter Scores in Boxes ↓	
A. Little interest or pleasure in doing things	☐	☐
B. Feeling or appearing down, depressed, or hopeless	☐	☐
C. Trouble falling or staying asleep, or sleeping too much	☐	☐
D. Feeling tired or having little energy	☐	☐
E. Poor appetite or overeating	☐	☐
F. Indicating that s/he feels bad about self, is a failure, or has let self or family down	☐	☐
G. Trouble concentrating on things, such as reading the newspaper or watching television	☐	☐
H. Moving or speaking so slowly that other people have noticed. Or the opposite - being so fidgety or restless that s/he has been moving around a lot more than usual	☐	☐
I. States that life isn't worth living, wishes for death, or attempts to harm self	☐	☐
J. Being short-tempered, easily annoyed	☐	☐

Item Rationale

Health-related Quality of Life

- PHQ-9© **Resident Mood Interview** is preferred as it improves the detection of a possible mood disorder. However, a small percentage of patients are unable or unwilling to complete the PHQ-9© **Resident Mood Interview**. Therefore, staff should complete the PHQ-9-OV© **Staff Assessment of Mood** in these instances so that any behaviors, signs, or symptoms of mood distress are identified.

- Persons unable to complete the PHQ-9© **Resident Mood Interview** may still have a mood disorder.

- Even if a resident was unable to complete the **Resident Mood Interview**, important insights may be gained from the responses that were obtained during the interview, as well as observations of the resident's behaviors and affect during the interview.

- The identification of symptom presence and frequency as well as staff observations are important in the detection of mood distress, as they may inform need for and type of treatment.

- It is important to note that coding the presence of indicators in Section D does not automatically mean that the resident has a diagnosis of depression or other mood disorder. Assessors do not make or assign a diagnosis in Section D; they simply record the presence or absence of specific clinical mood indicators.

D0500: Staff Assessment of Resident Mood (PHQ-9-OV©) (cont.)

- Alternate means of assessing mood must be used for residents who cannot communicate or refuse or are unable to participate in the PHQ-9© **Resident Mood Interview**. This ensures that information about their mood is not overlooked.

Planning for Care

- When the resident is not able to complete the PHQ-9©, scripted interviews with staff who know the resident well should provide critical information for understanding mood and making care planning decisions.

Steps for Assessment

Look-back period for this item is 14 days.

1. Interview staff from all shifts who know the resident best. Conduct interview in a location that protects resident privacy.
2. The same administration techniques outlined above for the PHQ-9© **Resident Mood Interview** (pages D-4–D-6) and Interviewing Tips & Techniques (pages D-6–D-8) should also be followed when staff are interviewed.
3. Encourage staff to report symptom frequency, even if the staff believes the symptom to be unrelated to depression.
4. Explore unclear responses, focusing the discussion on the specific symptom listed on the assessment rather than expanding into a lengthy clinical evaluation.
5. If frequency cannot be coded because the resident has been in the facility for less than 14 days, talk to family or significant other and review transfer records to inform the selection of a frequency code.

Examples of Staff Responses That Indicate Need for Follow-up Questioning with the Staff Member

1. **D0500A, Little Interest or Pleasure in Doing Things**
   - The resident doesn't really do much here.
   - The resident spends most of the time in his or her room.

2. **D0500B, Feeling or Appearing Down, Depressed, or Hopeless**
   - She's 95- what can you expect?
   - How would you feel if you were here?

3. **D0500C, Trouble Falling or Staying Asleep, or Sleeping Too Much**
   - Her back hurts when she lies down.
   - He urinates a lot during the night.

4. **D0500D, Feeling Tired or Having Little Energy**
   - She's 95—she's always saying she's tired.
   - He's having a bad spell with his COPD right now.

D0500: Staff Assessment of Resident Mood (PHQ-9-OV©) (cont.)

5. **D0500E, Poor Appetite or Overeating**
   - She has not wanted to eat much of anything lately.
   - He has a voracious appetite, more so than last week.

6. **D0500F, Indicating That S/he Feels Bad about Self, Is a Failure, or Has Let Self or Family Down**
   - She does get upset when there's something she can't do now because of her stroke.
   - He gets embarrassed when he can't remember something he thinks he should be able to.

7. **D0500G, Trouble Concentrating on Things, Such as Reading the Newspaper or Watching Television**
   - She says there's nothing good on TV.
   - She never watches TV.
   - He can't see to read a newspaper.

8. **D0500H, Moving or Speaking So Slowly That Other People Have Noticed. Or the Opposite— Being So Fidgety or Restless That S/he Has Been Moving Around a Lot More than Usual**
   - His arthritis slows him down.
   - He's bored and always looking for something to do.

9. **D0500I, States That Life Isn't Worth Living, Wishes for Death, or Attempts to Harm Self**
   - She says God should take her already.
   - He complains that man was not meant to live like this.

10. **D0500J, Being Short-Tempered, Easily Annoyed**
    - She's OK if you know how to approach her.
    - He can snap but usually when his pain is bad.
    - Not with me.
    - He's irritable.

Coding Instructions for Column 1. **Symptom Presence**

- **Code 0, no:** if symptoms listed are not present. Enter 0 in Column 2, **Symptom Frequency**.
- **Code 1, yes:** if symptoms listed are present. Enter 0, 1, 2, or 3 in Column 2, **Symptom Frequency**.

D0500: Staff Assessment of Resident Mood (PHQ-9-OV©) (cont.)

Coding Instructions for Column 2. **Symptom Frequency**

- **Code 0, never or 1 day:** if staff indicate that the resident has never or has experienced the symptom on only 1 day.
- **Code 1, 2-6 days (several days):** if staff indicate that the resident has experienced the symptom for 2-6 days.
- **Code 2, 7-11 days (half or more of the days):** if staff indicate that the resident has experienced the symptom for 7-11 days.
- **Code 3, 12-14 days (nearly every day):** if staff indicate that the resident has experienced the symptom for 12-14 days.

Coding Tips and Special Populations

- Ask the staff member being interviewed to select how often over the past 2 weeks the symptom occurred. Use the descriptive and/or numeric categories on the form (e.g., "nearly every day" or 3 = 12-14 days) to select a frequency response.
- If you separated a longer item into its component parts, select the **highest** frequency rating that is reported.
- If the staff member has difficulty selecting between two frequency responses, code for the **higher** frequency.
- If the resident has been in the facility for less than 14 days, also talk to the family or significant other and review transfer records to inform selection of the frequency code.

D0600: Total Severity Score

D0600. Total Severity Score	
☐☐ Enter Score	Add scores for all frequency responses in Column 2, Symptom Frequency. Total score must be between 00 and 30.

Item Rationale

Health-related Quality of Life

- Review Item Rationale for D0300, **Total Severity Score** (page D-8).
- The PHQ-9© Observational Version (PHQ-9-OV©) is adapted to allow the assessor to interview staff and identify a **Total Severity Score** for potential depressive symptoms.

Planning for Care

- The score can be communicated among health care providers and used to track symptoms and how they are changing over time.
- The score is useful for knowing when to request additional assessment by providers or mental health specialists for underlying depression.

D0600: Total Severity Score (cont.)

Steps for Assessment

After completing items D0500 A-J:

1. Add the numeric scores across all frequency items for **Staff Assessment of Mood, Symptom Frequency** (D0500) Column 2.

2. Maximum score is 30 (3 × 10).

Coding Instructions

The interview is successfully completed if the staff members were able to answer the frequency responses of at least 8 out of 10 items on the PHQ-9-OV©.

- The software will calculate the Total Severity Score. For detailed instructions on manual calculations and examples, see Appendix E: PHQ-9-OV© Total Severity Score Scoring Rules.

Coding Tips and Special Populations

- Responses to PHQ-9-OV© can indicate possible depression. Responses can be interpreted as follows:

  — Major Depressive Syndrome is suggested if—of the 10 items, 5 or more items are identified at a frequency of half or more of the days (7-11 days) during the look-back period and at least one of these, (1) little interest or pleasure in doing things, or (2) feeling down, depressed, or hopeless is identified at a frequency of half or more of the days (7-11 days) during the look-back period.

  — Minor Depressive Syndrome is suggested if—of the 10 items, (1) feeling down, depressed or hopeless, (2) trouble falling or staying asleep, or sleeping too much, or (3) feeling tired or having little energy are identified at a frequency of half or more of the days (7-11 days) during the look-back period and at least one of these, (1) little interest or pleasure in doing things, or (2) feeling down, depressed, or hopeless is identified at a frequency of half or more of the days (7-11 days).

  — In addition, PHQ-9© **Total Severity Score** can be used to track changes in severity over time. **Total Severity Score** can be interpreted as follows:

1-4:	minimal depression
5-9:	mild depression
10-14:	moderate depression
15-19:	moderately severe depression
20-30:	severe depression

D0650: Follow-up to D0500I

D0650. Safety Notification - Complete only if D0500I1 = 1 indicating possibility of resident self harm
Enter Code ⬜	**Was responsible staff or provider informed that there is a potential for resident self harm?** 0. No 1. Yes

Item Rationale

Health-related Quality of Life

- This item documents if appropriate clinical staff and/or mental health provider were informed that the resident expressed that they had thoughts of being better off dead, or hurting him or herself in some way.

- It is well known that untreated depression can cause significant distress and increased mortality in the geriatric population beyond the effects of other risk factors.

- Although rates of suicide have historically been lower in nursing homes than for comparable individuals living in the community, indirect self-harm and life-threatening behaviors, including poor nutrition and treatment refusal are common.

Planning for Care

- Recognition and treatment of depression in the nursing home can be lifesaving, reducing the risk of mortality within the nursing home and also for those discharged to the community (available at http://www.agingcare.com/Featured-Stories/125788/Suicide- and-the-Elderly.htm).

Steps for Assessment

1. Complete item D0650 only if item D0500I, **States That Life Isn't Worth Living, Wishes for Death, or Attempts to Harm Self** = 1 indicating the possibility of resident self-harm.

Coding Instructions

- **Code 0, no:** if responsible staff or provider was not informed that there is a potential for resident self-harm.
- **Code 1, yes:** if responsible staff or provider was informed that there is a potential for resident self-harm.

SECTION E: BEHAVIOR

Intent: The items in this section identify behavioral symptoms in the last seven days that may cause distress to the resident, or may be distressing or disruptive to facility residents, staff members or the care environment. These behaviors may place the resident at risk for injury, isolation, and inactivity and may also indicate unrecognized needs, preferences or illness. Behaviors include those that are potentially harmful to the resident himself or herself. The emphasis is identifying behaviors, which does not necessarily imply a medical diagnosis. Identification of the frequency and the impact of behavioral symptoms on the resident and on others is critical to distinguish behaviors that constitute problems from those that are not problematic. Once the frequency and impact of behavioral symptoms are accurately determined, follow-up evaluation and care plan interventions can be developed to improve the symptoms or reduce their impact.

This section focuses on the resident's actions, not the intent of his or her behavior. Because of their interactions with residents, staff may have become used to the behavior and may underreport or minimize the resident's behavior by presuming intent (e.g., "Mr. A. doesn't really mean to hurt anyone. He's just frightened."). Resident intent should **not** be taken into account when coding for items in this section.

E0100: Potential Indicators of Psychosis

E0100. Potential Indicators of Psychosis	
↓ Check all that apply	
☐	A. Hallucinations (perceptual experiences in the absence of real external sensory stimuli)
☐	B. Delusions (misconceptions or beliefs that are firmly held, contrary to reality)
☐	Z. None of the above

Item Rationale

Health-related Quality of Life

- Psychotic symptoms may be associated with
  - delirium,
  - dementia,
  - adverse drug effects,
  - psychiatric disorders, and
  - hearing or vision impairment.
- Hallucinations and delusions may
  - be distressing to residents and families,
  - cause disability,
  - interfere with delivery of medical, nursing, rehabilitative and personal care, and
  - lead to dangerous behavior or possible harm.

> **DEFINITIONS**
>
> **HALLUCINATION** The perception of the presence of something that is not actually there. It may be auditory or visual or involve smells, tastes or touch.
>
> **DELUSION** A fixed, false belief not shared by others that the resident holds even in the face of evidence to the contrary.

E0100: Potential Indicators of Psychosis (cont.)

Planning for Care

- Reversible and treatable causes should be identified and addressed promptly. When the cause is not reversible, the focus of management strategies should be to minimize the amount of disability and distress.

Steps for Assessment

1. Review the resident's medical record for the 7-day look-back period.
2. Interview staff members and others who have had the opportunity to observe the resident in a variety of situations during the 7-day look-back period.
3. Observe the resident during conversations and the structured interviews in other assessment sections and listen for statements indicating an experience of hallucinations, or the expression of false beliefs (delusions).
4. Clarify potentially false beliefs:

   - When a resident expresses a belief that is plausible but alleged by others to be false (e.g., history indicates that the resident's husband died 20 years ago, but the resident states her husband has been visiting her every day), try to verify the facts to determine whether there is reason to believe that it could have happened or whether it is likely that the belief is false.

   - When a resident expresses a clearly false belief, determine if it can be readily corrected by a simple explanation of verifiable (real) facts (which may only require a simple reminder or reorientation) or demonstration of evidence to the contrary. Do not, however, challenge the resident.

   - The resident's response to the offering of a potential alternative explanation is often helpful in determining whether the false belief is held strongly enough to be considered fixed.

Coding Instructions

Code based on behaviors observed and/or thoughts expressed in the last 7 days rather than the presence of a medical diagnosis. Check all that apply.

- **Check E0100A, hallucinations:** if hallucinations were present in the last 7 days. A hallucination is the perception of the presence of something that is not actually there. It may be auditory or visual or involve smells, tastes or touch.

- **Check E0100B, delusions:** if delusions were present in the last 7 days. A delusion is a fixed, false belief not shared by others that the resident holds true even in the face of evidence to the contrary.

- **Check E0100Z, none of the above:** if no hallucinations or delusions were present in the last 7 days.

E0100: Potential Indicators of Psychosis (cont.)

Coding Tips and Special Populations

- If a belief cannot be objectively shown to be false, or it is not possible to determine whether it is false, **do not** code it as a delusion.
- If a resident expresses a false belief but easily accepts a reasonable alternative explanation, **do not** code it as a delusion. If the resident continues to insist that the belief is correct despite an explanation or direct evidence to the contrary, **code as a delusion**.

Examples

1. A resident carries a doll which she believes is her baby and the resident appears upset. When asked about this, she reports she is distressed from hearing her baby crying and thinks she's hungry and wants to get her a bottle.

   Coding: E0100A would be **checked** and E0100B would be **checked.**
   Rationale: The resident believes the doll is a baby which is a delusion and she hears the doll crying which is an auditory hallucination.

2. A resident reports that he heard a gunshot. In fact, there was a loud knock on the door. When this is explained to him, he accepts the alternative interpretation of the loud noise.

   Coding: E0100Z would be **checked.**
   Rationale: He misinterpreted a real sound in the external environment. Because he is able to accept the alternative explanation for the cause of the sound, his report of a gunshot is not a fixed false belief and is therefore not a delusion.

3. A resident is found speaking aloud in her room. When asked about this, she states that she is answering a question posed to her by the gentleman in front of her. Staff note that no one is present and that no other voices can be heard in the environment.

   Coding: E0100A would be **checked.**
   Rationale: The resident reports an auditory sensation that occurs in the absence of any external stimulus. Therefore, this is a hallucination.

4. A resident announces that he must leave to go to work, because he is needed in his office right away. In fact, he has been retired for 15 years. When reminded of this, he continues to insist that he must get to his office.

   Coding: E0100B would be **checked.**
   Rationale: The resident adheres to the belief that he still works, even after being reminded about his retirement status. Because the belief is held firmly despite an explanation of the real situation, it is a delusion.

E0100: Potential Indicators of Psychosis (cont.)

5. A resident believes she must leave the facility immediately because her mother is waiting for her to return home. Staff know that, in reality, her mother is deceased and gently remind her that her mother is no longer living. In response to this reminder, the resident acknowledges, "Oh yes, I remember now. Mother passed away years ago."

> **Coding:** E0100Z would be **checked.**
>
> **Rationale:** The resident's initial false belief is readily altered with a simple reminder, suggesting that her mistaken belief is due to forgetfulness (i.e., memory loss) rather than psychosis. Because it is not a firmly held false belief, it does not fit the definition of a delusion.

E0200: Behavioral Symptom—Presence & Frequency

E0200. Behavioral Symptom - Presence & Frequency		
Note presence of symptoms and their frequency		
Coding: 0. **Behavior not exhibited** 1. **Behavior of this type occurred 1 to 3 days** 2. **Behavior of this type occurred 4 to 6 days, but less than daily** 3. **Behavior of this type occurred daily**	↓ Enter Codes in Boxes	
	☐	A. **Physical behavioral symptoms directed toward others** (e.g., hitting, kicking, pushing, scratching, grabbing, abusing others sexually)
	☐	B. **Verbal behavioral symptoms directed toward others** (e.g., threatening others, screaming at others, cursing at others)
	☐	C. **Other behavioral symptoms not directed toward others** (e.g., physical symptoms such as hitting or scratching self, pacing, rummaging, public sexual acts, disrobing in public, throwing or smearing food or bodily wastes, or verbal/vocal symptoms like screaming, disruptive sounds)

Item Rationale

Health-related Quality of Life

- New onset of behavioral symptoms warrants prompt evaluation, assurance of resident safety, relief of distressing symptoms, and compassionate response to the resident.
- Reversible and treatable causes should be identified and addressed promptly. When the cause is not reversible, the focus of management strategies should be to minimize the amount of disability and distress.

Planning for Care

- Identification of the frequency and the impact of behavioral symptoms on the resident and on others is critical to distinguish behaviors that constitute problems—and may therefore require treatment planning and intervention—from those that are not problematic.
- These behaviors may indicate unrecognized needs, preferences, or illness.
- Once the frequency and impact of behavioral symptoms are accurately determined, follow-up evaluation and interventions can be developed to improve the symptoms or reduce their impact.
- Subsequent assessments and documentation can be compared to baseline to identify changes in the resident's behavior, including response to interventions.

E0200: Behavioral Symptom-Presence & Frequency (cont.)

Steps for Assessment

1. Review the medical record for the 7-day look-back period.
2. Interview staff, across all shifts and disciplines, as well as others who had close interactions with the resident during the 7-day look-back period, including family or friends who visit frequently or have frequent contact with the resident.
3. Observe the resident in a variety of situations during the 7-day look-back period.

Coding Instructions

- **Code 0, behavior not exhibited:** if the behavioral symptoms were not present in the last 7 days. Use this code if the symptom has never been exhibited or if it previously has been exhibited but has been absent in the last 7 days.

- **Code 1, behavior of this type occurred 1-3 days:** if the behavior was exhibited 1-3 days of the last 7 days, regardless of the number or severity of episodes that occur on any one of those days.

- **Code 2, behavior of this type occurred 4-6 days, but less than daily:** if the behavior was exhibited 4-6 of the last 7 days, regardless of the number or severity of episodes that occur on any of those days.

- **Code 3, behavior of this type occurred daily:** if the behavior was exhibited daily, regardless of the number or severity of episodes that occur on any of those days.

Coding Tips and Special Populations

- Code based on whether the symptoms occurred and not based on an interpretation of the behavior's meaning, cause or the assessor's judgment that the behavior can be explained or should be tolerated.

- Code as present, even if staff have become used to the behavior or view it as typical or tolerable.

- Behaviors in these categories should be coded as present or not present, whether or not they might represent a rejection of care.

- Item E0200C does not include wandering.

Examples

1. Every morning, a nursing assistant tries to help a resident who is unable to dress himself. On the last 4 out of 6 mornings, the resident has hit or scratched the nursing assistant during attempts to dress him.

    Coding: E0200A would be **coded 2, behavior of this type occurred 4-6 days, but less than daily.**
    Rationale: Scratching the nursing assistant was a physical behavior directed toward others.

E0200: Behavioral Symptom-Presence & Frequency (cont.)

2. A resident has previously been found rummaging through the clothes in her roommate's dresser drawer. This behavior has not been observed by staff or reported by others in the last 7 days.

> **Coding:** E0200C would be **coded 0, behavior not exhibited.**
>
> **Rationale:** The behavior did not occur during the look-back period.

3. A resident throws his dinner tray at another resident who repeatedly spit food at him during dinner. This is a single, isolated incident.

> **Coding:** E0200A would be **coded 1, behavior of this type occurred 1-3 days of the last 7 days.**
>
> **Rationale:** Throwing a tray was a physical behavior directed toward others. Although a possible explanation exists, the behavior is noted as present because it occurred.

E0300: Overall Presence of Behavioral Symptoms

E0300. Overall Presence of Behavioral Symptoms	
Enter Code	Were any behavioral symptoms in questions E0200 coded 1, 2, or 3? 0. **No** → Skip to E0800, Rejection of Care 1. **Yes** → Considering all of E0200, Behavioral Symptoms, answer E0500 and E0600 below

Item Rationale

To determine whether or not additional items E0500, **Impact on Resident**, and E0600, **Impact on Others,** are required to be completed.

Steps for Assessment

1. Review coding for item E0200 and follow these coding instructions:

Coding Instructions

- **Code 0, no:** if E0200A, E0200B, and E0200C all are coded 0, not present. Skip to **Rejection of Care—Presence & Frequency** item (E0800).
- **Code 1, yes:** if any of E0200A, E0200B, or E0200C were coded 1, 2, or 3. Proceed to complete **Impact on Resident** item (E0500), and **Impact on Others** item (E0600).

E0500: Impact on Resident

E0500. Impact on Resident	

Enter Code [ ]	Did any of the identified symptom(s):
	 A. Put the resident at significant risk for physical illness or injury?
	    0. No
	    1. Yes

Enter Code [ ]	B. Significantly interfere with the resident's care?
	    0. No
	    1. Yes

Enter Code [ ]	C. Significantly interfere with the resident's participation in activities or social interactions?
	    0. No
	    1. Yes

Item Rationale

Health-related Quality of Life

- Behaviors identified in item E0200 impact the resident's risk for significant injury, interfere with care or their participation in activities or social interactions.

Planning for Care

- Identification of the impact of the behaviors noted in E0200 may require treatment planning and intervention.
- Subsequent assessments and documentation can be compared to a baseline to identify changes in the resident's behavior, including response to interventions.

Steps for Assessment

1. Consider the previous review of the medical record, staff interviews across all shifts and disciplines, interviews with others who had close interactions with the resident and previous observations of the behaviors identified in E0200 for the 7-day look-back period.
2. Code E0500A, E0500B, and E0500C based on **all** of the behavioral symptoms coded in E0200.
3. Determine whether those behaviors put the resident at significant risk of physical illness or injury, whether the behaviors significantly interfered with the resident's care, and/or whether the behaviors significantly interfered with the resident's participation in activities or social interactions.

Coding Instructions for E0500A. Did Any of the Identified Symptom(s) Put the Resident at Significant Risk for Physical Illness or Injury?

- **Code 0, no:** if none of the identified behavioral symptom(s) placed the resident at clinically significant risk for a physical illness or injury.
- **Code 1, yes:** if any of the identified behavioral symptom(s) placed the resident at clinically significant risk for a physical illness or injury, even if no injury occurred.

E0500: Impact on Resident (cont.)

Coding Instructions for E0500B. Did Any of the Identified Symptom(s) Significantly Interfere with the Resident's Care?

- **Code 0, no:** if none of the identified behavioral symptom(s) significantly interfered with the resident's care.

- **Code 1, yes:** if any of the identified behavioral symptom(s) impeded the delivery of essential medical, nursing, rehabilitative or personal care, including but not limited to assistance with activities of daily living, such as bathing, dressing, feeding, or toileting.

Coding Instructions for E0500C. Did Any of the Identified Symptom(s) Significantly Interfere with the Resident's Participation in Activities or Social Interactions?

- **Code 0, no:** if none of the identified symptom(s) significantly interfered with the resident's participation in activities or social interactions.

- **Code 1, yes:** if any of the identified behavioral symptom(s) significantly interfered with or decreased the resident's participation or caused staff not to include residents in activities or social interactions.

Coding Tips and Special Populations

- For E0500A, code based on whether the risk for physical injury or illness is known to occur commonly under similar circumstances (i.e., with residents who exhibit similar behavior in a similar environment). Physical injury is trauma that results in pain or other distressing physical symptoms, impaired organ function, physical disability, or other adverse consequences, regardless of the need for medical, surgical, nursing, or rehabilitative intervention.

- For E0500B, code if the impact of the resident's behavior is impeding the delivery of care to such an extent that necessary or essential care (medical, nursing, rehabilitative or personal that is required to achieve the resident's goals for health and well-being) cannot be received safely, completely, or in a timely way without more than a minimal accommodation, such as simple change in care routines or environment.

- For E0500C, code if the impact of the resident's behavior is limiting or keeping the resident from engaging in solitary activities or hobbies, joining groups, or attending programmed activities or having positive social encounters with visitors, other residents, or staff.

Examples

1. A resident frequently grabs and scratches staff when they attempt to change her soiled brief, digging her nails into their skin. This makes it difficult to complete the care task.

   Coding: E0500B would be **coded 1, yes.**
   Rationale: This behavior interfered with delivery of essential personal care.

E0500: Impact on Resident (cont.)

2. During the last 7 days, a resident with vascular dementia and severe hypertension, hits staff during incontinent care making it very difficult to change her. Six out of the last seven days the resident refuses all her medication including her antihypertensive. The resident closes her mouth and shakes her head and will not take it even if re-approached multiple times.

> **Coding:** E0500A and E0500B would both be **coded 1, yes.**
> **Rationale:** The behavior interfered significantly with delivery of her medical and nursing care and put her at clinically significant risk for physical illness.

3. A resident paces incessantly. When staff encourage him to sit at the dinner table, he returns to pacing after less than a minute, even after cueing and reminders. He is so restless that he cannot sit still long enough to feed himself or receive assistance in obtaining adequate nutrition.

> **Coding:** E0500A and E0500B would both be **coded 1, yes.**
> **Rationale:** This behavior significantly interfered with personal care (i.e., feeding) and put the resident at risk for malnutrition and physical illness.

4. A resident repeatedly throws his markers and card on the floor during bingo.

> **Coding:** E0500C would be **coded 1, yes.**
> **Rationale:** This behavior interfered with his ability to participate in the activity.

5. A resident with severe dementia has continuous outbursts while awake despite all efforts made by staff to address the issue, including trying to involve the resident in prior activities of choice.

> **Coding:** E0500C would be **coded 1, yes.**
> **Rationale:** The staff determined the resident's behavior interfered with the ability to participate in any activities.

E0600: Impact on Others

Enter Code	E0600. Impact on Others
	Did any of the identified symptom(s):
☐	A. Put others at significant risk for physical injury? 0. No 1. Yes
☐	B. Significantly intrude on the privacy or activity of others? 0. No 1. Yes
☐	C. Significantly disrupt care or living environment? 0. No 1. Yes

E0600: Impact on Others (cont.)

Item Rationale

Health-related Quality of Life

- Behaviors identified in item E0200 put others at risk for significant injury, intrude on their privacy or activities and/or disrupt their care or living environments. The impact on others is coded here in item E0600.

Planning for Care

- Identification of the behaviors noted in E0200 that have an impact on others may require treatment planning and intervention.
- Subsequent assessments and documentation can be compared with a baseline to identify changes in the resident's behavior, including response to interventions.

Steps for Assessment

1. Consider the previous review of the clinical record, staff interviews across all shifts and disciplines, interviews with others who had close interactions with the resident and previous observations of the behaviors identified in E0200 for the 7-day look-back period.

2. To code E0600, determine if the behaviors identified put others at significant risk of physical illness or injury, intruded on their privacy or activities, and/or interfered with their care or living environments.

Coding Instructions for E0600A. Did Any of the Identified Symptom(s) Put Others at Significant Risk for Physical Injury?

- **Code 0, no:** if none of the identified behavioral symptom(s) placed staff, visitors, or other residents at significant risk for physical injury.
- **Code 1, yes:** if any of the identified behavioral symptom(s) placed staff, visitors, or other residents at significant risk for physical injury.

Coding Instructions for E0600B. Did Any of the Identified Symptom(s) Significantly Intrude on the Privacy or Activity of Others?

- **Code 0, no:** if none of the identified behavioral symptom(s) significantly intruded on the privacy or activity of others.
- **Code 1, yes:** if any of the identified behavioral symptom(s) kept other residents from enjoying privacy or engaging in informal activities (not organized or run by staff). Includes coming in uninvited, invading, or forcing oneself on others' private activities.

E0600: Impact on Others (cont.)

Coding Instructions for E0600C. Did Any of the Identified Symptom(s) Significantly Disrupt Care or the Living Environment?

- **Code 0, no:** if none of the identified behavioral symptom(s) significantly disrupted delivery of care or the living environment.

- **Code 1, yes:** if any of the identified behavioral symptom(s) created a climate of excessive noise or interfered with the receipt of care or participation in organized activities by other residents.

Coding Tips and Special Populations

- For E0600A, code based on whether the behavior placed others at significant risk for physical injury. Physical injury is trauma that results in pain or other distressing physical symptoms, impaired organ function, physical disability or other adverse consequences, regardless of the need for medical, surgical, nursing, or rehabilitative intervention.

- For E0600B, code based on whether the behavior violates other residents' privacy or interrupts other residents' performance of activities of daily living or limits engagement in or enjoyment of informal social or recreational activities to such an extent that it causes the other residents to experience distress (e.g., displeasure or annoyance) or inconvenience, whether or not the other residents complain.

- For E0600C, code based on whether the behavior interferes with staff ability to deliver care or conduct organized activities, interrupts receipt of care or participation in organized activities by other residents, and/or causes other residents to experience distress or adverse consequences.

Examples

1. A resident appears to intentionally stick his cane out when another resident walks by.

   Coding: E0600A would be **coded 1, yes**; E0600B and E0600C would be **coded 0, no.**
   Rationale: The behavior put the other resident at risk for falling and physical injury. You may also need to consider coding B and C depending on the specific situation in the environment or care setting.

2. A resident, when sitting in the hallway outside the community activity room, continually yells, repeating the same phrase. The yelling can be heard by other residents in hallways and activity/recreational areas but not in their private rooms.

   Coding: E0600A would be **coded 0, no**; E0600B and E0600C would be **coded 1, yes.**
   Rationale: The behavior does not put others at risk for significant injury. The behavior does create a climate of excessive noise, disrupting the living environment and the activity of others.

E0600: Impact on Others (cont.)

3. A resident repeatedly enters the rooms of other residents and rummages through their personal belongings. The other residents do not express annoyance.

    Coding: E0600A and E0600C would be **coded 0, no**; E0600B would be **coded 1, yes.**

    Rationale: This is an intrusion and violates other residents' privacy regardless of whether they complain or communicate their distress.

4. When eating in the dining room, a resident frequently grabs food off the plates of other residents. Although the other resident's food is replaced, and the behavior does not compromise their nutrition, other residents become anxious in anticipation of this recurring behavior.

    Coding: E0600A would be **coded 0, no**; E0600B and E0600C would be **coded 1, yes.**

    Rationale: This behavior violates other residents' privacy as it is an intrusion on the personal space and property (food tray) . In addition, the behavior is pervasive and disrupts the staff's ability to deliver nutritious meals in dining room (an organized activity).

5. A resident tries to seize the telephone out of the hand of another resident who is attempting to complete a private conversation. Despite being asked to stop, the resident persists in grabbing the telephone and insisting that he wants to use it.

    Coding: E0600A and E0600C would be **coded 0, no**; E0600B would be **coded 1, yes.**

    Rationale: This behavior is an intrusion on another resident's private telephone conversation.

6. A resident begins taunting two residents who are playing an informal card game, yelling that they will "burn in hell" if they don't stop "gambling."

    Coding: E0600A and E0600C would be **coded 0, no**; E0600B would be **coded 1, yes.**

    Rationale: The behavior is intruding on the other residents' game. The game is not an organized facility event and does not involve care. It is an activity in which the two residents wanted to engage.

7. A resident yells continuously during an exercise group, diverting staff attention so that others cannot participate in and enjoy the activity.

    Coding: E0600A and E0600B would be **coded 0, no**; E0600C would be **coded 1, yes.**

    Rationale: This behavior disrupts the delivery of physical care (exercise) to the group participants and creates an environment of excessive noise.

E0600: Impact on Others (cont.)

8. A resident becomes verbally threatening in a group discussion activity, frightening other residents. In response to this disruption, staff terminate the discussion group early to avoid eliciting the behavioral symptom.

> **Coding:** E0600A and E0600B would be **coded 0, no**; E0600C would be **coded 1, yes.**
>
> **Rationale:** This behavior does not put other residents at risk for significant injury. However, the behavior restricts full participation in the organized activity, and limits the enjoyment of other residents. It also causes fear, thereby disrupting the living environment.

E0800: Rejection of Care—Presence & Frequency

E0800. Rejection of Care - Presence & Frequency	
Enter Code □	Did the resident reject evaluation or care (e.g., bloodwork, taking medications, ADL assistance) **that is necessary to achieve the resident's goals for health and well-being?** Do not include behaviors that have already been addressed (e.g., by discussion or care planning with the resident or family), and determined to be consistent with resident values, preferences, or goals. 0. **Behavior not exhibited** 1. **Behavior of this type occurred 1 to 3 days** 2. **Behavior of this type occurred 4 to 6 days,** but less than daily 3. **Behavior of this type occurred daily**

Item Rationale

Health-related Quality of Life

*   Goals for health and well-being reflect the resident's wishes and objectives for health, function, and life satisfaction that define an acceptable quality of life for that individual.

*   The resident's care preferences reflect desires, wishes, inclinations, or choices for care. Preferences do not have to appear logical or rational to the clinician. Similarly, preferences are not necessarily informed by facts or scientific knowledge and may not be consistent with "good judgment."

*   It is really a matter of resident choice. When rejection/decline of care is first identified, the team then investigates and determines the rejection/decline of care is really a matter of resident's choice. Education is provided and the resident's choices become part of the plan of care. On future assessments, this behavior would not be coded in this item.

*   A resident might reject/decline care because the care conflicts with his or her preferences and goals. In such cases, care rejection behavior is not considered a problem that warrants treatment to modify or eliminate the behavior.

*   Care rejection may be manifested by verbally declining, statements of refusal, or through physical behaviors that convey aversion to, result in avoidance of, or interfere with the receipt of care.

E0800: Rejection of Care—Presence & Frequency (cont.)

- This type of behavior interrupts or interferes with the delivery or receipt of care by disrupting the usual routines or processes by which care is given, or by exceeding the level or intensity of resources that are usually available for the provision of care.

- A resident's rejection of care might be caused by an underlying neuropsychiatric, medical, or dental problem. This can interfere with needed care that is consistent with the resident's preferences or established care goals. In such cases, care rejection behavior may be a problem that requires assessment and intervention.

Planning for Care

- Evaluation of rejection of care assists the nursing home in honoring the resident's care preferences in order to meet his or her desired health care goals.

- Follow-up assessment should consider:
  - whether established care goals clearly reflect the resident's preferences and goals and
  - whether alternative approaches could be used to achieve the resident's care goals.

DEFINITIONS

REJECTION OF CARE
Behavior that interrupts or interferes with the delivery or receipt of care. Care rejection may be manifested by verbally declining or statements of refusal or through physical behaviors that convey aversion to or result in avoidance of or interfere with the receipt of care.

INTERFERENCE WITH CARE
Hindering the delivery or receipt of care by disrupting the usual routines or processes by which care is given, or by exceeding the level or intensity of resources that are usually available for the provision of care.

- Determine whether a previous discussion identified an objection to the type of care or the way in which the care was provided. If so, determine approaches to accommodate the resident's preferences.

Steps for Assessment

1. Review the medical record.
2. Interview staff, across all shifts and disciplines, as well as others who had close interactions with the resident during the 7-day look-back period.
3. Review the record and consult staff to determine whether the rejected care is needed to achieve the resident's preferences and goals for health and well-being.
4. Review the medical record to find out whether the care rejection behavior was previously addressed and documented in discussions or in care planning with the resident, family, or significant other and determined to be an informed choice consistent with the resident's values, preferences, or goals; or whether that the behavior represents an objection to the way care is provided, but acceptable alternative care and/or approaches to care have been identified and employed.
5. If the resident exhibits behavior that appears to communicate a rejection of care (and that rejection behavior has not been previously determined to be consistent with the resident's values or goals), ask him or her directly whether the behavior is meant to decline or refuse care.

E0800: Rejection of Care—Presence & Frequency (cont.)

- If the resident indicates that the intention is to decline or refuse, then ask him or her about the reasons for rejecting care and about his or her goals for health care and well-being.
- If the resident is unable or unwilling to respond to questions about his or her rejection of care or goals for health care and well-being, then interview the family or significant other to ascertain the resident's health care preferences and goals.

Coding Instructions

- **Code 0, behavior not exhibited:** if rejection of care consistent with goals was not exhibited in the last 7 days.
- **Code 1, behavior of this type occurred 1-3 days:** if the resident rejected care consistent with goals 1-3 days during the 7-day look-back period, regardless of the number of episodes that occurred on any one of those days.
- **Code 2, behavior of this type occurred 4-6 days, but less than daily:** if the resident rejected care consistent with goals 4-6 days during the 7-day look-back period, regardless of the number of episodes that occurred on any one of those days.
- **Code 3, behavior of this type occurred daily:** if the resident rejected care consistent with goals daily in the 7-day look-back period, regardless of the number of episodes that occurred on any one of those days.

Coding Tips and Special Populations

- The intent of this item is to identify potential behavioral problems, not situations in which care has been rejected based on a choice that is consistent with the resident's preferences or goals for health and well-being or a choice made on behalf of the resident by a family member or other proxy decision maker.
- Do not include behaviors that have already been addressed (e.g., by discussion or care planning with the resident or family) and determined to be consistent with the resident's values, preferences, or goals. Residents who have made an informed choice about not wanting a particular treatment, procedure, etc., should not be identified as "rejecting care."

Examples

1. A resident with heart failure who recently returned to the nursing home after surgical repair of a hip fracture is offered physical therapy and declines. She says that she gets too short of breath when she tries to walk even a short distance, making physical therapy intolerable. She does not expect to walk again and does not want to try. Her physician has discussed this with her and has indicated that her prognosis for regaining ambulatory function is poor.

   Coding: E0800 would be **coded 0, behavior not exhibited.**

   Rationale: This resident has communicated that she considers physical therapy to be both intolerable and futile. The resident discussed this with her physician. Her choice to not accept physical therapy treatment is consistent with her values and goals for health care. Therefore, this would **not** be coded as rejection of care.

E0800: Rejection of Care—Presence & Frequency (cont.)

2. A resident informs the staff that he would rather receive care at home, and the next day he calls for a taxi and exits the nursing facility. When staff try to persuade him to return, he firmly states, "Leave me alone. I always swore I'd never go to a nursing home. I'll get by with my visiting nurse service at home again." He is not exhibiting signs of disorientation, confusion, or psychosis and has never been judged incompetent.

    Coding: E0800 would be **coded 0, behavior not exhibited.**

    Rationale: His departure is consistent with his stated preferences and goals for health care. Therefore, this is **not** coded as care rejection.

3. A resident goes to bed at night without changing out of the clothes he wore during the day. When a nursing assistant offers to help him get undressed, he declines, stating that he prefers to sleep in his clothes tonight. The clothes are wet with urine. This has happened 2 of the past 7 days. The resident was previously fastidious, recently has expressed embarrassment at being incontinent, and has care goals that include maintaining personal hygiene and skin integrity.

    Coding: E0800 would be **coded 1, behavior of this type occurred 1-3 days.**

    Rationale: The resident's care rejection behavior is not consistent with his values and goals for health and well-being. Therefore, this is classified as care rejection that occurred twice.

4. A resident chooses not to eat supper one day, stating that the food causes her diarrhea. She says she knows she needs to eat and does not wish to compromise her nutrition, but she is more distressed by the diarrhea than by the prospect of losing weight.

    Coding: E0800 would be **coded 1, behavior of this type occurred 1-3 days.**

    Rationale: Although choosing not to eat is consistent with the resident's desire to avoid diarrhea, it is also in conflict with her stated goal to maintain adequate nutrition.

5. A resident is given his antibiotic medication prescribed for treatment of pneumonia and immediately spits the pills out on the floor. This resident's assessment indicates that he does not have any swallowing problems. This happened on each of the last 4 days. The resident's advance directive indicates that he would choose to take antibiotics to treat a potentially life-threatening infection.

    Coding: E0800 would be **coded 2, behavior of this type occurred 4-6 days, but less than daily.**

    Rationale: The behavioral rejection of antibiotics prevents the resident from achieving his stated goals for health care listed in his advance directives. Therefore, the behavior is coded as care rejection.

E0800: Rejection of Care—Presence & Frequency (cont.)

6. A resident who recently returned to the nursing home after surgery for a hip fracture is offered physical therapy and declines. She states that she wants to walk again but is afraid of falling. This occurred on 4 days during the look-back period.

    Coding: E0800 would be **coded 2, behavior of this type occurred 4-6 days.**

    Rationale: Even though the resident's health care goal is to regain her ambulatory status, her fear of falling results in rejection of physical therapy and interferes with her rehabilitation. This would be coded as rejection of care.

7. A resident who previously ate well and prided herself on following a healthy diet has been refusing to eat every day for the past 2 weeks. She complains that the food is boring and that she feels full after just a few bites. She says she wants to eat to maintain her weight and avoid getting sick, but she cannot push herself to eat anymore.

    Coding: E0800 would be **coded 3, behavior of this type occurred daily.**

    Rationale: The resident's choice not to eat is not consistent with her goal of weight maintenance and health. Choosing not to eat may be related to a medical condition such as a disturbance of taste sensation, gastrointestinal illness, endocrine condition, depressive disorder, or medication side effects.

E0900: Wandering—Presence & Frequency

E0900. Wandering - Presence & Frequency	
Enter Code ☐	**Has the resident wandered?** 0. **Behavior not exhibited** → Skip to E1100, Change in Behavioral or Other Symptoms 1. **Behavior of this type occurred 1 to 3 days** 2. **Behavior of this type occurred 4 to 6 days**, but less than daily 3. **Behavior of this type occurred daily**

Item Rationale

Health-related Quality of Life

- Wandering may be a pursuit of exercise or a pleasurable leisure activity, or it may be related to tension, anxiety, agitation, or searching.

Planning for Care

- It is important to assess for reason for wandering. Determine the frequency of its occurrence, and any factors that trigger the behavior or that decrease the episodes.

- Assess for underlying tension, anxiety, psychosis, drug-induced psychomotor restlessness, agitation, or unmet need (e.g., for food, fluids, toileting, exercise, pain relief, sensory or cognitive stimulation, sense of security, companionship) that may be contributing to wandering.

E0900: Wandering—Presence & Frequency (cont.)

Steps for Assessment

1. Review the medical record and interview staff to determine whether wandering occurred during the 7-day look-back period.

    *   Wandering is the act of moving (walking or locomotion in a wheelchair) from place to place with or without a specified course or known direction. Wandering may or may not be aimless. The wandering resident may be oblivious to his or her physical or safety needs. The resident may have a purpose such as searching to find something, but he or she persists without knowing the exact direction or location of the object, person or place. The behavior may or may not be driven by confused thoughts or delusional ideas (e.g., when a resident believes she must find her mother, who staff know is deceased).

2. If wandering occurred, determine the frequency of the wandering during the 7-day look-back period.

Coding Instructions for E0900

*   **Code 0, behavior not exhibited:** if wandering was not exhibited during the 7-day look-back period. Skip to **Change in Behavioral or Other Symptoms** item (E1100).

*   **Code 1, behavior of this type occurred 1-3 days:** if the resident wandered on 1-3 days during the 7-day look-back period, regardless of the number of episodes that occurred on any one of those days. Proceed to answer **Wandering—Impact** item (E1000).

*   **Code 2, behavior of this type occurred 4-6 days, but less than daily:** if the resident wandered on 4-6 days during the 7-day look-back period, regardless of the number of episodes that occurred on any one of those days. Proceed to answer **Wandering—Impact** item (E1000).

*   **Code 3, behavior of this type occurred daily:** if the resident wandered daily during the 7-day look-back period, regardless of the number of episodes that occurred on any one of those days. Proceed to answer **Wandering—Impact** item (E1000).

Coding Tips and Special Populations

*   Pacing (repetitive walking with a driven/pressured quality) within a constrained space is not included in wandering.

*   Wandering may occur even if resident is in a locked unit.

*   Traveling via a planned course to another specific place (such as going to the dining room to eat a meal or to an activity) is not considered wandering.

E1000: Wandering—Impact

Answer this item only if E0900, Wandering—Presence & Frequency, was coded 1 (behavior of this type occurred 1-3 days), 2 (behavior of this type occurred 4-6 days, but less than daily), or 3 (behavior of this type occurred daily).

E1000. Wandering - Impact	
Enter Code ☐	**A.** Does the wandering place the resident at significant risk of getting to a potentially dangerous place (e.g., stairs, outside of the facility)? 0. **No** 1. **Yes**
Enter Code ☐	**B.** Does the wandering significantly intrude on the privacy or activities of others? 0. **No** 1. **Yes**

Item Rationale

Health-related Quality of Life

- Not all wandering is harmful.
- Some residents who wander are at potentially higher risk for entering an unsafe situation.
- Some residents who wander can cause significant disruption to other residents.

Planning for Care

- Care plans should consider the impact of wandering on resident safety and disruption to others.
- Care planning should be focused on minimizing these issues.
- Determine the need for environmental modifications (door alarms, door barriers, etc.) that enhance resident safety if wandering places the resident at risk.
- Determine when wandering requires interventions to reduce unwanted intrusions on other residents or disruption of the living environment.

Steps for Assessment

1. Consider the previous review of the resident's wandering behaviors identified in E0900 for the 7-day look-back period.
2. Determine whether those behaviors put the resident at significant risk of getting into potentially dangerous places and/or whether wandering significantly intrudes on the privacy or activities of others based on clinical judgement for the individual resident.

Coding Instructions for E1000A. Does the Wandering Place the Resident at Significant Risk of Getting to a Potentially Dangerous Place?

- **Code 0, no:** if wandering does not place the resident at significant risk.
- **Code 1, yes:** if the wandering places the resident at significant risk of getting to a dangerous place (e.g., wandering outside the facility where there is heavy traffic) or encountering a dangerous situation (e.g., wandering into the room of another resident with dementia who is known to become physically aggressive toward intruders).

E1000: Wandering-Impact (cont.)

Coding Instructions for E1000B. Does the Wandering Significantly Intrude on the Privacy or Activities of Others?

- **Code 0, no:** if the wandering does not intrude on the privacy or activity of others.
- **Code 1, yes:** if the wandering intrudes on the privacy or activities of others (i.e., if the wandering violates other residents' privacy or interrupts other residents' performance of activities of daily living or limits engagement in or enjoyment of social or recreational activities), whether or not the other resident complains or communicates displeasure or annoyance.

Examples

1. A resident wanders away from the nursing home in his pajamas at 3 a.m. When staff members talk to him, he insists he is looking for his wife. This elopement behavior had occurred when he was living at home, and on one occasion he became lost and was missing for 3 days, leading his family to choose nursing home admission for his personal safety.

    Coding: E1000A would be **coded 1, yes.**

    Rationale: Wandering that results in elopement from the nursing home places the resident at significant risk of getting into a dangerous situation.

2. A resident wanders away from the nursing facility at 7 a.m. Staff find him crossing a busy street against a red light. When staff try to persuade him to return, he becomes angry and says, "My boss called, and I have to get to the office." When staff remind him that he has been retired for many years, he continues to insist that he must get to work.

    Coding: E1000A would be **coded 1, yes.**

    Rationale: This resident's wandering is associated with elopement from the nursing home and into a dangerous traffic situation. Therefore, this is coded as placing the resident at significant risk of getting to a place that poses a danger. In addition, delusions would be checked in item E0100.

3. A resident propels himself in his wheelchair into the room of another resident, blocking the door to the other resident's bathroom.

    Coding: E1000B would be **coded 1, yes.**

    Rationale: Moving about in this manner with the use of a wheelchair meets the definition of wandering, and the resident has intruded on the privacy of another resident and has interfered with that resident's ability to use the bathroom.

E1100: Change in Behavioral or Other Symptoms

E1100. Change in Behavior or Other Symptoms	
Consider all of the symptoms assessed in items E0100 through E1000	
Enter Code ☐	How does resident's current behavior status, care rejection, or wandering **compare to prior assessment (OBRA or Scheduled PPS)?** 0. **Same** 1. **Improved** 2. **Worse** 3. **N/A** because no prior MDS assessment

E1100: Change in Behavioral or Other Symptoms (cont.)

Item Rationale

Health-related Quality of Life

- Change in behavior may be an important indicator of
  - a change in health status or a change in environmental stimuli,
  - positive response to treatment, and
  - adverse effects of treatment.

Planning for Care

- If behavior is worsening, assessment should consider whether it is related to
  - new health problems, psychosis, or delirium;
  - worsening of pre-existing health problems;
  - a change in environmental stimuli or caregivers that influences behavior; and
  - adverse effects of treatment.
- If behaviors are improved, assessment should consider what interventions should be continued or modified (e.g., to minimize risk of relapse or adverse effects of treatment).

Steps for Assessment

1. Review responses provided to items E0100-E1000 on the current MDS assessment.
2. Compare with responses provided on prior MDS assessment.
3. Taking all of these MDS items into consideration, make a global assessment of the change in behavior from the most recent to the current MDS.
4. Rate the overall behavior as same, improved, or worse.

Coding Instructions

- **Code 0, same:** if overall behavior is the same (unchanged).
- **Code 1, improved:** if overall behavior is improved.
- **Code 2, worse:** if overall behavior is worse.
- **Code 3, N/A:** if there was no prior MDS assessment of this resident.

Coding Tips

- For residents with multiple behavioral symptoms, it is possible that different behaviors will vary in different directions over time. That is, one behavior may improve while another worsens or remains the same. Using clinical judgment, this item should be rated to reflect the overall direction of behavior change, estimating the net effects of multiple behaviors.

E1100: Change in Behavioral or Other Symptoms (cont.)

Examples

1. On the prior assessment, the resident was reported to wander on 4 out of 7 days. Because of elopement, the behavior placed the resident at significant risk of getting to a dangerous place. On the current assessment, the resident was found to wander on 2 of the last 7 days. Because a door alarm system is now in use, the resident was not at risk for elopement and getting to a dangerous place. However, the resident is now wandering into the rooms of other residents, intruding on their privacy. This requires occasional redirection by staff.

    Coding: E1100 would be **coded 1, improved.**

    Rationale: Although one component of this resident's wandering behavior is worse because it has begun to intrude on the privacy of others, it is less frequent and less dangerous (without recent elopement) and is therefore improved overall since the last assessment. The fact that the behavior requires less intense surveillance or intervention by staff also supports the decision to rate the overall behavior as improved.

2. At the time of the last assessment, the resident was ambulatory and would threaten and hit other residents daily. He recently suffered a hip fracture and is not ambulatory. He is not approaching, threatening, or assaulting other residents. However, the resident is now combative when staff try to assist with dressing and bathing, and is hitting staff members daily.

    Coding: E1100 would be **coded 0, same.**

    Rationale: Although the resident is no longer assaulting other residents, he has begun to assault staff. Because the danger to others and the frequency of these behaviors is the same as before, the overall behavior is rated as unchanged.

3. On the prior assessment, a resident with Alzheimer's disease was reported to wander on 2 out of 7 days and has responded well to redirection. On the most recent assessment, it was noted that the resident has been wandering more frequently for 5 out of 7 days and has also attempted to elope from the building on two occasions.

    This behavior places the resident at significant risk of personal harm. The resident has been placed on more frequent location checks and has required additional redirection from staff. He was also provided with an elopement bracelet so that staff will be alerted if the resident attempts to leave the building. The intensity required of staff surveillance because of the dangerousness and frequency of the wandering behavior has significantly increased.

    Coding: E1100 would be **coded 2, worse.**

    Rationale: Because the danger and the frequency of the resident's wandering behavior have increased and there were two elopement attempts, the overall behavior is rated as worse.

SECTION F: PREFERENCES FOR CUSTOMARY ROUTINE AND ACTIVITIES

Intent: The intent of items in this section is to obtain information regarding the resident's preferences for his or her daily routine and activities. This is best accomplished when the information is obtained directly from the resident or through family or significant other, or staff interviews if the resident cannot report preferences. The information obtained during this interview is just a portion of the assessment. Nursing homes should use this as a guide to create an individualized plan based on the resident's preferences, and is not meant to be all-inclusive.

F0300: Should Interview for Daily and Activity Preferences Be Conducted?

F0300. Should Interview for Daily and Activity Preferences be Conducted? - Attempt to interview all residents able to communicate. If resident is unable to complete, attempt to complete interview with family member or significant other	
Enter Code [ ]	0. **No** (resident is rarely/never understood <u>and</u> family/significant other not available) → Skip to and complete F0800, Staff Assessment of Daily and Activity Preferences 1. **Yes** → Continue to F0400, Interview for Daily Preferences

Item Rationale

Health-related Quality of Life

- Most residents capable of communicating can answer questions about what they like.

- Obtaining information about preferences directly from the resident, sometimes called "hearing the resident's voice," is the most reliable and accurate way of identifying preferences.

- If a resident cannot communicate, then family or significant other who knows the resident well may be able to provide useful information about preferences.

Planning for Care

- Quality of life can be greatly enhanced when care respects the resident's choice regarding anything that is important to the resident.

- Interviews allow the resident's voice to be reflected in the care plan.

- Information about preferences that comes directly from the resident provides specific information for individualized daily care and activity planning.

Steps for Assessment

1. Determine whether or not resident is rarely/never understood and if family/significant other is available. If resident is rarely/never understood and family is not available, skip to item F0800, Staff Assessment of Daily and Activity Preferences.

2. Review **Language** item (A1100) to determine whether or not the resident needs or wants an interpreter.

   - If the resident needs or wants an interpreter, complete the interview with an interpreter.

3. The resident interview should be conducted if the resident can respond:

   - verbally,
   - by pointing to their answers on the cue card, <u>OR</u>
   - by writing out their answers.

F0300: Should Interview for Daily and Activity Preferences Be Conducted? (cont.)

Coding Instructions

Record whether the resident preference interview should be attempted.

- **Code 0, no:** if the interview should not be attempted with the resident. This option should be selected for residents who are rarely/never understood, who need an interpreter but one was not available, and who do not have a family member or significant other available for interview. Skip to F0800, (Staff Assessment of Daily and Activity Preferences).

- **Code 1, yes:** if the resident interview should be attempted. This option should be selected for residents who are able to be understood, for whom an interpreter is not needed or is present, or who have a family member or significant other available for interview. Continue to F0400 (Interview for Daily Preferences) and F0500 (Interview for Activity Preferences).

Coding Tips and Special Populations

- If the resident needs an interpreter, every effort should be made to have an interpreter present for the MDS clinical interview. If it is not possible for a needed interpreter to be present on the day of the interview, **and** a family member or significant other is not available for interview, **code F0300 = 0** to indicate interview not attempted, and complete the Staff Assessment of Daily and Activity Preferences (F0800) instead of the interview with the resident (F0400 and F0500).

F0400: Interview for Daily Preferences

F0400. Interview for Daily Preferences	
Show resident the response options and say: *"While you are in this facility..."*	

Coding: 1. Very important 2. Somewhat important 3. Not very important 4. Not important at all 5. Important, but can't do or no choice 9. No response or non-responsive	↓ Enter Codes in Boxes	
	☐	A. how important is it to you to **choose what clothes to wear?**
	☐	B. how important is it to you to **take care of your personal belongings or things?**
	☐	C. how important is it to you to **choose between a tub bath, shower, bed bath, or sponge bath?**
	☐	D. how important is it to you to **have snacks available between meals?**
	☐	E. how important is it to you to **choose your own bedtime?**
	☐	F. how important is it to you to **have your family or a close friend involved in discussions about your care?**
	☐	G. how important is it to you to **be able to use the phone in private?**
	☐	H. how important is it to you to **have a place to lock your things to keep them safe?**

F0400: Interview for Daily Preferences (cont.)

Item Rationale

Health-related Quality of Life

- Individuals who live in nursing homes continue to have distinct lifestyle preferences.
- A lack of attention to lifestyle preferences can contribute to depressed mood and increased behavior symptoms.
- Resident responses that something is important but that they can't do it or have no choice can provide clues for understanding pain, perceived functional limitations, and perceived environmental barriers.

Planning for Care

- Care planning should be individualized and based on the resident's preferences.
- Care planning and care practices that are based on resident preferences can lead to
  — improved mood,
  — enhanced dignity, and
  — increased involvement in daily routines and activities.
- Incorporating resident preferences into care planning is a dynamic, collaborative process. Because residents may adjust their preferences in response to events and changes in status, the preference assessment tool is intended as a first step in an ongoing dialogue between care providers and the residents. Care plans should be updated as residents' preferences change, paying special attention to preferences that residents state are important.

Steps for Assessment: Interview Instructions

1. Interview any resident not screened out by the **Should Interview for Daily and Activity Preferences Be Conducted?** item (F0300).
2. Conduct the interview in a private setting.
3. Sit so that the resident can see your face. Minimize glare by directing light sources away from the resident's face.
4. Be sure the resident can hear you.

   - Residents with hearing impairment should be interviewed using their usual communication devices/techniques, as applicable.
   - Try an external assistive device (headphones or hearing amplifier) if you have any doubt about hearing ability.
   - Minimize background noise.

5. Explain the reason for the interview before beginning.

   Suggested language: "I'd like to ask you a few questions about your daily routines. The reason I'm asking you these questions is that the staff here would like to know what's important to you. This helps us plan your care around your preferences so that you can have a comfortable stay with us. Even if you're only going to be here for a few days, we want to make your stay as personal as possible."

F0400: Interview for Daily Preferences (cont.)

6. Explain the interview response choices. While explaining, also show the resident a clearly written list of the response options, for example a cue card.

    Suggested language: "I am going to ask you how important various activities and routines are to you **while you are in this home.** I will ask you to answer using the choices you see on this card [read the answers while pointing to cue card]: 'Very Important,' 'Somewhat important,' 'Not very important,' 'Not important at all,' or 'Important, but can't do or no choice.'"

    Explain the "Important, but can't do or no choice" response option.

    Suggested language: "Let me explain the 'Important, but can't do or no choice' answer. You can select this answer if something would be important to you, but because of your health or because of what's available in this nursing home, you might not be able to do it. So, if I ask you about something that is important to you, but you don't think you're able to do it now, answer 'Important, but can't do or no choice.' If you choose this option, it will help us to think about ways we might be able to help you do those things."

7. Residents may respond to questions

    - verbally,

    - by pointing to their answers on the cue card, <u>OR</u>

    - by writing out their answers.

8. If resident cannot report preferences, then interview family or significant others.

Coding Instructions

- **Code 1, very important:** if resident, family, or significant other indicates that the topic is "very important."

- **Code 2, somewhat important:** if resident, family, or significant other indicates that the topic is "somewhat important."

- **Code 3, not very important:** if resident, family, or significant other indicates that the topic is "not very important."

> **DEFINITIONS**
>
> **NONSENSICAL RESPONSE**
> Any unrelated, incomprehensible, or incoherent response that is not informative with respect to the item being rated.

- **Code 4, not important at all:** if resident, family, or significant other indicates that the topic is "not important at all."

- **Code 5, important, but can't do or no choice:** if resident, family, or significant other indicates that the topic is "important," but that he or she is physically unable to participate, or has no choice about participating while staying in nursing home because of nursing home resources or scheduling.

F0400: Interview for Daily Preferences (cont.)

- **Code 9, no response or non-responsive:**
    - — If resident, family, or significant other refuses to answer or says he or she does not know.
    - — If resident does not give an answer to the question for several seconds and does not appear to be formulating an answer.
    - — If resident provides an incoherent or nonsensical answer that does not correspond to the question.

Coding Tips and Special Populations

- The interview is considered incomplete if the resident gives nonsensical responses or fails to respond to 3 or more of the 16 items in F0400 and F0500. If the interview is stopped because it is considered incomplete, fill the remaining F0400 and F0500 items with a 9 and proceed to F0600, Daily Activity Preferences Primary Respondent.
- No look-back is provided for resident. He or she is being asked about current preferences while in the nursing home but is not limited to a 7-day look-back period to convey what their preferences are.
- The facility is still obligated to complete the assessment within the 7-day look-back period.

Interviewing Tips and Techniques

- Sometimes respondents give long or indirect answers to interview items. To narrow the answer to the response choices available, it can be useful to summarize their longer answer and then ask them which response option best applies. This is known as echoing.
- For these questions, it is appropriate to explore residents' answers and try to understand the reason.

Examples for F0400A, How Important Is It to You to Choose What Clothes to Wear (including hospital gowns or other garments provided by the facility)?

1. Resident answers, "It's very important. I've always paid attention to my appearance."

    Coding: F0400A would be **coded 1, very important**.

2. Resident replies, "I leave that up to the nurse. You have to wear what you can handle if you have a stiff leg."

    Interviewer echoes, "You leave it up to the nurses. Would you say that, while you are here, choosing what clothes to wear is [pointing to cue card] very important, somewhat important, not very important, not important at all, or that it's important, but you can't do it because of your leg?"

    Resident responds, "Well, it would be important to me, but I just can't do it."

    Coding: F0400A would be **coded 5, important, but can't do or no choice**.

F0400: Interview for Daily Preferences (cont.)

Examples for F0400B, How Important Is It to You to Take Care of Your Personal Belongings or Things?

1. Resident answers, "It's somewhat important. I'm not a perfectionist, but I don't want to have to look for things."

   Coding: F0400B would be **coded 2, somewhat important**.

2. Resident answers, "All my important things are at home."

   Interviewer clarifies, "Your most important things are at home. Do you have any other things while you're here that you think are important to take care of yourself?"

   Resident responds, "Well, my son brought me this CD player so that I can listen to music. It is very important to me to take care of that."

   Coding: F0400B would be **coded 1, very important.**

> **DEFINITIONS**
>
> **PERSONAL BELONGINGS OR THINGS** Possessions such as eyeglasses, hearing aids, clothing, jewelry, books, toiletries, knickknacks, pictures.

Examples for F0400C, How Important Is It to You to Choose between a Tub Bath, Shower, Bed Bath, or Sponge Bath?

1. Resident answers, "I like showers."

   Interviewer clarifies, "You like showers. Would you say that choosing a shower instead of other types of bathing is very important, somewhat important, not very important, not important at all, or that it's important, but you can't do it or have no choice?"

   The resident responds, "It's very important."

   Coding: F0400C would be **coded 1, very important.**

2. Resident answers, "I don't have a choice. I like only sponge baths, but I have to take shower two times a week."

   The interviewer says, "So how important is it to you to be able to choose to have a sponge bath while you're here?"

   The resident responds, "Well, it is very important, but I don't always have a choice because that's the rule."

   Coding: F0400C would be **coded 5, important, but can't do or no choice.**

F0400: Interview for Daily Preferences (cont.)

Example for F0400D, How Important Is It to You to Have Snacks Available between Meals?

1. Resident answers, "I'm a diabetic, so it's very important that I get snacks."

    Coding: F0400D would be **coded 1, very important.**

Example for F0400E, How Important Is It to You to Choose Your Own Bedtime?

1. Resident answers, "At home I used to stay up and watch TV. But here I'm usually in bed by 8. That's because they get me up so early."

    Interviewer echoes and clarifies, "You used to stay up later, but now you go to bed before 8 because you get up so early. Would you say it's [pointing to cue card] very important, somewhat important, not very important, not important at all, or that it's important, but you don't have a choice about your bedtime?"

    Resident responds, "I guess it would be important, but I can't do it because they wake me up so early in the morning for therapy and by 8 o'clock at night, I'm tired."

    Coding: F0400E would be **coded 5, important, but can't do or no choice**.

> **DEFINITIONS**
>
> **BED BATH**
> Bath taken in bed using washcloths and water basin or other method in bed.
>
> **SHOWER**
> Bath taken standing or using gurney or shower chair in a shower room or stall.
>
> **SPONGE BATH**
> Bath taken sitting or standing at sink.
>
> **TUB BATH**
> Bath taken in bathtub.
>
> **SNACK**
> Food available between meals, including between dinner and breakfast.

Example for F0400F, How Important Is It to You to Have Your Family or a Close Friend Involved in Discussions about Your Care?

1. Resident responds, "They're not involved. They live in the city. They've got to take care of their own families."

    Interviewer replies, "You said that your family and close friends aren't involved right now. When you think about what you would prefer, would you say that it's very important, somewhat important, not very important, not important at all, or that it is important but you have no choice or can't have them involved in decisions about your care?"

    Resident responds, "It's somewhat important."

    Coding: F0400F would be **coded 2, somewhat important**.

F0400: Interview for Daily Preferences (cont.)

Example for F0400G, How Important Is It to You to Be Able to Use the Phone in Private?

1. Resident answers "That's not a problem for me, because I have my own room. If I want to make a phone call, I just shut the door."

   Interviewer echoes and clarifies, "So, you can shut your door to make a phone call. If you had to rate how important it is to be able to use the phone in private, would you say it's very important, somewhat important, not very important, or not important at all?"

   Resident responds, "Oh, it's very important."

   Coding: F0400G would be **coded 1, very important**.

> **DEFINITIONS**
>
> **PRIVATE TELEPHONE CONVERSATION**
> A telephone conversation on which no one can listen in, other than the resident.

Example for F0400H, How Important Is It to You to Have a Place to Lock Your Things to Keep Them Safe?

1. Resident answers, "I have a safe deposit box at my bank, and that's where I keep family heirlooms and personal documents."

   Interviewer says, "That sounds like a good service. While you are staying here, how important is it to you to have a drawer or locker here?"

   Resident responds, "It's not very important. I'm fine with keeping all my valuables at the bank."

   Coding: F0400H would be **coded 3, not very important.**

F0500: Interview for Activity Preferences

F0500. Interview for Activity Preferences		
Show resident the response options and say: "*While you are in this facility...*"		
Coding: 1. **Very important** 2. **Somewhat important** 3. **Not very important** 4. **Not important at all** 5. **Important, but can't do or no choice** 9. **No response or non-responsive**	↓ Enter Codes in Boxes	
	☐	A. *how important is it to you to **have books, newspapers, and magazines to read**?*
	☐	B. *how important is it to you to **listen to music you like**?*
	☐	C. *how important is it to you to **be around animals such as pets**?*
	☐	D. *how important is it to you to **keep up with the news**?*
	☐	E. *how important is it to you to **do things with groups of people**?*
	☐	F. *how important is it to you to **do your favorite activities**?*
	☐	G. *how important is it to you to **go outside to get fresh air when the weather is good**?*
	☐	H. *how important is it to you to **participate in religious services or practices**?*

F0500: Interview for Activity Preferences (cont.)

Item Rationale

Health-related Quality of Life

- Activities are a way for individuals to establish meaning in their lives, and the need for enjoyable activities and pastimes does not change on admission to a nursing home.

- A lack of opportunity to engage in meaningful and enjoyable activities can result in boredom, depression, and behavior disturbances.

- Individuals vary in the activities they prefer, reflecting unique personalities, past interests, perceived environmental constraints, religious and cultural background, and changing physical and mental abilities.

Planning for Care

- These questions will be useful for designing individualized care plans that facilitate residents' participation in activities they find meaningful.

- Preferences may change over time and extend beyond those included here. Therefore, the assessment of activity preferences is intended as a first step in an ongoing informal dialogue between the care provider and resident.

- As with daily routines, responses may provide insights into perceived functional, emotional, and sensory support needs.

Coding Instructions

- **See Coding Instructions on page F-5.**
  Coding approach is identical to that for daily preferences.

Coding Tips and Special Populations

- **See Coding Tips on page F-5.**
  Coding tips include those for daily preferences.

- Include Braille and or audio recorded material when coding items in F0500A.

Interviewing Tips and Techniques

- **See Interview Tips and Techniques on page F-5.**
  Coding tips and techniques are identical to those for daily preferences.

DEFINITIONS

READ
Script, Braille, or audio recorded written material.

NEWS
News about local, state, national, or international current events.

KEEP UP WITH THE NEWS
Stay informed by reading, watching, or listening.

NEWSPAPERS AND MAGAZINES
Any type, such as journalistic, professional, and trade publications in script, Braille, or audio recorded format.

F0500: Interview for Activity Preferences (cont.)

Examples for F0500A, How Important Is It to You to Have Books (Including Braille and Audio-recorded Format), Newspapers, and Magazines to Read?

1. Resident answers, "Reading is very important to me."

    Coding: F0500A would be **coded 1, very important**.

2. Resident answers, "They make the print so small these days. I guess they are just trying to save money."

    Interviewer replies, "The print is small. Would you say that having books, newspapers, and magazines to read is very important, somewhat important, not very important, not important at all, or that it is important but you can't do it because the print is so small?"

    Resident answers: "It would be important, but I can't do it because of the print."

    Coding: F0500A would be **coded 5, important, but can't do or no choice.**

Example for F0500B, How Important Is It to You to Listen to Music You Like?

1. Resident answers, "It's not important, because all we have in here is TV. They keep it blaring all day long."

    Interviewer echoes, "You've told me it's not important because all you have is a TV. Would you say it's not very important or not important at all to you to listen to music you like while you are here? Or are you saying that it's important, but you can't do it because you don't have a radio or CD player?"

    Resident responds, "Yeah. I'd enjoy listening to some jazz if I could get a radio."

    Coding: F0500B would be **coded 5, important, but can't do or no choice.**

Examples for F0500C, How Important Is It to You to Be Around Animals Such as Pets?

1. Resident answers, "It's very important for me NOT to be around animals. You get hair all around and I might inhale it."

    Coding: F0500C would be **coded 4, not important at all.**

2. Resident answers, "I'd love to go home and be around my own animals. I've taken care of them for years and they really need me."

    Interviewer probes, "You said you'd love to be at home with your own animals. How important is it to you to be around pets while you're staying here? Would you say it is [points to card] very important, somewhat important, not very important, not important at all, or is it important, but you can't do it or don't have a choice about it."

    Resident responds, "Well, it's important to me to be around my own dogs, but I can't be around them. I'd say important but can't do."

    Coding: F0500C would be **coded 5, Important, but can't do or no choice.**

    Rationale: Although the resident has access to therapeutic dogs brought to the nursing home, he does not have access to the type of pet that is important to him.

F0500: Interview for Activity Preferences (cont.)

Example for F0500D, How Important Is It to You to Keep Up with the News?

1. Resident answers, "Well, they are all so liberal these days, but it's important to hear what they are up to."

    Interviewer clarifies, "You think it is important to hear the news. Would you say it is [points to card] very important, somewhat important, or it's important but you can't do it or have no choice?"

    Resident responds, "I guess you can mark me somewhat important on that one."

    Coding: F0500D would be **coded 2, somewhat important.**

Example for F0500E, How Important Is It to You to Do Things with Groups of People?

1. Resident answers, "I've never really liked groups of people. They make me nervous."

    Interviewer echoes and clarifies, "You've never liked groups. To help us plan your activities, would you say that while you're here, doing things with groups of people is very important, somewhat important, not very important, not important at all, or would it be important to you but you can't do it because you feel nervous about it?"

    Resident responds, "At this point I'd say it's not very important."

    Coding: F0500E would be **coded 3, not very important.**

Examples for F0500F, How Important Is It to You to Do Your Favorite Activities?

1. Resident answers, "Well, it's very important, but I can't really do my favorite activities while I'm here. At home, I used to like to play board games, but you need people to play and make it interesting. I also like to sketch, but I don't have the supplies I need to do that here. I'd say important but no choice."

    Coding: F0500F would be **coded 5, important, but can't do or no choice.**

2. Resident answers, "I like to play bridge with my bridge club."

    Interviewer probes, "Oh, you like to play bridge with your bridge club. How important is it to you to play bridge while you are here in the nursing home?"

    Resident responds, "Well, I'm just here for a few weeks to finish my rehabilitation. It's not very important."

    Coding: F0500F would be **coded 3, not very important**.

F0500: Interview for Activity Preferences (cont.)

Example for F0500G, How Important Is It to You to Go Outside to Get Fresh Air When the Weather Is Good (Includes Less Temperate Weather if Resident Has Appropriate Clothing)?

1. Resident answers, "They have such a nice garden here. It's very important to me to go out there."

   Coding: F0500G would be **coded 1, very important.**

Examples for F0500H, How Important Is It to You to Participate in Religious Services or Practices?

1. Resident answers, "I'm Jewish. I'm Orthodox, but they have Reform services here. So I guess it's not important."

   Interviewer clarifies, "You're Orthodox, but the services offered here are Reform. While you are here, how important would it be to you to be able to participate in religious services? Would you say it is very important, somewhat important, not very important, not important at all, or would it be important to you but you can't or have no choice because they don't offer Orthodox services."

   Resident responds, "It's important for me to go to Orthodox services if they were offered, but they aren't. So, can't do or no choice."

   Coding: F0500I would be **coded 5, important, but can't do or no choice.**

2. Resident answers "My pastor sends taped services to me that I listen to in my room on Sundays. I don't participate in the services here."

   Interviewer probes, "You said your pastor sends you taped services. Would you say that it is very important, somewhat important, not very important, or not important at all, to you that you are able to listen to those tapes from your pastor?"

   Resident responds, "Oh, that's very important."

   Coding: F0500I would be **coded 1, very important**.

> **DEFINITIONS**
>
> **OUTSIDE**
> Any outdoor area in the proximity of the facility, including patio, porch, balcony, sidewalk, courtyard, or garden.
>
> **PARTICIPATE IN RELIGIOUS SERVICES**
> Any means of taking part in religious services or practices, such as listening to services on the radio or television, attending services in the facility or in the community, or private prayer or religious study.
>
> **RELIGIOUS PRACTICES**
> Rituals associated with various religious traditions or faiths, such as washing rituals in preparation for prayer, following kosher dietary laws, honoring holidays and religious festivals, and participating in communion or confession.

F0600: Daily and Activity Preferences Primary Respondent

F0600. Daily and Activity Preferences Primary Respondent	
Enter Code	**Indicate primary respondent** for Daily and Activity Preferences (F0400 and F0500) 1. **Resident** 2. **Family or significant other** (close friend or other representative) 9. **Interview could not be completed** by resident or family/significant other ("No response" to 3 or more items")

Item Rationale

- This item establishes the source of the information regarding the resident's preferences.

Coding Instructions

- **Code 1, resident:** if resident was the primary source for the preference questions in F0400 and F0500.

- **Code 2, family or significant other:** if a family member or significant other was the primary source of information for F0400 and F0500.

- **Code 9, interview could not be completed:** if F0400 and F0500 could not be completed by the resident, a family member, or a representative of the resident.

F0700: Should the Staff Assessment of Daily and Activity Preferences Be Conducted?

F0700. Should the Staff Assessment of Daily and Activity Preferences be Conducted?	
Enter Code	0. **No** (because Interview for Daily and Activity Preferences (F0400 and F0500) was completed by resident or family/significant other) → Skip to and complete G0110, Activities of Daily Living (ADL) Assistance 1. **Yes** (because 3 or more items in Interview for Daily and Activity Preferences (F0400 and F0500) were not completed by resident or family/significant other) → Continue to F0800, Staff Assessment of Daily and Activity Preferences

Item Rationale

Health-related Quality of Life

- Resident interview is preferred as it most accurately reflects what the resident views as important. However, a small percentage of residents are unable or unwilling to complete the interview for Daily and Activity Preferences.

- Persons unable to complete the preference interview should still have preferences evaluated and considered.

Planning for Care

- Even though the resident was unable to complete the interview, important insights may be gained from the responses that were obtained, observing behaviors, and observing the resident's affect during the interview.

Steps for Assessment

1. Review resident, family, or significant other responses to F0400A-H and F0500A-H.

F0700: Should the Staff Assessment of Daily and Activity Preferences Be Conducted? (cont.)

Coding Instructions

- **Code 0, no:** if **Interview for Daily and Activity Preferences** items (F0400 and F0500) was completed by resident, family or significant other. Skip to Section G, Functional Status.
- **Code 1, yes:** if **Interview for Daily and Activity Preferences** items (F0400 through F0500) were not completed because the resident, family, or significant other was unable to answer 3 or more items (i.e. 3 or more items in F0400 through F0500 were coded as **9** or **"-"**).

Coding Tips and Special Populations

- If the total number of unanswered questions in F0400 through F0500 is equal to 3 or more, the interview is considered incomplete.

F0800: Staff Assessment of Daily and Activity Preferences

F0800. Staff Assessment of Daily and Activity Preferences	
Do not conduct if Interview for Daily and Activity Preferences (F0400-F0500) was completed	
Resident Prefers:	
↓ Check all that apply	
☐	A. Choosing clothes to wear
☐	B. Caring for personal belongings
☐	C. Receiving tub bath
☐	D. Receiving shower
☐	E. Receiving bed bath
☐	F. Receiving sponge bath
☐	G. Snacks between meals
☐	H. Staying up past 8:00 p.m.
☐	I. Family or significant other involvement in care discussions
☐	J. Use of phone in private
☐	K. Place to lock personal belongings
☐	L. Reading books, newspapers, or magazines
☐	M. Listening to music
☐	N. Being around animals such as pets
☐	O. Keeping up with the news
☐	P. Doing things with groups of people
☐	Q. Participating in favorite activities
☐	R. Spending time away from the nursing home
☐	S. Spending time outdoors
☐	T. Participating in religious activities or practices
☐	Z. None of the above

F0800: Staff Assessment of Daily and Activity Preferences (cont.)

Item Rationale

Health-related Quality of Life

- Alternate means of assessing daily preferences must be used for residents who cannot communicate. This ensures that information about their preferences is not overlooked.
- Activities allow residents to establish meaning in their lives. A lack of meaningful and enjoyable activities can result in boredom, depression, and behavioral symptoms.

Planning for Care

- Caregiving staff should use observations of resident behaviors to understand resident likes and dislikes in cases where the resident, family, or significant other cannot report the resident's preferences. This allows care plans to be individualized to each resident.

Steps for Assessment

1. Observe the resident when the care, routines, and activities specified in these items are made available to the resident.
2. Observations should be made by staff across all shifts and departments and others with close contact with the resident.
3. If the resident appears happy or content (e.g., is involved, pays attention, smiles) during an activity listed in **Staff Assessment of Daily and Activity Preferences** item (F0800), then that item should be checked.

   If the resident seems to resist or withdraw when these are made available, then do not check that item.

Coding Instructions

Check all that apply in the last 7 days based on staff observation of resident preferences.

- **F0800A.** Choosing clothes to wear
- **F0800B.** Caring for personal belongings
- **F0800C.** Receiving tub bath
- **F0800D.** Receiving shower
- **F0800E.** Receiving bed bath
- **F0800F.** Receiving sponge bath
- **F0800G.** Snacks between meals
- **F0800H.** Staying up past 8:00 p.m.
- **F0800I.** Family or significant other involvement in care discussions
- **F0800J.** Use of phone in private
- **F0800K.** Place to lock personal belongings

F0800: Staff Assessment of Daily and Activity Preferences (cont.)

- **F0800L.** Reading books, newspapers, or magazines
- **F0800M.** Listening to music
- **F0800N.** Being around animals such as pets
- **F0800O.** Keeping up with the news
- **F0800P.** Doing things with groups of people
- **F0800Q.** Participating in favorite activities
- **F0800R.** Spending time away from the nursing home
- **F0800S.** Spending time outdoors
- **F0800T.** Participating in religious activities or practices
- **F0800Z.** None of the above

SECTION G: FUNCTIONAL STATUS

Intent: Items in this section assess the need for assistance with activities of daily living (ADLs), altered gait and balance, and decreased range of motion. In addition, on admission, resident and staff opinions regarding functional rehabilitation potential are noted.

G0110: Activities of Daily Living (ADL) Assistance

G0110. Activities of Daily Living (ADL) Assistance
Refer to the ADL flow chart in the RAI manual to facilitate accurate coding

Instructions for Rule of 3

- When an activity occurs three times at any one given level, code that level.
- When an activity occurs three times at multiple levels, code the most dependent, exceptions are total dependence (4), activity must require full assist every time, and activity did not occur (8), activity must not have occurred at all. Example, three times extensive assistance (3) and three times limited assistance (2), code extensive assistance (3).
- When an activity occurs at various levels, but not three times at any given level, apply the following:
  - When there is a combination of full staff performance, and extensive assistance, code extensive assistance.
  - When there is a combination of full staff performance, weight bearing assistance and/or non-weight bearing assistance code limited assistance (2).

If none of the above are met, code supervision.

1. ADL Self-Performance
Code for **resident's performance** over all shifts - not including setup. If the ADL activity occurred 3 or more times at various levels of assistance, code the most dependent - except for total dependence, which requires full staff performance every time

Coding:

Activity Occurred 3 or More Times
0. **Independent** - no help or staff oversight at any time
1. **Supervision** - oversight, encouragement or cueing
2. **Limited assistance** - resident highly involved in activity; staff provide guided maneuvering of limbs or other non-weight-bearing assistance
3. **Extensive assistance** - resident involved in activity, staff provide weight-bearing support
4. **Total dependence** - full staff performance every time during entire 7-day period

Activity Occurred 2 or Fewer Times
7. **Activity occurred only once or twice** - activity did occur but only once or twice
8. **Activity did not occur** - activity did not occur or family and/or non-facility staff provided care 100% of the time for that activity over the entire 7-day period

2. ADL Support Provided
Code for **most support provided** over all shifts; code regardless of resident's self-performance classification

Coding:
0. **No** setup or physical help from staff
1. **Setup** help only
2. **One** person physical assist
3. **Two+** persons physical assist
8. ADL activity itself **did not occur** or family and/or non-facility staff provided care 100% of the time for that activity over the entire 7-day period

	1. Self-Performance	2. Support
	↓ Enter Codes in Boxes ↓	
A. **Bed mobility** - how resident moves to and from lying position, turns side to side, and positions body while in bed or alternate sleep furniture	☐	☐
B. **Transfer** - how resident moves between surfaces including to or from: bed, chair, wheelchair, standing position (**excludes** to/from bath/toilet)	☐	☐
C. **Walk in room** - how resident walks between locations in his/her room	☐	☐
D. **Walk in corridor** - how resident walks in corridor on unit	☐	☐
E. **Locomotion on unit** - how resident moves between locations in his/her room and adjacent corridor on same floor. If in wheelchair, self-sufficiency once in chair	☐	☐
F. **Locomotion off unit** - how resident moves to and returns from off-unit locations (e.g., areas set aside for dining, activities or treatments). **If facility has only one floor**, how resident moves to and from distant areas on the floor. If in wheelchair, self-sufficiency once in chair	☐	☐
G. **Dressing** - how resident puts on, fastens and takes off all items of clothing, including donning/removing a prosthesis or TED hose. Dressing includes putting on and changing pajamas and housedresses	☐	☐
H. **Eating** - how resident eats and drinks, regardless of skill. Do not include eating/drinking during medication pass. Includes intake of nourishment by other means (e.g., tube feeding, total parenteral nutrition, IV fluids administered for nutrition or hydration)	☐	☐
I. **Toilet use** - how resident uses the toilet room, commode, bedpan, or urinal; transfers on/off toilet; cleanses self after elimination; changes pad; manages ostomy or catheter; and adjusts clothes. Do not include emptying of bedpan, urinal, bedside commode, catheter bag or ostomy bag	☐	☐
J. **Personal hygiene** - how resident maintains personal hygiene, including combing hair, brushing teeth, shaving, applying makeup, washing/drying face and hands (**excludes** baths and showers)	☐	☐

G0110: Activities of Daily Living (ADL) Assistance (cont.)

Item Rationale

Health-related Quality of Life

- Almost all nursing home residents need some physical assistance. In addition, most are at risk of further physical decline. The amount of assistance needed and the risk of decline vary from resident to resident.

- A wide range of physical, neurological, and psychological conditions and cognitive factors can adversely affect physical function.

- Dependence on others for ADL assistance can lead to feelings of helplessness, isolation, diminished self-worth, and loss of control over one's destiny.

- As inactivity increases, complications such as pressure ulcers, falls, contractures, depression, and muscle wasting may occur.

Planning for Care

- Individualized care plans should address strengths and weakness, possible reversible causes such as de-conditioning, and adverse side effects of medications or other treatments. These may contribute to needless loss of self-sufficiency. In addition, some neurologic injuries such as stroke may continue to improve for months after an acute event.

- For some residents, cognitive deficits can limit ability or willingness to initiate or participate in self-care or restrict understanding of the tasks required to complete ADLs.

> **DEFINITIONS**
>
> **ADL**
> Tasks related to personal care; any of the tasks listed in items G0110A-J and G0120.
>
> **ADL ASPECTS**
> Components of an ADL activity. These are listed next to the activity in the item set. For example, the components of G0110H (Eating) are eating, drinking, and intake of nourishment or hydration by other means, including tube feeding, total parenteral nutrition and IV fluids for hydration.
>
> **ADL SELF-PERFORMANCE**
> Measures what the resident **actually did** (not what he or she might be capable of doing) within each ADL category over the last 7 days according to a performance-based scale.

- A resident's potential for maximum function is often underestimated by family, staff, and the resident. Individualized care plans should be based on an accurate assessment of the resident's self-performance and the amount and type of support being provided to the resident.

- Many residents might require lower levels of assistance if they are provided with appropriate devices and aids, assisted with segmenting tasks, or are given adequate time to complete the task while being provided graduated prompting and assistance. This type of supervision requires skill, time, and patience.

G0110: Activities of Daily Living (ADL) Assistance (cont.)

- Most residents are candidates for nursing-based rehabilitative care that focuses on maintaining and expanding self-involvement in ADLs.

- Graduated prompting/task segmentation (helping the resident break tasks down into smaller components) and allowing the resident time to complete an activity can often increase functional independence.

<table>
<tr><td>DEFINITIONS

ADL SUPPORT PROVIDED
Measures the most support provided by staff over the last 7 days, even if that level of support only occurred once.</td></tr>
</table>

Steps for Assessment

1. Review the documentation in the medical record for the 7-day look-back period.

2. Talk with direct care staff from each shift that has cared for the resident to learn what the resident does for himself during each episode of each ADL activity definition as well as the type and level of staff assistance provided. Remind staff that the focus is on the 7-day look-back period only.

3. When reviewing records, interviewing staff, and observing the resident, be specific in evaluating each component as listed in the ADL activity definition. For example, when evaluating Bed Mobility, determine the level of assistance required for moving the resident to and from a lying position, for turning the resident from side to side, and/or for positioning the resident in bed.

To clarify your own understanding and observations about a resident's performance of an ADL activity (bed mobility, locomotion, transfer, etc.), ask probing questions, beginning with the general and proceeding to the more specific. See page G-9 for an example of using probes when talking to staff.

Coding Instructions

For each ADL activity:

- To assist in coding ADL self-performance items, please use the algorithm on page G-6.

- Consider each episode of the activity that occurred during the 7-day look-back period.

- In order to be able to promote the highest level of functioning among residents, clinical staff must first identify what the resident actually does for himself or herself, noting when assistance is received and clarifying the types of assistance provided (verbal cueing, physical support, etc.).

- Code based on the resident's level of assistance when using special adaptive devices such as a walker, device to assist with donning socks, dressing stick, long-handle reacher, or adaptive eating utensils.

- For the purposes of completing Section G, "facility staff" pertains to direct employees and facility-contracted employees (e.g. rehabilitation staff, nursing agency staff). Thus, does not include individuals hired, compensated or not, by individuals outside of the

G0110: Activities of Daily Living (ADL) Assistance (cont.)

facility's management and administration. Therefore, facility staff does not include, for example, hospice staff, nursing/CNA students, etc. Not including these individuals as facility staff supports the idea that the facility retains the primary responsibility for the care of the resident outside of the arranged services another agency may provide to facility residents.

- A resident's ADL self-performance may vary from day to day, shift to shift, or within shifts. There are many possible reasons for these variations, including mood, medical condition, relationship issues (e.g., willing to perform for a nursing assistant that he or she likes), and medications. The responsibility of the person completing the assessment, therefore, is to capture the total picture of the resident's ADL self-performance over the 7-day period, 24 hours a day (i.e., not only how the evaluating clinician sees the resident, but how the resident performs on other shifts as well).

- The ADL self-performance coding options are intended to reflect real world situations where slight variations in self-performance are common. Refer to the algorithm on page G-6 for assistance in determining the most appropriate self-performance code.

- Although it is not necessary to know the actual number of times the activity occurred, it is necessary to know whether or not the activity occurred three or more times within the last 7 days.

- Because this section involves a two-part evaluation (ADL Self-Performance and ADL Support), each using its own scale, it is recommended that the Self-Performance evaluation be completed for all ADL activities before beginning the ADL Support evaluation.

- **Instructions for the Rule of Three:**
  — When an activity occurs three times at any one given level, code that level.
  — When an activity occurs three times at multiple levels, **code the most dependent**.
    o Example, three times extensive assistance (3) and three times limited assistance (2)—code extensive assistance (3).

  Exceptions are as follows:
    o Total dependence (4)—activity must require full assist every time, and
    o Activity did not occur (8)—activity must not have occurred at all or family and/or non-facility staff provided care 100% of the time for the activity over the entire 7-day period.

  — When an activity occurs at more than one level, but not three times at any one level, apply the following:
    o Episodes of full staff performance are considered to be weight-bearing assistance (when every episode is full staff performance—this is total dependence).
    o When there are three or more episodes of a combination of full staff performance and weight-bearing assistance—code extensive assistance (3).

G0110: Activities of Daily Living (ADL) Assistance (cont.)

o When there are three or more episodes of a combination of full staff performance, weight-bearing assistance, and/or non-weight-bearing assistance—code limited assistance (2).

- **If none of the above are met, code supervision.**

Coding Instructions for G0110, Column 1, ADL-Self Performance

- **Code 0, independent:** if resident completed activity with no help or oversight every time during the 7-day look-back period.

- **Code 1, supervision:** if oversight, encouragement, or cueing was provided **three** or more times during the last 7 days.

- **Code 2, limited assistance:** if resident was highly involved in activity and received physical help in guided maneuvering of limb(s) or other non-weight-bearing assistance on **three** or more times during the last 7 days.

- **Code 3, extensive assistance:** if resident performed part of the activity over the last 7 days, help of the following type(s) was provided three or more times:

  — Weight-bearing support provided three or more times.

  — Full staff performance of activity during part but not all of the last 7 days.

- **Code 4, total dependence:** if there was full staff performance of an activity with no participation by resident for any aspect of the ADL activity. The resident must be unwilling or unable to perform any part of the activity over the entire 7-day look-back period.

- **Code 7, activity occurred only once or twice:** if the activity occurred but **not** three times or more.

- **Code 8, activity did not occur:** if the activity did not occur or family and/or non-facility staff provided care 100% of the time for that activity over the entire 7-day period.

Coding Instructions for G0110, Column 2, ADL Support

*Code for the **most** support provided over all shifts; code regardless of resident's self-performance classification.*

- **Code 0, no setup or physical help from staff:** if resident completed activity with no help or oversight.

- **Code 1, setup help only:** if resident is provided with materials or devices necessary to perform the ADL independently. This can include giving or holding out an item that the resident takes from the caregiver.

- **Code 2, one person physical assist:** if the resident was assisted by one staff person.

- **Code 3, two+ person physical assist:** if the resident was assisted by two or more staff persons.

- **Code 8, ADL activity itself did not occur during the entire period:** if the activity did not occur or family and/or non-facility staff provided care 100% of the time for that activity over the entire 7-day period.

G0110:   Activities of Daily Living (ADL) Assistance (cont.)

ADL Self Performance Algorithm

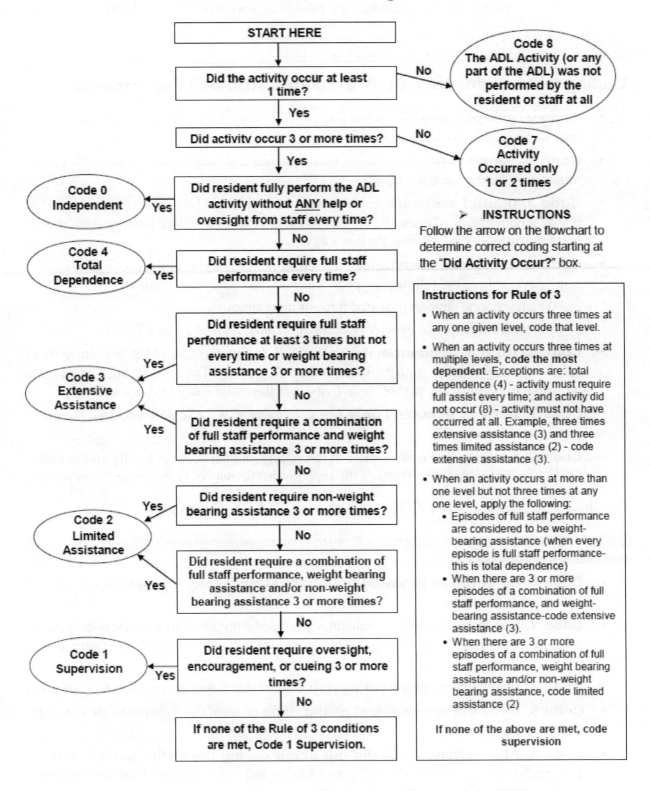

G0110: Activities of Daily Living (ADL) Assistance (cont.)

Coding Tips and Special Populations

- Some residents sleep on furniture other than a bed (for example, a recliner). Consider assistance received in this alternative bed when coding bed mobility.
- Do **NOT** include the emptying of bedpan, urinal, bedside commode, catheter bag or ostomy bag in G0110 I.
- **Differentiating between guided maneuvering and weight-bearing assistance:** determine **who** is supporting the weight of the resident's extremity or body. For example, if the staff member supports some of the weight of the resident's hand while helping the resident to eat (e.g., lifting a spoon or a cup to mouth), or performs part of the activity for the resident, this is "weight-bearing" assistance for this activity. If the resident can lift the utensil or cup, but staff assistance is needed to guide the resident's hand to his or her mouth, this is guided maneuvering.
- Do **NOT** record the staff's assessment of the resident's potential capability to perform the ADL activity. The assessment of potential capability is covered in **ADL Functional Rehabilitation Potential** Item (G0900).
- Do **NOT** record the type and level of assistance that the resident "should" be receiving according to the written plan of care. The level of assistance actually provided might be very different from what is indicated in the plan. Record what actually happened.
- Do **NOT** include assistance provided by family or other visitors.
- **Some examples for coding for ADL Support Setup Help when the activity involves the following:**
  - Bed Mobility—handing the resident the bar on a trapeze, staff raises the ½ rails for the resident's use and then provides no further help.
  - Transfer—giving the resident a transfer board or locking the wheels on a wheelchair for safe transfer.
  - Locomotion
    - o Walking—handing the resident a walker or cane.
    - o Wheeling—unlocking the brakes on the wheelchair or adjusting foot pedals to facilitate foot motion while wheeling.
  - Dressing—retrieving clothes from the closet and laying out on the resident's bed; handing the resident a shirt.
  - Eating—cutting meat and opening containers at meals; giving one food item at a time.
  - Toilet Use—handing the resident a bedpan or placing articles necessary for changing an ostomy appliance within reach.
  - Personal Hygiene—providing a washbasin and grooming articles.
- **Supervision**
  - **Code Supervision** for residents seated together or in close proximity of one another during a meal who receive individual supervision with eating.
  - General supervision of a dining room is not the same as individual supervision of a resident and **is not** captured in the coding for Eating.

G0110: Activities of Daily Living (ADL) Assistance (cont.)

- **Coding activity did not occur, 8:**
  - **Toileting** would be **coded 8, activity did not occur**: only if elimination did not occur during the entire look-back period, or if family and/or non-facility staff toileted the resident 100% of the time over the entire 7-day look-back period.
  - **Locomotion** would be **coded 8, activity did not occur**: if the resident was on bed rest and did not get out of bed, and there was no locomotion via bed, wheelchair, or other means during the look-back period.
  - **Eating** would be **coded 8, activity did not occur**: if the resident received no nourishment by any route (oral, IV, TPN, enteral) during the 7-day look-back period, if the resident was not fed by facility staff during the 7-day look-back period, or if family and/or non-facility staff fed the resident 100% of the time over the entire 7-day look-back period.
- **Coding activity occurred only once or twice, 7:**
  - Walk in corridor would be **coded 7, activity occurred only once or twice**: if the resident came out of the room and ambulated in the hallway for a weekly tub bath but otherwise stayed in the room during the 7-day look-back period.
  - Locomotion off unit would be **coded 7, activity occurred only once or twice**: if the resident left the vicinity of his or her room only one or two times to attend an activity in another part of the building.
- **Residents with tube feeding, TPN, or IV fluids**
  - **Code extensive assistance (1 or 2 persons):** if the resident with tube feeding, TPN, or IV fluids did not participate in management of this nutrition but did participate in receiving oral nutrition. This is the correct code because the staff completed a portion of the ADL activity for the resident (managing the tube feeding, TPN, or IV fluids).
  - **Code totally dependent in eating:** only if resident was assisted in eating all food items and liquids at all meals and snacks (including tube feeding delivered totally by staff) and did not participate in any aspect of eating (e.g., did not pick up finger foods, did not give self tube feeding or assist with swallow or eating procedure).

Example of a Probing Conversation with Staff

1. Example of a probing conversation between the RN Assessment Coordinator and a nursing assistant (NA) regarding a resident's bed mobility assessment:

   RN: "Describe to me how Mrs. L. moves herself in bed. By that I mean once she is in bed, how does she move from sitting up to lying down, lying down to sitting up, turning side to side and positioning herself?"

   NA: "She can lay down and sit up by herself, but I help her turn on her side."

   RN: "She lays down and sits up without any verbal instructions or physical help?"

   NA: "No, I have to remind her to use her trapeze every time. But once I tell her how to do things, she can do it herself."

   RN: "How do you help her turn side to side?"

   NA: "She can help turn herself by grabbing onto her side rail. I tell her what to do. But she needs me to lift her bottom and guide her legs into a good position."

   RN: "Do you lift her by yourself or does someone help you?"

   NA: "I do it by myself."

   RN: "How many times during the last 7 days did you give this type of help?"

   NA: "Every day, probably 3 times each day."

G0110: Activities of Daily Living (ADL) Assistance (cont.)

In this example, the assessor inquired specifically how Mrs. L. moves to and from a lying position, how she turns from side to side, and how the resident positions herself while in bed. A resident can be independent in one aspect of bed mobility, yet require extensive assistance in another aspect. If the RN did not probe further, he or she would not have received enough information to make an accurate assessment of actual assistance Mrs. L. received. Because accurate coding is important as a basis for reporting on the type and amount of care provided, be sure to consider each activity definition fully.

> **Coding:** Bed Mobility ADL assistance would be **coded 3 (self-performance) and 2 (support provided), extensive assistance with a one person assist.**

Examples for G0110A, Bed Mobility

1. Mrs. D. can easily turn and position herself in bed and is able to sit up and lie down without any staff assistance at any time during the 7-day look-back period. She requires use of a single side rail that staff place in the up position when she is in bed.

   > **Coding:** G0110A1 would be **coded 0, independent.**
   > G0110A2 would be **coded 1, setup help only.**
   > **Rationale:** Resident is independent at all times in bed mobility during the 7-day look-back period and needs only setup help.

2. Resident favors lying on her right side. Because she has had a history of skin breakdown, staff must verbally remind her to reposition off her right side daily during the 7-day look-back period.

   > **Coding:** G0110A1 would be **coded 1, supervision.**
   > G0110A2 would be **coded 0, no setup or physical help from staff.**
   > **Rationale:** Resident requires staff supervision, cueing, and reminders for repositioning more than three times during the look-back period.

3. Resident favors lying on her right side. Because she has had a history of skin breakdown, staff must sometimes cue the resident and guide (non-weight-bearing assistance) the resident to place her hands on the side rail and encourage her to change her position when in bed daily over the 7-day look-back period.

   > **Coding:** G0110A1 would be **coded 2, limited assistance.**
   > G0110A2 would be **coded 2, one person physical assist.**
   > **Rationale:** Resident requires cueing and encouragement with setup and non-weight-bearing physical help daily during the 7-day look-back period.

4. Mr. Q. has slid to the foot of the bed four times during the 7-day look-back period. Two staff members had to physically lift and reposition him toward the head of the bed. Mr. Q. was able to assist by bending his knees and pushing with legs when reminded by staff.

   > **Coding:** G0110A1 would be **coded 3, extensive assistance.**
   > G0110A2 would be **coded 3, two+ persons physical assist.**
   > **Rationale:** Resident required weight-bearing assistance of two staff members on four occasions during the 7-day look-back period with bed mobility.

G0110: Activities of Daily Living (ADL) Assistance (cont.)

5. Mrs. S. is unable to physically turn, sit up, or lie down in bed. Two staff members must physically turn her every 2 hours without any participation at any time from her at any time during the 7-day look-back period. She must be physically assisted to a seated position in bed when reading.

    Coding: G0110A1 would be **coded 4, total dependence**.

    G0110A2 would be **coded 3, two+ persons physical assist**.

    Rationale: Resident did not participate at any time during the 7-day look-back period and required two staff to position her in bed.

Examples for G0110B, Transfer

1. When transferring from bed to chair or chair back to bed, the resident is able to stand up from a seated position (without requiring any physical or verbal help) and walk from the bed to chair and chair back to the bed every day during the 7-day look back period.

    Coding: G0110B1 would be **coded 0, independent**.

    G0110B2 would be **coded 0, no setup or physical help from staff**.

    Rationale: Resident is independent each and every time she transferred during the 7-day look-back period and required no setup or physical help from staff.

2. Staff must supervise the resident as she transfers from her bed to wheelchair daily. Staff must bring the chair next to the bed and then remind her to hold on to the chair and position her body slowly.

    Coding: G0110B1 would be **coded 1, supervision**.

    G0110B2 would be **coded 1, setup help only**.

    Rationale: Resident requires staff supervision, cueing, and reminders for safe transfer. This activity happened daily over the 7-day look-back period.

3. Mrs. H. is able to transfer from the bed to chair when she uses her walker. Staff place the walker near her bed and then assist the resident with guided maneuvering as she transfers. The resident was noted to transfer from bed to chair six times during the 7-day look-back period.

    Coding: G0110B1 would be **coded 2, limited assistance**.

    G0110B2 would be **coded 2, one person physical assist**.

    Rationale: Resident requires staff to set up her walker and provide non-weight-bearing assistance when she is ready to transfer. The activity happened six times during the 7-day look-back period.

4. Mrs. B. requires weight-bearing assistance of one staff member to partially lift and support her when being transferred. The resident was noted to have been transferred 14 times in the 7-day look-back period and each time required weight-bearing assistance.

    Coding: G0110B1 would be **coded 3, extensive assistance**.

    G0110B2 would be **coded 2, one person physical assist**.

    Rationale: Resident partially participates in the task of transferring. The resident was noted to have transferred 14 times during the 7-day look-back period, each time requiring weight-bearing assistance of one staff member.

G0110: Activities of Daily Living (ADL) Assistance (cont.)

5. Mr. T. is in a physically debilitated state due to surgery. Two staff members must physically lift and transfer him to a reclining chair daily using a mechanical lift. Mr. T. is unable to assist or participate in any way.

> **Coding:** G0110B1 would be **coded 4, total dependence**.
> G0110B2 would be **coded 3, two+ persons physical assist**.
> **Rationale:** Resident did not participate and required two staff to transfer him out of his bed. The resident was transferred out of bed to the chair daily during the 7-day look-back period.

6. Mrs. D. is post-operative for extensive surgical procedures. Because of her ventilator dependent status in addition to multiple surgical sites, her physician has determined that she must remain on total bed rest. During the 7-day look-back period the resident was not moved from the bed.

> **Coding:** G0110B1 would be **coded 8, activity did not occur**.
> G0110B2 would be **coded 8, ADL activity itself did not occur during entire period**.
> **Rationale:** Activity did not occur.

7. Mr. M. has Parkinson's disease and needs weight-bearing assistance of two staff to transfer from his bed to his wheelchair. During the 7-day look-back period, Mr. M. was transferred once from the bed to the wheelchair and once from wheelchair to bed.

> **Coding:** G0110B1 would be **coded 7, activity occurred only once or twice**.
> G0110B2 would be **coded 3, two+ persons physical assist**.
> **Rationale:** The activity happened only twice during the look-back period, with the support of two staff members.

Examples for G0110C, Walk in Room

1. Mr. R. is able to walk freely in his room (obtaining clothes from closet, turning on TV) without any cueing or physical assistance from staff at all during the entire 7-day look-back period.

> **Coding:** G0110C1 would be **coded 0, independent**.
> G0110C2 would be **coded 0, no setup or physical help from staff**.
> **Rationale:** Resident is independent.

2. Mr. B. was able to walk in his room daily, but a staff member needed to cue and stand by during ambulation because the resident has had a history of an unsteady gait.

> **Coding:** G0110C1 would be **coded 1, supervision**.
> G0110C2 would be **coded 0, no setup or physical help from staff**.
> **Rationale:** Resident requires staff supervision, cueing, and reminders daily while walking in his room, but did not need setup or physical help from staff.

G0110: Activities of Daily Living (ADL) Assistance (cont.)

3. Mr. K. is able to walk in his room, and, with hand-held assist from one staff member, the resident was noted to ambulate daily during the 7-day look-back period.

   Coding: G0110C1 would be **coded 2, limited assistance**.
   G0110C2 would be **coded 2, one person physical assist**.

   Rationale: Resident requires hand-held (non-weight-bearing) assistance of one staff member daily for ambulation in his room.

4. Mr. A. has a bone spur on his heel and has difficulty ambulating in his room. He requires staff to help support him when he selects clothing from his closet. During the 7-day look-back period the resident was able to ambulate with weight-bearing assistance from one staff member in his room four times.

   Coding: G0110C1 would be **coded 3, extensive assistance**.
   G0110C2 would be **coded 2, one person physical assist**.

   Rationale: The resident was able to ambulate in his room four times during the 7-day look-back period with weight-bearing assistance of one staff member.

5. Mr. J. is attending physical therapy for transfer and gait training. He does not ambulate on the unit or in his room at this time. He calls for assistance to stand pivot to a commode next to his bed.

   Coding: G0110C1 would be **coded 8, activity did not occur**.
   G0110C2 would be **coded 8, ADL activity itself did not occur during entire period**.

   Rationale: Activity did not occur.

Examples for G0110D, Walk in Corridor

1. Mr. X. ambulated daily up and down the hallway on his unit with a cane and did not require any setup or physical help from staff at any time during the 7-day look-back period.

   Coding: G0110D1 would be **coded 0, independent**.
   G0110D2 would be **coded 0, no setup or physical help from staff**.

   Rationale: Resident requires no setup or help from the staff at any time during the entire 7-day look-back period.

2. Staff members provided verbal cueing while resident was walking in the hallway every day during the 7-day look-back period to ensure that the resident walked slowly and safely.

   Coding: G0110D1 would be **coded 1, supervision**.
   G0110D2 would be **coded 0, no setup or physical help from staff**.

   Rationale: Resident requires staff supervision, cueing, and reminders daily while ambulating in the hallway during the 7-day look-back period.

G0110: Activities of Daily Living (ADL) Assistance (cont.)

3. Mrs. Q. requires verbal cueing and physical guiding of her hand placement on the walker when walking down the unit hallway. She needs frequent verbal reminders of how to use her walker, where to place her hands, and to pick up her feet. Mrs. Q. needs to be physically guided to the day room. During the 7-day look-back period the resident was noted to ambulate in the hallway daily and required the above-mentioned support from one staff member.

    Coding: G0110D1 would be **coded 2, limited assistance**.

    G0110D2 would be **coded 2, one person physical assist**.

    Rationale: Resident requires non-weight-bearing assistance of one staff member for safe ambulation daily during the 7-day look-back period.

4. A resident had back surgery 2 months ago. Two staff members must physically support the resident as he is walking down the hallway because of his unsteady gait and balance problem. During the 7-day look-back period the resident was ambulated in the hallway three times with physical assist of two staff members.

    Coding: G0110D1 would be **coded 3, extensive assistance**.

    G0110D2 would be **coded 3, two+ persons physical assist**.

    Rationale: The resident was ambulated three times during the 7-day look-back period, with the resident partially participating in the task. Two staff members were required to physically support the resident so he could ambulate.

5. Mrs. J. ambulated in the corridor once with supervision and once with non-weight-bearing assistance of one staff member during the 7-day look-back period.

    Coding: G0110D1 would be **coded 7, activity occurred only once or twice**.

    G0110D2 would be **coded 2, one person physical assist**.

    Rationale: The activity occurred only twice during the look-back period. It does not matter that the level of assistance provided by staff was at different levels. During ambulation, the most support provided was physical help by one staff member.

Examples for G0110E, Locomotion on Unit

1. Mrs. L. is on complete bed rest. During the 7-day look-back period she did not get out of bed or leave the room.

    Coding: G0110E1 would be **coded 8, activity did not occur**.

    G0110E2 would be **coded 8, ADL activity itself did not occur during entire period**.

    Rationale: The resident was on bed rest during the look-back period and never left her room.

G0110: Activities of Daily Living (ADL) Assistance (cont.)

Examples for G0110F, Locomotion off Unit

1. Mr. R. does not like to go off his nursing unit. He prefers to stay in his room or the day room on his unit. He has visitors on a regular basis, and they visit with him in the day room on the unit. During the 7-day look-back period the resident did not leave the unit for any reason.

   > **Coding:** G0110F1 would be **coded 8, activity did not occur**.
   > G0110F2 would be **coded 8, ADL activity itself did not occur during entire period**.
   > **Rationale:** Activity did not occur at all.

2. Mr. Q. is a wheelchair-bound and is able to self-propel on the unit. On two occasions during the 7-day look-back period, he self-propelled off the unit into the courtyard.

   > **Coding:** G0110F1 would be **coded 7, activity occurred only once or twice**.
   > G0110F2 would be **coded 0, no setup or physical help from staff**.
   > **Rationale:** The activity of going off the unit happened only twice during the look-back period with no help or oversight from staff.

3. Mr. H. enjoyed walking in the nursing home garden when weather permitted. Due to inclement weather during the assessment period, he required various levels of assistance on the days he walked through the garden. On two occasions, he required limited assistance for balance of one staff person and on another occasion he only required supervision. On one day he was able to walk through the garden completely by himself.

   > **Coding:** G0110F1 would be **coded 1, supervision**.
   > G0110F2 would be **coded 2, one person physical assist**.
   > **Rationale:** Activity did not occur at any one level for three times and he did not require physical assistance for at least three times. The most support provided by staff was one person assist.

Examples for G0110G, Dressing

1. Mrs. C. did not feel well and chose to stay in her room. She requested to stay in night clothes and rest in bed for the entire 7-day look-back period. Each day, after washing up, Mrs. C. changed night clothes with staff assistance to guide her arms and assist in guiding her nightgown over her head and buttoning the front.

   > **Coding:** G0110G1 would be **coded 2, limited assistance**.
   > G0110G2 would be **coded 2, one person physical assist**.
   > **Rationale:** Resident was highly involved in the activity and changed clothing daily with non-weight-bearing assistance from one staff member during the 7-day look-back period.

G0110: Activities of Daily Living (ADL) Assistance (cont.)

Examples for G0110H, Eating

1. After staff deliver Mr. K.'s meal tray, he consumes all food and fluids without any cueing or physical help during the entire 7-day look-back period.

   Coding: G0110H1 would be **coded 0, independent**.

   G0110H2 would be **coded 0, no setup or physical help from staff**.

   Rationale: Resident is completely independent in eating during the entire 7-day look-back period.

2. One staff member had to verbally cue the resident to eat slowly and drink throughout each meal during the 7-day look-back period.

   Coding: G0110H1 would be **coded 1, supervision**.

   G0110H2 would be **coded 0, no setup or physical help from staff**.

   Rationale: Resident required staff supervision, cueing, and reminders for safe meal completion daily during the 7-day look-back period.

3. Mr. V. is able to eat by himself. Staff must set up the tray, cut the meat, open containers, and hand him the utensils. Each day during the 7-day look-back period, Mr. V. required more help during the evening meal, as he was tired and less interested in completing his meal. In the evening, in addition to encouraging the resident to eat and handing him his utensils and cups, staff must also guide the resident's hand so he will get the utensil to his mouth.

   Coding: G0110H1 would be **coded 2, limited assistance**.

   G0110H2 would be **coded 2, one person physical assist**.

   Rationale: Resident is unable to complete the evening meal without staff providing him non-weight-bearing assistance daily.

4. Mr. F. begins eating each meal daily by himself. During the 7-day look-back period, after he had eaten only his bread, he stated he was tired and unable to complete the meal. One staff member physically supported his hand to bring the food to his mouth and provided verbal cues to swallow the food. The resident was then able to complete the meal.

   Coding: G0110H1 would be **coded 3, extensive assistance**.

   G0110H2 would be **coded 2, one person physical assist**.

   Rationale: Resident partially participated in the task daily at each meal, but one staff member provided weight-bearing assistance with some portion of each meal.

5. Mrs. U. is severely cognitively impaired. She is unable to feed herself. She relied on one staff member for all nourishment during the 7-day look-back period.

   Coding: G0110H1 would be **coded 4, total dependence**.

   G0110H2 would be **coded 2, one person physical assist**.

   Rationale: Resident did not participate and required one staff person to feed her all of her meals during the 7-day look-back period.

G0110: Activities of Daily Living (ADL) Assistance (cont.)

6. Mrs. D. receives all of her nourishment via a gastrostomy tube. She did not consume any food or fluid by mouth. During the 7-day look-back period, she did not participate in the gastrostomy nourishment process.

> **Coding:** G0110H1 would be **coded 4, total dependence**.
> G0110H2 would be **coded 2, one person physical assist**.
> **Rationale:** During the 7-day look-back period, she did not participate in eating and/or receiving of her tube feed during the entire period. She required full staff performance of these functions.

Examples for G0110I, Toilet Use

1. Mrs. L. transferred herself to the toilet, adjusted her clothing, and performed the necessary personal hygiene after using the toilet without any staff assistance daily during the entire 7-day look-back period.

> **Coding:** G0110I1 would be **coded 0, independent**.
> G0110I2 would be **coded 0, no setup or physical help from staff**.
> **Rationale:** Resident was independent in all her toileting tasks.

2. Staff member must remind resident to toilet frequently during the day and to unzip and zip pants and to wash his hands after using the toilet. This occurred multiple times each day during the 7-day look-back period.

> **Coding:** G0110I1 would be **coded 1, supervision**.
> G0110I2 would be **coded 0, no setup or physical help from staff**.
> **Rationale:** Resident required staff supervision, cueing and reminders daily.

3. Staff must assist Mr. P. to zip his pants, hand him a washcloth, and remind him to wash his hands after using the toilet daily. This occurred multiple times each day during the 7-day look-back period.

> **Coding:** G0110I1 would be **coded 2, limited assistance**.
> G0110I2 would be **coded 2, one person physical assist**.
> **Rationale:** Resident required staff to perform non-weight-bearing activities to complete the task multiple times each day during the 7-day look-back period.

4. Mrs. M. has had recent bouts of vertigo. During the 7-day look-back period, the resident required one staff member to assist and provide weight-bearing support to her as she transferred to the bedside commode four times.

> **Coding:** G0110I1 would be **coded 3, extensive assistance**.
> G0110I2 would be **coded 2, one person physical assist**.
> **Rationale:** During the 7-day look-back period, the resident required weight-bearing assistance with the support of one staff member to use the commode four times.

G0110: Activities of Daily Living (ADL) Assistance (cont.)

5. Miss W. is cognitively and physically impaired. During the 7-day look-back period, she was on strict bed rest. Staff were unable to physically transfer her to toilet during this time. Miss W. is incontinent of both bowel and bladder. One staff member was required to provide all the care for her elimination and hygiene needs several times each day.

    Coding: G0110I1 would be **coded 4, total dependence**.

    G0110I2 would be **coded 2, one person physical assist**.

    Rationale: Resident did not participate and required one staff person to provide total care for toileting and hygiene each time during the entire 7-day look-back period.

Examples for G0110J, Personal Hygiene

1. The nurse assistant takes Mr. L.'s comb, toothbrush, and toothpaste from the drawer and places them at the bathroom sink. Mr. L. combs his own hair and brushes his own teeth daily. During the 7-day look-back period, he required cueing to brush his teeth on three occasions.

    Coding: G0110J1 would be **coded 1, supervision**.

    G0110J2 would be **coded 1, setup help only**.

    Rationale: Staff placed grooming devices at sink for his use, and during the 7-day look-back period staff provided cueing three times.

2. Mrs. J. normally completes all hygiene tasks independently. Three mornings during the 7-day look-back period, however, she was unable to brush and style her hair because of elbow pain, so a staff member did it for her.

    Coding: G0110J1 would be **coded 3, extensive assistance**.

    G0110J2 would be **coded 2, one person physical assist**.

    Rationale: A staff member had to complete part of the activity for the resident 3 days during the look-back period; the assistance was non-weight-bearing.

G0120: Bathing

G0120. Bathing	
How resident takes full-body bath/shower, sponge bath, and transfers in/out of tub/shower (**excludes** washing of back and hair). Code for **most dependent** in self-performance and support	
Enter Code ☐	**A. Self-performance** 0. **Independent** - no help provided 1. **Supervision** - oversight help only 2. **Physical help limited to transfer only** 3. **Physical help in part of bathing activity** 4. **Total dependence** 8. **Activity itself did not occur** or family and/or non-facility staff provided care 100% of the time for that activity over the entire 7-day period
Enter Code ☐	**B. Support provided** (Bathing support codes are as defined in item **G0110 column 2, ADL Support Provided**, above)

G0120: Bathing (cont.)

Item Rationale

Health-related Quality of Life

- The resident's choices regarding his or her bathing schedule should be accommodated when possible so that facility routine does not conflict with resident's desired routine.

Planning for Care

- The care plan should include interventions to address the resident's unique needs for bathing. These interventions should be periodically evaluated and, if objectives were not met, alternative approaches developed to encourage maintenance of bathing abilities.

> **DEFINITIONS**
>
> **BATHING**
> How the resident takes a full body bath, shower or sponge bath, including transfers in and out of the tub or shower. It does not include the washing of back or hair.

Coding Instructions for G0120A, Self Performance

Code for the maximum amount of assistance the resident received during the bathing episodes.

- **Code 0, independent:** if the resident required no help from staff.
- **Code 1, supervision:** if the resident required oversight help only.
- **Code 2, physical help limited to transfer only:** if the resident is able to perform the bathing activity, but required help with the transfer only.
- **Code 3, physical help in part of bathing activity:** if the resident required assistance with some aspect of bathing.
- **Code 4, total dependence:** if the resident is unable to participate in any of the bathing activity.
- **Code 8, ADL activity itself did not occur during entire period:** if the activity did not occur or family and/or non-facility staff provided care 100% of the time for that activity over the entire 7-day period.

Coding Instructions for G0120B, Support Provided

- Bathing support codes are as defined **ADL Support Provided** item (G0110), Column 2.

Coding Tips

- Bathing is the only ADL activity for which the ADL Self-Performance codes in Item G0110, **Column 1 (Self-Performance),** do not apply. A unique set of self-performance codes is used in the bathing assessment given that bathing may not occur as frequently as the other ADLs in the 7-day look-back period.
- If a nursing home has a policy that all residents are supervised when bathing (i.e., they are never left alone while in the bathroom for a bath or shower, regardless of resident capability), it is appropriate to code the resident self-performance as supervision, even if the supervision is precautionary because the resident is still being individually supervised. Support for bathing in this instance would be coded according to whether or not the staff had to actually assist the resident during the bathing activity.

G0120: Bathing (cont.)

Examples

1. Resident received verbal cueing and encouragement to take twice-weekly showers. Once staff walked resident to bathroom, he bathed himself with periodic oversight.

   Coding: G0120A would be **coded 1, supervision**.

   G0120B would be **coded 0, no setup or physical help from staff**.

   Rationale: Resident needed only supervision to perform the bathing activity with no setup or physical help from staff.

2. For one bath, the resident received physical help of one person to position self in bathtub. However, because of her fluctuating moods, she received total help for her other bath from one staff member.

   Coding: G0120A would be **coded 4, total dependence**.

   G0120B would be **coded 2, one person physical assist**.

   Rationale: Coding directions for bathing state, "code for most dependent in self performance and support." Resident's most dependent episode during the 7-day look-back period was total help with the bathing activity with assist from one staff person.

3. On Monday, one staff member helped transfer resident to tub and washed his legs. On Thursday, the resident had physical help of one person to get into tub but washed himself completely.

   Coding: G0120A would be **coded 3, physical help in part of bathing activity**.

   G0120B would be **coded 2, one person physical assist**.

   Rationale: Resident's most dependent episode during the 7-day look-back period was assistance with part of the bathing activity from one staff person.

G0300: Balance During Transitions and Walking

G0300. Balance During Transitions and Walking	
After observing the resident, **code the following walking and transition items for most dependent**	
Coding: 0. **Steady at all times** 1. **Not steady, but <u>able</u> to stabilize without staff assistance** 2. **Not steady, <u>only able</u> to stabilize with staff assistance** 8. **Activity did not occur**	↓ **Enter Codes in Boxes**
	☐ A. **Moving from seated to standing position**
	☐ B. **Walking** (with assistive device if used)
	☐ C. **Turning around** and facing the opposite direction while walking
	☐ D. **Moving on and off toilet**
	☐ E. **Surface-to-surface transfer** (transfer between bed and chair or wheelchair)

G0300: Balance During Transitions and Walking (cont.)

Item Rationale

Health-related Quality of Life

- Individuals with impaired balance and unsteadiness during transitions and walking
  - are at increased risk for falls;
  - often are afraid of falling;
  - may limit their physical and social activity, becoming socially isolated and despondent about limitations; and
  - can become increasingly immobile.

> **DEFINITIONS**
>
> **INTERDISCIPLINARY TEAM**
> Refers to a team that includes staff from multiple disciplines such as nursing, therapy, physicians, and other advanced practitioners.

Planning for Care

- Individuals with impaired balance and unsteadiness should be evaluated for the need for
  - rehabilitation or assistive devices;
  - supervision or physical assistance for safety; and/or
  - environmental modification.
- Care planning should focus on preventing further decline of function, and/or on return of function, depending on resident-specific goals.
- Assessment should identify all related risk factors in order to develop effective care plans to maintain current abilities, slow decline, and/or promote improvement in the resident's functional ability.

Steps for Assessment

1. Complete this assessment for all residents.
2. Throughout the 7-day look-back period, interdisciplinary team members should carefully observe and document observations of the resident during transitions from sitting to standing, walking, turning, transferring on and off toilet, and transferring from wheelchair to bed and bed to wheelchair (for residents who use a wheelchair).
3. If staff have not systematically documented the resident's stability in these activities at least once during the 7-day look-back period, use the following process to code these items:
   a. Before beginning the activity, explain what the task is and what you are observing for.
   b. Have assistive devices the resident normally uses available.
   c. Start with the resident sitting up on the edge of his or her bed, in a chair or in a wheelchair (if he or she generally uses one).
   d. Ask the resident to stand up and stay still for 3-5 seconds. **Moving from seated to standing position (G0300A) should be rated at this time.**
   e. Ask the resident to walk approximately 15 feet using his or her usual **assistive device**. **Walking (G0300B) should be rated at this time.**

G0300: Balance During Transitions and Walking (cont.)

f. Ask the resident to turn around. **Turning around (G0300C) should be rated at this time.**

g. Ask the **resident to walk or wheel** from a starting point in his or her room into the bathroom, **prepare for toileting** as he or she normally does (including taking down pants or other clothes; underclothes can be kept on for this observation), and sit on the toilet. **Moving on and off toilet (G0300D) should be rated at this time.**

h. Ask residents who are not ambulatory and who use a wheelchair for mobility to transfer from a seated position in the wheelchair to a seated position on the bed. **Surface-to-surface transfer should be rated at this time (G0300E).**

Balance During Transitions and Walking Algorithm

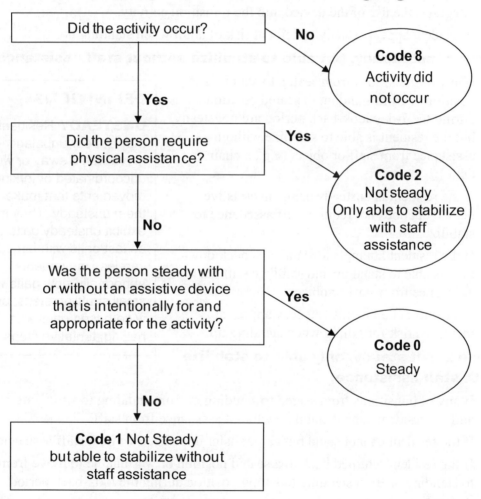

G0300: Balance During Transitions and Walking (cont.)

Coding Instructions G0300A, Moving from Seated to Standing Position

Code for the least steady episode, using assistive device if applicable.

- **Code 0, steady at all times:**
  - If all of the transitions from seated to standing position and from standing to seated position observed during the 7-day look-back period are steady.
  - If resident is stable when standing up using the arms of a chair or an assistive device identified for this purpose (such as a walker, locked wheelchair, or grab bar).
  - If an assistive device or equipment is used, the resident appropriately plans and integrates the use of the device into the transition activity.
  - If resident appears steady and not at risk of a fall when standing up.

- **Code 1, not steady, but able to stabilize without staff assistance:**
  - If any of transitions from seated to standing position or from standing to seated position during the 7-day look-back period are not steady, but the resident is able to stabilize without assistance from staff or object (e.g., a chair or table).
  - If the resident is unsteady using an assistive device but does not require staff assistance to stabilize.
  - If the resident attempts to stand, sits back down, then is able to stand up and stabilize without assistance from staff or object.
  - Residents coded in this category appear at increased risk for falling when standing up.

> **DEFINITIONS**
>
> **UNSTEADY** Residents may appear unbalanced or move with a sway or with uncoordinated or jerking movements that make them unsteady. They might exhibit unsteady gaits such as fast gaits with large, careless movements; abnormally slow gaits with small shuffling steps; or wide-based gaits with halting, tentative steps.

- **Code 2, not steady, only able to stabilize with staff assistance:**
  - If any of transitions from seated to standing or from standing to sitting are not steady, and the resident cannot stabilize without assistance from staff.
  - If the resident cannot stand but can transfer unassisted without staff assistance.
  - If the resident returned back to a seated position or was unable to move from a seated to standing or from standing to sitting position during the look-back period.
  - Residents coded in this category appear at high risk for falling during transitions.
  - If a lift device (a mechanical device operated by another person) is used because the resident requires staff assistance to stabilize, code as 2.

- **Code 8, activity did not occur:** if the resident did not move from seated to standing position during the 7-day look-back period.

G0300: Balance During Transitions and Walking (cont.)

Examples for G0300A, Moving from Seated to Standing Position

1. A resident sits up in bed, stands, and begins to sway, but steadies herself and sits down smoothly into her wheelchair.

    Coding: G0300A would be **coded 1, not steady, but able to stabilize without staff assistance**.

    Rationale: Resident was unsteady, but she was able to stabilize herself without assistance from staff.

2. A resident requires the use of a gait belt and physical assistance in order to stand.

    Coding: G0300A would be **coded 2, not steady, only able to stabilize with staff assistance**.

    Rationale: Resident required staff assistance to stand during the observation period.

3. A resident stands steadily by pushing himself up using the arms of a chair.

    Coding: G0300A would be **coded 0, steady at all times**.

    Rationale: Even though the resident used the arms of the chair to push himself up, he was steady at all times during the activity.

4. A resident locks his wheelchair and uses the arms of his wheelchair to attempt to stand. On the first attempt, he rises about halfway to a standing position then sits back down. On the second attempt, he is able to stand steadily.

    Coding: G0300A would be **coded 1, not steady, but able to stabilize without staff assistance**.

    Rationale: Even though the second attempt at standing was steady, the first attempt suggests he is unsteady and at risk for falling during this transition.

Coding Instructions G0300B, Walking (with Assistive Device if Used)

Code for the least steady episode, using assistive device if applicable.

- **Code 0, steady at all times:**
    — If during the 7-day look-back period the resident's walking (with assistive devices if used) is steady at all times.
    — If an assistive device or equipment is used, the resident appropriately plans and integrates the use of the device and is steady while walking with it.
    — Residents in this category do not appear at risk for falls.
    — Residents who walk with an abnormal gait and/or with an assistive device can be steady, and if they are they should be coded in this category.

- **Code 1, not steady, but able to stabilize without staff assistance:**
    — If during the 7-day look-back period the resident appears unsteady while walking (with assistive devices if used) but does not require staff assistance to stabilize.
    — Residents coded in this category appear at risk for falling while walking.

G0300: Balance During Transitions and Walking (cont.)

- **Code 2, not steady, only able to stabilize with staff assistance:**
  - If during the-7-day look-back period the resident at any time appeared unsteady and required staff assistance to be stable and safe while walking.
  - If the resident fell when walking during the look-back period.
  - Residents coded in this category appear at high risk for falling while walking.
- **Code 8, activity did not occur:**
  - If the resident did not walk during the 7-day look-back period.

Examples for G0300B, Walking (with Assistive Device if Used)

1. A resident with a recent stroke walks using a hemi-walker in her right hand because of left-sided weakness. Her gait is slow and short-stepped and slightly unsteady as she walks, she leans to the left and drags her left foot along the ground on most steps. She has not had to steady herself using any furniture or grab bars.

    Coding: G0300B would be **coded 1, not steady, but able to stabilize without staff assistance**.

    Rationale: Resident's gait is unsteady with or without an assistive device but does not require staff assistance.

2. A resident with Parkinson's disease ambulates with a walker. His posture is stooped, and he walks slowly with a short-stepped shuffling gait. On some occasions, his gait speeds up, and it appears he has difficulty slowing down. On multiple occasions during the 7-day observation period he has to steady himself using a handrail or a piece of furniture in addition to his walker.

    Coding: G0300B would be **coded 1, not steady, but able to stabilize without staff assistance**.

    Rationale: Resident has an unsteady gait but can stabilize himself using an object such as a handrail or piece of furniture.

3. A resident who had a recent total hip replacement ambulates with a walker. Although she is able to bear weight on her affected side, she is unable to advance her walker safely without staff assistance.

    Coding: G0300B would be **coded 2, not steady, only able to stabilize with staff assistance**.

    Rationale: Resident requires staff assistance to walk steadily and safely at any time during the observation period.

4. A resident with multi-infarct dementia walks with a short-stepped, shuffling-type gait. Despite the gait abnormality, she is steady.

    Coding: G0300B would be **coded 0, steady at all times**.

    Rationale: Resident walks steadily (with or without a normal gait and/or the use of an assistive device) at all times during the observation period.

G0300: Balance During Transitions and Walking (cont.)

Coding Instructions G0300C, Turning Around and Facing the Opposite Direction while Walking

Code for the least steady episode, using an assistive device if applicable.

- **Code 0, steady at all times:**
  - If all observed turns to face the opposite direction are steady without assistance of a staff during the 7-day look-back period.
  - If the resident is stable making these turns when using an assistive device.
  - If an assistive device or equipment is used, the resident appropriately plans and integrates the use of the device into the transition activity.
  - Residents coded as 0 should not appear to be at risk of a fall during a transition.

- **Code 1, not steady, but able to stabilize without staff assistance:**
  - If any transition that involves turning around to face the opposite direction is not steady, but the resident stabilizes without assistance from a staff.
  - If the resident is unstable with an assistive device but does not require staff assistance.
  - Residents coded in this category appear at increased risk for falling during transitions.

- **Code 2, not steady, only able to stabilize with staff assistance:**
  - If any transition that involves turning around to face the opposite direction is not steady, and the resident cannot stabilize without assistance from a staff.
  - If the resident fell when turning around to face the opposite direction during the look-back period.
  - Residents coded in this category appear at high risk for falling during transitions.

- **Code 8, activity did not occur:**
  - If the resident did not turn around to face the opposite direction while walking during the 7-day look-back period.

Examples for G0300C, Turning Around and Facing the Opposite Direction while Walking

1. A resident with Alzheimer's disease frequently wanders on the hallway. On one occasion, a nursing assistant noted that he was about to fall when turning around. However, by the time she got to him, he had steadied himself on the handrail.

   Coding: G0300C would be **coded 1, Not steady, but able to stabilize without staff assistance**.
   Rationale: The resident was unsteady when turning but able to steady himself on an object, in this instance, a handrail.

G0300: Balance During Transitions and Walking (cont.)

2. A resident with severe arthritis in her knee ambulates with a single-point cane. A nursing assistant observes her lose her balance while turning around to sit in a chair. The nursing assistant is able to get to her before she falls and lowers her gently into the chair.

> **Coding:** G0300C would be **coded 2, not steady, only able to stabilize with staff assistance**.
>
> **Rationale:** The resident was unsteady when turning around and would have fallen without staff assistance.

Coding for G0300D, Moving on and off Toilet

Code for the least steady episode of moving on and off a toilet or portable commode, using an assistive device if applicable. Include stability while manipulating clothing to allow toileting to occur in this rating.

- **Code 0, steady at all times:**
    - If all of the observed transitions on and off the toilet during the 7-day look-back period are steady without assistance of a staff.
    - If the resident is stable when transferring using an assistive device or object identified for this purpose.
    - If an assistive device is used (e.g., grab bar), the resident appropriately plans and integrates the use of the device into the transition activity.
    - Residents coded as 0 should not appear to be at risk of a fall during a transition.
- **Code 1, not steady, but able to stabilize without staff assistance:**
    - If any transitions on or off the toilet during the7-day look-back period are not steady, **but** the resident stabilizes **without** assistance from a staff.
    - If resident is unstable with an assistive device but does not require staff assistance.
    - Residents coded in this category appear at increased risk for falling during transitions.
- **Code 2, not steady, only able to stabilize with staff assistance:**
    - If any transitions on or off the toilet during the 7-day look-back period are not steady, and the resident cannot stabilize without assistance from a staff.
    - If the resident fell when moving on or off the toilet during the look-back period.
    - Residents coded in this category appear at high risk for falling during transitions.
    - If lift device is used.
- **Code 8, activity did not occur:**
    - If the resident did not transition on and off the toilet during the 7-day look-back period.

G0300: Balance During Transitions and Walking (cont.)

Examples for G0300D, Moving on and off Toilet

1. A resident sits up in bed, stands up, pivots and grabs her walker. She then steadily walks to the bathroom where she pivots, pulls down her underwear, uses the grab bar and smoothly sits on the commode using the grab bar to guide her. After finishing, she stands and pivots using the grab bar and smoothly ambulates out of her room with her walker.

    Coding: G0300D would be **coded 0, steady at all times**.

    Rationale: This resident's use of the grab bar was not to prevent a fall after being unsteady, but to maintain steadiness during her transitions. The resident was able to smoothly and steadily transfer onto the toilet, using a grab bar.

2. A resident wheels her wheelchair into the bathroom, stands up, begins to lift her dress, sways, and grabs onto the grab bar to steady herself. When she sits down on the toilet, she leans to the side and must push herself away from the towel bar to sit upright steadily.

    Coding: G0300D would be **coded 1, not steady, but able to stabilize without staff assistance**.

    Rationale: The resident was unsteady when disrobing to toilet but was able to steady herself with a grab bar.

3. A resident wheels his wheelchair into the bathroom, stands, begins to pull his pants down, sways, and grabs onto the grab bar to steady himself. When he sits down on the toilet, he leans to the side and must push himself away from the sink to sit upright steadily. When finished, he stands, sways, and then is able to steady himself with the grab bar.

    Coding: G0300D would be **coded 1, not steady, but able to stabilize without staff assistance**.

    Rationale: The resident was unsteady when disrobing to toilet but was able to steady himself with a grab bar.

Coding Instructions G0300E, Surface-to-Surface Transfer (Transfer between Bed and Chair or Wheelchair)

Code for the least steady episode.

*   **Code 0, steady at all times:**
    — If all of the observed transfers during the 7-day look-back period are steady without assistance of a staff.
    — If the resident is stable when transferring using an assistive device identified for this purpose.
    — If an assistive device or equipment is used, the resident uses it independently and appropriately plans and integrates the use of the device into the transition activity.
    — Residents **coded 0** should not appear to be at risk of a fall during a transition.

G0300: Balance During Transitions and Walking (cont.)

- **Code 1, not steady, but able to stabilize without staff assistance:**
  - If any transfers during the look-back period are not steady, but the resident stabilizes without assistance from a staff.
  - If the resident is unstable with an assistive device but does not require staff assistance.
  - Residents coded in this category appear at increased risk for falling during transitions.

- **Code 2, not steady, only able to stabilize with staff assistance:**
  - If any transfers during the 7-day look-back period are not steady, and the resident can only stabilize with assistance from a staff.
  - If the resident fell during a surface-to-surface transfer during the look-back period.
  - Residents coded in this category appear at high risk for falling during transitions.
  - If a lift device (a mechanical device that is completely operated by another person) is used, and this mechanical device is being used because the resident requires staff assistance to stabilize, **code 2**.

- **Code 8, activity did not occur:**
  - If the resident did not transfer between bed and chair or wheelchair during the 7-day look-back period.

Examples for G0300E, Surface-to-Surface Transfer (Transfer Between Bed and Chair or Wheelchair)

1. A resident who uses her wheelchair for mobility stands up from the edge of her bed, pivots, and sits in her locked wheelchair in a steady fashion.

   Coding: G0300E would be **coded 0, steady at all times**.
   Rationale: The resident was steady when transferring from bed to wheelchair.

2. A resident who needs assistance ambulating transfers to his chair from the bed. He is observed to stand halfway up and then sit back down on the bed. On a second attempt, a nursing assistant helps him stand up straight, pivot, and sit down in his chair.

   Coding: G0300E would be **coded 2, not steady, only able to stabilize with staff assistance**.
   Rationale: The resident was unsteady when transferring from bed to chair and required staff assistance to make a steady transfer.

3. A resident with an above-the-knee amputation sits on the edge of the bed and, using his locked wheelchair due to unsteadiness and the nightstand for leverage, stands and transfers to his wheelchair rapidly and almost misses the seat. He is able to steady himself using the nightstand and sit down into the wheelchair without falling to the floor.

   Coding: G0300E would be **coded 1, not steady, but able to stabilize without staff assistance**.

G0300: Balance During Transitions and Walking (cont.)

Rationale: The resident was unsteady when transferring from bed to wheelchair but did not require staff assistance to complete the activity.

4. A resident who uses her wheelchair for mobility stands up from the edge of her bed, sways to the right, but then is quickly able to pivot and sits in her locked wheelchair in a steady fashion.

> **Coding:** G0300E would be **coded 1, not steady, but able to stabilize without staff assistance**.
>
> **Rationale:** The resident was unsteady when transferring from bed to wheelchair but was able to steady herself without staff assistance or an object.

Additional examples for G0300A-E, Balance during Transitions and Walking

1. A resident sits up in bed, stands up, pivots and sits in her locked wheelchair. She then wheels her chair to the bathroom where she stands, pivots, lifts gown and smoothly sits on the commode.

> **Coding:** G0300A, G0300D, G0300E would be **coded 0, steady at all times**.
>
> **Rationale:** The resident was steady during each activity.

G0400: Functional Limitation in Range of Motion

G0400. Functional Limitation in Range of Motion	
Code for limitation that interfered with daily functions or placed resident at risk of injury	
Coding: 0. **No impairment** 1. **Impairment on one side** 2. **Impairment on both sides**	↓ **Enter Codes in Boxes** ☐ A. **Upper extremity** (shoulder, elbow, wrist, hand) ☐ B. **Lower extremity** (hip, knee, ankle, foot)

Intent: The intent of G0400 is to determine whether functional limitation in range of motion (ROM) interferes with the resident's activities of daily living or places him or her at risk of injury. When completing this item, staff should refer back to item G0110 and view the limitation in ROM taking into account activities that the resident is able to perform.

> **DEFINITIONS**
>
> **FUNCTIONAL LIMITATION IN RANGE OF MOTION** Limited ability to move a joint that interferes with daily functioning (particularly with activities of daily living) or places the resident at risk of injury.

Item Rationale

Health-related Quality of Life

- Functional impairment could place the resident at risk of injury or interfere with performance of activities of daily living.

Planning for Care

- Individualized care plans should address possible reversible causes such as de-conditioning and adverse side effects of medications or other treatments.

G0400: Functional Limitation in Range of Motion (cont.)

Steps for Assessment

1. Review the medical record for references to functional range of motion limitation during the 7-day look-back period.
2. Talk with staff members who work with the resident as well as family/significant others about any impairment in functional ROM.
3. Coding for functional ROM limitations is a 3 step process:

   - Test the resident's upper and lower extremity ROM (See #6 below for examples).
   - If the resident is noted to have limitation of upper and/or lower extremity ROM, review G0110 and/or directly observe the resident to determine if the limitation interferes with function or places the resident at risk for injury.
   - Code G0400 A/B as appropriate based on the above assessment.

4. Assess the resident's ROM bilaterally at the shoulder, elbow, wrist, hand, hip, knee, ankle, foot, and other joints unless contraindicated (e.g., recent fracture, joint replacement or pain).
5. Staff observations of various activities, including ADLs, may be used to determine if any ROM limitations impact the resident's functional abilities.
6. Although this item codes for the presence or absence of functional limitation related to ROM; thorough assessment ought to be comprehensive and follow standards of practice for evaluating ROM impairment. Below are some suggested assessment strategies:

   - Ask the resident to follow your verbal instructions for each movement.
   - Demonstrate each movement (e.g., ask the resident to do what you are doing).
   - Actively assist the resident with the movements by supporting his or her extremity and guiding it through the joint ROM.

Lower Extremity – includes hip, knee, ankle, and foot

While resident is lying supine in a flat bed, instruct the resident to flex (pull toes up towards head) and extend (push toes down away from head) each foot. Then ask the resident to lift his or her leg one at a time, bending it at the knee to a right angle (90 degrees) Then ask the resident to slowly lower his or her leg and extend it flat on the mattress. If assessing lower extremity ROM by observing the resident, the flexion and extension of the foot mimics the motion on the pedals of a bicycle. Extension might also be needed to don a shoe. If assessing bending at the knee, the motion would be similar to lifting of the leg when donning lower body clothing.

Upper Extremity – includes shoulder, elbow, wrist, and fingers

For each hand, instruct the resident to make a fist and then open the hand. With resident seated in a chair, instruct him or her to reach with both hands and touch palms to back of head. Then ask resident to touch each shoulder with the opposite hand. Alternatively, observe the resident donning or removing a shirt over the head. If assessing upper extremity ROM by observing the resident, making a fist mimics useful actions for grasping and letting go of utensils. When an individual reaches both hands to the back of the head, this mimics the action needed to comb hair.

G0400: Functional Limitation in Range of Motion (cont.)

Coding Tips

- Do not look at limited ROM in isolation. You must determine if the limited ROM impacts functional ability or places the resident at risk for injury. For example, if the resident has an amputation it does not automatically mean that they are limited in function. He/she may not have a particular joint in which certain range of motion can be tested, however, it does not mean that the resident with an amputation has a limitation in completing activities of daily living, nor does it mean that the resident is automatically at risk of injury. There are many amputees who function extremely well and can complete all activities of daily living either with or without the use of prosthetics. If the resident with an amputation does indeed have difficulty completing ADLs and is at risk for injury, the facility should code this item as appropriate. This item is coded in terms of function and risk of injury, not by diagnosis or lack of a limb or digit.

Coding Instructions for G0400A, Upper Extremity (Shoulder, Elbow, Wrist, Hand); G0400B, Lower Extremity (Hip, Knee, Ankle, Foot)

- **Code 0, no impairment:** if resident has full functional range of motion on the right and left side of upper/lower extremities.

- **Code 1, impairment on one side:** if resident has an upper and/or lower extremity impairment on one side that interferes with daily functioning or places the resident at risk of injury.

- **Code 2, impairment on both sides:** if resident has an upper and/or lower extremity impairment on both sides that interferes with daily functioning or places the resident at risk of injury.

Examples for G0400A, Upper Extremity (Shoulder, Elbow, Wrist, Hand); G0400B, Lower Extremity (Hip, Knee, Ankle, Foot)

1. The resident can perform all arm, hand, and leg motions on the right side, with smooth coordinated movements. She is able to perform grooming activities (e.g. brush teeth, comb her hair) with her right upper extremity, and is also able to pivot to her wheelchair with the assist of one person. She is, however, unable to voluntarily move her left side (limited arm, hand and leg motion) as she has a flaccid left hemiparesis from a prior stroke.

    Coding: G0400A would be **coded 1, upper extremity impairment on one side**. G0400B would be **coded 1, lower extremity impairment on one side**.

    Rationale: Impairment due to left hemiparesis affects both upper and lower extremities on one side. Even though this resident has limited ROM that impairs function on the left side, as indicated above, the resident can perform ROM fully on the right side. Even though there is impairment on one side, the facility should always attempt to provide the resident with assistive devices or physical assistance that allows for the resident to be as independent as possible.

G0400: Functional Limitation in Range of Motion (cont.)

2. The resident had shoulder surgery and can't brush her hair or raise her right arm above her head. The resident has no impairment on the lower extremities.

> **Coding:** G0400A would be **coded 1, upper extremity impairment on one side**. G0400B would be **coded 0, no impairment**.
>
> **Rationale:** Impairment due to shoulder surgery affects only one side of her upper extremities.

3. The resident has a diagnosis of Parkinson's and ambulates with a shuffling gate. The resident has had 3 falls in the past quarter and often forgets his walker which he needs to ambulate. He has tremors of both upper extremities that make it very difficult to feed himself, brush his teeth or write.

> **Coding**: G0400A would be **coded 2, upper extremity impairment on both sides**. G0400B would be **coded 2, lower extremity impairment on both sides**.
>
> **Rationale:** Impairment due to Parkinson's disease affects the resident at the upper and lower extremities on both sides.

G0600: Mobility Devices

G0600. Mobility Devices	
↓ Check all that were normally used	
☐	A. Cane/crutch
☐	B. Walker
☐	C. Wheelchair (manual or electric)
☐	D. Limb prosthesis
☐	Z. None of the above were used

Item Rationale

Health-related Quality of Life

- Maintaining independence is important to an individual's feelings of autonomy and self-worth. The use of devices may assist the resident in maintaining that independence.

Planning for Care

- Resident ability to move about his or her room, unit or nursing home may be directly related to the use of devices. It is critical that nursing home staff assure that the resident's independence is optimized by making available mobility devices on a daily basis, if needed.

Steps for Assessment

1. Review the medical record for references to locomotion during the 7-day look-back period.

G0600: Mobility Devices (cont.)

2. Talk with staff members who work with the resident as well as family/significant others about devices the resident used for mobility during the look-back period.

3. Observe the resident during locomotion.

Coding Instructions

Record the type(s) of mobility devices the resident normally uses for locomotion (in room and in facility). Check all that apply:

- **Check G0600A, cane/crutch:** if the resident used a cane or crutch, including single prong, tripod, quad cane, etc.

- **Check G0600B, walker:** if the resident used a walker or hemi-walker, including an enclosed frame-wheeled walker with/without a posterior seat and lap cushion. Also check this item if the resident walks while pushing a wheelchair for support.

- **Check G0600C, wheelchair (manual or electric):** if the resident normally sits in wheelchair when moving about. Include hand-propelled, motorized, or pushed by another person.

- **Check G0600D, limb prosthesis:** if the resident used an artificial limb to replace a missing extremity.

- **Check G0600Z, none of the above:** if the resident used none of the mobility devices listed in G0600 or locomotion did not occur during the look-back period.

Examples

1. The resident uses a quad cane daily to walk in the room and on the unit. The resident uses a standard push wheelchair that she self-propels when leaving the unit due to her issues with endurance.

> **Coding: G0600A, use of cane/crutch,** and **G0600C, wheelchair,** would be checked.
> **Rationale:** The resident uses a quad cane in her room and on the unit and a wheelchair off the unit.

2. The resident has an artificial leg that is applied each morning and removed each evening. Once the prosthesis is applied the resident is able to ambulate independently.

> **Coding: G0600D, limb prosthesis,** would be checked.
> **Rationale:** The resident uses a leg prosthesis for ambulating.

G0900: Functional Rehabilitation Potential

Complete only on OBRA Admission Assessment (A0310A = 1)

G0900. Functional Rehabilitation Potential Complete only if A0310A = 01	
Enter Code ☐	**A. Resident believes he or she is capable of increased independence** in at least some ADLs 0. **No** 1. **Yes** 9. **Unable to determine**
Enter Code ☐	**B. Direct care staff believe resident is capable of increased independence** in at least some ADLs 0. **No** 1. **Yes**

Item Rationale

Health-related Quality of Life

- Attaining and maintaining independence is important to an individual's feelings of autonomy and self-worth.

- Independence is also important to health status, as decline in function can trigger all of the complications of immobility, depression, and social isolation.

Planning for Care

- Beliefs held by the resident and staff that the resident has the capacity for greater independence and involvement in self-care in at least some ADL areas may be important clues to assist in setting goals.

- Even if highly independent in an activity, the resident or staff may believe the resident can gain more independence (e.g., walk longer distances, shower independently).

- Disagreement between staff beliefs and resident beliefs should be explored by the interdisciplinary team.

Steps for Assessment: Interview Instructions for G0900A, Resident Believes He or She Is Capable of Increased Independence in at Least Some ADLs

1. Ask if the resident thinks he or she could be more self-sufficient given more time.

2. Listen to and record what the resident believes, even if it appears unrealistic.

   - It is sometimes helpful to have a conversation with the resident that helps him/her break down this question. For example, you might ask the resident what types of things staff assist him with and how much of those activities the staff do for the resident. Then ask the resident, "Do you think that you could get to a point where you do more or all of the activity yourself?"

Coding Instructions for G0900A, Resident Believes He or She Is Capable of Increased Independence in at Least Some ADLs

- **Code 0, no:** if the resident indicates that he or she believes he or she will probably stay the same and continue with his or her current needs for assistance.

G0900: Functional Rehabilitation Potential (cont.)

- **Code 1, yes:** if the resident indicates that he or she thinks he or she can improve. Code even if the resident's expectation appears unrealistic.

- **Code 9, unable to determine:** if the resident cannot indicate any beliefs about his or her functional rehabilitation potential.

Example for G0900A, Resident Believes He or She Is Capable of Increased Independence in at Least Some ADLs

1. Mr. N. is cognitively impaired and receives limited physical assistance in locomotion for safety purposes. However, he believes he is capable of walking alone and often gets up and walks by himself when staff are not looking.

    Coding: G0900A would be **coded 1, yes**.
    Rationale: The resident believes he is capable of increased independence.

Steps for Assessment for G0900B, Direct Care Staff Believe Resident Is Capable of Increased Independence in at Least Some ADLs

1. Discuss in interdisciplinary team meeting.
2. Ask staff who routinely care for or work with the resident if they think he or she is capable of greater independence in at least some ADLs.

Coding Instructions for G0900B, Direct Care Staff Believe Resident Is Capable of Increased Independence in at Least Some ADLs

- **Code 0, no:** if staff believe the resident probably will stay the same and continue with current needs for assistance. Also **code 0** if staff believe the resident is likely to experience a decrease in his or her capacity for ADL care performance.

- **Code 1, yes:** if staff believe the resident can gain greater independence in ADLs or if staff indicate they are not sure about the potential for improvement, because that indicates some potential for improvement.

Example for G0900B, Direct Care Staff Believe Resident Is Capable of Increased Independence in at Least Some ADLs

1. The nurse assistant who totally feeds Mrs. W. has noticed in the past week that Mrs. W. has made several attempts to pick up finger foods. She believes Mrs. W. could become more independent in eating if she received close supervision and cueing in a small group for restorative care in eating.

    Coding: G0900B would be **coded 1, yes**.
    Rationale: Based upon observation of the resident, the nurse assistant believes Mrs. W. is capable of increased independence.

SECTION H: BLADDER AND BOWEL

Intent: The intent of the items in this section is to gather information on the use of bowel and bladder appliances, the use of and response to urinary toileting programs, urinary and bowel continence, bowel training programs, and bowel patterns. Each resident who is incontinent or at risk of developing incontinence should be identified, assessed, and provided with individualized treatment (medications, non-medicinal treatments and/or devices) and services to achieve or maintain as normal elimination function as possible.

H0100: Appliances

H0100. Appliances	
↓ Check all that apply	
☐	A. **Indwelling catheter** (including suprapubic catheter and nephrostomy tube)
☐	B. **External catheter**
☐	C. **Ostomy** (including urostomy, ileostomy, and colostomy)
☐	D. **Intermittent catheterization**
☐	Z. **None of the above**

Item Rationale

Health-related Quality of Life

- It is important to know what appliances are in use and the history and rationale for such use.

- External catheters should fit well and be comfortable, minimize leakage, maintain skin integrity, and promote resident dignity.

- Indwelling catheters should not be used unless there is valid medical justification. Assessment should include consideration of the risk and benefits of an indwelling catheter, the anticipated duration of use, and consideration of complications resulting from the use of an indwelling catheter. Complications can include an increased risk of urinary tract infection, blockage of the catheter with associated bypassing of urine, expulsion of the catheter, pain, discomfort, and bleeding.

- Ostomies (and periostomal skin) should be free of redness, tenderness, excoriation, and breakdown. Appliances should fit well, be comfortable, and promote resident dignity.

Planning for Care

- Care planning should include interventions that are consistent with the resident's goals and minimize complications associated with appliance use.

DEFINITIONS

INDWELLING CATHETER

A catheter that is maintained within the bladder for the purpose of continuous drainage of urine.

SUPRAPUBIC CATHETER

An indwelling catheter that is placed by a urologist directly into the bladder through the abdomen. This type of catheter is frequently used when there is an obstruction of urine flow through the urethra.

NEPHROSTOMY TUBE

A catheter inserted through the skin into the kidney in individuals with an abnormality of the ureter (the fibromuscular tube that carries urine from the kidney to the bladder) or the bladder.

H0100: Appliances (cont.)

- Care planning should be based on an assessment and evaluation of the resident's history, physical examination, physician orders, progress notes, nurses' notes and flow sheets, pharmacy and lab reports, voiding history, resident's overall condition, risk factors and information about the resident's continence status, catheter status, environmental factors related to continence programs, and the resident's response to catheter/continence services.

Steps for Assessment

1. Examine the resident to note the presence of any urinary or bowel appliances.
2. Review the medical record, including bladder and bowel records, for documentation of current or past use of urinary or bowel appliances.

Coding Instructions

Check next to each appliance that was used at any time in the past 7 days. Select none of the above if none of the appliances A-D were used in the past 7 days.

- **H0100A,** indwelling catheter (including suprapubic catheter and nephrostomy tube)
- **H0100B,** external catheter
- **H0100C,** ostomy (including urostomy, ileostomy, and colostomy)
- **H0100D,** intermittent catheterization
- **H0100Z,** none of the above

Coding Tips and Special Populations

- Suprapubic catheters and nephrostomy tubes should be coded as an indwelling catheter (H0100A) only and not as an ostomy (H0100C).
- Condom catheters (males) and external urinary pouches (females) are often used intermittently or at night only; these should be coded as external catheters.
- Do not code gastrostomies or other feeding ostomies in this section. Only appliances used for elimination are coded here.
- Do not include one time catheterization for urine specimen during look back period as intermittent catheterization.

DEFINITIONS

EXTERNAL CATHETER
Device attached to the shaft of the penis like a condom for males or a receptacle pouch that fits around the labia majora for females and connected to a drainage bag.

OSTOMY
Any type of surgically created opening of the gastrointestinal or genitourinary tract for discharge of body waste.

UROSTOMY
A stoma for the urinary system used in cases where long-term drainage of urine through the bladder and urethra is not possible, e.g., after extensive surgery or in case of obstruction.

ILEOSTOMY
A stoma that has been constructed by bringing the end or loop of small intestine (the ileum) out onto the surface of the skin.

COLOSTOMY
A stoma that has been constructed by connecting a part of the colon onto the anterior abdominal wall.

INTERMITTENT CATHETERIZATION
Sterile insertion and removal of a catheter through the urethra for bladder drainage.

H0200: Urinary Toileting Program

H0200. Urinary Toileting Program	
Enter Code ☐	**A. Has a trial of a toileting program (e.g., scheduled toileting, prompted voiding, or bladder training)** been attempted on admission/reentry or since urinary incontinence was noted in this facility? 0. **No** → Skip to H0300, Urinary Continence 1. **Yes** → Continue to H0200B, Response 9. **Unable to determine** → Skip to H0200C, Current toileting program or trial
Enter Code ☐	**B. Response** - What was the resident's response to the trial program? 0. **No improvement** 1. **Decreased wetness** 2. **Completely dry** (continent) 9. **Unable to determine** or trial in progress
Enter Code ☐	**C. Current toileting program or trial** - Is a toileting program (e.g., scheduled toileting, prompted voiding, or bladder training) currently being used to manage the resident's urinary continence? 0. **No** 1. **Yes**

Item Rationale

Health-related Quality of Life

- An individualized, resident-centered toileting program may decrease or prevent urinary incontinence, minimizing or avoiding the negative consequences of incontinence.
- Determining the type of urinary incontinence can allow staff to provide more individualized programming or interventions to enhance the resident's quality of life and functional status.
- Many incontinent residents (including those with dementia) respond to a toileting program, especially during the day.

Planning for Care

- The steps toward ensuring that the resident receives appropriate treatment and services to restore as much bladder function as possible are
  - determining if the resident is currently experiencing some level of incontinence or is at risk of developing urinary incontinence;
  - completing an accurate, thorough assessment of factors that may predispose the resident to having urinary incontinence; and
  - implementing appropriate, individualized interventions and modifying them as appropriate.
- If the toileting program or bladder retraining leads to a decrease or resolution of incontinence, the program should be maintained.
- Research has shown that one quarter to one third of residents will have a decrease or resolution of incontinence in response to a toileting program.
- If incontinence is not decreased or resolved with a toileting trial, consider whether other reversible or treatable causes are present.
- Residents may need to be referred to practitioners who specialize in diagnosing and treating conditions that affect bladder function.
- Residents who do not respond to a toileting trial and for whom other reversible or treatable causes are not found should receive supportive management (such as checking the resident for incontinence and changing his or her brief if needed and providing good skin care).

H0200: Urinary Toileting Program (cont.)

Steps for Assessment: H0200A, Trial of a Toileting Program

The look-back period for this item is since the most recent admission/entry or reentry or since urinary incontinence was first noted within the facility.

1. Review the medical record for evidence of a trial of an individualized, resident-centered toileting program. A toileting trial should include observations of at least 3 days of toileting patterns with prompting to toilet and of recording results in a bladder record or voiding diary. Toileting programs may have different names, e.g., habit training/scheduled voiding, bladder rehabilitation/bladder retraining.
2. Review records of voiding patterns (such as frequency, volume, duration, nighttime or daytime, quality of stream) over several days for those who are experiencing incontinence.
3. Voiding records help detect urinary patterns or intervals between incontinence episodes and facilitate providing care to avoid or reduce the frequency of episodes.
4. Simply tracking continence status using a bladder record or voiding diary should not be considered a trial of an individualized, resident-centered toileting program.
5. Residents should be reevaluated whenever there is a change in cognition, physical ability, or urinary tract function. Nursing home staff must use clinical judgment to determine when it is appropriate to reevaluate a resident's ability to participate in a toileting trial or, if the toileting trial was unsuccessful, the need for a trial of a different toileting program.

Steps for Assessment: H0200B, Response to Trial Toileting Program

1. Review the resident's responses as recorded during the toileting trial, noting any change in the number of incontinence episodes or degree of wetness the resident experiences.

DEFINITIONS

BLADDER REHABILITATION/ BLADDER RETRAINING

A behavioral technique that requires the resident to resist or inhibit the sensation of urgency (the strong desire to urinate), to postpone or delay voiding, and to urinate according to a timetable rather than to the urge to void.

PROMPTED VOIDING

Prompted voiding includes (1) regular monitoring with encouragement to report continence status, (2) using a schedule and prompting the resident to toilet, and (3) praise and positive feedback when the resident is continent and attempts to toilet.

HABIT TRAINING/ SCHEDULED VOIDING

A behavior technique that calls for scheduled toileting at regular intervals on a planned basis to match the resident's voiding habits or needs.

CHECK AND CHANGE

Involves checking the resident's dry/wet status at regular intervals and using incontinence devices and products.

H0200: Urinary Toileting Program (cont.)

Steps for Assessment: H0200C, Current Toileting Program or Trial

1. Review the medical record for evidence of a toileting program being used to manage incontinence during the 7-day look-back period. Note the number of days during the look-back period that the toileting program was implemented or carried out.

2. Look for documentation in the medical record showing that the following three requirements have been met:

   - implementation of an individualized, resident-specific toileting program that was based on an assessment of the resident's unique voiding pattern

   - evidence that the individualized program was communicated to staff and the resident (as appropriate) verbally and through a care plan, flow records, and a written report

   - notations of the resident's response to the toileting program and subsequent evaluations, as needed

3. Guidance for developing a toileting program may be obtained from sources found in Appendix C.

Coding Instructions H0200A, Toileting Program Trial

- **Code 0, no:** if for any reason the resident did not undergo a toileting trial. This includes residents who are continent of urine with or without toileting assistance, or who use a permanent catheter or ostomy, as well as residents who prefer not to participate in a trial. Skip to **Urinary Continence** item (H0300).

- **Code 1, yes:** for residents who underwent a trial of an individualized, resident-centered toileting program at least once since admission/readmission, prior assessment, or when urinary incontinence was first noted.

- **Code 9, unable to determine:** if records cannot be obtained to determine if a trial toileting program has been attempted. If code 9, skip H0200B and go to H0200C, **Current Toileting Program or Trial**.

Coding Instructions H0200B, Toileting Program Trial Response

- **Code 0, no improvement:** if the frequency of resident's urinary incontinence did not decrease during the toileting trial.

- **Code 1, decreased wetness:** if the resident's urinary incontinence frequency decreased, but the resident remained incontinent. There is no quantitative definition of improvement. However, the improvement should be clinically meaningful—for example, having at least one less incontinent void per day than before the toileting program was implemented.

- **Code 2, completely dry (continent):** if the resident becomes completely continent of urine, with no episodes of urinary incontinence during the toileting trial. (For residents who have undergone more than one toileting program trial during their stay, use the most recent trial to complete this item.)

- **Code 9, unable to determine or trial in progress:** if the response to the toileting trial cannot be determined because information cannot be found or because the trial is still in progress.

H0200: Urinary Toileting Program (cont.)

Coding Instructions H0200C, **Current Toileting Program**

- **Code 0, no:** if an individualized resident-centered toileting program (i.e., prompted voiding, scheduled toileting, or bladder training) is used less than 4 days of the 7-day look-back period to manage the resident's urinary continence.

- **Code 1, yes:** for residents who are being managed, during 4 or more days of the 7-day look-back period, with some type of systematic toileting program (i.e., bladder rehabilitation/bladder retraining, prompted voiding, habit training/scheduled voiding). Some residents prefer to not be awakened to toilet. If that resident, however, is on a toileting program during the day, code "yes."

Coding Tips for H0200A-C

- Toileting (or trial toileting) programs refer to a specific approach that is organized, planned, documented, monitored, and evaluated that is consistent with the nursing home's policies and procedures and current standards of practice. A toileting program does not refer to
  - simply tracking continence status,
  - changing pads or wet garments, and
  - random assistance with toileting or hygiene.

- For a resident currently undergoing a trial of a toileting program,
  - H0200A would be **coded 1, yes, a trial toileting program is attempted,**
  - H0200B would be **coded 9, unable to determine or trial in progress,** and
  - H0200C would be **coded 1, current toileting program**.

Example

1. Mrs. H. has a diagnosis of advanced Alzheimer's disease. She is dependent on the staff for her ADLs, does not have the cognitive ability to void in the toilet or other appropriate receptacle, and is totally incontinent. Her voiding assessment/diary indicates no pattern to her incontinence. Her care plan states that due to her total incontinence, staff should follow the facility standard policy for incontinence, which is to check and change every 2 hours while awake and apply a superabsorbent brief at bedtime so as not to disturb her sleep.

    Coding: H0200A would be **coded as 0, no** H0200B and H0200C would be skipped.

    Rationale: Based on this resident's voiding assessment/diary, there was no pattern to her incontinence. Therefore, H0200A would be coded as 0, no. Due to total incontinence a toileting program is not appropriate for this resident. Since H0200A is coded 0, no skip to H0300, Urinary Continence.

H0200: Urinary Toileting Program (cont.)

2. Mr. M., who has a diagnosis of congestive heart failure (CHF) and a history of left-sided hemiplegia from a previous stroke, has had an increase in urinary incontinence. The team has assessed him for a reversible cause of the incontinence and has evaluated his voiding pattern using a voiding assessment/diary. After completing the assessment, it was determined that incontinence episodes could be reduced. A plan was developed and implemented that called for toileting every hour for 4 hours after receiving his 8 a.m. diuretic, then every 3 hours until bedtime at 9 p.m. The team has communicated this approach to the resident and the care team and has placed these interventions in the care plan. The team will reevaluate the resident's response to the plan after 1 month and adjust as needed.

> **Coding**: H0200A would be **coded as 1, yes.**
>
> H0200B would be **coded as 9, unable to determine or trial in progress**
>
> H0200C would be **coded as 1, current toileting program or trial.**
>
> **Rationale:** Based on this resident's voiding assessment/diary, it was determined that this resident could benefit from a toileting program. Therefore H0200A is coded as 1, yes. Based on the assessment it was determined that incontinence episodes could be reduced, therefore H0200B is coded as 9, unable to determine or trial in progress. An individualized plan has been developed, implemented, and communicated to the resident and staff, therefore H0200C is coded as 1, current toileting program or trial.

H0300: Urinary Continence

H0300. Urinary Continence	
Enter Code	**Urinary continence -** Select the one category that best describes the resident 0. **Always continent** 1. **Occasionally incontinent** (less than 7 episodes of incontinence) 2. **Frequently incontinent** (7 or more episodes of urinary incontinence, but at least one episode of continent voiding) 3. **Always incontinent** (no episodes of continent voiding) 9. **Not rated,** resident had a catheter (indwelling, condom), urinary ostomy, or no urine output for the entire 7 days

Item Rationale

Health-related Quality of Life

- Incontinence can

  — interfere with participation in activities,

  — be socially embarrassing and lead to increased feelings of dependency,

  — increase risk of long-term institutionalization,

  — increase risk of skin rashes and breakdown,

  — increased risk of repeated urinary tract infections, and

  — increase the risk of falls and injuries resulting from attempts to reach a toilet unassisted.

> **DEFINITIONS**
>
> **URINARY INCONTINENCE**
> The involuntary loss of urine.
>
> **CONTINENCE**
> Any void into a commode, urinal, or bedpan that occurs voluntarily, or as the result of prompted toileting, assisted toileting, or scheduled toileting.

H0300: Urinary Continence (cont.)

Planning for Care

- For many residents, incontinence can be resolved or minimized by
    - identifying and treating underlying potentially reversible causes, including medication side effects, urinary tract infection, constipation and fecal impaction, and immobility (especially among those with the new or recent onset of incontinence);
    - eliminating environmental physical barriers to accessing commodes, bedpans, and urinals; and
    - bladder retraining, prompted voiding, or scheduled toileting.
- For residents whose incontinence does not have a reversible cause and who do not respond to retraining, prompted voiding, or scheduled toileting, the interdisciplinary team should establish a plan to maintain skin dryness and minimize exposure to urine.

Steps for Assessment

1. Review the medical record for bladder or incontinence records or flow sheets, nursing assessments and progress notes, physician history, and physical examination.
2. Interview the resident if he or she is capable of reliably reporting his or her continence. Speak with family members or significant others if the resident is not able to report on continence.
3. Ask direct care staff who routinely work with the resident on all shifts about incontinence episodes.

Coding Instructions

- **Code 0, always continent:** if throughout the 7-day look-back period the resident has been continent of urine, without any episodes of incontinence.
- **Code 1, occasionally incontinent:** if during the 7-day look-back period the resident was incontinent less than 7 episodes. This includes incontinence of any amount of urine sufficient to dampen undergarments, briefs, or pads during daytime or nighttime.
- **Code 2, frequently incontinent:** if during the 7-day look-back period, the resident was incontinent of urine during seven or more episodes but had at least one continent void. This includes incontinence of any amount of urine, daytime and nighttime.
- **Code 3, always incontinent:** if during the 7-day look-back period, the resident had no continent voids.
- **Code 9, not rated:** if during the 7-day look-back period the resident had an indwelling bladder catheter, condom catheter, ostomy, or no urine output (e.g., is on chronic dialysis with no urine output) for the entire 7 days.

Coding Tips and Special Populations

- If intermittent catheterization is used to drain the bladder, code continence level based on continence between catheterizations.

H0300: Urinary Continence (cont.)

Examples

1. An 86-year-old female resident has had longstanding stress-type incontinence for many years. When she has an upper respiratory infection and is coughing, she involuntarily loses urine. However, during the current 7-day look-back period, the resident has been free of respiratory symptoms and has not had an episode of incontinence.

   Coding: H0300 would be **coded 0, always continent.**

   Rationale: Even though the resident has known intermittent stress incontinence, she was continent during the current 7-day look-back period.

2. A resident with multi-infarct dementia is incontinent of urine on three occasions on day one of observation, continent of urine in response to toileting on days two and three, and has one urinary incontinence episode during each of the nights of days four, five, six, and seven of the look-back period.

   Coding: H0300 would be **coded as 2, frequently incontinent.**

   Rationale: The resident had seven documented episodes of urinary incontinence over the look-back period. The criterion for "frequent" incontinence has been set at seven or more episodes over the 7-day look-back period with at least one continent void.

3. A resident with Parkinson's disease is severely immobile, and cannot be transferred to a toilet. He is unable to use a urinal and is managed by adult briefs and bed pads that are regularly changed. He did not have a continent void during the 7-day look-back period.

   Coding: H0300 would be **coded as 3, always incontinent.**

   Rationale: The resident has no urinary continent episodes and cannot be toileted due to severe disability or discomfort. Incontinence is managed by a check and change in protocol.

4. A resident had one continent urinary void during the 7-day look-back period, after the nursing assistant assisted him to the toilet and helped with clothing. All other voids were incontinent.

   Coding: H0300 would be **coded as 2, frequently incontinent.**

   Rationale: The resident had at least one continent void during the look-back period. The reason for the continence does not enter into the coding decision.

H0400: Bowel Continence

H0400. Bowel Continence	
Enter Code ⬜	**Bowel continence -** Select the one category that best describes the resident 0. **Always continent** 1. **Occasionally incontinent** (one episode of bowel incontinence) 2. **Frequently incontinent** (2 or more episodes of bowel incontinence, but at least one continent bowel movement) 3. **Always incontinent** (no episodes of continent bowel movements) 9. **Not rated,** resident had an ostomy or did not have a bowel movement for the entire 7 days

H0400: Bowel Continence (cont.)

Item Rationale

Health-related Quality of Life

- Incontinence can
  - interfere with participation in activities,
  - be socially embarrassing and lead to increased feelings of dependency,
  - increase risk of long-term institutionalization,
  - increase risk of skin rashes and breakdown, and
  - increase the risk of falls and injuries resulting from attempts to reach a toilet unassisted.

Planning for Care

- For many residents, incontinence can be resolved or minimized by
  - identifying and managing underlying potentially reversible causes, including medication side effects, constipation and fecal impaction, and immobility (especially among those with the new or recent onset of incontinence); and
  - eliminating environmental physical barriers to accessing commodes, bedpans, and urinals.
- For residents whose incontinence does not have a reversible cause and who do not respond to retraining programs, the interdisciplinary team should establish a plan to maintain skin dryness and minimize exposure to stool.

Steps for Assessment

1. Review the medical record for bowel records and incontinence flow sheets, nursing assessments and progress notes, physician history and physical examination.
2. Interview the resident if he or she is capable of reliably reporting his or her bowel habits. Speak with family members or significant other if the resident is unable to report on continence.
3. Ask direct care staff who routinely work with the resident on all shifts about incontinence episodes.

Coding Instructions

- **Code 0, always continent:** if during the 7-day look-back period the resident has been continent of bowel on all occasions of bowel movements, without any episodes of incontinence.
- **Code 1, occasionally incontinent:** if during the 7-day look-back period the resident was incontinent of stool once. This includes incontinence of any amount of stool day or night.
- **Code 2, frequently incontinent:** if during the 7-day look-back period, the resident was incontinent of bowel more than once, but had at least one continent bowel movement. This includes incontinence of any amount of stool day or night.
- **Code 3, always incontinent:** if during the 7-day look-back period, the resident was incontinent of bowel for all bowel movements and had no continent bowel movements.

H0400: Bowel Continence (cont.)

- **Code 9, not rated:** if during the 7-day look-back period the resident had an ostomy or did not have a bowel movement for the entire 7 days. (Note that these residents should be checked for fecal impaction and evaluated for constipation.)

Coding Tips and Special Populations

- Bowel incontinence precipitated by loose stools or diarrhea from any cause (including laxatives) would count as incontinence.

H0500: Bowel Toileting Program

H0500. Bowel Toileting Program	
Enter Code	Is a toileting program currently being used to manage the resident's bowel continence? 0. No 1. Yes

Item Rationale

Health-related Quality of Life

- A systematically implemented bowel toileting program may decrease or prevent bowel incontinence, minimizing or avoiding the negative consequences of incontinence.

- Many incontinent residents respond to a bowel toileting program, especially during the day.

Planning for Care

- If the bowel toileting program leads to a decrease or resolution of incontinence, the program should be maintained.

- If bowel incontinence is not decreased or resolved with a bowel toileting trial, consider whether other reversible or treatable causes are present.

- Residents who do not respond to a bowel toileting trial and for whom other reversible or treatable causes are not found should receive supportive management (such as a regular check and change program with good skin care).

- Residents with a colostomy or colectomy may need their diet monitored to promote healthy bowel elimination and careful monitoring of skin to prevent skin irritation and breakdown.

- When developing a toileting program the provider may want to consider assessing the resident for adequate fluid intake, adequate fiber in the diet, exercise, and scheduled times to attempt bowel movement (Newman, 2009).

H0500: Bowel Toileting Program (cont.)

Steps for Assessment

1. Review the medical record for evidence of a bowel toileting program being used to manage bowel incontinence during the 7-day look-back period.
2. Look for documentation in the medical record showing that the following three requirements have been met:

   - implementation of an individualized, resident-specific bowel toileting program based on an assessment of the resident's unique bowel pattern;

   - evidence that the individualized program was communicated to staff and the resident (as appropriate) verbally and through a care plan, flow records, verbal and a written report; and

   - notations of the resident's response to the toileting program and subsequent evaluations, as needed.

Coding Instructions

- **Code 0, no:** if the resident is not currently on a toileting program targeted specifically at managing bowel continence.
- **Code 1, yes:** if the resident is currently on a toileting program targeted specifically at managing bowel continence.

H0600: Bowel Patterns

H0600. Bowel Patterns	
Enter Code	Constipation present? 0. No 1. Yes

Item Rationale

Health-related Quality of Life

- Severe constipation can cause abdominal pain, anorexia, vomiting, bowel incontinence, and delirium.
- If unaddressed, constipation can lead to fecal impaction.

Planning for Care

- This item identifies residents who may need further evaluation of and intervention on bowel habits.
- Constipation may be a manifestation of serious conditions such as
  — dehydration due to a medical condition or inadequate access to and intake of fluid, and
    — side effects of medications.

> **DEFINITIONS**
>
> **CONSTIPATION**
> If the resident has two or fewer bowel movements during the 7-day look-back period or if for most bowel movements their stool is hard and difficult for them to pass (no matter what the frequency of bowel movements).

H0600: Bowel Patterns (cont.)

Steps for Assessment

1. Review the medical record for bowel records or flow sheets, nursing assessments and progress notes, physician history and physical examination to determine if the resident has had problems with constipation during the 7- day look-back period.
2. Residents who are capable of reliably reporting their continence and bowel habits should be interviewed. Speak with family members or significant others if the resident is unable to report on bowel habits.
3. Ask direct care staff who routinely work with the resident on all shifts about problems with constipation.

> **DEFINITIONS**
>
> **FECAL IMPACTION**
> A large mass of dry, hard stool that can develop in the rectum due to chronic constipation. This mass may be so hard that the resident is unable to move it from the rectum. Watery stool from higher in the bowel or irritation from the impaction may move around the mass and leak out, causing soiling, often a sign of a fecal impaction.

Coding Instructions

- **Code 0, no:** if the resident shows no signs of constipation during the 7-day look-back period.
- **Code 1, yes:** if the resident shows signs of constipation during the 7-day look-back period.

Coding Tips and Special Populations

- Fecal impaction is caused by chronic constipation. Fecal impaction is not synonymous with constipation.

SECTION I: ACTIVE DIAGNOSES

Intent: The items in this section are intended to code diseases that have a direct relationship to the resident's current functional status, cognitive status, mood or behavior status, medical treatments, nursing monitoring, or risk of death. One of the important functions of the MDS assessment is to generate an updated, accurate picture of the resident's current health status.

Active Diagnoses in the Last 7 Days

Active Diagnoses in the last 7 days - Check all that apply
Diagnoses listed in parentheses are provided as examples and should not be considered as all-inclusive lists

Cancer
- [ ] I0100. Cancer (with or without metastasis)

Heart/Circulation
- [ ] I0200. Anemia (e.g., aplastic, iron deficiency, pernicious, and sickle cell)
- [ ] I0300. Atrial Fibrillation or Other Dysrhythmias (e.g., bradycardias and tachycardias)
- [ ] I0400. Coronary Artery Disease (CAD) (e.g., angina, myocardial infarction, and atherosclerotic heart disease (ASHD))
- [ ] I0500. Deep Venous Thrombosis (DVT), Pulmonary Embolus (PE), or Pulmonary Thrombo-Embolism (PTE)
- [ ] I0600. Heart Failure (e.g., congestive heart failure (CHF) and pulmonary edema)
- [ ] I0700. Hypertension
- [ ] I0800. Orthostatic Hypotension
- [ ] I0900. Peripheral Vascular Disease (PVD) or Peripheral Arterial Disease (PAD)

Gastrointestinal
- [ ] I1100. Cirrhosis
- [ ] I1200. Gastroesophageal Reflux Disease (GERD) or Ulcer (e.g., esophageal, gastric, and peptic ulcers)
- [ ] I1300. Ulcerative Colitis, Crohn's Disease, or Inflammatory Bowel Disease

Genitourinary
- [ ] I1400. Benign Prostatic Hyperplasia (BPH)
- [ ] I1500. Renal Insufficiency, Renal Failure, or End-Stage Renal Disease (ESRD)
- [ ] I1550. Neurogenic Bladder
- [ ] I1650. Obstructive Uropathy

Infections
- [ ] I1700. Multidrug-Resistant Organism (MDRO)
- [ ] I2000. Pneumonia
- [ ] I2100. Septicemia
- [ ] I2200. Tuberculosis
- [ ] I2300. Urinary Tract Infection (UTI) (LAST 30 DAYS)
- [ ] I2400. Viral Hepatitis (e.g., Hepatitis A, B, C, D, and E)
- [ ] I2500. Wound Infection (other than foot)

Metabolic
- [ ] I2900. Diabetes Mellitus (DM) (e.g., diabetic retinopathy, nephropathy, and neuropathy)
- [ ] I3100. Hyponatremia
- [ ] I3200. Hyperkalemia
- [ ] I3300. Hyperlipidemia (e.g., hypercholesterolemia)
- [ ] I3400. Thyroid Disorder (e.g., hypothyroidism, hyperthyroidism, and Hashimoto's thyroiditis)

Musculoskeletal
- [ ] I3700. Arthritis (e.g., degenerative joint disease (DJD), osteoarthritis, and rheumatoid arthritis (RA))
- [ ] I3800. Osteoporosis
- [ ] I3900. Hip Fracture - any hip fracture that has a relationship to current status, treatments, monitoring (e.g., sub-capital fractures, and fractures of the trochanter and femoral neck)
- [ ] I4000. Other Fracture

Neurological
- [ ] I4200. Alzheimer's Disease
- [ ] I4300. Aphasia
- [ ] I4400. Cerebral Palsy
- [ ] I4500. Cerebrovascular Accident (CVA), Transient Ischemic Attack (TIA), or Stroke
- [ ] I4800. Non-Alzheimer's Dementia (e.g. Lewy body dementia, vascular or multi-infarct dementia; mixed dementia; frontotemporal dementia such as Pick's disease; and dementia related to stroke, Parkinson's or Creutzfeldt-Jakob diseases)

Neurological Diagnoses continued on next page

I: Active Diagnoses in the Last 7 Days (cont.)

Active Diagnoses in the last 7 days - Check all that apply
Diagnoses listed in parentheses are provided as examples and should not be considered as all-inclusive lists

	Neurological - Continued
☐	I4900. Hemiplegia or Hemiparesis
☐	I5000. Paraplegia
☐	I5100. Quadriplegia
☐	I5200. Multiple Sclerosis (MS)
☐	I5250. Huntington's Disease
☐	I5300. Parkinson's Disease
☐	I5350. Tourette's Syndrome
☐	I5400. Seizure Disorder or Epilepsy
☐	I5500. Traumatic Brain Injury (TBI)
	Nutritional
☐	I5600. Malnutrition (protein or calorie) or at risk for malnutrition
	Psychiatric/Mood Disorder
☐	I5700. Anxiety Disorder
☐	I5800. Depression (other than bipolar)
☐	I5900. Manic Depression (bipolar disease)
☐	I5950. Psychotic Disorder (other than schizophrenia)
☐	I6000. Schizophrenia (e.g., schizoaffective and schizophreniform disorders)
☐	I6100. Post Traumatic Stress Disorder (PTSD)
	Pulmonary
☐	I6200. Asthma, Chronic Obstructive Pulmonary Disease (COPD), or Chronic Lung Disease (e.g., chronic bronchitis and restrictive lung diseases such as asbestosis)
☐	I6300. Respiratory Failure
	Vision
☐	I6500. Cataracts, Glaucoma, or Macular Degeneration
	None of Above
☐	I7900. None of the above active diagnoses within the last 7 days
	Other
	I8000. Additional active diagnoses

Enter diagnosis on line and ICD code in boxes. Include the decimal for the code in the appropriate box.

A. _____ ☐☐☐☐☐☐☐☐

B. _____ ☐☐☐☐☐☐☐☐

C. _____ ☐☐☐☐☐☐☐☐

D. _____ ☐☐☐☐☐☐☐☐

E. _____ ☐☐☐☐☐☐☐☐

F. _____ ☐☐☐☐☐☐☐☐

G. _____ ☐☐☐☐☐☐☐☐

H. _____ ☐☐☐☐☐☐☐☐

I. _____ ☐☐☐☐☐☐☐☐

J. _____ ☐☐☐☐☐☐☐☐

I: Active Diagnoses in the Last 7 Days (cont.)

Item Rationale

Health-Related Quality of Life

- Disease processes can have a significant adverse affect on an individual's health status and quality of life.

Planning for Care

- This section identifies active diseases and infections that drive the current plan of care.

Steps for Assessment

There are two look-back periods for this section:

- Diagnosis identification (Step 1) is a 60-day look-back period.
- Diagnosis status: Active or Inactive (Step 2) is a 7-day look-back period (except for Item I2300 UTI, which does not use the active 7-day look-back period).

1. **Identify diagnoses:** The disease conditions in this section require a physician-documented diagnosis (or by a nurse practitioner, physician assistant, or clinical nurse specialist if allowable under state licensure laws) in the **last 60 days.**

   Medical record sources for physician diagnoses include progress notes, the most recent history and physical, transfer documents, discharge summaries, diagnosis/problem list, and other resources as available. If a diagnosis/problem list is used, only diagnoses confirmed by the physician should be entered.

   - Although open communication regarding diagnostic information between the physician and other members of the interdisciplinary team is important, it is also essential that diagnoses communicated verbally be documented in the medical record by the physician to ensure follow-up.
   - Diagnostic information, including past history obtained from family members and close contacts, must also be documented in the medical record by the physician to ensure validity and follow-up.

2. **Determine whether diagnoses are active:** Once a diagnosis is identified, it must be determined if the diagnosis is **active.** Active diagnoses are diagnoses that have a **direct relationship** to the resident's current functional, cognitive, or mood or behavior status, medical treatments, nursing monitoring, or risk of death during the 7-day look-back period. Do not include conditions that have been resolved, do not affect the resident's current status, or do not drive the resident's plan of care during the 7-day look-back period, as these would be considered inactive diagnoses.

> **DEFINITIONS**
>
> **ACTIVE DIAGNOSES**
> Physician-documented diagnoses in the last 60 days that have a direct relationship to the resident's current functional status, cognitive status, mood or behavior, medical treatments, nursing monitoring, or risk of death during the 7-day look-back period.
>
> **FUNCTIONAL LIMITATIONS**
> Loss of range of motion, contractures, muscle weakness, fatigue, decreased ability to perform, ADLs, paresis, or paralysis.
>
> **NURSING MONITORING**
> Nursing Monitoring includes clinical monitoring by a licensed nurse (e.g., serial blood pressure evaluations, medication management, etc.).

I: Active Diagnoses in the Last 7 Days (cont.)

- Item I2300 UTI, has specific coding criteria and does not use the active 7-day look-back. Please refer to Page I-8 for specific coding instructions for Item I2300 UTI.

- Check the following information sources in the medical record for the last 7 days to identify "active" diagnoses: transfer documents, physician progress notes, recent history and physical, recent discharge summaries, nursing assessments, nursing care plans, medication sheets, doctor's orders, consults and official diagnostic reports, and other sources as available.

Coding Instructions

Code diseases that have a documented diagnosis in the last 60 days and have a direct relationship to the resident's current functional status, cognitive status, mood or behavior status, medical treatments, nursing monitoring, or risk of death during the 7-day look-back period (except Item I2300 UTI, which does not use the active diagnosis 7-day look-back. Please refer to Item I2300 UTI, Page I-8 for specific coding instructions).

- Document active diagnoses on the MDS as follows:
  — Diagnoses are listed by major disease category: Cancer; Heart/Circulation; Gastrointestinal; Genitourinary; Infections; Metabolic; Musculoskeletal; Neurological; Nutritional; Psychiatric/Mood Disorder; Pulmonary; and Vision.
  — Examples of diseases are included for some disease categories. Diseases to be coded in these categories are not meant to be limited to only those listed in the examples. For example, **I0200, Anemia,** includes anemia of any etiology, including those listed (e.g., aplastic, iron deficiency, pernicious, sickle cell).
- Check off each active disease. Check all that apply.
- If a disease or condition is **not** specifically listed, enter the diagnosis and ICD code in item I8000, Additional active diagnosis.
- Computer specifications are written such that the ICD code should be automatically justified. The important element is to ensure that the ICD code's decimal point is in its own box and should be right justified (aligned with the right margin so that any unused boxes and on the left.)
- If a diagnosis is a V-code, another diagnosis for the related primary medical condition should be checked in items I0100-I7900 or entered in I8000.

Cancer

- **I0100,** cancer (with or without metastasis)

Heart/Circulation

- **I0200,** anemia (e.g., aplastic, iron deficiency, pernicious, sickle cell)
- **I0300,** atrial fibrillation or other dysrhythmias (e.g., bradycardias, tachycardias)
- **I0400,** coronary artery disease (CAD) (e.g., angina, myocardial infarction, atherosclerotic heart disease [ASHD])

I: Active Diagnoses in the Last 7 Days (cont.)

- **I0500,** deep venous thrombosis (DVT), pulmonary embolus (PE), or pulmonary thrombo-embolism (PTE)
- **I0600,** heart failure (e.g., congestive heart failure [CHF], pulmonary edema)
- **I0700,** hypertension
- **I0800,** orthostatic hypotension
- **I0900,** peripheral vascular disease or peripheral arterial disease

Gastrointestinal

- **I1100,** cirrhosis
- **I1200,** gastroesophageal reflux disease (GERD) or ulcer (e.g., esophageal, gastric, and peptic ulcers)
- **I1300,** ulcerative colitis or Crohn's disease or inflammatory bowel disease

Genitourinary

- **I1400,** benign prostatic hyperplasia (BPH)
- **I1500,** renal insufficiency, renal failure, or end-stage renal disease (ESRD)
- **I1550,** neurogenic bladder
- **I1650,** obstructive uropathy

Infections

- **I1700,** multidrug resistant organism (MDRO)
- **I2000,** pneumonia
- **I2100,** septicemia
- **I2200,** tuberculosis
- **I2300,** urinary tract infection (UTI) (last 30 days)
- **I2400,** viral hepatitis (e.g., hepatitis A, B, C, D, and E)
- **I2500,** wound infection (other than foot)

Metabolic

- **I2900,** diabetes mellitus (DM) (e.g., diabetic retinopathy, nephropathy, neuropathy)
- **I3100,** hyponatremia
- **I3200,** hyperkalemia
- **I3300,** hyperlipidemia (e.g., hypercholesterolemia)
- **I3400,** thyroid disorder (e.g., hypothyroidism, hyperthyroidism, Hashimoto's thyroiditis)

I: Active Diagnoses in the Last 7 Days (cont.)

Musculoskeletal

- **I3700,** arthritis (e.g., degenerative joint disease [DJD], osteoarthritis, rheumatoid arthritis [RA])
- **I3800,** osteoporosis
- **I3900,** hip fracture (any hip fracture that has a relationship to current status, treatments, monitoring (e.g., subcapital fractures and fractures of the trochanter and femoral neck)
- **I4000,** other fracture

Neurological

- **I4200,** Alzheimer's disease
- **I4300,** aphasia
- **I4400,** cerebral palsy
- **I4500,** cerebrovascular accident (CVA), transient ischemic attack (TIA), or stroke
- **I4800,** dementia (e.g., Lewy-Body dementia; vascular or multi-infarct dementia; mixed dementia; frontotemporal dementia, such as Pick's disease; and dementia related to stroke, Parkinson's disease or Creutzfeldt-Jakob diseases)
- **I4900,** hemiplegia or hemiparesis
- **I5000,** paraplegia
- **I5100,** quadriplegia
- **I5200,** multiple sclerosis (MS)
- **I5250,** Huntington's disease
- **I5300,** Parkinson's disease
- **I5350,** Tourette's syndrome
- **I5400,** seizure disorder or epilepsy
- **I5500,** traumatic brain injury (TBI)

Nutritional

- **I5600,** malnutrition (protein or calorie) or at risk for malnutrition

Psychiatric/Mood Disorder

- **I5700,** anxiety disorder
- **I5800,** depression (other than bipolar)
- **I5900,** manic depression (bipolar disease)
- **I5950,** psychotic disorder (other than schizophrenia)
- **I6000,** schizophrenia (e.g., schizoaffective and schizophreniform disorders)
- **I6100,** post-traumatic stress disorder (PTSD)

I: Active Diagnoses in the Last 7 Days (cont.)

Pulmonary

- **I6200,** asthma, chronic obstructive pulmonary disease (COPD), or chronic lung disease (e.g., chronic bronchitis and restrictive lung diseases, such as asbestosis)
- **I6300,** respiratory failure

Vision

- **I6500,** cataracts, glaucoma, or macular degeneration

None of Above

- **I7900,** none of the above active diagnoses within the past 7 days

Other

- **I8000,** additional active diagnoses

Coding Tips

The following indicators may assist assessors in determining whether a diagnosis should be coded as active in the MDS.

- **There may be specific documentation in the medical record by a physician, nurse practitioner, physician assistant, or clinical nurse specialist of active diagnosis.**
  - The physician may specifically indicate that a condition is active. Specific documentation may be found in progress notes, most recent history and physical, transfer notes, hospital discharge summary, etc.
  - For example, the physician documents that the resident has inadequately controlled hypertension and will modify medications. This would be sufficient documentation of active disease and would require no additional confirmation.
- **In the absence of specific documentation that a disease is active, the following indicators may be used to confirm active disease:**
  - Recent onset or acute exacerbation of the disease or condition indicated by a positive study, test or procedure, hospitalization for acute symptoms and/or recent change in therapy in the last 7 days. Examples of a recent onset or acute exacerbation include the following: new diagnosis of pneumonia indicated by chest X-ray; hospitalization for fractured hip; or a blood transfusion for a hematocrit of 24. Sources may include radiological reports, hospital discharge summaries, doctor's orders, etc.
  - Symptoms and abnormal signs indicating ongoing or decompensated disease in the last 7 days. For example, intermittent claudication (lower extremity pain on exertion) in conjunction with a diagnosis of peripheral vascular disease would indicate active disease. Sometimes signs and symptoms can be nonspecific and could be caused by several disease processes. Therefore, a symptom must be specifically attributed to the disease. For example, a productive cough would confirm a diagnosis of pneumonia if specifically noted as such by a physician. Sources may include radiological reports, nursing assessments and care plans, progress notes, etc.

I: Active Diagnoses in the Last 7 Days (cont.)

— Listing a disease/diagnosis (e.g., arthritis) on the resident's medical record problem list is not sufficient for determining active or inactive status. To determine if arthritis, for example, is an "active" diagnosis, the reviewer would check progress notes (including the history and physical) during the 7-day look-back period for notation of treatment of symptoms of arthritis, doctor's orders for medications for arthritis, and documentation of physical or other therapy for functional limitations caused by arthritis.

— Ongoing therapy with medications or other interventions to manage a condition that requires monitoring for therapeutic efficacy or to monitor potentially severe side effects in the last 7 days. A medication indicates active disease if that medication is prescribed to manage an ongoing condition that requires monitoring or is prescribed to decrease active symptoms associated with a condition. This includes medications used to limit disease progression and complications. If a medication is prescribed for a condition that requires regular staff monitoring of the drug's effect on that condition (therapeutic efficacy), then the prescription of the medication would indicate active disease.

- **It is expected that nurses monitor all medications for adverse effects as part of usual nursing practice.** For coding purposes, this monitoring relates to management of pharmacotherapy and not to management or monitoring of the underlying disease.

- **Item I2300 Urinary tract infection (UTI):**

  — The UTI has a look-back period of 30 days for active disease instead of 7 days.

  — **Code only if all the following are met**

    1. Physician, nurse practitioner, physician assistant, or clinical nurse specialist or other authorized licensed staff as permitted by state law diagnosis of a UTI in last 30 days,

    2. Sign or symptom attributed to UTI, which may or may not include but not be limited to: fever, urinary symptoms (e.g., peri-urethral site burning sensation, frequent urination of small amounts), pain or tenderness in flank, confusion or change in mental status, change in character of urine (e.g., pyuria),

    3. "Significant laboratory findings" (The attending physician should determine the level of significant laboratory findings and whether or not a culture should be obtained), and

    4. Current medication or treatment for a UTI in the last 30 days.

In response to questions regarding the resident with colonized MRSA, we consulted with the Centers for Disease Control (CDC) who provided the following information:

A physician often prescribes empiric antimicrobial therapy for a suspected infection **after a culture is obtained, but prior to receiving the culture results**. The confirmed diagnosis of UTI will depend on the culture results and other clinical assessment to determine appropriateness and continuation of antimicrobial therapy. This should not be any different, even if the resident is known to be colonized with an antibiotic resistant

I: Active Diagnoses in the Last 7 Days (cont.)

organism. An appropriate culture will help to ensure the diagnosis of infection is correct, and the appropriate antimicrobial is prescribed to treat the infection. The CDC does not recommend routine antimicrobial treatment for the purposes of attempting to eradicate colonization of MRSA or any other antimicrobial resistant organism.

The CDC's Healthcare Infection Control Practices Advisory Committee (HICPAC) has released infection prevention and control guidelines that contain recommendations that should be applied in all healthcare settings. At this site you will find information related to UTIs and many other issues related to infections in LTC.
http://www.cdc.gov/ncidod/dhqp/gl_longterm_care.html

Examples of Active Disease

1. A resident is prescribed hydrochlorothiazide for hypertension. The resident requires regular blood pressure monitoring to determine whether blood pressure goals are achieved by the current regimen. Physician progress note documents hypertension.

   Coding: Hypertension item (I0700), would be **checked**.
   Rationale: This would be considered an active diagnosis because of the need for ongoing monitoring to ensure treatment efficacy.

2. Warfarin is prescribed for a resident with atrial fibrillation to decrease the risk of embolic stroke. The resident requires monitoring for change in heart rhythm, for bleeding, and for anticoagulation.

   Coding: Atrial fibrillation item (I0300), would be **checked**.
   Rationale: This would be considered an active diagnosis because of the need for ongoing monitoring to ensure treatment efficacy as well as to monitor for side effects related to the medication.

3. A resident with a past history of healed peptic ulcer is prescribed a non-steroidal anti-inflammatory (NSAID) medication for arthritis. The physician also prescribes a proton-pump inhibitor to decrease the risk of peptic ulcer disease (PUD) from NSAID treatment.

   Coding: Arthritis item (I3700), would be **checked**.
   Rationale: Arthritis would be considered an active diagnosis because of the need for medical therapy. Given that the resident has a history of a healed peptic ulcer without current symptoms, the proton-pump inhibitor prescribed is preventive and therefore PUD would not be coded as an active disease.

4. The resident had a stroke 4 months ago and continues to have left-sided weakness, visual problems, and inappropriate behavior. The resident is on aspirin and has physical therapy and occupational therapy three times a week. The physician's note 25 days ago lists stroke.

   Coding: Cerebrovascular Vascular Accident (CVA), Transient Ischemic Attack (TIA), or Stroke item (I4500), would be **checked**.

I: Active Diagnoses in the Last 7 Days (cont.)

Rationale: The physician note within the last 30 days indicates stroke, and the resident is receiving medication and therapies to manage continued symptoms from stroke.

Examples of Inactive Diagnoses (do not code)

1. The admission history states that the resident had pneumonia 2 months prior to this admission. The resident has recovered completely, with no residual effects and no continued treatment during the 7-day look back period.

   Coding: Pneumonia item (I2000), would **not be checked.**

   Rationale: The pneumonia diagnosis would not be considered active because of the resident's complete recovery and the discontinuation of any treatment during the look-back period.

2. The problem list includes a diagnosis of coronary artery disease (CAD). The resident had an angioplasty 3 years ago, is not symptomatic, and is not taking any medication for CAD.

   Coding: CAD item (I0400), would **not be checked.**

   Rationale: The resident has had no symptoms and no treatment during the 7-day look-back period; thus, the CAD would be considered inactive.

3. Mr. J fell and fractured his hip 2 years ago. At the time of the injury, the fracture was surgically repaired. Following the surgery, the resident received several weeks of physical therapy in an attempt to restore him to his previous ambulation status, which had been independent without any devices. Although he received therapy services at that time, he now requires assistance to stand from the chair and uses a walker. He also needs help with lower body dressing because of difficulties standing and leaning over.

   Coding: Hip Fracture item (I3900), would **not be checked.**

   Rationale: Although the resident has mobility and self-care limitations in ambulation and ADLs due to the hip fracture, he has not received therapy services during the 7-day look-back period; thus, Hip Fracture would be considered inactive.

SECTION J: HEALTH CONDITIONS

Intent: The intent of the items in this section is to document a number of health conditions that impact the resident's functional status and quality of life. The items include an assessment of pain which uses an interview with the resident or staff if the resident is unable to participate. The pain items assess the presence of pain, pain frequency, effect on function, intensity, management and control. Other items in the section assess dyspnea, tobacco use, prognosis, problem conditions, and falls.

J0100: Pain Management (5-Day Look Back)

J0100. Pain Management - Complete for all residents, regardless of current pain level	
At any time in the last 5 days, has the resident:	
Enter Code	A. Been on a scheduled pain medication regimen? 0. No 1. Yes
Enter Code	B. Received PRN pain medications? 0. No 1. Yes
Enter Code	C. Received non-medication intervention for pain? 0. No 1. Yes

Item Rationale

Health-related Quality of Life

- Pain can cause suffering and is associated with inactivity, social withdrawal, depression, and functional decline.
- Pain can interfere with participation in rehabilitation.
- Effective pain management interventions can help to avoid these adverse outcomes.

Planning for Care

- Goals for pain management for most residents should be to achieve a consistent level of comfort while maintaining as much function as possible.
- Identification of pain management interventions facilitates review of the effectiveness of pain management and revision of the plan if goals are not met.
- Residents may have more than one source of pain and will need a comprehensive, individualized management regimen.
- Most residents with moderate to severe pain will require regularly dosed pain medication, and some will require additional PRN (as-needed) pain medications for breakthrough pain.
- Some residents with intermittent or mild pain may have orders for PRN dosing only.

> **DEFINITIONS**
>
> **PAIN MEDICATION REGIMEN**
> Pharmacological agent(s) prescribed to relieve or prevent the recurrence of pain. Include all medications used for pain management by any route and any frequency during the look-back period. Include oral, transcutaneous, subcutaneous, intramuscular, rectal, intravenous injections or intraspinal delivery. This item does not include medications that primarily target treatment of the underlying condition, such as chemotherapy or steroids, although such treatments may lead to pain reduction.

J0100: Pain Management (cont.)

- Non-medication pain (non-pharmacologic) interventions for pain can be important adjuncts to pain treatment regimens.

- Interventions must be included as part of a care plan that aims to prevent or relieve pain and includes monitoring for effectiveness and revision of care plan if stated goals are not met. There must be documentation that the intervention was received and its effectiveness was assessed. It does not have to have been successful to be counted.

Steps for Assessment

1. Review medical record to determine if a pain regimen exists.
2. Review the medical record and interview staff and direct caregivers to determine what, if any, pain management interventions the resident received during the 5-day look-back period. Include information from all disciplines.

Coding Instructions for J0100A-C

Determine all interventions for pain provided to the resident during the 5-day look-back period. Answer these items even if the resident currently denies pain.

Coding Instructions for J0100A, **Been on a Scheduled Pain Medication Regimen**

- **Code 0, no:** if the medical record does not contain documentation that a scheduled pain medication was received.
- **Code 1, yes:** if the medical record contains documentation that a scheduled pain medication was received.

Coding Instructions for J0100B, **Received PRN Pain Medication**

- **Code 0, no:** if the medical record does not contain documentation that a PRN medication was received or offered.

- **Code 1, yes:** if the medical record contains documentation that a PRN medication was either received OR was offered but declined.

DEFINITIONS

SCHEDULED PAIN MEDICATION REGIMEN
Pain medication order that defines dose and specific time interval for pain medication administration. For example, "once a day," "every 12 hours."

PRN PAIN MEDICATIONS
Pain medication order that specifies dose and indicates that pain medication may be given on an as needed basis, including a time interval, such as "every 4 hours as needed for pain" or "every 6 hours as needed for pain."

NON-MEDICATION PAIN INTERVENTION
Scheduled and implemented non-pharmacological interventions include, but are not limited to: bio-feedback, application of heat/cold, massage, physical therapy, nerve block, stretching and strengthening exercises, chiropractic, electrical stimulation, radiotherapy, ultrasound and acupuncture. Herbal medications are not included in this category.

J0100: Pain Management (cont.)

Coding Instructions for J0100C, Received Non-medication Intervention for Pain

- **Code 0, no:** if the medical record does not contain documentation that a non-medication pain intervention was received.
- **Code 1, yes:** if the medical record contains documentation that a non-medication pain intervention was scheduled as part of the care plan and it is documented that the intervention was actually received and assessed for efficacy.

Coding Tips

- Code only pain medication regimens without PRN pain medications in J0100A. Code receipt of PRN pain medications in J0100B.
- For coding J0100B code only residents with PRN pain medication regimens here. If the resident has a scheduled pain medication J0100A should be coded.

Examples

1. The resident's medical record documents that she received the following pain management in the past 5 days:

   - Hydrocodone/acetaminophen 5/500 1 tab PO every 6 hours. Discontinued on day 1 of look-back period.
   - Acetaminophen 500mg PO every 4 hours. Started on day 2 of look-back period.
   - Cold pack to left shoulder applied by PT BID. PT notes that resident reports significant pain improvement after cold pack applied.

     Coding: J0100A would be **coded 1, yes**.
     Rationale: Medical record indicated that resident received a scheduled pain medication during the 5-day look-back period.
     Coding: J0100B would be **coded 0, no**.
     Rationale: No documentation was found in the medical record that resident received or was offered and declined any PRN medications during the 5-day look-back period.
     Coding: J0100C would be **coded 1, yes**.
     Rationale: The medical record indicates that the resident received scheduled non-medication pain intervention (cold pack to the left shoulder) during the 5-day look-back period.

2. The resident's medical record includes the following pain management documentation:

   - Morphine sulfate controlled-release 15 mg PO Q 12 hours: Resident refused every dose of medication during the 5-day look-back period. No other pain management interventions were documented.

J0100: Pain Management (cont.)

Coding: J0100A would be **coded 0, no.**
Rationale: The medical record documented that the resident did not receive scheduled pain medication during the 5-day look-back period. Residents may refuse scheduled medications; however, medications are not considered "received" if the resident refuses the dose.

Coding: J0100B would be **coded 0, no.**
Rationale: The medical record contained no documentation that the resident received or was offered and declined any PRN medications during the 5-day look-back period.

Coding: J0100C would be **coded 0, no.**
Rationale: The medical record contains no documentation that the resident received non-medication pain intervention during the 5-day look-back period.

J0200: Should Pain Assessment Interview Be Conducted?

J0200. Should Pain Assessment Interview be Conducted?
Attempt to conduct interview with all residents. If resident is comatose, skip to J1100, Shortness of Breath (dyspnea)
Enter Code [ ]   0. **No** (resident is rarely/never understood) → Skip to and complete J0800, Indicators of Pain or Possible Pain 1. **Yes** → Continue to J0300, Pain Presence

Item Rationale

Health-related Quality of Life

- Most residents who are capable of communicating can answer questions about how they feel.
- Obtaining information about pain directly from the resident, sometimes called "hearing the resident's voice," is more reliable and accurate than observation alone for identifying pain.
- If a resident cannot communicate (e.g., verbal, gesture, written), then staff observations for pain behavior (J0800 and J0850) will be used.

Planning for Care

- Interview allows the resident's voice to be reflected in the care plan.
- Information about pain that comes directly from the resident provides symptom-specific information for individualized care planning.

Steps for Assessment

1. Determine whether the resident is understood at least sometimes. Review **Language** item (A1100), to determine whether the resident needs or wants an interpreter.

   - If an interpreter is needed or requested, every effort should be made to have an interpreter present for the MDS clinical interview.

J0200: Should Pain Assessment Interview Be Conducted? (cont.)

Coding Instructions

*Attempt to complete the interview if the resident is at least sometimes understood and an **interpreter is present** or not required.*

- **Code 0, no:** if the resident is rarely/never understood or an interpreter is required but not available. Skip to **Indicators of Pain or Possible Pain** item (J0800).
- **Code 1, yes:** if the resident is at least sometimes understood and an interpreter is present or not required. Continue to **Pain Presence** item (J0300).

Coding Tips and Special Populations

- If it is not possible for an interpreter to be present during the look-back period, code J0200 = 0 to indicate interview not attempted and complete **Staff Assessment of Pain** item (J0800), instead of the **Pain Interview** items (J0300-J0600).

J0300-J0600: Pain Assessment Interview

Pain Assessment Interview
J0300. Pain Presence

Enter Code   Ask resident: *"Have you had pain or hurting at any time in the last 5 days?"*
     0. **No** → Skip to J1100, Shortness of Breath
     1. **Yes** → Continue to J0400, Pain Frequency
     9. **Unable to answer** → Skip to J0800, Indicators of Pain or Possible Pain

J0400. Pain Frequency

Enter Code   Ask resident: *"How much of the time have you experienced pain or hurting over the last 5 days?"*
     1. **Almost constantly**
     2. **Frequently**
     3. **Occasionally**
     4. **Rarely**
     9. **Unable to answer**

J0500. Pain Effect on Function

Enter Code   **A.** Ask resident: *"Over the past 5 days, has pain made it hard for you to sleep at night?"*
     0. **No**
     1. **Yes**
     9. **Unable to answer**

Enter Code   **B.** Ask resident: *"Over the past 5 days, have you limited your day-to-day activities because of pain?"*
     0. **No**
     1. **Yes**
     9. **Unable to answer**

J0600. Pain Intensity - Administer **ONLY ONE** of the following pain intensity questions (A or B)

Enter Rating   **A. Numeric Rating Scale (00-10)**
     Ask resident: *"Please rate your worst pain over the last 5 days on a zero to ten scale, with zero being no pain and ten as the worst pain you can imagine."* (Show resident 00-10 pain scale)
     Enter two-digit response. Enter 99 if unable to answer.

Enter Code   **B. Verbal Descriptor Scale**
     Ask resident: *"Please rate the intensity of your worst pain over the last 5 days."* (Show resident verbal scale)
     1. **Mild**
     2. **Moderate**
     3. **Severe**
     4. **Very severe, horrible**
     9. **Unable to answer**

J0300-J0600: Pain Assessment Interview (cont.)

Item Rationale

Health-related Quality of Life

- The effects of unrelieved pain impact the individual in terms of functional decline, complications of immobility, skin breakdown and infections.
- Pain significantly adversely affects a person's quality of life and is tightly linked to depression, diminished self-confidence and self-esteem, as well as an increase in behavior problems, particularly for cognitively-impaired residents.
- Some older adults limit their activities in order to avoid having pain. Their report of lower pain frequency may reflect their avoidance of activity more than it reflects adequate pain management.

Planning for Care

- Directly asking the resident about pain rather than relying on the resident to volunteer the information or relying on clinical observation significantly improves the detection of pain.
- Resident self-report is the most reliable means for assessing pain.
- Pain assessment provides a basis for evaluation, treatment need, and response to treatment.
- Assessing whether pain interferes with sleep or activities provides additional understanding of the functional impact of pain and potential care planning implications.
- Assessment of pain provides insight into the need to adjust the timing of pain interventions to better cover sleep or preferred activities.
- Pain assessment prompts discussion about factors that aggravate and alleviate pain.
- Similar pain stimuli can have varying impact on different individuals.
- Consistent use of a standardized pain intensity scale improves the validity and reliability of pain assessment. Using the same scale in different settings may improve continuity of care.
- Pain intensity scales allow providers to evaluate whether pain is responding to pain medication regimen(s) and/or non-pharmacological intervention(s).

Steps for Assessment: Basic Interview Instructions for Pain Assessment Interview (J0300-J0600)

1. Interview any resident not screened out by the **Should Pain Assessment Interview be Conducted?** item (J0200).
2. The Pain Assessment Interview for residents consists of four items: the primary question **Pain Presence** item (J0300), and three follow-up questions **Pain Frequency** item (J0400); **Pain Effect on Function** item (J0500); and **Pain Intensity** item (J0600). If the resident is unable to answer the primary question on **Pain Presence** item J0300, skip to the **Staff Assessment for Pain** beginning with **Indicators of Pain or Possible Pain** item (J0800).

J0300-J0600: Pain Assessment Interview (cont.)

3. The look-back period on these items is 5 days. Because this item asks the resident to recall pain during the past 5 days, this assessment should be conducted close to the end of the 5-day look-back period; preferably on the day before, or the day of the ARD. This should more accurately capture pain episodes that occur during the 5-day look-back period.
4. Conduct the interview in a private setting.
5. Be sure the resident can hear you.
   - Residents with hearing impairment should be tested using their usual communication devices/techniques, as applicable.
   - Try an external assistive device (headphones or hearing amplifier) if you have any doubt about hearing ability.
   - Minimize background noise.
6. Sit so that the resident can see your face. Minimize glare by directing light sources away from the resident's face.
7. Give an introduction before starting the interview.
   Suggested language: "I'd like to ask you some questions about pain. The reason I am asking these questions is to understand how often you have pain, how severe it is, and how pain affects your daily activities. This will help us to develop the best plan of care to help manage your pain."
8. Directly ask the resident each item in J0300 through J0600 in the order provided.
   - Use other terms for pain or follow-up discussion if the resident seems unsure or hesitant. Some residents avoid use of the term "pain" but may report that they "hurt." Residents may use other terms such as "aching" or "burning" to describe pain.
9. If the resident chooses not to answer a particular item, accept his/her refusal, **code 9**, and move on to the next item.
10. If the resident is unsure about whether the pain occurred in the 5-day time interval, prompt the resident to think about the most recent episode of pain and try to determine whether it occurred within the look-back period.

> **DEFINITIONS**
>
> **PAIN** Any type of physical pain or discomfort in any part of the body. It may be localized to one area or may be more generalized. It may be acute or chronic, continuous or intermittent, or occur at rest or with movement. Pain is very subjective; pain is whatever the experiencing person says it is and exists whenever he or she says it does.

J0300: Pain Presence (5-Day Look Back)

Pain Assessment Interview
J0300. Pain Presence

Enter Code ☐   Ask resident: "*Have you had pain or hurting at any time in the last 5 days?*"
    0. **No** → Skip to J1100, Shortness of Breath
    1. **Yes** → Continue to J0400, Pain Frequency
    9. **Unable to answer** → Skip to J0800, Indicators of Pain or Possible Pain

J0300: Pain Presence (cont.)

Steps for Assessment

1. Ask the resident: "Have you had pain or hurting at any time in the last 5 days?"

Coding Instructions for J0300, Pain Presence

> DEFINITIONS
>
> **NONSENSICAL RESPONSE**
> Any unrelated, incomprehensible, or incoherent response that is not informative with respect to the item being coded.

Code for the presence or absence of pain regardless of pain management efforts during the 5-day look-back period.

- **Code 0, no:** if the resident responds "no" to any pain in the 5-day look-back period. **Code 0, no:** even if the reason for no pain is that the resident received pain management interventions. If coded 0, the pain interview is complete. Skip to **Shortness of Breath** item (J1100).

- **Code 1, yes:** if the resident responds "yes" to pain at any time during the look-back period. If coded 1, proceed to items J0400, J0500, J0600 AND J0700.

- **Code 9, unable to answer:** if the resident is unable to answer, does not respond, or gives a nonsensical response. If coded 9, skip to the **Staff Assessment for Pain** beginning with **Indicators of Pain or Possible Pain** item (J0800).

Coding Tips

- Rates of self-reported pain are higher than observed rates. Although some observers have expressed concern that residents may not complain and may deny pain, the regular and objective use of self-report pain scales enhances residents' willingness to report.

Examples

1. When asked about pain, Mrs. S. responds, "No. I have been taking the pain medication regularly, so fortunately I have had no pain."

    Coding: J0300 would be **coded 0, no**. The assessor would skip to **Shortness of Breath** item (J1100).
    Rationale: Mrs. S. reports having no pain during the look-back period. Even though she received pain management interventions during the look-back period, the item is coded "No," because there was no pain.

2. When asked about pain, Mr. T. responds, "No pain, but I have had a terrible burning sensation all down my leg."

    Coding: J0300 would be **coded 1, yes**. The assessor would proceed to **Pain Frequency** item (J0400).
    Rationale: Although Mr. T.'s initial response is "no," the comments indicate that he has experienced pain (burning sensation) during the look-back period.

J0300: Pain Presence (cont.)

3. When asked about pain, Ms. G. responds, "I was on a train in 1905."

   Coding: J0300 would be **coded 9, unable to respond.** The assessor would skip to **Indicators of Pain** item (J0800).

   Rationale: Ms. G. has provided a nonsensical answer to the question. The assessor will complete the **Staff Assessment for Pain** beginning with **Indicators of Pain** item (J0800).

J0400: Pain Frequency (5-Day Look Back)

J0400. Pain Frequency	
Enter Code	Ask resident: *"How much of the time have you experienced pain or hurting over the last 5 days?"* 1. Almost constantly 2. Frequently 3. Occasionally 4. Rarely 9. Unable to answer

Steps for Assessment

1. Ask the resident: "How much of the time have you experienced pain or hurting over the last 5 days?" Staff may present response options on a written sheet or cue card. This can help the resident respond to the items.

2. If the resident provides a related response but does not use the provided response scale, help clarify the best response by echoing (repeating) the resident's own comment and providing related response options. This interview approach frequently helps the resident clarify which response option he or she prefers.

3. If the resident, despite clarifying statement and repeating response options, continues to have difficulty selecting between two of the provided responses, then select the more frequent of the two.

Coding Instructions

Code for pain frequency during the 5-day look-back period.

- **Code 1, almost constantly:** if the resident responds "almost constantly" to the question.

- **Code 2, frequently:** if the resident responds "frequently" to the question.

- **Code 3, occasionally:** if the resident responds "occasionally" to the question.

- **Code 4, rarely:** if the resident responds "rarely" to the question.

- **Code 9, unable to answer:** if the resident is unable to respond, does not respond, or gives a nonsensical response. Proceed to items J0500, J0600 AND J0700.

J0400: Pain Frequency (cont.)

Coding Tips

- No predetermined definitions are offered to the resident related to frequency of pain.
  - The response should be based on the resident's interpretation of the frequency options.
  - Facility policy should provide standardized tools to use throughout the facility in assessing pain to ensure consistency in interpretation and documentation of the resident's pain.

Examples

1. When asked about pain, Mrs. C. responds, "All the time. It has been a terrible week. I have not been able to get comfortable for more than 10 minutes at a time since I started physical therapy four days ago."

   Coding: J0400 would be **coded 1, almost constantly**.

   Rationale: Mrs. C. describes pain that has occurred "all the time."

2. When asked about pain, Mr. J. responds, "I don't know if it is frequent or occasional. My knee starts throbbing every time they move me from the bed or the wheelchair."

   The interviewer says: "Your knee throbs every time they move you. If you had to choose an answer, would you say that you have pain frequently or occasionally?"

   Mr. J. is still unable to choose between frequently and occasionally.

   Coding: J0400 would be **coded 2, frequently**.

   Rationale: The interviewer appropriately echoed Mr. J.'s comment and provided related response options to help him clarify which response he preferred. Mr. J. remained unable to decide between frequently and occasionally. The interviewer therefore coded for the higher frequency of pain.

3. When asked about pain, Miss K. responds: "I can't remember. I think I had a headache a few times in the past couple of days, but they gave me acetaminophen and the headaches went away."

   The interviewer clarifies by echoing what Miss K. said: "You've had a headache a few times in the past couple of days and the headaches went away when you were given acetaminophen. If you had to choose from the answers, would you say you had pain occasionally or rarely?"

   Miss K. replies "Occasionally."

   Coding: J0400 would be **coded 3, occasionally**.

   Rationale: After the interviewer clarified the resident's choice using echoing, the resident selected a response option.

J0400: Pain Frequency (cont.)

4. When asked about pain, Ms. M. responds, "I would say rarely. Since I started using the patch, I don't have much pain at all, but four days ago the pain came back. I think they were a bit overdue in putting on the new patch, so I had some pain for a little while that day."

> **Coding:** J0400 would be **coded 4, rarely**.
> **Rationale:** Ms. M. selected the "rarely" response option.

J0500: Pain Effect on Function (5-Day Look Back)

J0500. Pain Effect on Function	
Enter Code	**A.** Ask resident: *"Over the past 5 days, has pain made it hard for you to sleep at night?"* 0. **No** 1. **Yes** 9. **Unable to answer**
Enter Code	**B.** Ask resident: *"Over the past 5 days, have you limited your day-to-day activities because of pain?"* 0. **No** 1. **Yes** 9. **Unable to answer**

Steps for Assessment

1. Ask the resident each of the two questions exactly as they are written.
2. If the resident's response does not lead to a clear "yes" or "no" answer, repeat the resident's response and then try to narrow the focus of the response. For example, if the resident responded to the question, "Has pain made it hard for you to sleep at night?" by saying, "I always have trouble sleeping," then the assessor might reply, "You always have trouble sleeping. Is it your pain that makes it hard for you to sleep?

Coding Instructions for J0500A, Over the Past 5 Days, Has Pain Made It Hard for You to Sleep at Night?

- **Code 0, no:** if the resident responds "no," indicating that pain did not interfere with sleep.
- **Code 1, yes:** if the resident responds "yes," indicating that pain interfered with sleep.
- **Code 9, unable to answer:** if the resident is unable to answer the question, does not respond or gives a nonsensical response. Proceed to items J0500B, J0600 AND J0700.

Coding Instructions for J0500B, Over the Past 5 Days, Have You Limited Your Day-to-day Activities because of Pain?

- **Code 0, no:** if the resident indicates that pain did not interfere with daily activities.
- **Code 1, yes:** if the resident indicates that pain interfered with daily activities.
- **Code 9, unable to answer:** if the resident is unable to answer the question, does not respond or gives a nonsensical response. Proceed to items J0600 AND J0700.

J0500: Pain Effect on Function (5-Day Look Back) (cont.)

Examples for J0500A, Over the Past 5 Days, Has Pain Made It Hard for You to Sleep at Night?

1. Mrs. D. responds, "I had a little back pain from being in the wheelchair all day, but it felt so much better when I went to bed. I slept like a baby."

   Coding: J0500A would be **coded 0, no.**

   Rationale: Mrs. D. reports no sleep problems related to pain.

2. Mr. E. responds, "I can't sleep at all in this place."
   The interviewer clarifies by saying, "You can't sleep here. Would you say that was because pain made it hard for you to sleep at night?"
   Mr. E. responds, "No. It has nothing to do with me. I have no pain. It is because everyone is making so much noise."

   Coding: J0500A would be **coded 0, no.**

   Rationale: Mr. E. reports that his sleep problems are not related to pain.

3. Miss G. responds, "Yes, the back pain makes it hard to sleep. I have to ask for extra pain medicine, and I still wake up several times during the night because my back hurts so much."

   Coding: J0500A would be **coded 1, yes.**

   Rationale: The resident reports pain-related sleep problems.

Examples for J0500B, Over the Past 5 Days, Have You Limited Your Day-to-day Activities because of Pain?

1. Ms. L. responds, "No, I had some pain on Wednesday, but I didn't want to miss the shopping trip, so I went."

   Coding: J0500B would be **coded 0, no.**

   Rationale: Although Ms. L. reports pain, she did not limit her activity because of it.

2. Mrs. N. responds, "Yes, I haven't been able to play the piano, because my shoulder hurts."

   Coding: J0500B would be **coded 1, yes.**

   Rationale: Mrs. N. reports limiting her activities because of pain.

3. Mrs. S. responds, "I don't know. I have not tried to knit since my finger swelled up yesterday, because I am afraid it might hurt even more than it does now."

   Coding: J0500B would be **coded 1, yes.**

   Rationale: Resident avoided a usual activity because of fear that her pain would increase.

4. Mr. Q. responds, "I don't like painful activities."
   Interviewer repeats question and Mr. Q. responds, "I designed a plane one time."

   Coding: J0500B would be **coded 9, unable to answer**.

   Rationale: Resident has provided a nonsensical answer to the question. Proceed to items J0600 AND J0700.

J0600: Pain Intensity (5-Day Look Back)

J0600. Pain Intensity - Administer **ONLY ONE** of the following pain intensity questions (A or B)

Enter Rating	**A. Numeric Rating Scale (00-10)**
	Ask resident: *"Please rate your worst pain over the last 5 days on a zero to ten scale, with zero being no pain and ten as the worst pain you can imagine."* (Show resident 00 -10 pain scale)
	Enter two-digit response. Enter 99 if unable to answer.

Enter Code	**B. Verbal Descriptor Scale**
	Ask resident: *"Please rate the intensity of your worst pain over the last 5 days."* (Show resident verbal scale)
	1. **Mild**
	2. **Moderate**
	3. **Severe**
	4. **Very severe, horrible**
	9. **Unable to answer**

Steps for Assessment

1. You may use either **Numeric Rating Scale** item (J0600A) or **Verbal Descriptor Scale** item (J0600B) to interview the resident about pain intensity.

   - For each resident, try to use the same scale used on prior assessments.

2. If the resident is unable to answer using one scale, the other scale should be attempted.
3. Record **either** the **Numeric Rating Scale** item (J0600A) **or** the **Verbal Descriptor Scale** item (J0600B). Leave the response for the unused scale blank.
4. Read the question and item choices slowly. While reading, you may show the resident the response options (the **Numeric Rating Scale** or **Verbal Descriptor Scale**) clearly printed on a piece of paper, such as a cue card. Use large, clear print.

   - For the **Numeric Rating Scale**, say, "Please rate your worst pain over the last 5 days with zero being no pain, and ten as the worst pain you can imagine."
   - For **Verbal Descriptor Scale**, say, "Please rate the intensity of your worst pain over the last 5 days."

5. The resident may provide a verbal response, point to the written response, or both.

Coding Instructions for J0600A. Numeric Rating Scale (00-10)

Enter the two digit number (00-10) indicated by the resident as corresponding to the intensity of his or her worst pain during the 5-day look-back period, where zero is no pain, and 10 is the worst pain imaginable.

- Enter 99 if unable to answer.
- If the Numeric Rating Scale is not used, leave the response box blank.

Coding Instructions for J0600B. Verbal Descriptor Scale

- **Code 1, mild:** if resident indicates that his or her pain is "mild."
- **Code 2, moderate:** if resident indicates that his or her pain is "moderate."
- **Code 3, severe:** if resident indicates that his or her pain is "severe."
- **Code 4, very severe, horrible:** if resident indicates that his or her pain is "very severe or horrible."

J0600: Pain Intensity (cont.)

- **Code 9, unable to answer:** if resident is unable to answer, chooses not to respond, does not respond or gives a nonsensical response. Proceed to item J0700.
- If the **Verbal Descriptor Scale** is not used, leave the response box blank.

Examples for J0600A. Numeric Rating Scale (00-10)

1. The nurse asks Ms. T. to rate her pain on a scale of 0 to 10. Ms. T. states that she is not sure, because she has shoulder pain and knee pain, and sometimes it is really bad, and sometimes it is OK. The nurse reminds Ms. T. to think about all the pain she had during the last 5 days and select the number that describes her worst pain. She reports that her pain is a "6."

    Coding: J0600A would be **coded 06**.

    Rationale: The resident said her pain was 6 on the 0 to 10 scale. Because a 2-digit number is required, it is entered as 06.

2. The nurse asks Mr. S. to rate his pain, reviews use of the scale, and provides the 0 to 10 visual aid. Mr. S. says, "My pain doesn't have any numbers." The nurse explains that the numbers help the staff understand how severe his pain is, and repeats that the "0" end is no pain and the "10" end is the worst pain imaginable. Mr. S. replies, "I don't know where it would fall."

    Coding: Item J0600A would be **coded 99, unable to answer.** The interviewer would go on to ask about pain intensity using the **Verbal Descriptor Scale** item (J0600B).

    Rationale: The resident was unable to select a number or point to a location on the 0-10 scale that represented his level of pain intensity.

Examples for J0600B. Verbal Descriptor Scale

1. The nurse asks Mr. R. to rate his pain using the verbal descriptor scale. He looks at the response options presented using a cue card and says his pain is "severe" sometimes, but most of the time it is "mild."

    Coding: J0600B would be **coded 3, severe.**

    Rationale: The resident said his worst pain was "Severe."

2. The nurse asks Ms. U. to rate her pain, reviews use of the verbal descriptor scale, and provides a cue card as a visual aid. Ms. U. says, "I'm not sure whether it's mild or moderate." The nurse reminds Ms. U. to think about her worst pain during the last 5 days. Ms. U. says "At its worst, it was moderate."

    Coding: Item J0600B would be **coded 2, moderate.**

    Rationale: The resident indicated that her worst pain was "Moderate."

J0700: Should the Staff Assessment for Pain be Conducted? (5-Day Look Back)

J0700. Should the Staff Assessment for Pain be Conducted?	
Enter Code ☐	0. No (J0400 = 1 thru 4) → Skip to J1100, Shortness of Breath (dyspnea)
	1. Yes (J0400 = 9) → Continue to J0800, Indicators of Pain or Possible Pain

Item Rationale

Item J0700 closes the pain interview and determines if the resident interview was complete or incomplete and based on this determination, whether a staff assessment needs to be completed.

Health-related Quality of Life

- Resident interview for pain is preferred because it improves the detection of pain. However, a small percentage of residents are unable or unwilling to complete the pain interview.
- Persons unable to complete the pain interview may still have pain.

Planning for Care

- Resident self-report is the most reliable means of assessing pain. However, when a resident is unable to provide the information, staff assessment is necessary.

> **DEFINITIONS**
>
> **COMPLETED INTERVIEW**
> The pain interview is successfully completed if the resident reported no pain (answered No to J0300), or if the resident reported pain (J0300=yes) and the follow-up question J0400 is answered.

- Even though the resident was unable to complete the interview, important insights may be gained from the responses that were obtained, observing behaviors and observing the resident's affect during the interview.

Steps for Assessment

1. Review the resident's responses to items J0200-J0400.
2. The **Staff Assessment for Pain** should only be completed if the **Pain Assessment Interview** (J0200-J0600) was not completed.

Coding Instructions for J0700. Should the Staff Assessment for Pain be Conducted? This item is to be coded at the completion of items J0400-J0600.

- **Code 0, no:** if the resident completed the **Pain Assessment Interview** item (J0400 = 1, 2, 3, or 4). Skip to **Shortness of Breath (dyspnea)** item (J1100).
- **Code 1, yes:** if the resident was unable to complete the **Pain Assessment Interview** (J0400 = 9). Continue to **Indicators of Pain or Possible Pain** item (J0800).

J0800: Indicators of Pain (5-Day Look Back)

*Complete this item only if the **Pain Assessment Interview** (J0200-J0600) was not completed.*

Staff Assessment for Pain	
J0800. Indicators of Pain or Possible Pain in the last 5 days	
↓ Check all that apply	
☐	A. **Non-verbal sounds** (e.g., crying, whining, gasping, moaning, or groaning)
☐	B. **Vocal complaints of pain** (e.g., that hurts, ouch, stop)
☐	C. **Facial expressions** (e.g., grimaces, winces, wrinkled forehead, furrowed brow, clenched teeth or jaw)
☐	D. **Protective body movements or postures** (e.g., bracing, guarding, rubbing or massaging a body part/area, clutching or holding a body part during movement)
☐	Z. **None of these signs observed or documented** → If checked, skip to J1100, Shortness of Breath (dyspnea)

Item Rationale

Health-related Quality of Life

- Residents who cannot verbally communicate about their pain are at particularly high risk for underdetection and undertreatment of pain.

- Severe cognitive impairment may affect the ability of residents to verbally communicate, thus limiting the availability of self-reported information about pain. In this population, fewer complaints may not mean less pain.

- Individuals who are unable to verbally communicate may be more likely to use alternative methods of expression to communicate their pain.

- Even in this population some verbal complaints of pain may be made and should be taken seriously.

Planning for Care

- Consistent approach to observation improves the accuracy of pain assessment for residents who are unable to verbally communicate their pain.

- Particular attention should be paid to using the indicators of pain during activities when pain is most likely to be demonstrated (e.g., bathing, transferring, dressing, walking and potentially during eating).

- Staff must carefully monitor, track, and document any possible signs and symptoms of pain.

- Identification of these pain indicators can:
  - provide a basis for more comprehensive pain assessment,
  - provide a basis for determining appropriate treatment, and
  - provide a basis for ongoing monitoring of pain presence and treatment response.

- If pain indicators are present, assessment should identify aggravating/alleviating factors related to pain.

J0800: Indicators of Pain (cont.)

Steps for Assessment

1. **Review the medical record** for documentation of each indicator of pain listed in J0800 that occurred during the 5-day look-back period. If the record documents the presence of any of the signs and symptoms listed, confirm your record review with the direct care staff on all shifts who work most closely with the resident during activities of daily living (ADL).

2. **Interview staff** because the medical record may fail to note all observable pain behaviors. For any indicators that were not noted as present in medical record review, interview direct care staff on all shifts who work with the resident during ADL. Ask directly about the presence of each indicator that was not noted as being present in the record.

3. **Observe resident** during care activities. If you observe additional indicators of pain during the 5-day look-back period, code the corresponding items.

   - Observations for pain indicators may be more sensitive if the resident is observed during ADL, or wound care.

Coding Instructions

Check all that apply in the past 5 days based on staff observation of pain indicators.

- If the medical record review and the interview with direct care providers and observation on all shifts provide no evidence of pain indicators, Check J0800Z, None of these **signs observed or documented**, and proceed to **Shortness of Breath** item (J1100).

- **Check J0800A, nonverbal sounds:** included but not limited to if crying, whining, gasping, moaning, or groaning were observed or reported during the look-back period.

- **Check J0800B, vocal complaints of pain:** included but not limited to if the resident was observed to make vocal complaints of pain (e.g. "that hurts," "ouch," or "stop").

- **Check J0800C, facial expressions:** included but not limited to if grimaces, winces, wrinkled forehead, furrowed brow, clenched teeth or jaw were observed or reported during the look-back period.

- **Check J0800D, protective body movements or postures:** included but not limited to if bracing, guarding, rubbing or massaging a body part/area, or clutching or holding a body part during movement were observed or reported during the look-back period.

> **DEFINITIONS**
>
> **NON VERBAL SOUNDS**
> e.g., crying, whining, gasping, moaning, groaning or other audible indications associated with pain.
>
> **VOCAL COMPLAINTS OF PAIN**
> e.g., "That hurts," "ouch," "stop," etc.
>
> **FACIAL EXPRESSIONS THAT MAY BE INDICATORS OF PAIN**
> e.g., grimaces, winces, wrinkled forehead, furrowed brow, clenched teeth or jaw, etc.
>
> **PROTECTIVE BODY MOVEMENTS OR POSTURES**
> e.g., bracing, guarding, rubbing or massaging a body part/area, clutching or holding a body part during movement, etc.

J0800: Indicators of Pain (cont.)

- **Check J0800Z, none of these signs observed or documented:** if none of these signs were observed or reported during the look-back period.

Coding Tips

- Behavior change, depressed mood, rejection of care and decreased activity participation may be related to pain. These behaviors and symptoms are identified in other sections and not reported here as pain screening items. However, the contribution of pain should be considered when following up on those symptoms and behaviors.

Examples

1. Mr. P. has advanced dementia and is unable to verbally communicate. A note in his medical record documents that he has been awake during the last night crying and rubbing his elbow. When you go to his room to interview the certified nurse aide (CNA) caring for him, you observe Mr. P. grimacing and clenching his teeth. The CNA reports that he has been moaning and said "ouch" when she tried to move his arm.

   Coding: **Nonverbal Sounds** item (J0800A); **Vocal Complaints of Pain** item (J0800B); **Facial Expressions** item (J0800C); and **Protective Body Movements or Postures** item (J0800D), would be **checked**.

   Rationale: Mr. P. has demonstrated vocal complaints of pain (ouch), nonverbal sounds (crying and moaning), facial expression of pain (grimacing and clenched teeth), and protective body movements (rubbing his elbow).

2. Mrs. M. has end-stage Parkinson's disease and is unable to verbally communicate. There is no documentation of pain in her medical record during the 5-day look-back period. The CNAs caring for her report that on some mornings she moans and winces when her arms and legs are moved during morning care. During direct observation, you note that Mrs. M. cries and attempts to pull her hand away when the CNA tries to open the contracted hand to wash it.

   Coding: **Nonverbal Sounds** items (J0800A); **Facial Expressions** item (J0800C); and **Protective Body Movements or Postures** item (J0800D), would be **checked**.

   Rationale: Mrs. M. has demonstrated nonverbal sounds (crying, moaning); facial expression of pain (wince), and protective body movements (attempt to withdraw).

3. Mrs. E. has been unable to verbally communicate following a massive cerebrovascular accident (CVA) several months ago and has a Stage 3 pressure ulcer. There is no documentation of pain in her medical record. The CNA who cares for her reports that she does not seem to have any pain. You observe the resident during her pressure ulcer dressing change. During the treatment, you observe groaning, facial grimaces, and a wrinkled forehead.

   Coding: **Nonverbal Sounds** item (J0800A), and **Facial Expressions** item (J0800C), would be **checked**.

   Rationale: The resident has demonstrated nonverbal sounds (groaning) and facial expression of pain (wrinkled forehead and grimacing).

J0800: Indicators of Pain (cont.)

Examples (cont.)

4. Mr. S. is in a persistent vegetative state following a traumatic brain injury. He is unable to verbally communicate. There is no documentation of pain in his medical record during the 5-day look-back period. The CNA reports that he appears comfortable whenever she cares for him. You observe the CNA providing morning care and transferring him from bed to chair. No pain indicators are observed at any time.

> **Coding: None of These Signs Observed or Documented** item (J0800Z), would be **checked**.
>
> **Rationale:** All steps for the assessment have been followed and no pain indicators have been documented, reported or directly observed.

J0850: Frequency of Indicator of Pain or Possible Pain (5-Day Look Back)

J0850. Frequency of Indicator of Pain or Possible Pain in the last 5 days	
Enter Code	Frequency with which resident complains or shows evidence of pain or possible pain 1. **Indicators of pain** or possible pain observed **1 to 2 days** 2. **Indicators of pain** or possible pain observed **3 to 4 days** 3. **Indicators of pain** or possible pain observed **daily**

Item Rationale

Health-related Quality of Life

- Unrelieved pain adversely affects function and mobility contributing to dependence, skin breakdown, contractures, and weight loss.
- Pain significantly adversely affects a person's quality of life and is tightly linked to depression, diminished self-confidence and self-esteem, as well as to an increase in behavior problems, particularly for cognitively impaired residents.

Planning for Care

- Assessment of pain frequency provides:
  — A basis for evaluating treatment need and response to treatment.
  — Information to aide in identifying optimum timing of treatment.

Steps for Assessment

1. Review medical record and interview staff and direct caregivers to determine the number of days the resident either complained of pain or showed evidence of pain as described in J0800 over the past 5 days.

J0850: Frequency of Indicator of Pain or Possible Pain (cont.)

Coding Instructions

Code for pain frequency over the last 5 days.

- **Code 1:** if based on staff observation, the resident complained or showed evidence of pain 1 to 2 days.
- **Code 2:** if based on staff observation, the resident complained or showed evidence of pain on 3 to 4 of the last 5 days.
- **Code 3:** if based on staff observation, the resident complained or showed evidence of pain on a daily basis.

Examples

1. Mr. M. is an 80-year old male with advanced dementia. During the 5-day look-back period, Mr. M. was noted to be grimacing and verbalizing "ouch" over the past 2 days when his right shoulder was moved.

   Coding: Item J0850 would be **coded 1, indicators of pain observed 1 to 2 days.**
   Rationale: He has demonstrated vocal complaints of pain ("ouch"), facial expression of pain (grimacing) on 2 of the last 5 days.

2. Mrs. C. is a 78-year old female with a history of CVA with expressive aphasia and dementia. During the 5-day look-back period, the resident was noted on a daily basis to be rubbing her right knee and grimacing.

   Coding: Item J0850 would be **coded 3, indicators of pain observed daily.**
   Rationale: The resident was observed with a facial expression of pain (grimacing) and protective body movements (rubbing her knee) every day during the look-back period.

J1100: Shortness of Breath (dyspnea)

J1100. Shortness of Breath (dyspnea)
↓ Check all that apply
☐ A. Shortness of breath or trouble breathing with exertion (e.g., walking, bathing, transferring)
☐ B. Shortness of breath or trouble breathing when sitting at rest
☐ C. Shortness of breath or trouble breathing when lying flat
☐ Z. None of the above

Item Rationale

Health-related Quality of Life

- Shortness of breath can be an extremely distressing symptom to residents and lead to decreased interaction and quality of life.
- Some residents compensate for shortness of breath by limiting activity. They sometimes compensate for shortness of breath when lying flat by elevating the head of the bed and do not alert caregivers to the problem.

J1100: Shortness of Breath (dyspnea) (cont.)

Planning for Care

- Shortness of breath can be an indication of a change in condition requiring further assessment and should be explored.
- The care plan should address underlying illnesses that may exacerbate symptoms of shortness of breath as well as symptomatic treatment for shortness of breath when it is not quickly reversible.

Steps for Assessment

Interview the resident about shortness of breath. Many residents, including those with mild to moderate dementia, may be able to provide feedback about their own symptoms.

1. If the resident is not experiencing shortness of breath or trouble breathing during the interview, ask the resident if shortness of breath occurs when he or she engages in certain activities.
2. Review the medical record for staff documentation of the presence of shortness of breath or trouble breathing. Interview staff on all shifts, and family/significant other regarding resident history of shortness of breath, allergies or other environmental triggers of shortness of breath.
3. Observe the resident for shortness of breath or trouble breathing. Signs of shortness of breath include: increased respiratory rate, pursed lip breathing, a prolonged expiratory phase, audible respirations and gasping for air at rest, interrupted speech pattern (only able to say a few words before taking a breath) and use of shoulder and other accessory muscles to breathe.
4. If shortness of breath or trouble breathing is observed, note whether it occurs with certain positions or activities.

Coding Instructions

Check all that apply during the 7-day look-back period.

Any evidence of the presence of a symptom of shortness of breath should be captured in this item. A resident may have any combination of these symptoms.

- **Check J1100A:** if shortness of breath or trouble breathing is present when the resident is engaging in activity. Shortness of breath could be present during activity as limited as turning or moving in bed during daily care or with more strenuous activity such as transferring, walking, or bathing. If the resident avoids activity or is unable to engage in activity because of shortness of breath, then code this as present.
- **Check J1100B:** if shortness of breath or trouble breathing is present when the resident is sitting at rest.
- **Check J1100C:** if shortness of breath or trouble breathing is present when the resident attempts to lie flat. Also code this as present if the resident avoids lying flat because of shortness of breath.
- **Check J1100Z:** if the resident reports no shortness of breath or trouble breathing and the medical record and staff interviews indicate that shortness of breath appears to be absent or well controlled with current medication.

J1100: Shortness of Breath (dyspnea) (cont.)

Examples

1. Mrs. W. has diagnoses of chronic obstructive pulmonary disease (COPD) and heart failure. She is on 2 liters of oxygen and daily respiratory treatments. With oxygen she is able to ambulate and participate in most group activities. She reports feeling "winded" when going on outings that require walking one or more blocks and has been observed having to stop to rest several times under such circumstances. Recently, she describes feeling "out of breath" when she tries to lie down.

    Coding: J1100A and J1100C would be **checked.**
    Rationale: Mrs. W. reported being short of breath when lying down as well as during outings that required ambulating longer distances.

2. Mr. T. has used an inhaler for years. He is not typically noted to be short of breath. Three days ago, during a respiratory illness, he had mild trouble with his breathing, even when sitting in bed. His shortness of breath also caused him to limit group activities.

    Coding: J1100A and J1100B would be **checked.**
    Rationale: Mr. T. was short of breath at rest and was noted to avoid activities because of shortness of breath.

J1300: Current Tobacco Use

J1300. Current Tobacco Use	
Enter Code	Tobacco use 0. No 1. Yes

Item Rationale

Health-related Quality of Life

-   The negative effects of smoking can shorten life expectancy and create health problems that interfere with daily activities and adversely affect quality of life.

Planning for Care

-   This item opens the door to negotiation of a plan of care with the resident that includes support for smoking cessation.
-   If cessation is declined, a care plan that allows safe and environmental accommodation of resident preferences is needed.

Steps for Assessment

1. Ask the resident if he or she used tobacco in any form during the 7-day look-back period.
2. If the resident states that he or she used tobacco in some form during the 7-day look-back period, **code 1, yes**.

DEFINITIONS

TOBACCO USE
Includes tobacco used in any form.

J1300: Current Tobacco Use (cont.)

3. If the resident is unable to answer or indicates that he or she did not use tobacco of any kind during the look-back period, review the medical record and interview staff for any indication of tobacco use by the resident during the look-back period.

Coding Instructions

- **Code 0, no:** if there are no indications that the resident used any form of tobacco.

- **Code 1, yes:** if the resident or any other source indicates that the resident used tobacco in some form during the look-back period.

J1400: Prognosis

J1400. Prognosis	
Enter Code	Does the resident have a condition or chronic disease that may result in a **life expectancy of less than 6 months?** (Requires physician documentation) 0. No 1. Yes

Item Rationale

Health-related Quality of Life

- Residents with conditions or diseases that may result in a life expectancy of less than 6 months have special needs and may benefit from palliative or hospice services in the nursing home.

Planning for Care

- If life expectancy is less than 6 months, interdisciplinary team care planning should be based on the resident's preferences for goals and interventions of care whenever possible.

Steps for Assessment

1. Review the medical record for documentation by the physician that the resident's condition or chronic disease may result in a life expectancy of less than 6 months, or that they have a terminal illness.
2. If the physician states that the resident's life expectancy may be less than 6 months, request that he or she document this in the medical record. Do not code until there is documentation in the medical record.
3. Review the medical record to determine whether the resident is receiving hospice services.

> **DEFINITIONS**
>
> **CONDITION OR CHRONIC DISEASE THAT MAY RESULT IN A LIFE EXPECTANCY OF LESS THAN 6 MONTHS** In the physician's judgment, the resident has a diagnosis or combination of clinical conditions that have advanced (or will continue to deteriorate) to a point that the average resident with that level of illness would not be expected to survive more than 6 months.
>
> This judgment should be substantiated by a physician note. It can be difficult to pinpoint the exact life expectancy for a single resident. Physician judgment should be based on typical or average life expectancy of residents with similar level of disease burden as this resident.

J1400: Prognosis (cont.)

Coding Instructions

- **Code 0, no:** if the medical record does not contain physician documentation that the resident is terminally ill and the resident is not receiving hospice services.
- **Code 1, yes:** if the medical record includes physician documentation: 1) that the resident is terminally ill; or 2) the resident is receiving hospice services.

Examples

1. Mrs. T. has a diagnosis of heart failure. During the past few months, she has had three hospital admissions for acute heart failure. Her heart has become significantly weaker despite maximum treatment with medications and oxygen. Her physician has discussed her deteriorating condition with her and her family and has documented that her prognosis for survival beyond the next couple of months is poor.

   Coding: J1400 would be **coded 1, yes**.
   Rationale: The physician documented that her life expectancy is likely to be less than 6 months.

2. Mr. J. was diagnosed with non-small cell lung cancer that is metastatic to his bone. He is not a candidate for surgical or curative treatment. With his consent, Mr. J. has been referred to hospice by his physician, who documented that his life expectancy was less than 6 months.

   Coding: J1400 would be **coded 1, yes**.
   Rationale: The physician referred the resident to hospice and documented that his life expectancy is likely to be less than 6 months.

J1550: Problem Conditions

J1550. Problem Conditions	
↓ Check all that apply	
☐	A. Fever
☐	B. Vomiting
☐	C. Dehydrated
☐	D. Internal bleeding
☐	Z. None of the above

> **DEFINITIONS**
>
> **HOSPICE SERVICES**
> A program for terminally ill persons where an array of services is provided for the palliation and management of terminal illness and related conditions. The hospice must be licensed by the state as a hospice provider and/or certified under the Medicare program as a hospice provider. Under the hospice program benefit regulations, a physician is required to document in the medical record a life expectancy of less than 6 months, so if a resident is on hospice the expectation is that the documentation is in the medical record.
>
> **TERMINALLY ILL**
> "Terminally ill" means that the individual has a medical prognosis that his or her life expectancy is 6 months or less if the illness runs its normal course.

J1550: Problem Conditions (cont.)

Intent: This item provides an opportunity for screening in the areas of fever, vomiting, fluid deficits, and internal bleeding. Clinical screenings provide indications for further evaluation, diagnosis and clinical care planning.

Item Rationale

Health-related Quality of Life

- Timely assessment is needed to identify underlying causes and risk for complications.

Planning for Care

- Implementation of care plans to treat underlying causes and avoid complications is critical.

Steps for Assessment

1. Review the medical record, interview staff on all shifts and observe the resident for any indication that the resident had vomiting, fever, potential signs of dehydration, or internal bleeding during the 7-day look-back period.

Coding Instructions

Check all that apply (blue box)

- **J1550A,** fever
- **J1550B,** vomiting
- **J1550C,** dehydrated
- **J1550D,** internal bleeding
- **J1550Z,** none of the above

Coding Tips

- **Fever:** Fever is defined as a temperature 2.4 degrees F higher than baseline. The resident's baseline temperature should be established prior to the Assessment Reference Date.
- **Fever assessment prior to establishing base line temperature:** A temperature of 100.4 degrees F (38 degrees C) on admission (i.e., prior to the establishment of the baseline temperature) would be considered a fever.
- **Vomiting:** Regurgitation of stomach contents; may be caused by many factors (e.g., drug toxicity, infection, psychogenic).

J1550: Problem Conditions (cont.)

- **Dehydrated:** Check this item if the resident presents with two or more of the following potential indicators for dehydration:

  1. Resident takes in less than the recommended 1,500 ml of fluids daily (water or liquids in beverages and water in foods with high fluid content, such as gelatin and soups). Note: The recommended intake level has been changed from 2,500 ml to 1,500 ml to reflect current practice standards.
  2. Resident has one or more potential clinical signs (indicators) of dehydration, **including but not limited to** dry mucous membranes, poor skin turgor, cracked lips, thirst, sunken eyes, dark urine, new onset or increased confusion, fever, or abnormal laboratory values (e.g., elevated hemoglobin and hematocrit, potassium chloride, sodium, albumin, blood urea nitrogen, or urine specific gravity).
  3. Resident's fluid loss exceeds the amount of fluids he or she takes in (e.g., loss from vomiting, fever, diarrhea that exceeds fluid replacement).

- **Internal Bleeding:** Bleeding may be frank (such as bright red blood) or occult (such as guaiac positive stools). Clinical indicators include black, tarry stools, vomiting "coffee grounds," hematuria (blood in urine), hemoptysis (coughing up blood), and severe epistaxis (nosebleed) that requires packing. However, nose bleeds that are easily controlled, menses, or a urinalysis that shows a small amount of red blood cells should not be coded as internal bleeding.

J1700: Fall History on Admission/Entry or Reentry

J1700. Fall History on Admission/Entry or Reentry Complete only if A0310A = 01 or A0310E = 1	

Enter Code
☐
	A. Did the resident have a fall any time in the **last month** prior to admission/entry or reentry?
	  0. No
	  1. Yes
	  9. Unable to determine

Enter Code
☐
	B. Did the resident have a fall any time in the **last 2-6 months** prior to admission/entry or reentry?
	  0. No
	  1. Yes
	  9. Unable to determine

Enter Code
☐
	C. Did the resident have any **fracture related to a fall in the 6 months** prior to admission/entry or reentry?
	  0. No
	  1. Yes
	  9. Unable to determine

Item Rationale

Health-related Quality of Life

- Falls are a leading cause of injury, morbidity, and mortality in older adults.
- A previous fall, especially a recent fall, recurrent falls, and falls with significant injury are the most important predictors of risk for future falls and injurious falls.
- Persons with a history of falling may limit activities because of a fear of falling and should be evaluated for reversible causes of falling.

J1700: Fall History on Admission (cont.)

Planning for Care

- Determine the potential need for further assessment and intervention, including evaluation of the resident's need for rehabilitation or assistive devices.
- Evaluate the physical environment as well as staffing needs for residents who are at risk for falls.

Steps for Assessment

The period of review is 180 days (6 months) prior to admission, looking back from the resident's entry date (A1600).

1. Ask the resident and family or significant other about a history of falls in the month prior to admission and in the 6 months prior to admission. This would include any fall, no matter where it occurred.
2. Review inter-facility transfer information (if the resident is being admitted from another facility) for evidence of falls.
3. Review all relevant medical records received from facilities where the resident resided during the previous 6 months; also review any other medical records received for evidence of one or more falls.

Coding Instructions for J1700A, Did the Resident Have a Fall Any Time in the Last Month Prior to Admission/Entry or Reentry?

> **DEFINITIONS**
>
> **FALL**
> Unintentional change in position coming to rest on the ground, floor or onto the next lower surface (e.g., onto a bed, chair, or bedside mat). The fall may be witnessed, reported by the resident or an observer or identified when a resident is found on the floor or ground. Falls include any fall, no matter whether it occurred at home, while out in the community, in an acute hospital or a nursing home. Falls are not a result of an overwhelming external force (e.g., a resident pushes another resident).
>
> An intercepted fall occurs when the resident would have fallen if he or she had not caught him/herself or had not been intercepted by another person – this is still considered a fall.

- **Code 0, no:** if resident and family report no falls and transfer records and medical records do not document a fall in the month preceding the resident's entry date item (A1600).

- **Code 1, yes:** if resident or family report or transfer records or medical records document a fall in the month preceding the resident's entry date item (A1600).

- **Code 9, unable to determine:** if the resident is unable to provide the information or if the resident and family are not available or do not have the information and medical record information is inadequate to determine whether a fall occurred.

J1700: Fall History on Admission (cont.)

Coding Instructions for J1700B, Did the Resident Have a Fall Any Time in the Last 2-6 Months prior to Admission/Entry or Reentry?

- **Code 0, no:** if resident and family report no falls and transfer records and medical records do not document a fall in the 2-6 months prior to the resident's entry date item (A1600).

- **Code 1, yes:** if resident or family report or transfer records or medical records document a fall in the 2-6 months prior to the resident's entry date item (A1600).

- **Code 9, unable to determine:** if the resident is unable to provide the information, **or** if the resident and family are not available or do not have the information, and medical record information is inadequate to determine whether a fall occurred.

Coding Instructions for J1700C. Did the Resident Have Any Fracture Related to a Fall in the 6 Months prior to Admission/Entry or Reentry?

- **Code 0, no:** if resident and family report no fractures related to falls and transfer records and medical records do not document a fracture related to fall in the 6 months (0-180 days) preceding the resident's entry date item (A1600).

- **Code 1, yes:** if resident or family report or transfer records or medical records document a fracture related to fall in the 6 months (0-180 days) preceding the resident's entry date item (A1600).

- **Code 9, unable to determine:** if the resident is unable to provide the information, **or** if the resident and family are not available or do not have the information, and medical record information is inadequate to determine whether a fall occurred.

> **DEFINITIONS**
>
> **FRACTURE RELATED TO A FALL**
> Any documented bone fracture (in a problem list from a medical record, an x-ray report, or by history of the resident or caregiver) that occurred as a direct result of a fall or was recognized and later attributed to the fall. Do not include fractures caused by trauma related to car crashes or pedestrian versus car accidents or impact of another person or object against the resident.

Examples

1. On admission interview, Mrs. J. is asked about falls and says she has "not really fallen." However, she goes on to say that when she went shopping with her daughter about 2 weeks ago, her walker got tangled with the shopping cart and she slipped down to the floor.

    Coding: J1700A would be **coded 1, yes**.
    Rationale: Falls caused by slipping meet the definition of falls.

J1700: Fall History on Admission (cont.)

2. On admission interview a resident denies a history of falling. However, her daughter says that she found her mother on the floor near her toilet twice about 3-4 months ago.

   Coding: J1700B would be **coded 1, yes**.

   Rationale: If the individual is found on the floor, a fall is assumed to have occurred.

3. On admission interview, Mr. M. and his family deny any history of falling. However, nursing notes in the transferring hospital record document that Mr. M. repeatedly tried to get out of bed unassisted at night to go to the bathroom and was found on a mat placed at his bedside to prevent injury the week prior to nursing home transfer.

   Coding: J1700A would be **coded 1, yes**.

   Rationale: Medical records from an outside facility document that Mr. M. was found on a mat on the floor. This is defined as a fall.

4. Medical records note that Miss K. had hip surgery 5 months prior to admission to the nursing home. Miss K.'s daughter says the surgery was needed to fix a broken hip due to a fall.

   Coding: Both J1700B and J1700C would be **coded 1, yes**.

   Rationale: Miss K. had a fall related fracture 1-6 months prior to nursing home entry.

5. Mr. O.'s hospital transfer record includes a history of osteoporosis and vertebral compression fractures. The record does not mention falls, and Mr. O. denies any history of falling.

   Coding: J1700C would be **coded 0, no**.

   Rationale: The fractures were not related to a fall.

6. Ms. P. has a history of a "Colles' fracture" of her left wrist about 3 weeks before nursing home admission. Her son recalls that the fracture occurred when Ms. P. tripped on a rug and fell forward on her outstretched hands.

   Coding: Both J1700A and J1700C would be **coded 1, yes**.

   Rationale: Ms. P. had a fall-related fracture less than 1 month prior to entry.

J1800: Any Falls Since Admission/Entry or Reentry or Prior Assessment (OBRA or Scheduled PPS), whichever is more recent

J1800. Any Falls Since Admission/Entry or Reentry or Prior Assessment (OBRA or Scheduled PPS), whichever is more recent	
Enter Code	Has the resident had any falls since admission/entry or reentry or the prior assessment (OBRA or Scheduled PPS), whichever is more recent? 0. No → Skip to K0100, Swallowing Disorder 1. Yes → Continue to J1900, Number of Falls Since Admission/Entry or Reentry or Prior Assessment (OBRA or Scheduled PPS)

Item Rationale

Health-related Quality of Life

- Falls are a leading cause of morbidity and mortality among nursing home residents.
- Falls result in serious injury, especially hip fractures.
- Fear of falling can limit an individual's activity and negatively impact quality of life.

> **DEFINITIONS**
>
> **PRIOR ASSESSMENT**
> Most recent MDS assessment that reported on falls.

J1800: Any Falls Since Admission/Entry or Reentry or Prior Assessment (OBRA or Scheduled PPS), whichever is more recent (cont.)

Planning for Care

- Identification of residents who are at high risk of falling is a top priority for care planning. A previous fall is the most important predictor of risk for future falls.
- Falls may be an indicator of functional decline and development of other serious conditions such as delirium, adverse drug reactions, dehydration, and infections.
- External risk factors include medication side effects, use of appliances and restraints, and environmental conditions.
- A fall should stimulate evaluation of the resident's need for rehabilitation, ambulation aids, modification of the physical environment, or additional monitoring (e.g., toileting, to avoid incontinence).

Steps for Assessment

1. If this is the first assessment (A0310E = 1), review the medical record for the time period from the admission date to the ARD.
2. If this is not the first assessment (A0310E = 0), the review period is from the day after the ARD of the last MDS assessment to the ARD of the current assessment.
3. Review all available sources for any fall since the last assessment, no matter whether it occurred while out in the community, in an acute hospital, or in the nursing home. Include medical records generated in any health care setting since last assessment.
4. Review nursing home incident reports, fall logs and the medical record (physician, nursing, therapy, and nursing assistant notes).
5. Ask the resident and family about falls during the look-back period. Resident and family reports of falls should be captured here whether or not these incidents are documented in the medical record.

Coding Instructions

- **Code 0, no:** if the resident has not had any fall since the last assessment. Skip to **Swallowing Disorder** item (K0100).
- **Code 1, yes:** if the resident has fallen since the last assessment. Continue to **Number of Falls Since Admission/Entry or Reentry or Prior Assessment (OBRA or Scheduled PPS)** item (J1900), whichever is more recent.

Examples

1. An incident report describes an event in which Mr. S. was walking down the hall and appeared to slip on a wet spot on the floor. He lost his balance and bumped into the wall, but was able to grab onto the hand rail and steady himself.

    Coding: J1800 would be **coded 1, yes**.
    Rationale: An intercepted fall is considered a fall.

J1900: Number of Falls Since Admission/Entry or Reentry or Prior Assessment (OBRA or Scheduled PPS), whichever is more recent

J1900. Number of Falls Since Admission/Entry or Reentry or Prior Assessment (OBRA or Scheduled PPS), whichever is more recent		
Coding: 0. None 1. One 2. Two or more	↓ Enter Codes in Boxes	
	☐	**A. No injury** - no evidence of any injury is noted on physical assessment by the nurse or primary care clinician; no complaints of pain or injury by the resident; no change in the resident's behavior is noted after the fall
	☐	**B. Injury (except major)** - skin tears, abrasions, lacerations, superficial bruises, hematomas and sprains; or any fall-related injury that causes the resident to complain of pain
	☐	**C. Major injury** - bone fractures, joint dislocations, closed head injuries with altered consciousness, subdural hematoma

Item Rationale

Health-related Quality of Life

- Falls are a leading cause of morbidity and mortality among nursing home residents.
- Falls result in serious injury, especially hip fractures.
- Previous falls, especially recurrent falls and falls with injury, are the most important predictor of future falls and injurious falls.

Planning for Care

- Identification of residents who are at high risk of falling is a top priority for care planning.
- Falls indicate functional decline and other serious conditions such as delirium, adverse drug reactions, dehydration, and infections.
- External risk factors include medication side effects, use of appliances and restraints, and environmental conditions.
- A fall should stimulate evaluation of the resident's need for rehabilitation or ambulation aids and of the need for monitoring or modification of the physical environment.

Steps for Assessment

1. If this is the first assessment (A0310E = 1), review the medical record for the time period from the admission date to the ARD.
2. If this is not the first assessment (A0310E = 0), the review period is from the day after the ARD of the last MDS assessment to the ARD of the current assessment.

> **DEFINITIONS**
>
> **INJURY RELATED TO A FALL**
> Any documented injury that occurred as a result of, or was recognized within a short period of time (e.g., hours to a few days) after the fall and attributed to the fall.

> **DEFINITIONS**
>
> **INJURY (EXCEPT MAJOR)**
> Includes skin tears, abrasions, lacerations, superficial bruises, hematomas, and sprains; or any fall-related injury that causes the resident to complain of pain.
>
> **MAJOR INJURY**
> Includes bone fractures, joint dislocations, closed head injuries with altered consciousness, subdural hematoma.

J1900: Number of Falls Since Admission/Entry or Reentry or Prior Assessment (OBRA or Scheduled PPS), whichever is more recent (cont.)

3. Review all available sources for any fall since the last assessment, no matter whether it occurred while out in the community, in an acute hospital, or in the nursing home. Include medical records generated in any health care setting since last assessment. All relevant records received from acute and post-acute facilities where the resident was admitted during the look-back period should be reviewed for evidence of one or more falls.

4. Review nursing home incident reports and medical record (physician, nursing, therapy, and nursing assistant notes) for falls and level of injury.

5. Ask the resident, staff, and family about falls during the look-back period. Resident and family reports of falls should be captured here, whether or not these incidents are documented in the medical record.

Coding Instructions for J1900

Determine the number of falls that occurred since admission/entry or reentry or prior assessment (OBRA or Scheduled PPS) and code the level of fall-related injury for each. Code each fall only once. If the resident has multiple injuries in a single fall, code the fall for the highest level of injury.

Coding Instructions for J1900A, No Injury

- **Code 0, none:** if the resident had no injurious fall since the admission/entry or reentry or prior assessment (OBRA or Scheduled PPS).
- **Code 1, one:** if the resident had one non-injurious fall since admission/entry or reentry or prior assessment (OBRA or Scheduled PPS).
- **Code 2, two or more:** if the resident had two or more non-injurious falls since admission/entry or reentry or prior assessment (OBRA or Scheduled PPS).

Coding Instructions for J1900B, Injury (Except Major)

- **Code 0, none:** if the resident had no injurious fall (except major) since admission/entry or reentry or prior assessment (OBRA or Scheduled PPS).
- **Code 1, one:** if the resident had one injurious fall (except major) since admission/entry or reentry or prior assessment (OBRA or Scheduled PPS).
- **Code 2, two or more:** if the resident had two or more injurious falls (except major) since admission/entry or reentry or prior assessment (OBRA or Scheduled PPS).

Coding Instructions for J1900C, Major Injury

- **Code 0, none:** if the resident had no major injurious fall since admission/entry or reentry or prior assessment (OBRA or Scheduled PPS).
- **Code 1, one:** if the resident had one major injurious fall since admission/entry or reentry or prior assessment (OBRA or Scheduled PPS).

J1900: Number of Falls Since Admission/Entry or Reentry or Prior Assessment (OBRA or Scheduled PPS), whichever is more recent (cont.)

- **Code 2, two or more:** if the resident had two or more major injurious falls since admission/entry or reentry or prior assessment (OBRA or Scheduled PPS).

Examples

1. A nursing note states that Mrs. K. slipped out of her wheelchair onto the floor while at the dining room table. Before being assisted back into her chair, an assessment was completed that indicated no injury.

   Coding: J1900A would be **coded 1, one**
   Rationale: Slipping to the floor is a fall. No injury was noted.

2. Nurse's notes describe a situation in which Ms. Z. went out with her family for dinner. When they returned, her son stated that while at the restaurant, she fell in the bathroom. No injury was noted when she returned from dinner.

   Coding: J1900A would be **coded 1, one**
   Rationale: Falls during the nursing home stay, even if on outings, are captured here.

3. A nurse's note describes a resident who, while being treated for pneumonia, climbed over his bedrails and fell to the floor. He had a cut over his left eye and some swelling on his arm. He was sent to the emergency room, where X-rays revealed no injury and neurological checks revealed no changes in mental status.

   Coding: J1900B would be **coded 1, one**
   Rationale: Lacerations and swelling without fracture are classified as injury (except major).

4. A resident fell, lacerated his head, and head CT scan indicated a subdural hematoma.

   Coding: J1900C would be **coded 1, one**
   Rationale: Subdural hematoma is a major injury. The injury occurred as a result of a fall.

SECTION K: SWALLOWING/NUTRITIONAL STATUS

Intent: The items in this section are intended to assess the many conditions that could affect the resident's ability to maintain adequate nutrition and hydration. This section covers swallowing disorders, height and weight, weight loss, and nutritional approaches. The assessor should collaborate with the dietitian and dietary staff to ensure that items in this section have been assessed and calculated accurately.

K0100: Swallowing Disorder

K0100. Swallowing Disorder
Signs and symptoms of possible swallowing disorder
↓ Check all that apply
☐ A. Loss of liquids/solids from mouth when eating or drinking
☐ B. Holding food in mouth/cheeks or residual food in mouth after meals
☐ C. Coughing or choking during meals or when swallowing medications
☐ D. Complaints of difficulty or pain with swallowing
☐ Z. None of the above

Item Rationale

Health-related Quality of Life

- The ability to swallow safely can be affected by many disease processes and functional decline.
- Alterations in the ability to swallow can result in choking and aspiration, which can increase the resident's risk for malnutrition, dehydration, and aspiration pneumonia.

Planning for Care

- Care planning should include provisions for monitoring the resident during mealtimes and during functions/activities that include the consumption of food and liquids.
- When necessary, the resident should be evaluated by the physician, speech language pathologist and/or occupational therapist to assess for any need for swallowing therapy and/or to provide recommendations regarding the consistency of food and liquids.
- Assess for signs and symptoms that suggest a swallowing disorder that has not been successfully treated or managed with diet modifications or other interventions (e.g., tube feeding, double swallow, turning head to swallow, etc.) and therefore represents a functional problem for the resident.
- Care plan should be developed to assist resident to maintain safe and effective swallow using compensatory techniques, alteration in diet consistency, and positioning during and following meals.

Steps for Assessment

1. Ask the resident if he or she has had any difficulty swallowing during the 7-day look-back period. Ask about each of the symptoms in K0100A through K0100D.

   Observe the resident during meals or at other times when he or she is eating, drinking, or swallowing to determine whether any of the listed symptoms of possible swallowing disorder are exhibited.

2. Interview staff members on all shifts who work with the resident and ask if any of the four listed symptoms were evident during the 7-day look-back period.

K0100: Swallowing/Nutritional Status (cont.)

3. Review the medical record, including nursing, physician, dietician, and speech language pathologist notes, and any available information on dental history or problems. Dental problems may include poor fitting dentures, dental caries, edentulous, mouth sores, tumors and/or pain with food consumption.

Coding Instructions

Check all that apply.

- **K0100A, loss of liquids/solids from mouth when eating or drinking.** When the resident has food or liquid in his or her mouth, the food or liquid dribbles down chin or falls out of the mouth.

- **K0100B, holding food in mouth/cheeks or residual food in mouth after meals.** Holding food in mouth or cheeks for prolonged periods of time (sometimes labeled pocketing) or food left in mouth because resident failed to empty mouth completely.

- **K0100C, coughing or choking during meals or when swallowing medications.** The resident may cough or gag, turn red, have more labored breathing, or have difficulty speaking when eating, drinking, or taking medications. The resident may frequently complain of food or medications "going down the wrong way."

- **K0100D, complaints of difficulty or pain with swallowing.** Resident may refuse food because it is painful or difficult to swallow.

- **K0100Z, none of the above:** if none of the K0100A through K0100D signs or symptoms were present during the look-back.

Coding Tips

- Do not code a swallowing problem when interventions have been successful in treating the problem and therefore the signs/symptoms of the problem (K0100A through K0100D) did not occur during the 7-day look-back period.
- Code even if the symptom occurred only once in the 7-day look-back period.

K0200: Height and Weight

K0200. Height and Weight - While measuring, if the number is X.1 - X.4 round down; X.5 or greater round up	
☐☐ inches	**A. Height** (in inches). Record most recent height measure since the most recent admission/entry or reentry
☐☐☐ pounds	**B. Weight** (in pounds). Base weight on most recent measure in last 30 days; measure weight consistently, according to standard facility practice (e.g., in a.m. after voiding, before meal, with shoes off, etc.)

K0200: Height and Weight (cont.)

Item Rationale

Health-related Quality of Life

- Diminished nutritional and hydration status can lead to debility that can adversely affect health and safety as well as quality of life.

Planning for Care

- Height and weight measurements assist staff with assessing the resident's nutrition and hydration status by providing a mechanism for monitoring stability of weight over a period of time. The measurement of weight is one guide for determining nutritional status.

Steps for Assessment for K0200A, Height

1. Base height on the most recent height since the most recent admission/entry or reentry. Measure and record height in inches.
2. Measure height consistently over time in accordance with the facility policy and procedure, which should reflect current standards of practice (shoes off, etc.).
3. For subsequent assessments, check the medical record. If the last height recorded was more than one year ago, measure and record the resident's height again.

Coding Instructions for K0200A, Height

- Record height to the nearest whole inch.
- Use mathematical rounding (i.e., if height measurement is X.5 inches or greater, round height upward to the nearest whole inch. If height measurement number is X.1 to X.4 inches, round down to the nearest whole inch). For example, a height of 62.5 inches would be rounded to 63 inches and a height of 62.4 inches would be rounded to 62 inches.

Steps for Assessment for K0200B, Weight

1. Base weight on the most recent measure in the last 30 days.
2. Measure weight consistently over time in accordance with facility policy and procedure, which should reflect current standards of practice (shoes off, etc.).
3. For subsequent assessments, check the medical record and enter the weight taken within 30 days of the ARD of this assessment.
4. If the last recorded weight was taken more than 30 days prior to the ARD of this assessment or previous weight is not available, weigh the resident again.
5. If the resident's weight was taken more than once during the preceding month, record the most recent weight.

Coding Instructions for K0200B, Weight

- Use mathematical rounding (i.e., If weight is X.5 pounds [lbs] or more, round weight upward to the nearest whole pound. If weight is X.1 to X.4 lbs, round down to the nearest whole pound). For example, a weight of 152.5 lbs would be rounded to 153 lbs and a weight of 152.4 lbs would be rounded to 152 lbs.

K0200: Height and Weight (cont.)

- If a resident cannot be weighed, for example because of extreme pain, immobility, or risk of pathological fractures, use the standard no-information code (-) and document rationale on the resident's medical record.

K0300: Weight Loss

K0300. Weight Loss	
Enter Code ☐	**Loss of 5% or more in the last month or loss of 10% or more in last 6 months** 0. **No** or unknown 1. **Yes, on** physician-prescribed weight-loss regimen 2. **Yes, not on** physician-prescribed weight-loss regimen

Item Rationale

Health-related Quality of Life

- Weight loss can result in debility and adversely affect health, safety, and quality of life.
- For persons with morbid obesity, controlled and careful weight loss can improve mobility and health status.
- For persons with a large volume (fluid) overload, controlled and careful diuresis can improve health status.

Planning for Care

- Weight loss may be an important indicator of a change in the resident's health status or environment.
- If significant weight loss is noted, the interdisciplinary team should review for possible causes of changed intake, changed caloric need, change in medication (e.g., diuretics), or changed fluid volume status.
- Weight loss should be monitored on a continuing basis; weight loss should be assessed and care planned at the time of detection and not delayed until the next MDS assessment.

> **DEFINITIONS**
>
> **5% WEIGHT LOSS IN 30 DAYS**
> Start with the resident's weight closest to 30 days ago and multiply it by .95 (or 95%). The resulting figure represents a 5% loss from the weight 30 days ago. If the resident's current weight is equal to or less than the resulting figure, the resident has lost more than 5% body weight.
>
> **10% WEIGHT LOSS IN 180 DAYS**
> Start with the resident's weight closest to 180 days ago and multiply it by .90 (or 90%). The resulting figure represents a 10% loss from the weight 180 days ago. If the resident's current weight is equal to or less than the resulting figure, the resident has lost 10% or more body weight.

Steps for Assessment

This item compares the resident's weight in the current observation period with his or her weight at two snapshots in time:

- At a point closest to 30-days preceding the current weight.
- At a point closest to 180-days preceding the current weight.

K0300: Weight Loss (cont.)

This item does not consider weight fluctuation outside of these two time points, although the resident's weight should be monitored on a continual basis and weight loss assessed and addressed on the care plan as necessary.

For a New Admission

1. Ask the resident, family, or significant other about weight loss over the past 30 and 180 days.
2. Consult the resident's physician, review transfer documentation, and compare with admission weight.
3. If the admission weight is less than the previous weight, calculate the percentage of weight loss.
4. Complete the same process to determine and calculate weight loss comparing the admission weight to the weight 30 and 180 days ago.

For Subsequent Assessments

1. From the medical record, compare the resident's weight in the current observation period to his or her weight in the observation period 30 days ago.
2. If the current weight is less than the weight in the observation period 30 days ago, calculate the percentage of weight loss.
3. From the medical record, compare the resident's weight in the current observation period to his or her weight in the observation period 180 days ago.
4. If the current weight is less than the weight in the observation period 180 days ago, calculate the percentage of weight loss.

> **DEFINITIONS**
>
> **PHYSICIAN-PRESCRIBED WEIGHT-LOSS REGIMEN**
> A weight reduction plan ordered by the resident's physician with the care plan goal of weight reduction. May employ a calorie-restricted diet or other weight loss diets and exercise. Also includes planned diuresis. It is important that weight loss is intentional.
>
> **BODY MASS INDEX (BMI)**
> Number calculated from a person's weight and height. BMI is used as a screening tool to identify possible weight problems for adults. Visit http://www.cdc.gov/healthyweight/assessing/bmi/adult_bmi/index.html.

Coding Instructions

Mathematically round weights as described in Section K0200B before completing the weight loss calculation.

- **Code 0, no or unknown:** if the resident has not experienced weight loss of 5% or more in the past 30 days or 10% or more in the last 180 days or if information about prior weight is not available.

- **Code 1, yes on physician-prescribed weight-loss regimen:** if the resident has experienced a weight loss of 5% or more in the past 30 days or 10% or more in the last 180 days, and the weight loss was planned and pursuant to a physician's order. In cases where a resident has a weight loss of 5% or more in 30 days or 10% or more in 180 days as a result of any physician ordered diet plan or expected weight loss due to loss of fluid with physician orders for diuretics, K0300 can be coded as **1**.

K0300: Weight Loss (cont.)

- **Code 2, yes, not on physician-prescribed weight-loss regimen:** if the resident has experienced a weight loss of 5% or more in the past 30 days or 10% or more in the last 180 days, and the weight loss was not planned and prescribed by a physician.

Coding Tips

- A resident may experience weight variances in between the snapshot time periods. Although these require follow up at the time, they are not captured on the MDS.
- If the resident is losing a significant amount of weight, the facility should not wait for the 30- or 180-day timeframe to address the problem. Weight changes of 5% in 1 month, 7.5% in 3 months, or 10% in 6 months should prompt a thorough assessment of the resident's nutritional status.
- To code K0300 as **1, yes**, the expressed goal of the weight loss diet or the expected weight loss of edema through the use of diuretics must be documented.
- On occasion, a resident with normal BMI or even low BMI is placed on a diabetic or otherwise calorie-restricted diet. In this instance, the intent of the diet is not to induce weight loss, and it would not be considered a physician-ordered weight-loss regimen.

Examples

1. Mrs. J has been on a physician ordered calorie-restricted diet for the past year. She and her physician agreed to a plan of weight reduction. Her current weight is 169 lbs. Her weight 30 days ago was 172 lbs. Her weight 180 days ago was 192 lbs.

   > **Coding:** K0300 would be **coded 1, yes, on physician-prescribed weight-loss regimen.**
   > **Rationale:**
   > - 30-day calculation: $172 \times 0.95 = 163.4$. Since the resident's current weight of 169 lbs is more than 163.4 lbs, which is the 5% point, she **has not** lost 5% body weight in the last 30 days.
   > - 180-day calculation: $192 \times .90 = 172.8$. Since the resident's current weight of 169 lbs **is** less than 172.8 lbs, which is the 10% point, she **has** lost 10% or more of body weight in the last 180 days.

K0300: Weight Loss (cont.)

2. Mr. S has had increasing need for assistance with eating over the past 6 months. His current weight is 195 lbs. His weight 30 days ago was 197 lbs. His weight 180 days ago was 185 lbs.

> **Coding:** K0300 would be **coded 0, No.**
>
> **Rationale:**
>
> - 30-day calculation: 197 x 0.95 = 187.15. Because the resident's current weight of 195 lbs is more than 187.15 lbs, which is the 5% point, he **has not** lost 5% body weight in the last 30 days.
> - 180-day calculation: Mr. S's current weight of 195 lbs is greater than his weight 180 days ago, so there is no need to calculate his weight loss. He has gained weight over this time period.

3. Ms. K underwent a BKA (below the knee amputation). Her preoperative weight 30 days ago was 130 lbs. Her most recent postoperative weight is 102 lbs. The amputated leg weighed 8 lbs. Her weight 180 days ago was 125 lbs.

Was the change in weight significant? Calculation of change in weight must take into account the weight of the amputated limb (which in this case is 6% of 130 lbs = 7.8 lbs).

> - 30-day calculation:
>   Step 1: Add the weight of the amputated limb to the current weight to obtain the weight if no amputation occurred:
>   102 lbs (current weight) + 8 lbs (weight of leg) = 110 lbs (current body weight taking the amputated leg into account)
>   Step 2: Calculate the difference between the most recent weight (including weight of the limb) and the previous weight (at 30 days)
>   130 lbs (preoperative weight) - 110 lbs (present weight if had two legs) = 20 lbs (weight lost)
>   Step 3: Calculate the percent weight change relative to the initial weight:
>   20 lbs (weight change) /130 lbs (preoperative weight) = 15% weight loss
>   Step 4: The percent weight change is significant if >5% at 30 days
>   Therefore, the most recent postoperative weight of 102 lbs (110 lbs, taking the amputated limb into account) is >5% weight loss (significant at 30 days).
>
> - 180-day calculation:
>   Step 1: Add the weight of the amputated limb to the current weight to obtain the weight if no amputation occurred:
>   102 lbs (current weight) + 8 lbs (weight of leg) = 110 lbs (current body weight taking the amputated leg into account)
>   Step 2: Calculate the difference between the most recent weight (including weight of the limb) and the previous weight (at 180 days):
>   125 lbs (preoperative weight 180 days ago) - 110 lbs (present weight if had two legs) = 15 lbs (weight lost)
>   Step 3: Calculate the percent weight change relative to the initial weight:
>   15 lbs (weight change) / 130 lbs (preoperative weight) = 12% weight loss
>   Step 4: The percent weight change is significant if >10% at 180 days

K0300: Weight Loss (cont.)

The most recent postoperative weight of 110 lbs (110 lbs, taking the amputated limb into account) is >10% weight loss (significant at 180 days).

Present weight of 110 lbs >10% weight loss (significant at 180 days).

Coding: K0300 would be **coded 2, yes, weight change is significant; not on physician-prescribed weight-loss regimen.**

Rationale: The resident had a significant weight loss of >5% in 30 days and did have a weight loss of >10% in 180 days, the item would be coded as 2, yes weight change is significant; not on physician-prescribed weight–loss regime, with one of the items being triggered. This item is coded for either a 5% 30-day weight loss or a 10% 180-day weight loss. In this example both items, the criteria are met but the coding does not change as long as one of them are met.

K0310: Weight Gain

K0310. Weight Gain	
Enter Code	**Gain of 5% or more in the last month or gain of 10% or more in last 6 months** 0. **No** or unknown 1. **Yes, on** physician-prescribed weight-gain regimen 2. **Yes, not on** physician-prescribed weight-gain regimen

Item Rationale

Health-related Quality of Life

- Weight gain can result in debility and adversely affect health, safety, and quality of life.

Planning for Care

- Weight gain may be an important indicator of a change in the resident's health status or environment.

- If significant weight gain is noted, the interdisciplinary team should review for possible causes of changed intake, changed caloric need, change in medication (e.g., steroidals), or changed fluid volume status.

- Weight gain should be monitored on a continuing basis; weight gain should be assessed and care planned at the time of detection and not delayed until the next MDS assessment.

Steps for Assessment

This item compares the resident's weight in the current observation period with his or her weight at two snapshots in time:

- At a point closest to 30-days preceding the current weight.
- At a point closest to 180-days preceding the current weight.

DEFINITIONS

5% WEIGHT GAIN IN 30 DAYS

Start with the resident's weight closest to 30 days ago and multiply it by 1.05 (or 105%). The resulting figure represents a 5% gain from the weight 30 days ago. If the resident's current weight is equal to or more than the resulting figure, the resident has gained more than 5% body weight.

10% WEIGHT GAIN IN 180 DAYS

Start with the resident's weight closest to 180 days ago and multiply it by 1.10 (or 110%). The resulting figure represents a 10% gain from the weight 180 days ago. If the resident's current weight is equal to or more than the resulting figure, the resident has gained more than 10% body weight.

K0310: Weight Gain (cont.)

This item does not consider weight fluctuation outside of these two time points, although the resident's weight should be monitored on a continual basis and weight gain assessed and addressed on the care plan as necessary.

For a New Admission

1. Ask the resident, family, or significant other about weight gain over the past 30 and 180 days.
2. Consult the resident's physician, review transfer documentation, and compare with admission weight.
3. If the admission weight is more than the previous weight, calculate the percentage of weight gain.
4. Complete the same process to determine and calculate weight gain comparing the admission weight to the weight 30 and 180 days ago.

For Subsequent Assessments

1. From the medical record, compare the resident's weight in the current observation period to his or her weight in the observation period 30 days ago.
2. If the current weight is more than the weight in the observation period 30 days ago, calculate the percentage of weight gain.
3. From the medical record, compare the resident's weight in the current observation period to his or her weight in the observation period 180 days ago.
4. If the current weight is more than the weight in the observation period 180 days ago, calculate the percentage of weight gain.

Coding Instructions

Mathematically round weights as described in Section K0200B before completing the weight gain calculation.

- **Code 0, no or unknown:** if the resident has not experienced weight gain of 5% or more in the past 30 days or 10% or more in the last 180 days or if information about prior weight is not available.

- **Code 1, yes on physician-prescribed weight-gain regimen:** if the resident has experienced a weight gain of 5% or more in the past 30 days or 10% or more in the last 180 days, and the weight gain was planned and pursuant to a physician's order. In cases where a resident has a weight gain of 5% or more in 30 days or 10% or more in 180 days as a result of any physician ordered diet plan, K0310 can be coded as **1**.

- **Code 2, yes, not on physician-prescribed weight-gain regimen:** if the resident has experienced a weight gain of 5% or more in the past 30 days or 10% or more in the last 180 days, and the weight gain was not planned and prescribed by a physician.

Coding Tips

- A resident may experience weight variances in between the snapshot time periods. Although these require follow up at the time, they are not captured on the MDS.

K0310: Weight Gain (cont.)

- If the resident is gaining a significant amount of weight, the facility should not wait for the 30- or 180-day timeframe to address the problem. Weight changes of 5% in 1 month, 7.5% in 3 months, or 10% in 6 months should prompt a thorough assessment of the resident's nutritional status.
- To code K0310 as **1, yes**, the expressed goal of the weight gain diet must be documented.

K0510: Nutritional Approaches

K0510. Nutritional Approaches		
Check all of the following nutritional approaches that were performed during the last **7 days**		
1. While NOT a Resident Performed *while NOT a resident* of this facility and within the *last 7 days*. Only check column 1 if resident entered (admission or reentry) IN THE LAST 7 DAYS. If resident last entered 7 or more days ago, leave column 1 blank **2. While a Resident** Performed *while a resident* of this facility and within the *last 7 days*	**1.** While NOT a Resident	**2.** While a Resident
	↓ Check all that apply ↓	
A. **Parenteral/IV feeding**	☐	☐
B. **Feeding tube** - nasogastric or abdominal (PEG)	☐	☐
C. **Mechanically altered diet** - require change in texture of food or liquids (e.g., pureed food, thickened liquids)	☐	☐
D. **Therapeutic diet** (e.g., low salt, diabetic, low cholesterol)	☐	☐
Z. **None of the above**	☐	☐

Item Rationale

Health-related Quality of Life

- Nutritional approaches that vary from the normal (e.g., mechanically altered food) or that rely on alternative methods (e.g., parenteral/IV or feeding tubes) can diminish an individual's sense of dignity and self-worth as well as diminish pleasure from eating.
- The resident's clinical condition may potentially benefit from the various nutritional approaches included here. It is important to work with the resident and family members to establish nutritional support goals that balance the resident's preferences and overall clinical goals.

Planning for Care

- Alternative nutritional approaches should be monitored to validate effectiveness.
- Care planning should include periodic reevaluation of the appropriateness of the approach.

DEFINITIONS

PARENTERAL/IV FEEDING Introduction of a nutritive substance into the body by means other than the intestinal tract (e.g., subcutaneous, intravenous).

FEEDING TUBE Presence of any type of tube that can deliver food/ nutritional substances/ fluids/ medications directly into the gastrointestinal system. Examples include, but are not limited to, nasogastric tubes, gastrostomy tubes, jejunostomy tubes, percutaneous endoscopic gastrotomy (PEG) tubes.

K0510: Nutritional Approaches (cont.)

Steps for Assessment

- Review the medical record to determine if any of the listed nutritional approaches were performed during the 7-day look-back period.

Coding Instructions for Column 1

Check all nutritional approaches performed **prior** to admission/entry or reentry to the facility and within the 7-day look-back period. Leave Column 1 blank if the resident was admitted/entered or reentered the facility more than 7 days ago.

Coding Instructions for Column 2

Check all nutritional approaches performed **after** admission/entry or reentry to the facility and within the 7-day look-back period.

Check all that apply. If none apply, check K0510Z, None of the above

- **K0510A,** parenteral/IV feeding
- **K0510B,** feeding tube – nasogastric or abdominal (PEG)
- **K0510C,** mechanically altered diet – require change in texture of food or liquids (e.g., pureed food, thickened liquids)
- **K0510D,** therapeutic diet (e.g., low salt, diabetic, low cholesterol)
- **K0510Z,** none of the above

> ### DEFINITIONS
>
> **MECHANICALLY ALTERED DIET**
>
> A diet specifically prepared to alter the texture or consistency of food to facilitate oral intake. Examples include soft solids, puréed foods, ground meat, and thickened liquids. A mechanically altered diet should not automatically be considered a therapeutic diet.
>
> **THERAPEUTIC DIET**
>
> A therapeutic diet is a diet intervention ordered by a health care practitioner as part of the treatment for a disease or clinical condition manifesting an altered nutritional status, to eliminate, decrease, or increase certain substances in the diet (e.g. sodium, potassium) (ADA, 2011).

Coding Tips for K0510A

K0510A includes any and all nutrition and hydration received by the nursing home resident in the last 7 days either at the nursing home, at the hospital as an outpatient or an inpatient, provided they were administered for nutrition or hydration.

- Parenteral/IV feeding—The following fluids may be included **when there is supporting documentation that reflects the need for additional fluid intake specifically addressing a nutrition or hydration need. This supporting documentation should be noted in the resident's medical record according to State and/or internal facility policy:**
  - IV fluids or hyperalimentation, including total parenteral nutrition (TPN), administered continuously or intermittently
  - IV fluids running at KVO (Keep Vein Open)
  - IV fluids contained in IV Piggybacks
  - Hypodermoclysis and subcutaneous ports in hydration therapy

K0510: Nutritional Approaches (cont.)

- — IV fluids can be coded in K0510A if needed to prevent dehydration if the additional fluid intake is specifically needed for nutrition and hydration. Prevention of dehydration should be clinically indicated and supporting documentation should be provided in the medical record.
- **The following items are NOT to be coded in K0510A:**
  - — IV Medications—**Code these when appropriate in O0100H, IV Medications.**
  - — IV fluids used to reconstitute and/or dilute medications for IV administration.
  - — IV fluids administered as a routine part of an operative or diagnostic procedure or recovery room stay.
  - — IV fluids administered solely as flushes.
  - — Parenteral/IV fluids administered in conjunction with chemotherapy or dialysis.
- Guidelines on basic fluid and electrolyte replacement can be found online at http://guidelines.gov/content.aspx?id=15590&search=fluid+and+electrolyte+replacement+amda.
- Enteral feeding formulas:
  - — Should not be coded as a mechanically altered diet.
  - — Should only be coded as **K0510D, Therapeutic Diet** when the enteral formula is altered to manage problematic health conditions, e.g. enteral formulas specific to diabetics.

Coding Tips for K0510D

- Therapeutic diets are not defined by the content of what is provided or when it is served, but _why_ the diet is required. Therapeutic diets provide the corresponding treatment that addresses a particular disease or clinical condition which is manifesting an altered nutritional status by providing the specific nutritional requirements to remedy the alteration.
- A nutritional supplement (house supplement or packaged) given as part of the treatment for a disease or clinical condition manifesting an altered nutrition status, does not constitute a therapeutic diet, but may be _part_ of a therapeutic diet. Therefore, supplements (whether given with, in-between, or instead of meals) are only coded in K0510D, Therapeutic Diet when they are being administered as part of a therapeutic diet to manage problematic health conditions (e.g. supplement for protein-calorie malnutrition).

Examples

1. Mrs. H is receiving an antibiotic in 100 cc of normal saline via IV. She has a urinary tract infection (UTI), fever, abnormal lab results (e.g., new pyuria, microscopic hematuria, urine culture with growth >100,000 colony forming units of a urinary pathogen), and documented inadequate fluid intake (i.e., output of fluids far exceeds fluid intake) with signs and symptoms of dehydration. She is placed on the nursing home's hydration plan to ensure adequate hydration. Documentation shows IV fluids are being administered as part of the already identified need for additional hydration.

K0510: Nutritional Approaches (cont.)

Coding: K0510A would **be checked.** The IV medication would be coded at **IV Medications** item (O0100H).

Rationale: The resident received 100 cc of IV fluid **and** there is supporting documentation that reflected an identified need for additional fluid intake for hydration.

2. Mr. J is receiving an antibiotic in 100 cc of normal saline via IV. He has a UTI, no fever, and documented adequate fluid intake. He is placed on the nursing home's hydration plan to ensure adequate hydration.

Coding: K0510A would **NOT be checked.** The IV medication would be coded at **IV Medications** item (O0100H).

Rationale: Although the resident received the additional fluid, there is no documentation to support a need for additional fluid intake.

K0700: Percent Intake by Artificial Route

Complete K0700 only if Column 1 and/or Column 2 are checked for K0510A and/or K0510B.

	K0700. Percent Intake by Artificial Route - Complete K0700 only if Column 1 and/or Column 2 are checked for K0510A and/or K0510B
Enter Code ☐	A. Proportion of total calories the resident received through parenteral or tube feeding 　1. 25% or less 　2. 26-50% 　3. 51% or more
Enter Code ☐	B. Average fluid intake per day by IV or tube feeding 　1. 500 cc/day or less 　2. 501 cc/day or more

Item Rationale

Health-related Quality of Life

- Nutritional approaches that vary from the normal, such as parenteral/IV or feeding tubes, can diminish an individual's sense of dignity and self-worth as well as diminish pleasure from eating.

Planning for Care

- The proportion of calories received through artificial routes should be monitored with periodic reassessment to ensure adequate nutrition and hydration.
- Periodic reassessment is necessary to facilitate transition to increased oral intake as indicated by the resident's condition.

K0700A, Proportion of Total Calories the Resident Received through Parental or Tube Feedings in the Last 7 Days

Steps for Assessment

1. Review intake records to determine actual intake through parenteral or tube feeding routes.
2. Calculate proportion of total calories received through these routes.
   - If the resident took no food or fluids by mouth or took just sips of fluid, stop here and **code 3, 51% or more.**
   - If the resident had more substantial oral intake than this, consult with the dietician.

K0700: Percent Intake by Artificial Route (cont.)

Coding Instructions

- Select the best response:
  1. 25% or less
  2. 26% to 50%
  3. 51% or more

Example

1. Calculation for Proportion of Total Calories from IV or Tube Feeding

   Mr. H has had a feeding tube since his surgery. He is currently more alert and feeling much better. He is very motivated to have the tube removed. He has been taking soft solids by mouth, but only in small to medium amounts. For the past 7 days, he has been receiving tube feedings for nutritional supplementation. The dietitian has totaled his calories per day as follows:

Oral and Tube Feeding Intake		
	Oral	Tube
Sun.	500	2,000
Mon.	250	2,250
Tues.	250	2,250
Wed.	350	2,250
Thurs.	500	2,000
Fri.	250	2,250
Sat.	350	2,000
Total	2,450	15,000

Coding: K0700A would be coded **3, 51% or more.**

Rationale: Total Oral intake is 2,450 calories

Total Tube intake is 15,000 calories

Total calories is 2,450 + 15,000 = 17,450

Calculation of the percentage of total calories by tube feeding:

15,000/17,450 = .859 X 100 = 85.9%

Mr. H received 85.9% of his calories by tube feeding, therefore K0700A **code 3, 51% or more** is correct.

K0700B, Average Fluid Intake per Day by IV or Tube Feeding in the Last 7 Days.

Steps for Assessment

1. Review intake records from the last 7 days.
2. Add up the total amount of fluid received each day by IV and/or tube feedings only.
3. Divide the week's total fluid intake by 7 to calculate the average of fluid intake per day.
4. Divide by 7 even if the resident did not receive IV fluids and/or tube feeding on each of the 7 days.

K0700: Percent Intake by Artificial Route (cont.)

Coding Instructions

Code for the average number of cc per day of fluid the resident received via IV or tube feeding. Record what was actually received by the resident, not what was ordered.

- **Code 1:** 500 cc/day or less
- **Code 2:** 501 cc/day or more

Examples

1. **Calculation for Average Daily Fluid Intake**

   Ms. A has swallowing difficulties secondary to Huntington's disease. She is able to take oral fluids by mouth with supervision, but not enough to maintain hydration. She received the following daily fluid totals by supplemental tube feedings (including water, prepared nutritional supplements, juices) during the last 7 days.

IV Fluid Intake	
Sun.	1250 cc
Mon.	775 cc
Tues.	925 cc
Wed.	1200 cc
Thurs.	1200 cc
Fri.	500 cc
Sat.	450 cc
Total	6,300 cc

   Coding: K0700B would be coded **2, 501cc/day or more**.

   Rationale: The total fluid intake by supplemental tube feedings = 6,300 cc
   6,300 cc divided by 7 days = 900 cc/day
   900 cc is greater than 500 cc, therefore **code 2, 501 cc/day or more** is correct.

2. **Calculation for Average Daily Fluid Intake**

   Mrs. G. received 1 liter of IV fluids during the 7-day assessment period. She received no other intake via IV or tube feeding during the assessment period.

IV Fluid Intake	
Sun.	0 cc
Mon.	0 cc
Tues.	1,000 cc
Wed.	0 cc
Thurs.	0 cc
Fri.	0 cc
Sat.	0 cc
Total	1,000 cc

K0700: Percent Intake by Artificial Route (cont.)

Coding: K0700b would be coded **1, 500 cc/day or less**.

Rationale: The total fluid intake by supplemental tube feedings = 1000 cc

1000 cc divided by 7 days = 142.9 cc/day

142.9 cc is less than 500 cc, therefore **code 1, 500 cc/day or less** is correct.

SECTION L: ORAL/DENTAL STATUS

Intent: This item is intended to record any dental **problems** present in the 7-day look-back period.

L0200: Dental

	L0200. Dental	
	↓ Check all that apply	
☐	A.	**Broken or loosely fitting full or partial denture** (chipped, cracked, uncleanable, or loose)
☐	B.	**No natural teeth or tooth fragment(s)** (edentulous)
☐	C.	**Abnormal mouth tissue** (ulcers, masses, oral lesions, including under denture or partial if one is worn)
☐	D.	**Obvious or likely cavity or broken natural teeth**
☐	E.	**Inflamed or bleeding gums or loose natural teeth**
☐	F.	**Mouth or facial pain, discomfort or difficulty with chewing**
☐	G.	**Unable to examine**
☐	Z.	**None of the above were present**

Item Rationale

Health-related Quality of Life

- Poor oral health has a negative impact on:
  - quality of life
  - overall health
  - nutritional status
- Assessment can identify periodontal disease that can contribute to or cause systemic diseases and conditions, such as aspiration, malnutrition, pneumonia, endocarditis, and poor control of diabetes.

Planning for Care

- Assessing dental status can help identify residents who may be at risk for aspiration, malnutrition, pneumonia, endocarditis, and poor control of diabetes.

DEFINITIONS

CAVITY

A tooth with a discolored hole or area of decay that may have debris in it.

BROKEN NATURAL TEETH OR TOOTH FRAGMENT

Very large cavity, tooth broken off or decayed to gum line, or broken teeth (from a fall or trauma).

ORAL LESIONS

A discolored area of tissue (red, white, yellow, or darkened) on the lips, gums, tongue, palate, cheek lining, or throat.

L0200: Dental (cont.)

Steps for Assessment

> **DEFINITIONS**
>
> **ORAL MASS**
> A swollen or raised lump, bump, or nodule on any oral surface. May be hard or soft, and with or without pain.
>
> **ULCER**
> Mouth sore, blister or eroded area of tissue on any oral surface.

1. Ask the resident about the presence of chewing problems or mouth or facial pain/discomfort.
2. Ask the resident, family, or significant other whether the resident has or recently had dentures or partials. (If resident or family/significant other reports that the resident recently had dentures or partials, but they do not have them at the facility, ask for a reason.)
3. If the resident has dentures or partials, examine for loose fit. Ask him or her to remove, and examine for chips, cracks, and cleanliness. Removal of dentures and/or partials is necessary for adequate assessment.
4. Conduct exam of the resident's lips and oral cavity with dentures or partials removed, if applicable. Use a light source that is adequate to visualize the back of the mouth. Visually observe and feel all oral surfaces including lips, gums, tongue, palate, mouth floor, and cheek lining. Check for abnormal mouth tissue, abnormal teeth, or inflamed or bleeding gums. The assessor should use his or her gloved fingers to adequately feel for masses or loose teeth.
5. If the resident is unable to self-report, then observe him or her while eating with dentures or partials, if indicated, to determine if chewing problems or mouth pain are present.
6. Oral examination of residents who are uncooperative and do not allow for a thorough oral exam may result in medical conditions being missed. Referral for dental evaluation should be considered for these residents and any resident who exhibits dental or oral issues.

Coding Instructions

- **Check L0200A, broken or loosely fitting full or partial denture:** if the denture or partial is chipped, cracked, uncleanable, or loose. A denture is coded as loose if the resident complains that it is loose, the denture visibly moves when the resident opens his or her mouth, or the denture moves when the resident tries to talk.

- **Check L0200B, no natural teeth or tooth fragment(s) (edentulous):** if the resident is edentulous or lacks all natural teeth or parts of teeth.

- **Check L0200C, abnormal mouth tissue (ulcers, masses, oral lesions):** select if any ulcer, mass, or oral lesion is noted on any oral surface.

- **Check L0200D, obvious or likely cavity or broken natural teeth:** if any cavity or broken tooth is seen.

- **Check L0200E, inflamed or bleeding gums or loose natural teeth:** if gums appear irritated, red, swollen, or bleeding. Teeth are coded as loose if they readily move when light pressure is applied with a fingertip.

- **Check L0200F, mouth or facial pain or discomfort with chewing:** if the resident reports any pain in the mouth or face, or discomfort with chewing.

- **Check L0200G, unable to examine:** if the resident's mouth cannot be examined.

- **Check L0200Z, none of the above:** if none of conditions A through F is present.

L0200: Dental (cont.)

Coding Tips

- Mouth or facial pain coded for this item should also be coded in Section J, items J0100 through J0850, in any items in which the coding requirements of Section J are met.

SECTION M: SKIN CONDITIONS

Intent: The items in this section document the risk, presence, appearance, and change of pressure ulcers. This section also notes other skin ulcers, wounds, or lesions, and documents some treatment categories related to skin injury or avoiding injury. It is important to recognize and evaluate each resident's risk factors and to identify and evaluate all areas at risk of constant pressure. A complete assessment of skin is essential to an effective pressure ulcer prevention and skin treatment program. Be certain to include in the assessment process, a holistic approach. It is imperative to determine the etiology of all wounds and lesions, as this will determine and direct the proper treatment and management of the wound.

M0100: Determination of Pressure Ulcer Risk

M0100. Determination of Pressure Ulcer Risk	
↓ Check all that apply	
☐	A. Resident has a stage 1 or greater, a scar over bony prominence, or a non-removable dressing/device
☐	B. Formal assessment instrument/tool (e.g., Braden, Norton, or other)
☐	C. Clinical assessment
☐	Z. None of the above

Item Rationale

Health-related Quality of Life

- Pressure ulcers occur when tissue is compressed between a bony prominence and an external surface. In addition to pressure, shear force, and friction are important contributors to pressure ulcer development.

- The underlying health of a resident's soft tissue affects how much pressure, shear force, or friction is needed to damage tissue. Skin and soft tissue changes associated with aging, illness, small blood vessel disease, and malnutrition increase vulnerability to pressure ulcers.

- Additional external factors, such as excess moisture, and tissue exposure to urine or feces, can increase risk.

Planning for Care

- The care planning process should include efforts to stabilize, reduce, or remove underlying risk factors; to monitor the impact of the interventions; and to modify the interventions as appropriate based on the individualized needs of the resident.
- Throughout this section, terminology referring to "healed" vs. "unhealed" ulcers refers to whether or not the ulcer is "closed" vs. "open." When considering this, recognize that Stage 1, Suspected Deep Tissue Injury (sDTI), and unstageable pressure ulcers although "closed," (i.e. may be covered with tissue, eschar, slough, etc.) would not be considered "healed."
- Facilities should be aware that the resident is at higher risk of having the area of a closed pressure ulcer open up due to damage, injury, or pressure, because of the loss of tensile strength of the overlying tissue. Tensile strength of the skin overlying a closed pressure ulcer is 80% of normal skin tensile strength. Facilities should put preventative measures in place that will mitigate the opening of a closed ulcer due to the fragility of the overlying tissue.

M0100: Determination of Pressure Ulcer Risk (cont.)

Steps for Assessment

1. Review the medical record, including skin care flow sheets or other skin tracking forms, nurses' notes, and pressure ulcer risk assessments.
2. Speak with the treatment nurse and direct care staff on all shifts to confirm conclusions from the medical record review and observations of the resident.
3. Examine the resident and determine whether any ulcers, scars, or non-removable dressings/devices are present. Assess key areas for pressure ulcer development (e.g., sacrum, coccyx, trochanters, ischial tuberosities, and heels). Also assess bony prominences (e.g., elbows and ankles) and skin that is under braces or subjected to pressure (e.g., ears from oxygen tubing).

Coding Instructions

For this item, check all that apply:

- **Check A if resident has a Stage 1 or greater pressure ulcer, a scar over bony prominence, or a non-removable dressing/device.** Review descriptions of pressure ulcer stages and information obtained during physical examination and medical record review. Examples of non-removable dressings/devices include a primary surgical dressing, a cast, or a brace.

- **Check B if a formal assessment has been completed.** An example of an established pressure ulcer risk tool is the *Braden Scale for Predicting Pressure Sore Risk©*. Other tools may be used.

- **Check C if the resident's risk for pressure ulcer development is based on clinical assessment.** A clinical assessment could include a head-to-toe physical examination of the skin and observation or medical record review of pressure ulcer risk factors. Examples of risk factors include the following:
  - impaired/decreased mobility and decreased functional ability
  - co-morbid conditions, such as end stage renal disease, thyroid disease, or diabetes mellitus;
  - drugs, such as steroids, that may affect wound healing;
  - impaired diffuse or localized blood flow (e.g., generalized atherosclerosis or lower extremity arterial insufficiency);

> **DEFINITIONS**
>
> **PRESSURE ULCER RISK FACTOR**
> Examples of risk factors include immobility and decreased functional ability; co-morbid conditions such as end-stage renal disease, thyroid disease, or diabetes; drugs such as steroids; impaired diffuse or localized blood flow; resident refusal of care and treatment; cognitive impairment; exposure of skin to urinary and fecal incontinence; under nutrition, malnutrition, and hydration deficits; and a healed ulcer.
>
> **PRESSURE ULCER RISK TOOLS**
> Screening tools that are designed to help identify residents who might develop a pressure ulcer. A common risk assessment tool is the Braden Scale for Predicting Pressure Sore Risk©.

M0100: Determination of Pressure Ulcer Risk (cont.)

— resident refusal of some aspects of care and treatment;
— cognitive impairment;
— urinary and fecal incontinence;
— under nutrition, malnutrition, and hydration deficits; and
— healed pressure ulcers, especially Stage 3 or 4 which are more likely to have recurrent breakdown.

- **Check Z if none of the above apply.**

M0150: Risk of Pressure Ulcers

M0150. Risk of Pressure Ulcers	
Enter Code	Is this resident at risk of developing pressure ulcers? 0. No 1. Yes

Item Rationale

Health-related Quality of Life

- It is important to recognize and evaluate each resident's risk factors and to identify and evaluate all areas at risk of constant pressure.

Planning for Care

- The care process should include efforts to stabilize, reduce, or remove underlying risk factors; to monitor the impact of the interventions; and to modify the interventions as appropriate.

Steps for Assessment

1. Based on the item(s) reviewed for M0100, determine if the resident is at risk for developing a pressure ulcer.
2. If the medical record reveals that the resident currently has a Stage 1 or greater pressure ulcer, a scar over a bony prominence, or a non-removable dressing or device, the resident is at risk for worsening or new pressure ulcers.
3. Review formal risk assessment tools to determine the resident's "risk score."
4. Review the components of the clinical assessment conducted for evidence of pressure ulcer risk.

Coding Instructions

- **Code 0, no:** if the resident is not at risk for developing pressure ulcers based on a review of information gathered for M0100.

- **Code 1, yes:** if the resident is at risk for developing pressure ulcers based on a review of information gathered for M0100.

M0210: Unhealed Pressure Ulcer(s)

M0210. Unhealed Pressure Ulcer(s)	
Enter Code ☐	**Does this resident have one or more unhealed pressure ulcer(s) at Stage 1 or higher?** 0. **No** → Skip to M0900, Healed Pressure Ulcers 1. **Yes** → Continue to M0300, Current Number of Unhealed (non-epithelialized) Pressure Ulcers at Each Stage

Item Rationale

Health-related Quality of Life

- Pressure ulcers and other wounds or lesions affect quality of life for residents because they may limit activity, may be painful, and may require time-consuming treatments and dressing changes.

Planning for Care

- The pressure ulcer definitions used in the RAI Manual have been adapted from those recommended by the National Pressure Ulcer Advisory Panel (NPUAP) 2007 Pressure Ulcer Stages.

- An existing pressure ulcer identifies residents at risk for further complications or skin injury. Risk factors described in M0100 should be addressed.

- For MDS assessment, initial numerical staging of pressure ulcers and the initial numerical staging of ulcers after debridement, or sDTI that declares itself, should be coded in terms of what is assessed (seen or palpated, i.e. visible tissue, palpable bone) during the look-back period. Nursing homes may adopt the NPUAP guidelines in their clinical practice and nursing documentation. However, since CMS has adapted the NPUAP guidelines for MDS purposes, the definitions do not perfectly correlate with each stage as described by NPUAP. Therefore, you cannot use the NPUAP definitions to code the MDS. You must code the MDS according to the instructions in this manual.

- Pressure ulcer staging is an assessment system that provides a description and classification based on anatomic depth of soft tissue damage. This tissue damage can be visible or palpable in the ulcer bed. Pressure ulcer staging also informs expectations for healing times.

> **DEFINITIONS**
>
> **PRESSURE ULCER**
> A pressure ulcer is localized injury to the skin and/or underlying tissue usually over a bony prominence, as a result of pressure, or pressure in combination with shear and/or friction.

Steps for Assessment

1. Review the medical record, including skin care flow sheets or other skin tracking forms.
2. Speak with direct care staff and the treatment nurse to confirm conclusions from the medical record review.
3. Examine the resident and determine whether any skin ulcers are present.
   - Key areas for pressure ulcer development include the sacrum, coccyx, trochanters, ischial tuberosities, and heels. Other areas, such as bony deformities, skin under braces, and skin subjected to excess pressure, shear or friction, are also at risk for pressure ulcers.
   - Without a full body skin assessment, a pressure ulcer can be missed.
   - Examine the resident in a well-lit room. Adequate lighting is important for detecting skin changes. For any pressure ulcers identified, measure and record the deepest anatomical stage.
4. Identify any known or likely unstageable pressure ulcers.

M0210: Unhealed Pressure Ulcer(s) (cont.)

Coding Instructions

Code based on the presence of any pressure ulcer (regardless of stage) in the past 7 days.

- **Code 0, no:** if the resident did not have a pressure ulcer in the 7-day look-back period. Then skip Items M0300–M0800.
- **Code 1, yes:** if the resident had any pressure ulcer (Stage 1, 2, 3, 4, or unstageable) in the 7-day look-back period. Proceed to **Current Number of Unhealed Pressure Ulcers at Each Stage** item (M0300).

Coding Tips

- If an ulcer arises from a combination of factors which are primarily caused by pressure, then the ulcer should be included in this section as a pressure ulcer.
- Oral Mucosal ulcers caused by pressure should not be coded in Section M. These ulcers are captured in item **L0200C, Abnormal mouth tissue**. Mucosal ulcers are not staged using the skin pressure ulcer staging system because anatomical tissue comparisons cannot be made.
- If a pressure ulcer is surgically closed with a flap or graft, it should be coded as a surgical wound and not as a pressure ulcer. If the flap or graft fails, continue to code it as a surgical wound until healed.
- Residents with diabetes mellitus (DM) can have a pressure, venous, arterial, or diabetic neuropathic ulcer. The primary etiology should be considered when coding whether the diabetic has an ulcer that is caused by pressure or other factors.
- If a resident with DM has a heel ulcer from pressure and the ulcer is present in the 7-day look-back period, **code 1** and proceed to code items M0300–M0900 as appropriate for the pressure ulcer.
- If a resident with DM has an ulcer on the plantar (bottom) surface of the foot closer to the metatarsal and the ulcer is present in the 7-day look-back period, **code 0** and proceed to M1040 to code the ulcer as a diabetic foot ulcer.
- Scabs and eschar are different both physically and chemically. Eschar is a collection of dead tissue within the wound that is flush with the surface of the wound. A scab is made up of dried blood cells and serum, sits on the top of the skin, and forms over exposed wounds such as wounds with granulating surfaces (like pressure ulcers, lacerations, evulsions, etc.). A scab is evidence of wound healing. A pressure ulcer that was staged as a 2 and now has a scab indicates it is a healing stage 2, and therefore, staging should not change. Eschar characteristics and the level of damage it causes to tissues is what makes it easy to distinguish from a scab. It is extremely important to have staff who are trained in wound assessment and who are able to distinguish scabs from eschar.
- If a resident had a pressure ulcer on the last assessment and it is now healed, complete **Healed Pressure Ulcers** item (M0900).
- If a pressure ulcer healed during the look-back period, and was not present on prior assessment, **code 0**.

M0300: Current Number of Unhealed Pressure Ulcers at Each Stage

Steps for completing M0300A–G

Step 1: Determine Deepest Anatomical Stage

For each pressure ulcer, determine the deepest anatomical stage. Do not reverse or back stage. Consider current and historical levels of tissue involvement.

1. Observe and palpate the base of any identified pressure ulcers present to determine the anatomic depth of soft tissue damage involved.
2. Ulcer staging should be based on the ulcer's deepest anatomic soft tissue damage that is visible or palpable. If a pressure ulcer's tissues are obscured such that the depth of soft tissue damage cannot be observed, it is considered to be unstageable (see Step 2 below). Review the history of each pressure ulcer in the medical record. If the pressure ulcer has ever been classified at a higher numerical stage than what is observed now, it should continue to be classified at the higher numerical stage. Nursing homes that carefully document and track pressure ulcers will be able to more accurately code this item.

Step 2: Identify Unstageable Pressure Ulcers

1. Visualization of the wound bed is necessary for accurate staging.
2. Pressure ulcers that have eschar (tan, black, or brown) or slough (yellow, tan, gray, green or brown) tissue present such that the anatomic depth of soft tissue damage cannot be visualized or palpated in the wound bed, should be classified as unstageable, as illustrated at http://www.npuap.org/wp-content/uploads/2012/03/NPUAP-Unstage2.jpg
3. If the wound bed is only partially covered by eschar or slough, and the anatomical depth of tissue damage can be visualized or palpated, numerically stage the ulcer, and do not code this as unstageable.
4. A pressure ulcer with intact skin that is a suspected deep tissue injury (sDTI) should not be coded as a Stage 1 pressure ulcer. It should be coded as unstageable, as illustrated at http://www.npuap.org/images/NPUAP-SuspectDTI.jpg
5. Known pressure ulcers covered by a non-removable dressing/device (e.g., primary surgical dressing, cast) should be coded as unstageable.

M0300: Current Number of Unhealed Pressure Ulcers at Each Stage (cont.)

Step 3: Determine "Present on Admission"

*For **each** pressure ulcer, determine if the pressure ulcer was present at the time of admission/entry or reentry and **<u>not</u>** acquired while the resident was in the care of the nursing home. Consider current and historical levels of tissue involvement.*

DEFINITIONS

ON ADMISSION
As close to the actual time of admission as possible.

1. Review the medical record for the history of the ulcer.
2. Review for location and stage at the time of admission/entry or reentry. If the pressure ulcer was present on admission/entry or reentry and subsequently increased in numerical stage during the resident's stay, the pressure ulcer is coded at that higher stage, and that higher stage **should not be considered as "present on admission."**
3. If the pressure ulcer was unstageable on admission/entry or reentry, but becomes numerically stageable later, it should be considered as "present on admission" at the stage at which it first becomes numerically stageable. If it subsequently increases in numerical stage, that higher stage **should not be considered "present on admission."**
4. If a resident who has a pressure ulcer is hospitalized and returns with that pressure ulcer at the same numerical stage, the pressure ulcer **should not be coded as "present on admission"** because it was present at the facility prior to the hospitalization.
5. If a current pressure ulcer increases in numerical stage during a hospitalization, it is coded at the higher stage upon reentry and **should be coded as "present on admission."**

M0300A: Number of Stage 1 Pressure Ulcers

M0300. Current Number of Unhealed (non-epithelialized) **Pressure Ulcers at Each Stage**	
Enter Number ☐	**A. Number of Stage 1 pressure ulcers** **Stage 1:** Intact skin with non-blanchable redness of a localized area usually over a bony prominence. Darkly pigmented skin may not have a visible blanching; in dark skin tones only it may appear with persistent blue or purple hues

Item Rationale

Health-related Quality of Care

- Stage 1 pressure ulcers may deteriorate to more severe pressure ulcers without adequate intervention; as such, they are an important risk factor for further tissue damage.

Planning for Care

- Development of a Stage 1 pressure ulcer should be one of multiple factors that initiate pressure ulcer prevention interventions.

M0300A: Number of Stage 1 Pressure Ulcers (cont.)

Steps for Assessment

1. Perform head-to-toe assessment. Conduct a full body skin assessment focusing on bony prominences and pressure-bearing areas (sacrum, buttocks, heels, ankles, etc).

2. For the purposes of coding, determine that the lesion being assessed is **primarily** related to pressure and that other conditions have been ruled out. If pressure is **not** the **primary** cause, do **not** code here.

3. Reliance on only one descriptor is inadequate to determine the staging of the pressure ulcer between Stage 1 and suspected deep tissue ulcers. The descriptors are similar for these two types of ulcers (e.g., temperature (warmth or coolness); tissue consistency (firm or boggy).

4. Check any reddened areas for ability to blanch by firmly pressing a finger into the reddened tissues and then removing it. In non-blanchable reddened areas, there is no loss of skin color or pressure-induced pallor at the compressed site.

5. Search for other areas of skin that differ from surrounding tissue that may be painful, firm, soft, warmer, or cooler compared to adjacent tissue. Stage 1 may be difficult to detect in individuals with dark skin tones. Visible blanching may not be readily apparent in darker skin tones. Look for temperature or color changes.

> **DEFINITIONS**
>
> **STAGE 1 PRESSURE ULCER**
> An observable, pressure-related alteration of intact skin, whose indicators as compared to an adjacent or opposite area on the body may include changes in one or more of the following parameters: skin temperature (warmth or coolness); tissue consistency (firm or boggy); sensation (pain, itching); and/or a defined area of persistent redness in lightly pigmented skin, whereas in darker skin tones, the ulcer may appear with persistent red, blue, or purple hues.
>
> **NON-BLANCHABLE**
> Reddened areas of tissue that do not turn white or pale when pressed firmly with a finger or device.

Coding Instructions for M0300A

- **Enter the number** of Stage 1 pressure ulcers that are currently present.
- **Enter 0** if no Stage 1 pressure ulcers are present.

Coding Tips

- If a resident had a pressure ulcer on the last assessment and it is now healed, complete **Healed Pressure Ulcers** item (M0900).
- If a pressure ulcer healed during the look-back period, and was not present on prior assessment, **code 0**.

M0300B: Stage 2 Pressure Ulcers

B. Stage 2: Partial thickness loss of dermis presenting as a shallow open ulcer with a red or pink wound bed, without slough. May also present as an intact or open/ruptured blister

Enter Number

1. **Number of Stage 2 pressure ulcers** - If 0 ⟶ Skip to M0300C, Stage 3

Enter Number

2. **Number of these Stage 2 pressure ulcers that were present upon admission/entry or reentry** - enter how many were noted at the time of admission/entry or reentry

3. **Date of oldest Stage 2 pressure ulcer** - Enter dashes if date is unknown:

   ☐☐ – ☐☐ – ☐☐☐☐
   Month   Day   Year

Item Rationale

Health-related Quality of Life

- Stage 2 pressure ulcers may worsen without proper interventions.
- These residents are at risk for further complications or skin injury.

Planning for Care

- **Most Stage 2** pressure ulcers should heal in a reasonable time frame (e.g., 60 days).

> **DEFINITIONS**
>
> **STAGE 2 PRESSURE ULCER**
> Partial thickness loss of dermis presenting as a shallow open ulcer with a red-pink wound bed, **without slough.**
>
> May also present as an intact or open/ruptured blister.

- If a pressure ulcer fails to show some evidence toward healing within 14 days, the pressure ulcer (including potential complications) and the patient's overall clinical condition should be reassessed.
- Stage 2 pressure ulcers are often related to friction and/or shearing force, and the care plan should incorporate efforts to limit these forces on the skin and tissues.
- Stage 2 pressure ulcers may be more likely to heal with treatment than higher stage pressure ulcers.
- The care plan should include individualized interventions and evidence that the interventions have been monitored and modified as appropriate.

Steps for Assessment

1. Perform head-to-toe assessment. Conduct a full body skin assessment focusing on bony prominences and pressure-bearing areas (sacrum, buttocks, heels, ankles, etc).
2. For the purposes of coding, determine that the lesion being assessed is primarily related to pressure and that other conditions have been ruled out. If pressure is **not** the primary cause, do **not** code here.

M0300B: Stage 2 Pressure Ulcers (cont.)

3. **Examine the area adjacent to or surrounding an intact blister for evidence of tissue damage. If other conditions are ruled out and the tissue adjacent to, or surrounding the blister demonstrates signs of tissue damage, (e.g., color change, tenderness, bogginess or firmness, warmth or coolness) these characteristics suggest a suspected deep tissue injury (sDTI) rather than a Stage 2 Pressure Ulcer.**

4. Stage 2 pressure ulcers will **generally** lack the surrounding characteristics found with a deep tissue injury.

5. Identify the number of **these** pressure ulcers that were present on admission/entry or reentry (see instructions on page M-6).

6. Identify the oldest Stage 2 pressure ulcer and the date it was first noted at that stage.

Coding Instructions for M0300B

- **Enter the number** of pressure ulcers that are currently present and whose deepest anatomical stage is Stage 2.

- **Enter 0** if no Stage 2 pressure ulcers are present and skip to **Current Number of Unhealed Pressure Ulcers at Each Stage** item (M0300C).

- **Enter the number** of Stage 2 pressure ulcers that were first noted at the time of admission/entry AND—for residents who are reentering the facility after a hospital stay, enter the number of Stage 2 pressure ulcers that were acquired during the hospitalization (i.e., the Stage 2 pressure ulcer was not acquired in the nursing facility prior to admission to the hospital).

- **Enter 0** if no Stage 2 pressure ulcers were first noted at the time of admission/entry or reentry.

- **Enter the date of the oldest Stage 2 pressure ulcer.** The facility should make every effort to determine the actual date that the Stage 2 pressure ulcer was first identified whether or not it was acquired in the facility. If the facility is unable to determine the actual date that the Stage 2 pressure ulcer was first identified (i.e., the date is unknown), enter a dash in every block. Do not leave any boxes blank. If the month or day contains only a single digit, fill the first box in with a "0." For example, January 2, 2012, should be entered as 01-02-2012.

Coding Tips

- A Stage 2 pressure ulcer presents as a shiny or dry shallow ulcer without slough or bruising.

- If the oldest Stage 2 pressure ulcer was present on admission/entry or reentry and the date it was first noted is unknown, enter a dash in every block.

- Do **not** code skin tears, tape burns, moisture associated skin damage, or excoriation here.

- When a pressure ulcer presents as an intact blister, examine the adjacent and surrounding area for signs of deep tissue injury. When a deep tissue injury **is** determined, do **not** code as a Stage 2.

M0300C: Stage 3 Pressure Ulcers

> **C. Stage 3:** Full thickness tissue loss. Subcutaneous fat may be visible but bone, tendon or muscle is not exposed. Slough may be present but does not obscure the depth of tissue loss. May include undermining and tunneling
>
> Enter Number ☐
>
> **1. Number of Stage 3 pressure ulcers** - If 0 → Skip to M0300D, Stage 4
>
> Enter Number ☐
>
> **2. Number of <u>these</u> Stage 3 pressure ulcers that were present upon admission/entry or reentry** - enter how many were noted at the time of admission/entry or reentry

Item Rationale

Health-related Quality of Life

- Pressure ulcers affect quality of life for residents because they may limit activity, may be painful, and may require time-consuming treatments and dressing changes.

Planning for Care

- Pressure ulcers at more advanced stages typically require more aggressive interventions, including more frequent repositioning, attention to nutritional status, and care that may be more time or staff intensive.

- An existing pressure ulcer may put residents at risk for further complications or skin injury.

- If a pressure ulcer fails to show some evidence toward healing within 14 days, the pressure ulcer (including potential complications) and the resident's overall clinical condition should be reassessed.

> **DEFINITIONS**
>
> **STAGE 3 PRESSURE ULCER**
> Full thickness tissue loss. Subcutaneous fat may be visible but bone, tendon or muscle is not exposed. Slough may be present but does not obscure the depth of tissue loss. May include undermining or tunneling.

Steps for Assessment

1. Perform head-to-toe assessment. Conduct a full body skin assessment focusing on bony prominences and pressure-bearing areas (sacrum, buttocks, heels, ankles, etc).
2. For the purposes of coding, determine that the lesion being assessed is primarily related to pressure and that other conditions have been ruled out. If pressure is **not** the primary cause, do **not** code here.
3. Identify all Stage 3 pressure ulcers currently present.
4. Identify the number of **these** pressure ulcers that were present on admission/entry or reentry.

Coding Instructions for M0300C

- **Enter the number** of pressure ulcers that are currently present and whose deepest anatomical stage is Stage 3.

- **Enter 0** if no Stage 3 pressure ulcers are present and skip to **Current Number of Unhealed Pressures Ulcers at Each Stage** item (M0300D).

- **Enter the number** of Stage 3 pressure ulcers that were first noted at Stage 3 at the time of admission/entry AND—for residents who are reentering the facility after a hospital stay, enter the number of Stage 3 pressure ulcers that were acquired during the

M0300C: Stage 3 Pressure Ulcers (cont.)

hospitalization (i.e., the Stage 3 pressure ulcer was not acquired in the nursing facility prior to admission to the hospital).

- **Enter 0** if no Stage 3 pressure ulcers were first noted at the time of admission/entry or reentry.

Coding Tips

- The depth of a Stage 3 pressure ulcer varies by anatomical location. Stage 3 pressure ulcers can be shallow, particularly on areas that do not have subcutaneous tissue, such as the bridge of the nose, ear, occiput, and malleolus.

- In contrast, areas of significant adiposity can develop extremely deep Stage 3 pressure ulcers. Therefore, observation and assessment of skin folds should be part of overall skin assessment.

- Bone/tendon/muscle is not visible or directly palpable in a Stage 3 pressure ulcer.

Examples

1. A pressure ulcer described as a Stage 2 was noted and documented in the resident's medical record on admission. On a later assessment, the wound is noted to be a full thickness ulcer without exposed bone, tendon, or muscle, thus it is now a Stage 3 pressure ulcer.

   Coding: The current Stage 3 pressure ulcer would be coded at **M0300C1 as Code 1, and at M0300C2 as 0, not present on admission/entry or reentry.**

   Rationale: The designation of "present on admission" requires that the pressure ulcer be at the same location **and** not have increased in numerical stage. This pressure ulcer worsened after admission.

2. A resident develops a Stage 2 pressure ulcer while at the nursing facility. The resident is hospitalized due to pneumonia for 8 days and returns with a Stage 3 pressure ulcer in the same location.

   Coding: The pressure ulcer would be coded at **M0300C1 as Code 1, and at M0300C2 as 1, present on admission/entry or reentry.**

   Rationale: Even though the resident had a pressure ulcer in the same anatomical location prior to transfer, because the pressure ulcer increased in numerical stage to Stage 3 during hospitalization, it should be coded as a Stage 3, present on admission/entry or reentry.

M0300C: Stage 3 Pressure Ulcers (cont.)

3. On admission, the resident has three small Stage 2 pressure ulcers on her coccyx. Two weeks later, the coccyx is assessed. Two of the Stage 2 pressure ulcers have merged and the third has increased in numerical stage to a Stage 3 pressure ulcer.

> **DEFINITIONS**
>
> **STAGE 4 PRESSURE ULCER**
> Full thickness tissue loss with exposed bone, tendon or muscle. Slough or eschar may be present on some parts of the wound bed. Often includes undermining and tunneling.

> **Coding:** The two merged pressure ulcers would be coded at **M0300B1 as 1, and at M0300B2 as 1, present on admission/entry or reentry**. The **Stage 3 pressure ulcer** would be **coded at M0300C1 as 1, and at M0300C2 as 0, not present on admission/entry or reentry.**
>
> **Rationale:** Two of the pressure ulcers on the coccyx have merged, but have remained at the same stage as they were at the time of admission; the one that increased in numerical stage to a Stage 3 cannot be coded in M0300C2 as present on admission/entry or reentry since the Stage 3 ulcer was not present on admission/entry or reentry.

4. A resident developed two Stage 2 pressure ulcers during her stay; one on the coccyx and the other on the left lateral malleolus. At some point she is hospitalized and returns with two pressure ulcers. One is the previous Stage 2 on the coccyx, which has not changed; the other is a new Stage 3 on the left trochanter. The Stage 2 previously on the left lateral malleolus has healed.

> **Coding:** The **Stage 2** pressure ulcer would be coded at **M0300B1 as 1, and at M0300B2 as 0, not present on admission; the Stage 3** would be coded at **M0300C1 as 1, and at M0300C2 as 1, present on admission/entry or reentry.**
>
> **Rationale:** The Stage 2 pressure ulcer on the coccyx was present prior to hospitalization; the Stage 3 pressure ulcer developed during hospitalization and is coded in M0300C2 as present on admission/entry or reentry. The Stage 2 pressure ulcer on the left lateral malleolus has healed and is therefore no longer coded here but in Item M0900, Healed Pressure Ulcers.

M0300D: Stage 4 Pressure Ulcers

> **D. Stage 4:** Full thickness tissue loss with exposed bone, tendon or muscle. Slough or eschar may be present on some parts of the wound bed. Often includes undermining and tunneling
>
> Enter Number
> ☐
>
> 1. **Number of Stage 4 pressure ulcers** - If 0 → Skip to M0300E, Unstageable: Non-removable dressing
>
> Enter Number
> ☐
>
> 2. **Number of these Stage 4 pressure ulcers that were present upon admission/entry or reentry** - enter how many were noted at the time of admission/entry or reentry

Item Rationale

Health-related Quality of Life

- Pressure ulcers affect quality of life for residents because they may limit activity, may be painful, and may require time-consuming treatments and dressing changes.

M0300D: Stage 4 Pressure Ulcers (cont.)

Planning for Care

- Pressure ulcers at more advanced stages typically require more aggressive interventions, including more frequent repositioning, attention to nutritional status, more frequent dressing changes, and treatment that is more time-consuming than with routine preventive care.

- An existing pressure ulcer may put residents at risk for further complications or skin injury.

- If a pressure ulcer fails to show some evidence toward healing within 14 days, the pressure ulcer (including potential complications) and the resident's overall clinical condition should be reassessed.

> **DEFINITIONS**
>
> **TUNNELING**
> A passage way of tissue destruction under the skin surface that has an opening at the skin level from the edge of the wound.
>
> **UNDERMINING**
> The destruction of tissue or ulceration extending under the skin edges (margins) so that the pressure ulcer is larger at its base than at the skin surface.

Steps for Assessment

1. Perform head-to-toe assessment. Conduct a full body skin assessment focusing on bony prominences and pressure-bearing areas (sacrum, buttocks, heels, ankles, etc.).
2. For the purposes of coding, determine that the lesion being assessed is primarily related to pressure and that other conditions have been ruled out. If pressure is **not** the primary cause, do **not** code here.
3. Identify all Stage 4 pressure ulcers currently present.
4. Identify the number of **these** pressure ulcers that were present on admission/entry or reentry.

Coding Instructions for M0300D

- **Enter the number** of pressure ulcers that are currently present and whose deepest anatomical stage is Stage 4.

- **Enter 0** if no Stage 4 pressure ulcers are present and skip to **Current Number of Unhealed Pressure Ulcers at Each Stage** item (M0300E).

- **Enter the number** of Stage 4 pressure ulcers that were first noted at Stage 4 at the time of admission/entry AND—for residents who are reentering the facility after a hospital stay, enter the number of Stage 4 pressure ulcers that were acquired during the hospitalization (i.e., the Stage 4 pressure ulcer was not acquired in the nursing facility prior to admission to the hospital).

- **Enter 0** if no Stage 4 pressure ulcers were first noted at the time of admission/entry or reentry.

M0300D: Stage 4 Pressure Ulcers (cont.)

Coding Tips

- The depth of a Stage 4 pressure ulcer varies by anatomical location. The bridge of the nose, ear, occiput, and malleolus do not have subcutaneous tissue, and these ulcers can be shallow.
- Stage 4 pressure ulcers can extend into muscle and/or supporting structures (e.g., fascia, tendon, or joint capsule) making osteomyelitis possible.
- Exposed bone/tendon/muscle is visible or directly palpable.
- Cartilage serves the same anatomical function as bone. Therefore, pressure ulcers that have exposed cartilage should be classified as a Stage 4.

M0300E: Unstageable Pressure Ulcers Related to Non-removable Dressing/Device

Enter Number [ ]	**E. Unstageable - Non-removable dressing:** Known but not stageable due to non-removable dressing/device
	1. Number of unstageable pressure ulcers due to non-removable dressing/device - If 0 → Skip to M0300F, Unstageable: Slough and/or eschar
Enter Number [ ]	**2. Number of _these_ unstageable pressure ulcers that were present upon admission/entry or reentry** - enter how many were noted at the time of admission/entry or reentry

Item Rationale

Health-related Quality of Life

- Although the wound bed cannot be visualized, and hence the pressure ulcer cannot be staged, the pressure ulcer may affect quality of life for residents because it may limit activity and may be painful.

Planning for Care

- Although the pressure ulcer itself cannot be observed, the surrounding area is monitored for signs of redness, swelling, increased drainage, or tenderness to touch, and the resident is monitored for adequate pain control.

> **DEFINITIONS**
>
> **NON-REMOVABLE DRESSING/ DEVICE**
> Includes, for example, a primary surgical dressing that cannot be removed, an orthopedic device, or cast.

Steps for Assessment

1. Review the medical record for documentation of a pressure ulcer covered by a non-removable dressing.
2. Determine the number of pressure ulcers unstageable related to a non-removable dressing/device. Examples of non-removable dressings/devices include a dressing that is not to be removed per physician's order, an orthopedic device, or a cast.
3. Identify the number of these pressure ulcers that were present on admission/entry or reentry (see page M-6 for assessment process).

M0300E: Unstageable Pressure Ulcers Related to Non-removable Dressing/Device (cont.)

Coding Instructions for M0300E

- **Enter the number** of pressure ulcers that are unstageable related to non-removable dressing/device.

- **Enter 0** if no unstageable pressure ulcers related to non-removable dressing/device are present and skip to **Current Number of Unhealed Pressure Ulcers at Each Stage** item (M0300F).

- **Enter the number** of unstageable pressure ulcers related to a non-removable dressing/device that were first noted at the time of admission/entry AND—for residents who are reentering the facility after a hospital stay, that were acquired during the hospitalization (i.e., the unstageable pressure ulcer related to a non-removable dressing/device was not acquired in the nursing facility prior to admission to the hospital).

- **Enter 0** if no unstageable pressure ulcers related to non-removable dressing/device were first noted at the time of admission/entry or reentry.

M0300F: Unstageable Pressure Ulcers Related to Slough and/or Eschar

	F. Unstageable - Slough and/or eschar: Known but not stageable due to coverage of wound bed by slough and/or eschar
Enter Number [ ]	**1. Number of unstageable pressure ulcers due to coverage of wound bed by slough and/or eschar** - If 0 → Skip to M0300G, Unstageable: Deep tissue
Enter Number [ ]	**2. Number of these unstageable pressure ulcers that were present upon admission/entry or reentry** - enter how many were noted at the time of admission/entry or reentry

Item Rationale

Health-related Quality of Life

- Although the wound bed cannot be visualized, and hence the pressure ulcer cannot be staged, the pressure ulcer may affect quality of life for residents because it may limit activity, may be painful, and may require time-consuming treatments and dressing changes.

Planning for Care

- Visualization of the wound bed is necessary for accurate staging.
- The presence of pressure ulcers and other skin changes should be accounted for in the interdisciplinary care plan.

DEFINITIONS

SLOUGH TISSUE
Non-viable yellow, tan, gray, green or brown tissue; usually moist, can be soft, stringy and mucinous in texture. Slough may be adherent to the base of the wound or present in clumps throughout the wound bed.

ESCHAR TISSUE
Dead or devitalized tissue that is hard or soft in texture; usually black, brown, or tan in color, and may appear scab-like. Necrotic tissue and eschar are usually firmly adherent to the base of the wound and often the sides/edges of the wound.

M0300F: Unstageable Pressure Ulcers Related to Slough and/or Eschar (cont.)

- Pressure ulcers that present as unstageable require care planning that includes, in the absence of ischemia, debridement of necrotic and dead tissue and restaging once this tissue is removed.

Steps for Assessment

1. Determine the number of pressure ulcers that are unstageable due to slough and/or eschar.
2. Identify the number of **these** pressure ulcers that were present on admission/entry or reentry (see page M-6 for assessment process).

Coding Instructions for M0300F

- **Enter the number** of pressure ulcers that are unstageable related to slough and/or eschar.

- **Enter 0** if no unstageable pressure ulcers related to slough and/or eschar are present and skip to **Current Number of Unhealed Pressure Ulcers at Each Stage** item (M0300G).

- **Enter the number** of unstageable pressure ulcers related to slough and/or eschar that were first noted at the time of admission/entry AND—for residents who are reentering the facility after a hospital stay that were acquired during the hospitalization (i.e., the unstageable pressure ulcer related to slough and/or eschar was not acquired in the nursing facility prior to admission to the hospital).

- **Enter 0** if no unstageable pressure ulcers related to slough and/or eschar were first noted at the time of admission/entry or reentry.

Coding Tips

- Pressure ulcers that are covered with slough and/or eschar should be coded as unstageable because the true anatomic depth of soft tissue damage (and therefore stage) cannot be determined. Only until enough slough and/or eschar is removed to expose the anatomic depth of soft tissue damage involved, can the stage of the wound be determined.

> **DEFINITIONS**
>
> **FLUCTUANCE**
> Used to describe the texture of wound tissue indicative of underlying unexposed fluid.

- Stable eschar (i.e., dry, adherent, intact without erythema or fluctuance) on the heels serves as "the body's natural (biological) cover" and should only be removed after careful clinical consideration, including ruling out ischemia, and consultation with the resident's physician, or nurse practitioner, physician assistant, or clinical nurse specialist if allowable under state licensure laws.

- Once the pressure ulcer is debrided of slough and/or eschar such that the anatomic depth of soft tissue damage involved can be determined, then code the ulcer for the reclassified stage. The pressure ulcer does not have to be completely debrided or free of all slough and/or eschar tissue in order for reclassification of stage to occur.

M0300F: Unstageable Pressure Ulcers Related to Slough and/or Eschar (cont.)

Examples

1. A resident is admitted with a sacral pressure ulcer that is 100% covered with black eschar.

    Coding: The pressure ulcer would be coded at **M0300F1 as 1, and at M0300F2 as 1, present on admission/entry or reentry.**

    Rationale: The pressure ulcer depth is not observable because the pressure ulcer is covered with eschar. This pressure ulcer is unstageable and was present on admission.

2. A pressure ulcer on the sacrum was present on admission and was 100% covered with black eschar. On the admission assessment, it was coded as unstageable and present on admission. The pressure ulcer is later debrided using conservative methods and after 4 weeks the ulcer has 50% to 75% eschar present. The assessor can now see that the damage extends down to the bone.

    Coding: The ulcer is reclassified as a Stage 4 pressure ulcer. On the subsequent MDS, it is coded at **M0300D1 as 1, and at M0300D2 as 1, present on admission/entry or reentry.**

    Rationale: After debridement, the pressure ulcer is no longer unstageable because bone is visible in the wound bed. Therefore, this ulcer can be classified as a Stage 4 pressure ulcer and should be coded at M0300D. If this pressure ulcer has the largest surface area of all Stage 3 or 4 pressure ulcers for this resident, the pressure ulcer's dimensions would also be entered at M0610, Dimensions of Unhealed Stage 3 or 4 Pressure Ulcers or Unstageable Pressure Ulcer Due to Slough or Eschar.

3. Miss J. was admitted with one small Stage 2 pressure ulcer. Despite treatment, it is not improving. In fact, it now appears deeper than originally observed, and the wound bed is covered with slough.

    Coding: Code at **M0300F1 as 1, and at M0300F2 as 0**, not present on admission/entry or reentry.

    Rationale: The pressure ulcer depth is not observable because it is covered with slough. This pressure ulcer is unstageable and is not coded in M0300F2 as present on admission/entry or reentry because it can no longer be coded as a Stage 2.

M0300G: Unstageable Pressure Ulcers Related to Suspected Deep Tissue Injury

> **G. Unstageable - Deep tissue:** Suspected deep tissue injury in evolution
>
> Enter Number
> 1. **Number of unstageable pressure ulcers with suspected deep tissue injury in evolution** - If 0 → Skip to M0610, Dimension of Unhealed Stage 3 or 4 Pressure Ulcers or Eschar
>
> Enter Number
> 2. **Number of these unstageable pressure ulcers that were present upon admission/entry or reentry** - enter how many were noted at the time of admission/entry or reentry

M0300G: Unstageable Pressure Ulcers Related to Suspected Deep Tissue Injury (cont.)

Item Rationale

> **DEFINITIONS**
>
> **SUSPECTED DEEP TISSUE INJURY**
> Purple or maroon area of discolored intact skin due to damage of underlying soft tissue. The area may be preceded by tissue that is painful, firm, mushy, boggy, warmer or cooler as compared to adjacent tissue.

Health-related Quality of Life

- Deep tissue injury may precede the development of a Stage 3 or 4 pressure ulcer even with optimal treatment.
- Quality health care begins with prevention and risk assessment, and care planning begins with prevention. Appropriate care planning is essential in optimizing a resident's ability to avoid, as well as recover from, pressure (as well as all) wounds. Deep tissue injuries may sometimes indicate severe damage. Identification and management of suspected deep tissue injury (sDTI) is imperative.

Planning for Care

- Suspected deep tissue injury requires vigilant monitoring because of the potential for rapid deterioration. Such monitoring should be reflected in the care plan.

Steps for Assessment

1. Perform head-to-toe assessment. Conduct a full body skin assessment focusing on bony prominences and pressure-bearing areas (sacrum, buttocks, heels, ankles, etc.).
2. For the purposes of coding, determine that the lesion being assessed is primarily a result of pressure and that other conditions have been ruled out. If pressure is **not** the primary cause, do **not** code here.
3. Examine the area adjacent to, or surrounding, an intact blister for evidence of tissue damage. If the tissue adjacent to, or surrounding, the blister **does not show** signs of tissue damage (e.g., color change, tenderness, bogginess or firmness, warmth or coolness), do **not** code as a suspected deep tissue injury.
4. In dark-skinned individuals, the area of injury is probably not purple/maroon, but rather darker than the surrounding tissue.
5. Determine the number of pressure ulcers that are unstageable related to suspected deep tissue injury.
6. Identify the number of **these** pressure ulcers that were present on admission/entry or reentry (see page M-6 for instructions).
7. Clearly document assessment findings in the resident's medical record, and track and document appropriate wound care planning and management.

M0300G: Unstageable Pressure Ulcers Related to Suspected Deep Tissue Injury (cont.)

Coding Instructions for M0300G

- **Enter the number** of unstageable pressure ulcers related to suspected deep tissue injury. Based on skin tone, the injured tissue area may present as a darker tone than the surrounding intact skin. These areas of discoloration are potentially areas of suspected deep tissue injury.

- **Enter 0** if no unstageable pressure ulcers related to suspected deep tissue injury are present and skip to **Dimensions of Unhealed Stage 3 or Stage 4 Pressure Ulcers or Eschar** item (M0610).

- **Enter the number** of unstageable pressure ulcers related to suspected deep tissue injury that were first noted at the time of admission/entry AND—for residents who are reentering the facility after a hospital stay, that were acquired during the hospitalization (i.e., the unstageable pressure ulcer related to suspected deep tissue injury was not acquired in the nursing facility prior to admission to the hospital).

- **Enter 0** if no unstageable pressure ulcers related to suspected deep tissue injury were first noted at the time of admission/entry or reentry.

Coding Tips

- Once suspected deep tissue injury has opened to an ulcer, reclassify the ulcer into the appropriate stage. Then code the ulcer for the reclassified stage.
- Deep tissue injury may be difficult to detect in individuals with dark skin tones.
- Evolution may be rapid, exposing additional layers of tissue even with optimal treatment.
- When a lesion due to pressure presents with an intact blister AND the surrounding or adjacent soft tissue does NOT have the characteristics of deep tissue injury, do **not** code here.

M0610: Dimensions of Unhealed Stage 3 or 4 Pressure Ulcers or Unstageable Pressure Ulcer Due to Slough and/or Eschar

M0610. Dimensions of Unhealed Stage 3 or 4 Pressure Ulcers or Eschar	
Complete only if M0300C1, M0300D1 or M0300F1 is greater than 0	
If the resident has one or more unhealed (non-epithelialized) Stage 3 or 4 pressure ulcers or an unstageable pressure ulcer due to slough or eschar, identify the pressure ulcer with the largest surface area (length x width) and record in centimeters:	
☐☐.☐ cm	**A. Pressure ulcer length:** Longest length from head to toe
☐☐.☐ cm	**B. Pressure ulcer width:** Widest width of the same pressure ulcer, side-to-side perpendicular (90-degree angle) to length
☐☐.☐ cm	**C. Pressure ulcer depth:** Depth of the same pressure ulcer from the visible surface to the deepest area (if depth is unknown, enter a dash in each box)

M0610: Dimensions of Unhealed Stage 3 or 4 Pressure Ulcers or Unstageable Pressure Ulcer Due to Slough and/or Eschar (cont.)

Item Rationale

Health-related Quality of Life

- Pressure ulcer dimensions are an important characteristic used to assess and monitor healing.

Planning for Care

- Evaluating the dimensions of the pressure ulcer is one aspect of the process of monitoring response to treatment.
- Pressure ulcer measurement findings are used to plan interventions that will best prepare the wound bed for healing.

Steps for Assessment

*If the resident has **one or more** unhealed Stage 3 or 4 pressure ulcers or an unstageable pressure ulcer due to slough and/or eschar, **identify the pressure ulcer with the largest surface area** (length × width) and record in centimeters. **Complete only if a pressure ulcer is coded in M0300C1, M0300D1, or M0300F1.** The Figure (right) illustrates the measurement process.*

1. Measurement is based on observation of the Stage 3, Stage 4, or unstageable pressure ulcer due to slough and/or eschar **after** the dressing and any exudate are removed.

2. Use a disposable measuring device or a cotton-tipped applicator.
3. Determine longest length (white arrow line) head to toe and greatest width (black arrow line) of each Stage 3, Stage 4, or unstageable pressure ulcer due to slough and/or eschar.
4. Measure the longest length of the pressure ulcer. If using a cotton-tipped applicator, mark on the applicator the distance between healthy skin tissue at each margin and lay the applicator next to a centimeter ruler to determine length.
5. Using a similar approach, measure the longest width (perpendicular to the length forming a "+," side to side).
6. Measure every Stage 3, Stage 4, and unstageable pressure ulcer due to slough and/or eschar that is present. **The clinician must be aware of all pressure ulcers present in order to determine which pressure ulcer is the largest.** Use a skin tracking sheet or other worksheet to record the dimensions for each pressure ulcer. Select the largest one by comparing the surface areas (length x width) of each.

M0610: Dimensions of Unhealed Stage 3 or 4 Pressure Ulcers or Unstageable Pressure Ulcer Due to Slough and/or Eschar (cont.)

7. Considering **only** the largest Stage 3 or 4 pressure ulcer due to slough or eschar, determine the deepest area and record the depth in centimeters. To measure wound depth, moisten a sterile, cotton-tipped applicator with 0.9% sodium chloride (NaCl) solution or sterile water. Place the applicator tip in the deepest aspect of the ulcer and measure the distance to the skin level. If the depth is uneven, measure several areas and document the depth of the ulcer that is the deepest. If depth cannot be assessed due to slough and/or eschar, enter dashes in M0610C.

8. If two pressure ulcers occur on the same bony prominence and are separated, at least superficially, by skin, then count them as two separate pressure ulcers. Stage and measure each pressure ulcer separately.

Coding Instructions for M0610 Dimensions of Unhealed Stage 3 or 4 Pressure Ulcers or Unstageable Due to Slough and/or Eschar

-   **Enter the current longest length** of the largest Stage 3, Stage 4, or unstageable pressure ulcer due to slough and/or eschar in centimeters to one decimal point (e.g., 2.3 cm).

-   **Enter the widest width** in centimeters of the largest Stage 3, Stage 4, or unstageable pressure ulcer due to slough and/or eschar. Record the width in centimeters to one decimal point.

-   **Enter the depth** measured in centimeters of the largest Stage 3 or 4. Record the depth in centimeters to one decimal point. Note that depth cannot be assessed if wound bed is unstageable due to being covered with slough and/or eschar. If a pressure ulcer covered with slough and/or eschar is the largest unhealed pressure ulcer identified for measurement, enter dashes in item M0610C.

Coding Tips

-   Place the resident in the most appropriate position which will allow for accurate wound measurement.

-   Select a uniform, consistent method for measuring wound length, width, and depth to facilitate meaningful comparisons of wound measurements across time.

-   Assessment of the pressure ulcer for tunneling and undermining is an important part of the complete pressure ulcer assessment. Measurement of tunneling and undermining is not recorded on the MDS but should be assessed, monitored, and treated as part of the comprehensive care plan.

M0700: Most Severe Tissue Type for Any Pressure Ulcer

M0700. Most Severe Tissue Type for Any Pressure Ulcer

Enter Code [ ]

Select the best description of the most severe type of tissue present in any pressure ulcer bed
1. **Epithelial tissue** - new skin growing in superficial ulcer. It can be light pink and shiny, even in persons with darkly pigmented skin
2. **Granulation tissue** - pink or red tissue with shiny, moist, granular appearance
3. **Slough** - yellow or white tissue that adheres to the ulcer bed in strings or thick clumps, or is mucinous
4. **Necrotic tissue (Eschar)** - black, brown, or tan tissue that adheres firmly to the wound bed or ulcer edges, may be softer or harder than surrounding skin
9. **None of the Above**

Item Rationale

Health-related Quality of Life

- The presence of a pressure ulcer may affect quality of life for residents because it may limit activity, may be painful, and may require time-consuming treatments and dressing changes.
- Identify tissue type.

Planning for Care

- Tissue characteristics of pressure ulcers should be considered when determining treatment options and choices.
- Changes in tissue characteristics over time are indicative of wound healing or degeneration.

Steps for Assessment

1. Examine the wound bed or base of each pressure ulcer. Adequate lighting is important to detect skin changes.
2. Determine the type(s) of tissue in the wound bed (e.g., epithelial, granulation, slough, eschar).

Coding Instructions for M0700

- **Code 1, Epithelial tissue:** if the wound is superficial and is re-epithelializing.
- **Code 2, Granulation tissue:** if the wound is clean (e.g., free of slough and eschar tissue) and contains granulation tissue.
- **Code 3, Slough:** if there is any amount of slough tissue present and eschar tissue is absent.
- **Code 4, Necrotic tissue (eschar):** if there is any eschar tissue present.
- **Code 9, None of the above:** if none of the above apply.

DEFINITIONS

EPITHELIAL TISSUE
New skin that is light pink and shiny (even in person's with darkly pigmented skin). In Stage 2 pressure ulcers, epithelial tissue is seen in the center and edges of the ulcer. In full thickness Stage 3 and 4 pressure ulcers, epithelial tissue advances from the edges of the wound.

GRANULATION TISSUE
Red tissue with "cobblestone" or bumpy appearance, bleeds easily when injured.

SLOUGH TISSUE
Non-viable yellow, tan, gray, green or brown tissue; usually moist, can be soft, stringy and mucinous in texture. Slough may be adherent to the base of the wound or present in clumps throughout the wound bed.

NECROTIC TISSUE (ESCHAR)
Dead or devitalized tissue that is hard or soft in texture; usually black, brown, or tan in color, and may appear scab-like. Necrotic tissue and eschar are usually firmly adherent to the base of the wound and often the sides/edges of the wound.

M0700: Most Severe Tissue Type for Any Pressure Ulcer (cont.)

Coding Tips and Special Populations

- Stage 2 pressure ulcers by definition have partial-thickness loss of the dermis. Granulation tissue, slough or eschar are not present in Stage 2 pressure ulcers. Therefore, Stage 2 pressure ulcers should **not** be coded as having granulation, slough, or eschar tissue and should be **coded as 1** for this item.

- Code for the most severe type of tissue present in the pressure ulcer wound bed.

- If the wound bed is covered with a mix of different types of tissue, code for the most severe type. For example, if a mixture of necrotic tissue (eschar and slough) is present, code for eschar.

- Code this item with **Code 9, None of the above**, in the following situations:
  - Stage 1 pressure ulcer
  - Stage 2 pressure ulcer with intact blister
  - Unstageable pressure ulcer related to non-removable dressing/device
  - Unstageable pressure ulcer related to suspected deep tissue injury

  Code 9 is being used in these instances because the wound bed cannot be visualized and therefore cannot be assessed.

Examples

1. A resident has a Stage 2 pressure ulcer on the right ischial tuberosity that is healing and a Stage 3 pressure ulcer on the sacrum that is also healing with red granulation tissue that has filled 75% of the ulcer and epithelial tissue that has resurfaced 25% of the ulcer.

   Coding: Code **M0700 as 2, Granulation tissue.**

   Rationale: Coding for M0700 is based on the sacral ulcer, because it is the pressure ulcer with the most severe tissue type. Code 2, (Granulation tissue), is selected because this is the most severe tissue present in the wound.

2. A resident has a Stage 2 pressure ulcer on the right heel and no other pressure ulcers.

   Coding: Code **M0700 as 1, Epithelial tissue**.

   Rationale: Coding for M0700 is Code 1, (Epithelial tissue) because epithelial tissue is consistent with identification of this pressure ulcer as a Stage 2 pressure ulcer.

3. A resident has a pressure ulcer on the left trochanter that has 25% black eschar tissue present, 75% granulation tissue present, and some epithelialization at the edges of the wound.

   Coding: Code **M0700 as 4, Necrotic tissue (eschar).**

   Rationale: Coding is for the most severe tissue type present, which is not always the majority of type of tissue. Therefore, Coding for M0700 is Code 4, [Necrotic tissue (eschar)].

M0800: Worsening in Pressure Ulcer Status Since Prior Assessment (OBRA or scheduled PPS) or Last Admission/Entry or Reentry

M0800. Worsening in Pressure Ulcer Status Since Prior Assessment (OBRA or Scheduled PPS) or Last Admission/Entry or Reentry Complete only if A0310E = 0	
Indicate the number of current pressure ulcers that were **not present or were at a lesser stage** on prior assessment (OBRA or scheduled PPS) or last entry. If no current pressure ulcer at a given stage, enter 0.	
Enter Number ☐	A. Stage 2
Enter Number ☐	B. Stage 3
Enter Number ☐	C. Stage 4

Item Rationale

Health-related Quality of Life

- This item documents whether skin status, overall, has worsened since the last assessment. To track increasing skin damage, this item documents the number of new pressure ulcers and whether any pressure ulcers have "worsened" or increased in numerical stage since the last assessment. Such tracking of pressure ulcers is consistent with good clinical care.

Planning for Care

- The interdisciplinary care plan should be reevaluated to ensure that appropriate preventative measures and pressure ulcer management principles are being adhered to when new pressure ulcers develop or when pressure ulcers worsen.

Steps for Assessment

*Look-back period for this item is back to the ARD of the prior assessment. **If there was no prior assessment (i.e., if this is the first OBRA or scheduled PPS assessment), do not complete this item.** Skip to M1030, **Number of Venous and Arterial Ulcers**.*

> **DEFINITIONS**
>
> **PRESSURE ULCER "WORSENING"**
> Pressure ulcer "worsening" is defined as a pressure ulcer that has progressed to a deeper level of tissue damage and is therefore staged at a higher number using a numerical scale of 1-4 (using the staging assessment system classifications assigned to each stage; starting at stage 1, and increasing in severity to stage 4) on an assessment as compared to the previous assessment. For the purposes of identifying the absence of a pressure ulcer, zero pressure ulcers is used when there is no skin breakdown or evidence of damage.

1. Review the history of each current pressure ulcer. Specifically, compare the current stage to past stages to determine whether any pressure ulcer on the current assessment is new or at an increased numerical stage when compared to the last MDS assessment. This allows a more accurate assessment than simply comparing total counts on the current and prior MDS assessment.

M0800: Worsening in Pressure Ulcer Status Since Prior Assessment (OBRA or scheduled PPS) or Last Admission/Entry or Reentry (cont.)

2. For each current stage, count the number of current pressure ulcers that are new or have increased in numerical stage since the last MDS assessment was completed.

Coding Instructions for M0800

- **Enter the number** of pressure ulcers that were not present OR were at a lesser numerical stage on prior assessment.

- **Code 0:** if no pressure ulcers have increased in numerical stage OR there are no new pressure ulcers.

Coding Tips

- Coding this item will be easier for nursing homes that document and follow pressure ulcer status on a routine basis.
- If a numerically staged pressure ulcer increases in numerical staging it is considered worsened.
- Coding worsening of unstageable pressure ulcers:
  - If a pressure ulcer was unstageable on admission/entry or reentry, do not consider it to be worsened on the first assessment that it is able to be numerically staged. However, if the pressure ulcer subsequently increases in numerical stage after that assessment, it should be considered worsened.
  - If a pressure ulcer was numerically staged and becomes unstageable due to slough or eschar, do not consider this pressure ulcer as worsened. The only way to determine if this pressure ulcer has worsened is to remove enough slough or eschar so that the wound bed becomes visible. Once enough of the wound bed can be visualized and/or palpated such that the tissues can be identified and the wound restaged, the determination of worsening can be made.
  - If a pressure ulcer was numerically staged and becomes unstageable, and is subsequently debrided sufficiently to be numerically staged, compare its numerical stage before and after it was unstageable. If the pressure ulcer's current numerical stage has increased, consider this pressure ulcer as worsened.
  - If two pressure ulcers merge, do not code as worsened. Although two merged pressure ulcers might increase the overall surface area of the ulcer, there would need to be an increase in numerical stage in order for it to be considered as worsened.
  - If a pressure ulcer is acquired during a hospital admission, its stage should be coded on admission and is considered as present on admission/entry or reentry. It is **not** included or coded in this item.

M0800: Worsening in Pressure Ulcer Status Since Prior Assessment (OBRA or scheduled PPS) or Last Admission/Entry or Reentry (cont.)

— If a pressure ulcer increases in numerical stage during a hospital admission, its stage should be coded on admission and is considered as present on admission/entry or reentry. It is **not** included or coded in this item. While not included in this item, it is important to recognize clinically on reentry that the resident's overall skin status deteriorated while in the hospital. In either case, if the pressure ulcer deteriorates further and increases in numerical stage on a subsequent MDS assessment, it would be considered as worsened and would be coded in this item.

Examples

1. A resident has a pressure ulcer on the right ischial tuberosity that was Stage 2 on the previous MDS assessment and has now increased in numerical stage to a Stage 3 pressure ulcer.

    Coding: Code **M0800A as 0, M0800B as 1**, and **M0800C as 0.**

    Rationale: The pressure ulcer was at a lesser numerical stage on the prior assessment.

2. A resident is admitted with an unstageable pressure ulcer on the sacrum, which is debrided and reclassified as a Stage 4 pressure ulcer 3 weeks later. The initial MDS assessment listed the pressure ulcer as unstageable.

    Coding: Code **M0800A as 0**, **M0800B as 0**, and **M0800C as 0.**

    Rationale: The unstageable pressure ulcer was present on the initial MDS assessment. After debridement it numerically staged as a Stage 4 pressure ulcer. This is the first numerical staging since debridement and therefore, should not be considered or coded as worsening on the MDS assessment.

3. A resident has previous medical record and MDS documentation of a Stage 2 pressure ulcer on the sacrum and a Stage 3 pressure ulcer on the right heel. Current skin care flow sheets indicate a Stage 3 pressure ulcer on the sacrum, a Stage 4 pressure ulcer on the right heel, as well as a new Stage 2 pressure ulcer on the left trochanter.

    Coding: Code **M0800A as 1, M0800B as 1,** and **M0800C as 1.**

    Rationale: M0800A would be coded 1 because the new Stage 2 pressure ulcer on the left trochanter was not present on the prior assessment. M0800B would be coded 1 and M0800C would be coded 1 for the increased numerical staging of both the sacrum and right heel pressure ulcers.

M0800: Worsening in Pressure Ulcer Status Since Prior Assessment (OBRA or scheduled PPS) or Last Admission/Entry or Reentry (cont.)

4. A resident develops a Stage 3 pressure ulcer while at the nursing home. The wound bed is subsequently covered with slough and is coded on the next assessment as unstageable due to slough. After debridement, the wound bed is clean and the pressure ulcer is reassessed and determined to still be a Stage 3 pressure ulcer.

> **Coding:** Code **M0800A as 0**, **M0800B as 0**, and **M0800C as 0**.
>
> **Rationale:** M0800B would be coded 0 because the numerical stage of the pressure ulcer is the same numerical stage as it was prior to the period it became unstageable.

M0900: Healed Pressure Ulcers

M0900. Healed Pressure Ulcers	
Complete only if A0310E = 0	

Enter Code ☐	A. **Were pressure ulcers present on the prior assessment (OBRA or scheduled PPS)?**
	  0. **No** → Skip to M1030, Number of Venous and Arterial Ulcers
	  1. **Yes** → Continue to M0900B, Stage 2

	Indicate the number of pressure ulcers that were noted on the prior assessment (OBRA or scheduled PPS) that have completely closed (resurfaced with epithelium). If no healed pressure ulcer at a given stage since the prior assessment (OBRA or scheduled PPS), enter 0.
Enter Number ☐	B. **Stage 2**
Enter Number ☐	C. **Stage 3**
Enter Number ☐	D. **Stage 4**

Item Rationale

Health-related Quality of Life

- Pressure ulcers do not heal in a reverse sequence, that is, the body does not replace the types and layers of tissue (e.g., muscle, fat, and dermis) that were lost during pressure ulcer development before they re-epithelialize. Stage 3 and 4 pressure ulcers fill with granulation tissue. This replacement tissue is never as strong as the tissue that was lost and hence is more prone to future breakdown.

> **DEFINITIONS**
>
> **HEALED PRESSURE ULCER**
> Completely closed, fully epithelialized, covered completely with epithelial tissue, or resurfaced with new skin, *even if* the area continues to have some surface discoloration.

M0900: Healed Pressure Ulcers (cont.)

Planning for Care

- Pressure ulcers that heal require continued prevention interventions as the site is always at risk for future damage.

- **Most Stage 2** pressure ulcers should heal within a reasonable timeframe (e.g., 60 days). Full thickness Stage 3 and 4 pressure ulcers may require longer healing times.

- Clinical standards do not support reverse staging or backstaging as a way to document healing as it does not accurately characterize what is physiologically occurring as the ulcer heals. For example, over time, even though a Stage 4 pressure ulcer has been healing and contracting such that it is less deep, wide, and long, the tissues that were lost (muscle, fat, dermis) will never be replaced with the same type of tissue. Previous standards using reverse or backstaging would have permitted identification of this pressure ulcer as a Stage 3, then a Stage 2, and so on, when it reached a depth consistent with these stages. Clinical standards now would require that this ulcer continue to be documented as a Stage 4 pressure ulcer until it has completely healed. Nursing homes can document the healing of pressure ulcers using descriptive characteristics of the wound (i.e. depth, width, presence or absence of granulation tissue, etc.) or by using a validated pressure ulcer healing tool. Once a pressure ulcer has healed, it is documented as a healed pressure ulcer at its highest numerical stage – in this example, a healed Stage 4 pressure ulcer. For care planning purposes, this healed Stage 4 pressure ulcer would remain at increased risk for future breakdown or injury and would require continued monitoring and preventative care.

Steps for Assessment

Complete on all residents, including those without a current pressure ulcer. Look-back period for this item is the ARD of the prior assessment. ***If no prior assessment (i.e., if this is the first OBRA or scheduled PPS assessment), do not complete this item. Skip to M1030.***

1. Review medical records to identify whether any pressure ulcers that were noted on the prior MDS assessment have healed by the ARD (A2300) of the current assessment.

2. Identify the deepest anatomical stage (see definition on page M-5) of each healed pressure ulcer.

3. Count the number of healed pressure ulcers for each stage.

M0900: Healed Pressure Ulcers (cont.)

Coding Instructions for M0900A

*Complete on **all** residents (even if M0210 = 0)*

- **Enter 0:** if there were no pressure ulcers on the prior assessment and skip to **Number of Venous and Arterial Ulcers** item (M1030).

- **Enter 1:** if there were pressure ulcers noted on the prior assessment.

Coding Instructions for M0900B, C, and D

- **Enter the number** of pressure ulcers that have healed since the last assessment for each Stage, 2 through 4.

- **Enter 0:** if there were no pressure ulcers at the given stage or no pressure ulcers that have healed.

Coding Tips

- Coding this item will be easier for nursing homes that systematically document and follow pressure ulcer status.

- If the prior assessment documents that a pressure ulcer healed between MDS assessments, but another pressure ulcer occurred at the same anatomical location, do **not** consider this pressure ulcer as healed. The re-opened pressure ulcer should be staged at its highest numerical stage until fully healed.

M1030: Number of Venous and Arterial Ulcers

M1030. Number of Venous and Arterial Ulcers	
Enter Number ☐	Enter the total number of venous and arterial ulcers present

Item Rationale

Health-related Quality of Life

- Skin wounds and lesions affect quality of life for residents because they may limit activity, may be painful, and may require time-consuming treatments and dressing changes.

M1030: Number of Venous and Arterial Ulcers (cont.)

Planning for Care

- The presence of venous and arterial ulcers should be accounted for in the interdisciplinary care plan.
- This information identifies residents at risk for further complications or skin injury.

Steps for Assessment

1. Review the medical record, including skin care flow sheet or other skin tracking form.
2. Speak with direct care staff and the treatment nurse to confirm conclusions from the medical record review.
3. Examine the resident and determine whether any venous or arterial ulcers are present.

    - Key areas for venous ulcer development include the area proximal to the lateral and medial malleolus (e.g., above the inner and outer ankle area).

    - Key areas for arterial ulcer development include the distal part of the foot, dorsum or tops of the foot, or tips and tops of the toes.

    - Venous ulcers may or may not be painful and are typically shallow with irregular wound edges, a red granular (e.g., bumpy) wound bed, minimal to moderate amounts of yellow fibrinous material, and moderate to large amounts of exudate. The surrounding tissues may be erythematous or reddened, or appear brown-tinged due to hemosiderin staining. Leg edema may also be present.

    - Arterial ulcers are often painful and have a pale pink wound bed, necrotic tissue, minimal exudate, and minimal bleeding.

Coding Instructions

Check all that apply in the last 7 days.
*Pressure ulcers coded in M0210 through M0900 should **not** be coded here.*

- **Enter the number** of venous and arterial ulcers present.
- **Enter 0:** if there were no venous or arterial ulcers present.

DEFINITIONS

VENOUS ULCERS
Ulcers caused by peripheral venous disease, which most commonly occur proximal to the medial or lateral malleolus, above the inner or outer ankle, or on the lower calf area of the leg.

ARTERIAL ULCERS
Ulcers caused by peripheral arterial disease, which commonly occur on the tips and tops of the toes, tops of the foot, or distal to the medial malleolus.

DEFINITIONS

HEMOSIDERIN
An intracellular storage form of iron; the granules consist of an ill-defined complex of ferric hydroxides, polysaccharides, and proteins having an iron content of approximately 33% by weight. It appears as a dark yellow-brown pigment.

M1030: Number of Venous and Arterial Ulcers (cont.)

Coding Tips

Arterial Ulcers

- Trophic skin changes (e.g., dry skin, loss of hair growth, muscle atrophy, brittle nails) may also be present. The wound may start with some kind of minor trauma, such as hitting the leg on a wheelchair. The wound does not typically occur over a bony prominence, however, can occur on the tops of the toes. Pressure forces play virtually no role in the development of the ulcer, however, for some residents, pressure may play a part. Ischemia is the major etiology of these ulcers. Lower extremity and foot pulses may be diminished or absent.

Venous Ulcers

- The wound may start with some kind of minor trauma, such as hitting the leg on a wheelchair. The wound does not typically occur over a bony prominence, and pressure forces play virtually **no** role in the development of the ulcer.

Example

1. A resident has three toes on her right foot that have black tips. She does not have diabetes, but has been diagnosed with peripheral vascular disease.

    Coding: Code **M1030 as 3.**

    Rationale: Ischemic changes point to the ulcer being vascular.

M1040: Other Ulcers, Wounds and Skin Problems

M1040. Other Ulcers, Wounds and Skin Problems	
↓ Check all that apply	
	Foot Problems
☐	**A. Infection of the foot** (e.g., cellulitis, purulent drainage)
☐	**B. Diabetic foot ulcer(s)**
☐	**C. Other open lesion(s) on the foot**
	Other Problems
☐	**D. Open lesion(s) other than ulcers, rashes, cuts** (e.g., cancer lesion)
☐	**E. Surgical wound(s)**
☐	**F. Burn(s)** (second or third degree)
☐	**G. Skin tear(s)**
☐	**H. Moisture Associated Skin Damage (MASD)** (i.e. incontinence (IAD), perspiration, drainage)
	None of the Above
☐	**Z. None of the above** were present

M1040: Other Ulcers, Wounds and Skin Problems (cont.)

Item Rationale

Health-related Quality of Life

- Skin wounds and lesions affect quality of life for residents because they may limit activity, may be painful, and may require time-consuming treatments and dressing changes.

- Many of these ulcers, wounds and skin problems can worsen or increase risk for local and systemic infections.

Planning for Care

- This list represents only a subset of skin conditions or changes that nursing homes will assess and evaluate in residents.

- The presence of wounds and skin changes should be accounted for in the interdisciplinary care plan.

- This information identifies residents at risk for further complications or skin injury.

Steps for Assessment

1. Review the medical record, including skin care flow sheets or other skin tracking forms.
2. Speak with direct care staff and the treatment nurse to confirm conclusions from the medical record review.
3. Examine the resident and determine whether any ulcers, wounds, or skin problems are present.

   - Key areas for diabetic foot ulcers include the plantar (bottom) surface of the foot, especially the metatarsal heads (the ball of the foot).

Coding Instructions

*Check all that apply in the last 7 days. If there is no evidence of such problems in the last 7 days, check none of the above. Pressure ulcers coded in M0200 through M0900 should **not** be coded here.*

- **M1040A,** Infection of the foot (e.g., cellulitis, purulent drainage)

- **M1040B,** Diabetic foot ulcer(s)

- **M1040C,** Other open lesion(s) on the foot (e.g., cuts, fissures)

> ## DEFINITIONS
>
> ### DIABETIC FOOT ULCERS
> Ulcers caused by the neuropathic and small blood vessel complications of diabetes. Diabetic foot ulcers typically occur over the plantar (bottom) surface of the foot on load bearing areas such as the ball of the foot. Ulcers are usually deep, with necrotic tissue, moderate amounts of exudate, and callused wound edges. The wounds are very regular in shape and the wound edges are even with a punched-out appearance. These wounds are typically not painful.
>
> ### SURGICAL WOUNDS
> Any healing and non-healing, open or closed surgical incisions, skin grafts or drainage sites.
>
> ### OPEN LESION OTHER THAN ULCERS, RASHES, CUTS
> Most typically skin ulcers that develop as a result of diseases and conditions such as syphilis and cancer.
>
> ### BURNS (SECOND OR THIRD DEGREE)
> Skin and tissue injury caused by heat or chemicals and may be in any stage of healing.

M1040: Other Ulcers, Wounds and Skin Problems (cont.)

- **M1040D,** Open lesion(s) other than ulcers, rashes, cuts (e.g., cancer lesion)

- **M1040E,** Surgical wound(s)

- **M1040F,** Burn(s)(second or third degree)

- **M1040G,** Skin tear(s)

- **M1040H,** Moisture Associated Skin Damage (MASD) (i.e., incontinence (IAD), perspiration, drainage)

- **M1040Z,** None of the above were present

Coding Tips

M1040B Diabetic Foot Ulcers

- Diabetic neuropathy affects the lower extremities of individuals with diabetes. Individuals with diabetic neuropathy can have decreased awareness of pain in their feet. This means they are at high risk for foot injury, such as burns from hot water or heating pads, cuts or scrapes from stepping on foreign objects, and blisters from inappropriate or tight-fitting shoes. Because of decreased circulation and sensation, the resident may not be aware of the wound.

- Neuropathy can also cause changes in the structure of the bones and tissue in the foot. This means the individual with diabetes experiences pressure on the foot in areas not meant to bear pressure. Neuropathy can also cause changes in normal sweating, which means the individual with diabetes can have dry, cracked skin on his other foot.

- Do **not** include pressure ulcers that occur on residents with diabetes mellitus here. For example, an ulcer caused by pressure on the heel of a diabetic resident is a pressure ulcer and not a diabetic foot ulcer.

M1040D Open Lesion Other than Ulcers, Rashes, Cuts

- Do **not** code rashes, skin tears, cuts/lacerations here. Although not recorded on the MDS assessment, these skin conditions should be considered in the plan of care.

M1040E Surgical Wounds

- This category does not include healed surgical sites and healed stomas or lacerations that require suturing or butterfly closure as surgical wounds. PICC sites, central line sites, and peripheral IV sites are not coded as surgical wounds.

- Surgical debridement of a pressure ulcer does not create a surgical wound. Surgical debridement is used to remove necrotic or infected tissue from the pressure ulcer in order to facilitate healing. A pressure ulcer that has been surgically debrided should continue to be coded as a pressure ulcer.

M1040: Other Ulcers, Wounds and Skin Problems (cont.)

- Code pressure ulcers that require surgical intervention for closure with graft and/or flap procedures in this item (e.g., excision of pressure ulcer with myocutaneous flap). Once a pressure ulcer is excised and a graft and/or flap is applied, it is no longer considered a pressure ulcer, but a surgical wound

M1040F Burns (Second or Third Degree)

- Do **not** include first degree burns (changes in skin color only).

M1040G Skin Tear(s)

- Skin tears are a result of shearing, friction or trauma to the skin that causes a separation of the skin layers. They can be partial or full thickness. Code all skin tears in this item, even if already coded in Item J1900B.

M1040H Moisture Associated Skin Damage (MASD)

- Moisture associated skin damage (MASD) is a result of skin damage caused by moisture rather than pressure. It is caused by sustained exposure to moisture which can be caused, for example, by incontinence, wound exudate and perspiration. It is characterized by inflammation of the skin, and occurs with or without skin erosion and/or infection. MASD is also referred to as incontinence-associated dermatitis and can cause other conditions such as intertriginous dermatitis, periwound moisture-associated dermatitis, and peristomal moisture-associated dematitis. Provision of optimal skin care and early identification and treatment of minor cases of MASD can help avoid progression and skin breakdown.

Examples

1. A resident with diabetes mellitus presents with an ulcer on the heel that is due to pressure.

    Coding: This ulcer is **not checked at M1040B. This ulcer should be coded where appropriate under the Pressure Ulcers items (M0210-M0900).**
    Rationale: Persons with diabetes can still develop pressure ulcers.

2. A resident is readmitted from the hospital after myocutaneous flap surgery to excise and close his sacral pressure ulcer.

    Coding: Check **M1040E**, Surgical Wound.
    Rationale: A surgical flap procedure was used to close the resident's pressure ulcer. The pressure ulcer is now considered a surgical wound.

3. Mrs. J. was reaching over to get a magazine off of her bedside table and sustained a skin tear on her wrist from the edge of the table when she pulled the magazine back towards her.

    Coding: Check **M1040G**, Skin Tear(s).
    Rationale: The resident sustained a skin tear while reaching for a magazine.

M1040: Other Ulcers, Wounds and Skin Problems (cont.)

4. Mr. S. who is incontinent, is noted to have a large, red and excoriated area on his buttocks and interior thighs with serous exudate which is starting to cause skin glistening.

    Coding: Check **M1040H**, Moisture Associated Skin Damage (MASD).

    Rationale: Mr. S. skin assessment reveals characteristics of incontinence-associated dermatitis.

5. Mrs. F. complained of discomfort of her right great toe and when her stocking and shoe was removed, it was noted that her toe was red, inflamed and had pus draining from the edge of her nail bed. The podiatrist determined that Mrs. F. has an infected ingrown toenail.

    Coding: Check **M1040A**, Infection of the foot.

    Rationale: Mrs. F. has an infected right great toe due to an ingrown toenail.

6. Mr. G. has bullous pemphigoid and requires the application of sterile dressings to the open and weeping blistered areas.

    Coding: Check **M1040D**, Open lesion other than ulcers, rashes, cuts.

    Rationale: Mr. G. has open bullous pemphigoid blisters.

7. Mrs. A. was just admitted to the nursing home from the hospital burn unit after sustaining second and third degree burns in a house fire. She is here for continued treatment of her burns and for rehabilitative therapy.

    Coding: Check **M1040F**, Burns (second or third degree).

    Rationale: Mrs. A. has second and third degree burns, therefore, burns (second or third degree) should be checked.

M1200: Skin and Ulcer Treatments

M1200. Skin and Ulcer Treatments	
↓ Check all that apply	
☐	A. **Pressure reducing device for chair**
☐	B. **Pressure reducing device for bed**
☐	C. **Turning/repositioning program**
☐	D. **Nutrition or hydration intervention** to manage skin problems
☐	E. **Pressure ulcer care**
☐	F. **Surgical wound care**
☐	G. **Application of nonsurgical dressings** (with or without topical medications) other than to feet
☐	H. **Applications of ointments/medications** other than to feet
☐	I. **Application of dressings to feet** (with or without topical medications)
☐	Z. **None of the above** were provided

M1200: Skin and Ulcer Treatments (cont.)

Item Rationale

Health-related Quality of Life

- Appropriate prevention and treatment of skin changes and ulcers reduce complications and promote healing.

Planning for Care

- These general skin treatments include basic pressure ulcer prevention and skin health interventions that are a part of providing quality care and consistent with good clinical practice for those with skin health problems.
- These general treatments should guide more individualized and specific interventions in the care plan.
- If skin changes are not improving or are worsening, this information may be helpful in determining more appropriate care.

> **DEFINITIONS**
>
> **PRESSURE REDUCING DEVICE(S)**
> Equipment that aims to relieve pressure away from areas of high risk. May include foam, air, water gel, or other cushioning placed on a chair, wheelchair, or bed. Include pressure relieving, pressure reducing, and pressure redistributing devices. Devices are available for use with beds and seating.

Steps for Assessment

1. Review the medical record, including treatment records and health care provider orders for documented skin treatments during the past 7 days. Some skin treatments may be part of routine standard care for residents, so check the nursing facility's policies and procedures and indicate here if administered during the look-back period.
2. Speak with direct care staff and the treatment nurse to confirm conclusions from the medical record review.
3. Some skin treatments can be determined by observation. For example, observation of the resident's wheelchair and bed will reveal if the resident is using pressure-reducing devices for the bed or wheelchair.

Coding Instructions

Check all that apply in the last 7 days. Check Z, None of the above were provided, if none applied in the past 7 days.

- **M1200A,** Pressure reducing device for chair
- **M1200B,** Pressure reducing device for bed
- **M1200C,** Turning/repositioning program
- **M1200D,** Nutrition or hydration intervention to manage skin problems
- **M1200E,** Pressure ulcer care
- **M1200F,** Surgical wound care

CMS's RAI Version 3.0 Manual

CH 3: MDS Items [M]

M1200: Skin and Ulcer Treatments (cont.)

- **M1200G,** Application of non-surgical dressings (with or without topical medications) other than to feet. Non-surgical dressings do not include Band-Aids.
- **M1200H,** Application of ointments/medications other than to feet
- **M1200I,** Application of dressings to feet (with or without topical medications)
- **M1200Z,** None of the above were provided

Coding Tips

M1200A/M1200B Pressure Reducing Devices

- Pressure reducing devices redistribute pressure so that there is some relief on or near the area of the ulcer. The appropriate reducing (redistribution) device should be selected based on the individualized needs of the resident.
- Do **not** include egg crate cushions of any type in this category.
- Do **not** include doughnut or ring devices in chairs.

M1200C Turning/Repositioning Program

- The turning/repositioning program is specific as to the approaches for changing the resident's position and realigning the body. The program should specify the intervention (e.g., reposition on side, pillows between knees) and frequency (e.g., every 2 hours).
- Progress notes, assessments, and other documentation (as dictated by facility policy) should support that the turning/repositioning program is monitored and reassessed to determine the effectiveness of the intervention.

M1200D Nutrition or Hydration Intervention to Manage Skin Problems

- The determination as to whether or not one should receive nutritional or hydration interventions for skin problems should be based on an individualized nutritional assessment. The interdisciplinary team should review the resident's diet and determine if the resident is taking in sufficient amounts of nutrients and fluids or are already taking supplements that are fortified with the US Recommended Daily Intake (US RDI) of nutrients.

> **DEFINITIONS**
>
> **TURNING/ REPOSITIONING PROGRAM**
> Includes a consistent program for changing the resident's position and realigning the body. "Program" is defined as a specific approach that is organized, planned, documented, monitored, and evaluated based on an assessment of the resident's needs.
>
> **NUTRITION OR HYDRATION INTERVENTION TO MANAGE SKIN PROBLEMS**
> Dietary measures received by the resident for the purpose of preventing or treating specific skin conditions, e.g., wheat-free diet to prevent allergic dermatitis, high calorie diet with added supplementation to prevent skin breakdown, high-protein supplementation for wound healing.

May 2013

Page M-38

M1200: Skin and Ulcer Treatments (cont.)

- Additional supplementation above the US RDI has not been proven to provide any further benefits for management of skin problems including pressure ulcers. Vitamin and mineral supplementation should only be employed as an intervention for managing skin problems, including pressure ulcers, when nutritional deficiencies are confirmed or suspected through a thorough nutritional assessment (AMDA PU Guideline, page 6). If it is determined that nutritional supplementation, i.e. adding additional protein, calories, or nutrients is warranted, the facility should document the nutrition or hydration factors that are influencing skin problems and/or wound healing and "tailor nutritional supplementation to the individual's intake, degree of under-nutrition, and relative impact of nutrition as a factor overall; and obtain dietary consultation as needed," (AMDA PU Therapy Companion, page 4).

- It is important to remember that additional supplementation is not automatically required for pressure ulcer management. Any interventions should be specifically tailored to the resident's needs, condition, and prognosis (AMDA PU Therapy Companion, page 11).

M1200E Pressure Ulcer Care

- Pressure ulcer care includes **any** intervention for treating pressure ulcers coded in **Current Number of Unhealed Pressure Ulcers at Each Stage (M0300A-G)**. Examples may include the use of topical dressings, enzymatic, mechanical or surgical debridement, wound irrigations, negative pressure wound therapy (NPWT), and/or hydrotherapy.

M1200F Surgical Wound Care

- Does not include post-operative care following eye or oral surgery.

- Surgical debridement of a pressure ulcer does not create a surgical wound. Surgical debridement is used to remove necrotic or infected tissue from the pressure ulcer in order to facilitate healing, and thus, any wound care associated with pressure ulcer debridement would be coded in **M1200E, Pressure Ulcer Care**. The only time a surgical wound would be created is if the pressure ulcer itself was excised and a flap and/or graft used to close the pressure ulcer.

- Surgical wound care may include any intervention for treating or protecting any type of surgical wound. Examples may include topical cleansing, wound irrigation, application of antimicrobial ointments, application of dressings of any type, suture/staple removal, and warm soaks or heat application.

- Surgical wound care for pressure ulcers that require surgical intervention for closure (e.g., excision of pressure ulcer with flap and/or graft coverage) can be coded in this item, as once a pressure ulcer is excised and flap and/or graft applied, it is no longer considered a pressure ulcer, but a surgical wound.

M1200: Skin and Ulcer Treatments (cont.)

M1200G Application of Non-surgical Dressings (with or without Topical Medications) Other than to Feet

- Do **not** code application of non-surgical dressings for pressure ulcer(s) other than to feet in this item; use **M1200E, Pressure Ulcer Care**.
- Dressings do not have to be applied daily in order to be coded on the MDS assessment. If any dressing meeting the MDS definitions was applied even once during the 7-day look-back period, the assessor should check that MDS item.
- This category may include but is not limited to: dry gauze dressings, dressings moistened with saline or other solutions, transparent dressings, hydrogel dressings, and dressings with hydrocolloid or hydroactive particles used to treat a skin condition, compression bandages, etc. Non-surgical dressings do not include adhesive bandages (e.g., BAND-AID® bandages).

M1200H Application of Ointments/Medications Other than to Feet

- Do **not** code application of ointments/medications (e.g., chemical or enzymatic debridement) for pressure ulcers here; use **M1200E, Pressure Ulcer Care**.
- This category may include ointments or medications used to treat a skin condition (e.g., cortisone, antifungal preparations, chemotherapeutic agents).
- Ointments/medications may include topical creams, powders, and liquid sealants used to treat or prevent skin conditions.
- This category does not include ointments used to treat non-skin conditions (e.g., nitropaste for chest pain, testosterone cream).

M1200I Application of Dressings to the Feet (with or without Topical Medications)

- Includes interventions to treat any foot wound or ulcer **other than a pressure ulcer**.
- Do **not** code application of dressings to pressure ulcers on the foot, use **M1200E, Pressure Ulcer Care**.
- Do not code application of dressings to the ankle. The ankle is not considered part of the foot.

Examples

1. A resident is admitted with a Stage 3 pressure ulcer on the sacrum. Care during the last 7 days has included one debridement by the wound care consultant, application of daily dressings with enzymatic ointment for continued debridement, nutritional supplementation, and use of a pressure reducing (redistribution) pad on the wheelchair. The medical record documents delivery of care and notes that the resident is on a 2-hour turning/repositioning

M1200: Skin and Ulcer Treatments (cont.)

program that is organized, planned, documented, monitored and evaluated based on an individualized assessment of her needs. The physician documents that after reviewing the resident's nutritional intake, healing progress of the resident's pressure ulcer, dietician's nutritional assessment and laboratory results, that the resident has protein-calorie undernutrition. In order to support proper wound healing, the physician orders an oral supplement that provides all recommended daily allowances for protein, calories, nutrients and micronutrients. All mattresses in the nursing home are pressure reducing (redistribution) mattresses.

> **Coding:** Check items **M1200A, M1200B, M1200C, M1200D, and M1200E.**
>
> **Rationale:** Interventions include pressure reducing (redistribution) pad in the wheelchair (M1200A) and pressure reducing (redistribution) mattress on the bed (M1200B), turning and repositioning program (M1200C), nutritional supplementation (M1200D), enzymatic debridement and application of dressings (M1200E).

2. A resident has a venous ulcer on the right leg. During the past 7 days the resident has had a three layer compression bandaging system applied once (orders are to reapply the compression bandages every 5 days). The resident also has a pressure redistributing mattress and pad for the wheelchair.

> **Coding:** Check items **M1200A, M1200B, and M1200G.**
>
> **Rationale:** Treatments include pressure reducing (redistribution) mattress (M1200B) and pad (M1200A) in the wheelchair and application of the compression bandaging system (M1200G).

3. Mrs. S. has a diagnosis of right-sided hemiplegia from a previous stroke. As part of her assessment, it was noted that while in bed Mrs. S. is able to tolerate pressure on each side for approximately 3 hours before showing signs of the effects of pressure on her skin. Staff assist her to turn every 3 hours while in bed. When she is in her wheelchair, it is difficult for her to offload the pressure to her buttocks. Her assessment indicates that her skin cannot tolerate pressure for more than 1 hour without showing signs of the effect of the pressure when she is sitting, and therefore, Mrs. S. is assisted hourly by staff to stand for at least 1 full minute to relieve pressure. Staff document all of these interventions in the medical record and note the resident's response to the interventions.

> **Coding:** Check **M1200C.**
>
> **Rationale:** Treatments meet the criteria for a turning/repositioning program (i.e., it is organized, planned, documented, monitored, and evaluated), that is based on an assessment of the resident's unique needs.

M1200: Skin and Ulcer Treatments (cont.)

4. Mr. J. has a diagnosis of Advanced Alzheimer's and is totally dependent on staff for all of his care. His care plan states that he is to be turned and repositioned, per facility policy, every 2 hours.

> **Coding:** Do **not** check item **M1200C**.
>
> **Rationale:** Treatments provided do not meet the criteria for a turning/repositioning program. There is no notation in the medical record about an assessed need for turning/repositioning, nor is there a specific approach or plan related to positioning and realigning of the body. There is no reassessment of the resident's response to turning and repositioning. There are not any skin or ulcer treatments being provided.

Scenarios for Pressure Ulcer Coding

Examples M0300, M0610, M0700 and M0800

1. Mr. S was admitted to the nursing home on January 22, 2011 with a Stage 2 pressure ulcer. The pressure ulcer history was not available due to resident being admitted to the hospital from home prior to coming to the nursing home. On Mr. S' quarterly assessment, it was noted that the Stage 2 pressure ulcer had neither worsened nor improved. On the second quarterly assessment the Stage 2 pressure ulcer was noted to have worsened to a Stage 3. The current dimensions of the Stage 3 pressure ulcer are L 3.0cm, W 2.4cm, and D 0.2cm with 100% granulation tissue noted in the wound bed.

> **Admission Assessment:**
> **Coding:**
> - **M0300A** (Number of Stage 1 pressure ulcers), Code 0.
> - **M0300B1** (Number of Stage 2 pressure ulcers), Code 1.
> - **M0300B2** (Number of these Stage 2 pressure ulcers present on admission/entry or reentry), Code 1.
> - **M0300B3** (Date of the oldest Stage 2 pressure ulcer), code with dashes.
>
> **Rationale:** The resident had one Stage 2 pressure ulcer on admission and the date of the oldest pressure ulcer was unknown.

M0300. Current Number of Unhealed (non-epithelialized) Pressure Ulcers at Each Stage	
Enter Number `0`	**A. Number of Stage 1 pressure ulcers** **Stage 1:** Intact skin with non-blanchable redness of a localized area usually over a bony prominence. Darkly pigmented skin may not have a visible blanching; in dark skin tones only it may appear with persistent blue or purple hues
Enter Number `1` Enter Number `1`	**B. Stage 2:** Partial thickness loss of dermis presenting as a shallow open ulcer with a red or pink wound bed, without slough. May also present as an intact or open/ruptured blister 1. **Number of Stage 2 pressure ulcers** - If 0 → Skip to M0300C, Stage 3 2. **Number of these Stage 2 pressure ulcers that were present upon admission/entry or reentry** - enter how many were noted at the time of admission/entry or reentry 3. **Date of oldest Stage 2 pressure ulcer** - Enter dashes if date is unknown: `-` `-` – `-` `-` – `-` `-` `-` `-` Month Day Year

Scenarios for Pressure Ulcer Coding (cont.)

Quarterly Assessment #1:

Coding:
- **M0300A** (Number of Stage 1 pressure ulcers), Code 0.
- **M0300B1** (Number of Stage 2 pressure ulcers), Code 1.
- **M0300B2** (Number of these Stage 2 pressure ulcers present upon admission/entry or reentry), Code 1.
- **M0300B3** (Date of the oldest Stage 2 pressure ulcer), code with dashes.

Rationale: On the quarterly assessment the Stage 2 pressure ulcer is still present and date was unknown. Therefore, **M0300B3** is still coded with dashes.

M0300. Current Number of Unhealed (non-epithelialized) Pressure Ulcers at Each Stage	
Enter Number `0`	**A. Number of Stage 1 pressure ulcers** **Stage 1:** Intact skin with non-blanchable redness of a localized area usually over a bony prominence. Darkly pigmented skin may not have a visible blanching; in dark skin tones only it may appear with persistent blue or purple hues
	B. Stage 2: Partial thickness loss of dermis presenting as a shallow open ulcer with a red or pink wound bed, without slough. May also present as an intact or open/ruptured blister
Enter Number `1`	**1. Number of Stage 2 pressure ulcers** - If 0 → Skip to M0300C, Stage 3
Enter Number `1`	**2. Number of these Stage 2 pressure ulcers that were present upon admission/entry or reentry** - enter how many were noted at the time of admission/entry or reentry
	3. Date of oldest Stage 2 pressure ulcer - Enter dashes if date is unknown: `- -` – `- -` – `- - - -` Month Day Year

Quarterly Assessment #2:
Coding:
- **M0300A** (Number of Stage 1 pressure ulcers), Code 0.
- **M0300B1** (Number of Stage 2 pressure ulcers), Code 0 and skip to **M0300C**, Stage 3 pressure ulcers.
- **M0300C1** (Number of Stage 3 pressure ulcers). Code 1.
- **M0300C2** (Number of these Stage 3 pressure ulcers that were present upon admission//entry or reentry). Code 0.
- **M0300D1, M0300E1, M0300F1,** and **M0300G1** Code 0's and proceed to code **M0610** (Dimensions of unhealed Stage 3 or 4 pressure ulcers or unstageable pressure ulcer related to slough or eschar) with the dimensions of the Stage 3 ulcer.
- **M0610A** (Pressure ulcer length), Code 03.0, **M0610B** (Pressure ulcer width), Code 02.4, **M0610C** (Pressure ulcer depth) Code 00.2.
- **M0700** (Most severe tissue type for any pressure ulcer), Code 2, Granulation tissue.
- **M0800** (Worsening in pressure ulcer status since prior assessment – (OBRA or scheduled PPS or Last Admission/Entry or Reentry) – **M0800A** (Stage 2) Code 0, **M0800B** (Stage 3) Code 1, **M0800C** (Stage 4) Code 0.

Scenarios for Pressure Ulcer Coding (cont.)

Rationale:

- **M0300B1** is coded 0 due to the fact that the resident now has a Stage 3 pressure ulcer and no longer has a Stage 2 pressure ulcer. Therefore, you are required to skip to **M0300C** (Stage 3 pressure ulcer).
- **M0300C1** is coded as 1 due to the fact the resident has one Stage 3 pressure ulcer.
- **M0300C2** is coded as 0 due to the fact that the Stage 3 pressure ulcer was not present on admission, but worsened from a Stage 2 to a Stage 3 in the facility.
- **M0300D1, M0300E1, M0300F1,** and **M0300G1** are coded as zeros (due to the fact the resident does not have any Stage 4 or unstageable ulcers). Proceed to code **M0610** with the dimensions of the Stage 3 ulcer.
- **M0610A** is coded, 03.0 for length, **M0610B** is coded 02.4 for width, and **M0610C** is coded 00.2 for depth. Since this resident only had one Stage 3 pressure ulcer at the time of second quarterly assessment, these are the dimensions that would be coded here as the largest ulcer.
- **M0700** is coded as 2 (Granulation tissue) because this is the most severe type of tissue present.
- **M0800A** is coded as 0, **M0800B** is coded as 1, and **M0800C** is coded as 0 because the Stage 2 pressure ulcer that was present on admission has now worsened to a Stage 3 pressure ulcer since the last assessment.

M0300. Current Number of Unhealed (non-epithelialized) **Pressure Ulcers at Each Stage**

Enter Number [0]
A. **Number of Stage 1 pressure ulcers**
Stage 1: Intact skin with non-blanchable redness of a localized area usually over a bony prominence. Darkly pigmented skin may not have a visible blanching; in dark skin tones only it may appear with persistent blue or purple hues

Enter Number [0]
B. **Stage 2:** Partial thickness loss of dermis presenting as a shallow open ulcer with a red or pink wound bed, without slough. May also present as an intact or open/ruptured blister

Enter Number [0]
1. **Number of Stage 2 pressure ulcers -** If 0 → Skip to M0300C, Stage 3

2. **Number of these Stage 2 pressure ulcers that were present upon admission/entry or reentry -** enter how many were noted at the time of admission/entry or reentry

3. **Date of oldest Stage 2 pressure ulcer -** Enter dashes if date is unknown:
[ ][ ] – [ ][ ] – [ ][ ][ ][ ]
Month   Day   Year

Enter Number [1]
C. **Stage 3:** Full thickness tissue loss. Subcutaneous fat may be visible but bone, tendon or muscle is not exposed. Slough may be present but does not obscure the depth of tissue loss. May include undermining and tunneling

1. **Number of Stage 3 pressure ulcers -** If 0 → Skip to M0300D, Stage 4

Enter Number [0]
2. **Number of these Stage 3 pressure ulcers that were present upon admission/entry or reentry -** enter how many were noted at the time of admission/entry or reentry

Enter Number [0]
D. **Stage 4:** Full thickness tissue loss with exposed bone, tendon or muscle. Slough or eschar may be present on some parts of the wound bed. Often includes undermining and tunneling

1. **Number of Stage 4 pressure ulcers -** If 0 → Skip to M0300E, Unstageable: Non-removable dressing

2. **Number of these Stage 4 pressure ulcers that were present upon admission/entry or reentry -** enter how many were noted at the time of admission/entry or reentry

M0300 continued on next page

Scenarios for Pressure Ulcer Coding (cont.)

	M0300. Current Number of Unhealed (non-epithelialized) **Pressure Ulcers at Each Stage** - Continued
	E. Unstageable - Non-removable dressing: Known but not stageable due to non-removable dressing/device
Enter Number **0** Enter Number ☐	1. **Number of unstageable pressure ulcers due to non-removable dressing/device** - If 0 → Skip to M0300F, Unstageable: Slough and/or eschar 2. **Number of** <u>these</u> **unstageable pressure ulcers that were present upon admission/entry or reentry** - enter how many were noted at the time of admission/entry or reentry
	F. Unstageable - Slough and/or eschar: Known but not stageable due to coverage of wound bed by slough and/or eschar
Enter Number **0** Enter Number ☐	1. **Number of unstageable pressure ulcers due to coverage of wound bed by slough and/or eschar** - If 0 → Skip to M0300G, Unstageable: Deep tissue 2. **Number of** <u>these</u> **unstageable pressure ulcers that were present upon admission/entry or reentry** - enter how many were noted at the time of admission/entry or reentry
	G. Unstageable - Deep tissue: Suspected deep tissue injury in evolution
Enter Number **0** Enter Number ☐	1. **Number of unstageable pressure ulcers with suspected deep tissue injury in evolution** - If 0 → Skip to M0610, Dimension of Unhealed Stage 3 or 4 Pressure Ulcers or Eschar 2. **Number of** <u>these</u> **unstageable pressure ulcers that were present upon admission/entry or reentry** - enter how many were noted at the time of admission/entry or reentry

	M0610. Dimensions of Unhealed Stage 3 or 4 Pressure Ulcers or Eschar
	Complete only if M0300C1, M0300D1 or M0300F1 is greater than 0
	If the resident has one or more unhealed (non-epithelialized) Stage 3 or 4 pressure ulcers or an unstageable pressure ulcer due to slough or eschar, identify the pressure ulcer with the largest surface area (length x width) and record in centimeters:
0 3 . 0 cm	**A. Pressure ulcer length:** Longest length from head to toe
0 2 . 4 cm	**B. Pressure ulcer width:** Widest width of the same pressure ulcer, side-to-side perpendicular (90-degree angle) to length
0 0 . 2 cm	**C. Pressure ulcer depth:** Depth of the same pressure ulcer from the visible surface to the deepest area (if depth is unknown, enter a dash in each box)

	M0700. Most Severe Tissue Type for Any Pressure Ulcer
Enter Code **2**	Select the best description of the most severe type of tissue present in any pressure ulcer bed 1. **Epithelial tissue** - new skin growing in superficial ulcer. It can be light pink and shiny, even in persons with darkly pigmented skin 2. **Granulation tissue** - pink or red tissue with shiny, moist, granular appearance 3. **Slough** - yellow or white tissue that adheres to the ulcer bed in strings or thick clumps, or is mucinous 4. **Necrotic tissue (Eschar)** - black, brown, or tan tissue that adheres firmly to the wound bed or ulcer edges, may be softer or harder than surrounding skin 9. **None of the Above**

	M0800. Worsening in Pressure Ulcer Status Since Prior Assessment (OBRA or Scheduled PPS) or Last Admission/Entry or Reentry
	Complete only if A0310E = 0
	Indicate the number of current pressure ulcers that were **not present or were at a lesser stage** on prior assessment (OBRA or scheduled PPS) or last entry. If no current pressure ulcer at a given stage, enter 0.
Enter Number **0**	**A. Stage 2**
Enter Number **1**	**B. Stage 3**
Enter Number **0**	**C. Stage 4**

Scenarios for Pressure Ulcer Coding (cont.)

Example M0100-M1200

1. Mrs. P is admitted to the nursing home on 10/23/2010 for a Medicare stay. In completing the PPS 5-day assessment, it was noted that the resident had a head-to-toe skin assessment and her skin was intact, but upon assessment using the Braden scale, was found to be at risk for skin break down. On the 14-day PPS (ARD of 11/5/2010), the resident was noted to have a Stage 2 pressure ulcer that was identified on her coccyx on 11/1/2010. This Stage 2 pressure ulcer was noted to have pink tissue with some epithelialization present in the wound bed. Dimensions of the ulcer were length 01.1 cm, width 00.5 cm, and no measurable depth. Mrs. P does not have any arterial or venous ulcers, wounds, or skin problems. She is receiving ulcer care with application of a dressing applied to the coccygeal ulcer. Mrs. P. also has pressure redistribution devices on both her bed and chair, and has been placed on a 1½ hour turning and repositioning schedule per tissue tolerance. On 11/13/2010 the resident was discharged return anticipated and reentered the facility on 11/15/2010. Upon reentry the 5-day PPS ARD was set at 11/19/2010. In reviewing the record for this 5-day PPS assessment, it was noted that the resident had the same Stage 2 pressure ulcer on her coccyx, however, the measurements were now length 01.2 cm, width 00.6 cm, and still no measurable depth. It was also noted upon reentry that the resident had a suspected deep tissue injury of the right heel that was measured at length 01.9cm, width 02.5cm, and no visible depth.

   5-Day PPS #1:
   Coding:
   - **M0100B** (Formal assessment instrument), Check box.
   - **M0100C** (Clinical assessment), Check box.
   - **M0150** (Risk of Pressure Ulcers), Code 1.
   - **M0210** (One or more unhealed pressure ulcer(s) at Stage 1 or higher), Code 0 and skip to **M0900** (Healed pressure ulcers).
   - **M0900** (Healed pressure ulcers). Skip to **M1030** since this item is only completed if **A0310E=0**. The 5-Day PPS Assessment is the first assessment since the most recent admission/entry or reentry, therefore, **A0310E=1**.
   - **M1030** (Number of Venous and Arterial ulcers), Code 0.
   - **M1040** (Other ulcers, wounds and skin problems), Check Z (None of the above).
   - **M1200** (Skin and Ulcer Treatments), Check Z (None of the above were provided).

   Rationale: The resident had a formal assessment using the Braden scale and also had a head-to-toe skin assessment completed. Pressure ulcer risk was identified via formal assessment. Upon assessment the resident's skin was noted to be intact, therefore, **M0210** was coded 0, **M0900** was skipped because the 5-Day PPS is the first assessment. **M1030** was coded 0 due to the resident not having any of these conditions. **M1040Z** was checked since none of these problems were noted. **M1200Z** was checked because none of these treatments were provided.

Scenarios for Pressure Ulcer Coding (cont.)

M1030. Number of Venous and Arterial Ulcers	
Enter Number **0**	Enter the total number of venous and arterial ulcers present

M1040. Other Ulcers, Wounds and Skin Problems

↓ Check all that apply

Foot Problems

☐	**A. Infection of the foot** (e.g., cellulitis, purulent drainage)
☐	**B. Diabetic foot ulcer(s)**
☐	**C. Other open lesion(s) on the foot**

Other Problems

☐	**D. Open lesion(s) other than ulcers, rashes, cuts** (e.g., cancer lesion)
☐	**E. Surgical wound(s)**
☐	**F. Burn(s)** (second or third degree)
☐	**G. Skin tear(s)**
☐	**H. Moisture Associated Skin Damage (MASD)** (i.e. incontinence (IAD), perspiration, drainage)

None of the Above

☒	**Z. None of the above** were present

M1200. Skin and Ulcer Treatments

↓ Check all that apply

☐	**A. Pressure reducing device for chair**
☐	**B. Pressure reducing device for bed**
☐	**C. Turning/repositioning program**
☐	**D. Nutrition or hydration intervention** to manage skin problems
☐	**E. Pressure ulcer care**
☐	**F. Surgical wound care**
☐	**G. Application of nonsurgical dressings** (with or without topical medications) other than to feet
☐	**H. Applications of ointments/medications** other than to feet
☐	**I. Application of dressings to feet** (with or without topical medications)
☒	**Z. None of the above** were provided

Scenarios for Pressure Ulcer Coding (cont.)

14-Day PPS:

Coding:

- **M0100A** (Resident has a Stage 1 or greater, a scar over bony prominence, or a non-removable dressing/device), Check box.
- **M0100B** (Formal assessment instrument), Check box.
- **M0100C** (Clinical assessment), Check box.
- **M0150** (Risk of Pressure Ulcers), Code 1.
- **M0210** (One or more unhealed pressure ulcer(s) at Stage 1 or higher), Code 1.
- **M0300A** (Number of Stage 1 pressure ulcers), Code 0.
- **M0300B1** (Number of Stage 2 pressure ulcers), Code 1.
- **M0300B2** (Number of these Stage 2 pressure ulcers present on admission/entry or reentry), Code 0.
- **M0300B3** (Date of the oldest Stage 2 pressure ulcer), Enter 11-01-2010.
- **M0300C1** (Number of Stage 3 pressure ulcers), Code 0 and skip to **M0300D** (Stage 4).
- **M0300D1** (Number of Stage 4 pressure ulcers), Code 0 and skip to M0300E (Unstageable: Non-removable dressing).
- **M0300E1** (Unstageable: Non-removable dressing), Code 0 and skip to M0300F (Unstageable: Slough and/or eschar).
- **M0300F1** (Unstageable: Slough and/or eschar), Code 0 and skip to M0300G (Unstageable: Deep tissue).
- **M0300G1** (Unstageable: Deep tissue), Code 0 and skip to M0610 (Dimension of Unhealed Stage 3 or 4 Pressure Ulcers or Eschar).
- **M0610** (Dimension of Unhealed Stage 3 or 4 Pressure Ulcers or Eschar), is **not** completed, as the resident has a Stage 2 pressure ulcer.
- **M0700** (Most severe tissue type for any pressure ulcer), Code 1 (Epithelial tissue).
- **M0800** (Worsening in pressure ulcer status since prior assessment (OBRA or scheduled PPS or Last Admission/Entry or Reentry)), **M0800A**, Code 1; **M0800B**, Code 0; **M0800C**, Code 0. This item is completed because the 14-Day PPS is **not** the first assessment since the most recent admission/entry or reentry. Therefore, A0310E=0. **M0800A** is coded 1 because the resident has a new Stage 2 pressure ulcer that was not present on the prior assessment.
- **M0900A** (Healed pressure ulcers), Code 0. This is completed because the 14-Day PPS is **not** the first assessment since the most recent admission/entry or reentry. Therefore A0310E=0. Since there were no pressure ulcers noted on the 5-Day PPS assessment, this is coded 0, and skip to **M1030**.
- **M1030** (Number of Venous and Arterial ulcers), Code 0.
- **M1040** (Other ulcers, wounds and skin problems), Check Z (None of the above).

Scenarios for Pressure Ulcer Coding (cont.)

- **M1200A** (Pressure reducing device for chair), **M1200B** (Pressure reducing device for bed), **M1200C** (Turning/repositioning program), and **M1200E** (Pressure ulcer care) are all checked.

Rationale: The resident had a formal assessment using the Braden scale and also had a head-to-toe skin assessment completed. Pressure ulcer risk was identified via formal assessment. On the 5-Day PPS assessment the resident's skin was noted to be intact, however, on the 14-Day PPS assessment, it was noted that the resident had a new Stage 2 pressure ulcer. Since the resident has had both a 5-day and 14-Day PPS completed, the 14-Day PPS would be coded 0 at **A0310E**. This is because the 14-Day PPS is **not** the first assessment since the most recent admission/entry or reentry. Since **A0310E=0**, items **M0800** (Worsening in pressure ulcer status) and **M0900** (Healed pressure ulcers) would be completed. Since the resident did not have a pressure ulcer on the 5-Day PPS and did have one on the 14-Day PPS, the new Stage 2 pressure ulcer is documented under **M0800** (Worsening in pressure ulcer status). **M0900** (Healed pressure ulcers) is coded as 0 because there were no pressure ulcers noted on the prior assessment (5-Day PPS). There were no other skin problems noted. However the resident, since she is at an even higher risk of breakdown since the development of a new ulcer, has preventative measures put in place with pressure redistribution devices for her chair and bed. She was also placed on a turning and repositioning program based on tissue tolerance. Therefore **M1200A, M1200B, and M1200C** were all checked. She also now requires ulcer care and application of a dressing to the coccygeal ulcer, so **M1200E** is also checked.

M1200G (Application of nonsurgical dressings – with or without topical medications) would **not** be coded here because **any** intervention for treating pressure ulcers is coded in **M1200E** (Pressure ulcer care).

Scenarios for Pressure Ulcer Coding (cont.)

M0100. Determination of Pressure Ulcer Risk	
↓ Check all that apply	
X	A. Resident has a stage 1 or greater, a scar over bony prominence, or a non-removable dressing/device
X	B. Formal assessment instrument/tool (e.g., Braden, Norton, or other)
X	C. Clinical assessment
☐	Z. None of the above

M0150. Risk of Pressure Ulcers

Enter Code **[1]**

Is this resident at risk of developing pressure ulcers?
0. No
1. Yes

M0210. Unhealed Pressure Ulcer(s)

Enter Code **[1]**

Does this resident have one or more unhealed pressure ulcer(s) at Stage 1 or higher?
0. No → Skip to M0900, Healed Pressure Ulcers
1. Yes → Continue to M0300, Current Number of Unhealed (non-epithelialized) Pressure Ulcers at Each Stage

M0300. Current Number of Unhealed (non-epithelialized) **Pressure Ulcers at Each Stage**

Enter Number **[0]**

A. **Number of Stage 1 pressure ulcers**
Stage 1: Intact skin with non-blanchable redness of a localized area usually over a bony prominence. Darkly pigmented skin may not have a visible blanching; in dark skin tones only it may appear with persistent blue or purple hues

B. **Stage 2:** Partial thickness loss of dermis presenting as a shallow open ulcer with a red or pink wound bed, without slough. May also present as an intact or open/ruptured blister

Enter Number **[1]**

1. **Number of Stage 2 pressure ulcers** - If 0 → Skip to M0300C, Stage 3

Enter Number **[0]**

2. **Number of these Stage 2 pressure ulcers that were present upon admission/entry or reentry** - enter how many were noted at the time of admission/entry or reentry

3. **Date of oldest Stage 2 pressure ulcer** - Enter dashes if date is unknown:

☐☐ – ☐☐ – ☐☐☐☐
Month   Day   Year

C. **Stage 3:** Full thickness tissue loss. Subcutaneous fat may be visible but bone, tendon or muscle is not exposed. Slough may be present but does not obscure the depth of tissue loss. May include undermining and tunneling

Enter Number **[0]**

1. **Number of Stage 3 pressure ulcers** - If 0 → Skip to M0300D, Stage 4

Enter Number **[ ]**

2. **Number of these Stage 3 pressure ulcers that were present upon admission/entry or reentry** - enter how many were noted at the time of admission/entry or reentry

D. **Stage 4:** Full thickness tissue loss with exposed bone, tendon or muscle. Slough or eschar may be present on some parts of the wound bed. Often includes undermining and tunneling

Enter Number **[0]**

1. **Number of Stage 4 pressure ulcers** - If 0 → Skip to M0300E, Unstageable: Non-removable dressing

Enter Number **[ ]**

2. **Number of these Stage 4 pressure ulcers that were present upon admission/entry or reentry** - enter how many were noted at the time of admission/entry or reentry

M0300 continued on next page

Scenarios for Pressure Ulcer Coding (cont.)

M0300. Current Number of Unhealed (non-epithelialized) **Pressure Ulcers at Each Stage** - Continued	

E. Unstageable - Non-removable dressing: Known but not stageable due to non-removable dressing/device

Enter Number
`0`

   1. **Number of unstageable pressure ulcers due to non-removable dressing/device** - If 0 ➞ Skip to M0300F, Unstageable: Slough and/or eschar

Enter Number
`☐`

   2. **Number of these unstageable pressure ulcers that were present upon admission/entry or reentry** - enter how many were noted at the time of admission/entry or reentry

F. Unstageable - Slough and/or eschar: Known but not stageable due to coverage of wound bed by slough and/or eschar

Enter Number
`0`

   1. **Number of unstageable pressure ulcers due to coverage of wound bed by slough and/or eschar** - If 0 ➞ Skip to M0300G, Unstageable: Deep tissue

Enter Number
`☐`

   2. **Number of these unstageable pressure ulcers that were present upon admission/entry or reentry** - enter how many were noted at the time of admission/entry or reentry

G. Unstageable - Deep tissue: Suspected deep tissue injury in evolution

Enter Number
`0`

   1. **Number of unstageable pressure ulcers with suspected deep tissue injury in evolution** - If 0 ➞ Skip to M0610, Dimension of Unhealed Stage 3 or 4 Pressure Ulcers or Eschar

Enter Number
`☐`

   2. **Number of these unstageable pressure ulcers that were present upon admission/entry or reentry** - enter how many were noted at the time of admission/entry or reentry

---

M0700. Most Severe Tissue Type for Any Pressure Ulcer

Enter Code
`1`

Select the best description of the most severe type of tissue present in any pressure ulcer bed
1. **Epithelial tissue** - new skin growing in superficial ulcer. It can be light pink and shiny, even in persons with darkly pigmented skin
2. **Granulation tissue** - pink or red tissue with shiny, moist, granular appearance
3. **Slough** - yellow or white tissue that adheres to the ulcer bed in strings or thick clumps, or is mucinous
4. **Necrotic tissue (Eschar)** - black, brown, or tan tissue that adheres firmly to the wound bed or ulcer edges, may be softer or harder than surrounding skin
9. **None of the Above**

M0800. Worsening in Pressure Ulcer Status Since Prior Assessment (OBRA or Scheduled PPS) or Last Admission/Entry or Reentry
Complete only if A0310E = 0

Indicate the number of current pressure ulcers that were **not present or were at a lesser stage** on prior assessment (OBRA or scheduled PPS) or last entry. If no current pressure ulcer at a given stage, enter 0.

Enter Number	
`1`	**A. Stage 2**
Enter Number	
`0`	**B. Stage 3**
Enter Number	
`0`	**C. Stage 4**

Scenarios for Pressure Ulcer Coding (cont.)

M0900. Healed Pressure Ulcers Complete only if A0310E = 0	

Enter Code `0`	**A. Were pressure ulcers present on the prior assessment (OBRA or scheduled PPS)?** 0. **No** → Skip to M1030, Number of Venous and Arterial Ulcers 1. **Yes** → Continue to M0900B, Stage 2
	Indicate the number of pressure ulcers that were noted on the prior assessment (OBRA or scheduled PPS) that have completely closed (resurfaced with epithelium). If no healed pressure ulcer at a given stage since the prior assessment (OBRA or scheduled PPS), enter 0.
Enter Number ☐	**B. Stage 2**
Enter Number ☐	**C. Stage 3**
Enter Number ☐	**D. Stage 4**

M1030. Number of Venous and Arterial Ulcers	
Enter Number `0`	**Enter the total number of venous and arterial ulcers present**

M1040. Other Ulcers, Wounds and Skin Problems	
↓	**Check all that apply**
	Foot Problems
☐	**A. Infection of the foot** (e.g., cellulitis, purulent drainage)
☐	**B. Diabetic foot ulcer(s)**
☐	**C. Other open lesion(s) on the foot**
	Other Problems
☐	**D. Open lesion(s) other than ulcers, rashes, cuts** (e.g., cancer lesion)
☐	**E. Surgical wound(s)**
☐	**F. Burn(s)** (second or third degree)
☐	**G. Skin tear(s)**
☐	**H. Moisture Associated Skin Damage (MASD)** (i.e. incontinence (IAD), perspiration, drainage)
	None of the Above
☒	**Z. None of the above** were present

M1200. Skin and Ulcer Treatments	
↓	**Check all that apply**
☒	**A. Pressure reducing device for chair**
☒	**B. Pressure reducing device for bed**
☒	**C. Turning/repositioning program**
☐	**D. Nutrition or hydration intervention** to manage skin problems
☒	**E. Pressure ulcer care**
☐	**F. Surgical wound care**
☐	**G. Application of nonsurgical dressings** (with or without topical medications) other than to feet
☐	**H. Applications of ointments/medications** other than to feet
☐	**I. Application of dressings to feet** (with or without topical medications)
☐	**Z. None of the above** were provided

SECTION N: MEDICATIONS

Intent: The intent of the items in this section is to record the number of days, during the last 7 days (or since admission/entry or reentry if less than 7 days) that any type of injection (subcutaneous, intramuscular or intradermal), insulin, and/or select medications were received by the resident.

N0300: Injections

N0300. Injections	
Enter Days [ ]	**Record the number of days that injections of any type** were received during the last 7 days or since admission/entry or reentry if less than 7 days. If 0 → Skip to N0410, Medications Received

Item Rationale

Health-related Quality of Life

- Frequency of administration of medication via injection can be an indication of stability of a resident's health status and/or complexity of care needs.

Planning for Care

- Monitor for adverse effects of injected medications.
- Although antigens and vaccines are not considered to be medications per se, it is important to track when they are given to monitor for localized or systemic reactions.

Steps for Assessment

1. Review the resident's medication administration records for the 7-day look-back period (or since admission/entry or reentry if less than 7 days).
2. Review documentation from other health care locations where the resident may have received injections while a resident of the nursing home (e.g., flu vaccine in a physician's office, in the emergency room – as long as the resident was not admitted).
3. Determine if any medications were received by the resident via injection. If received, determine the number of days during the look-back period they were received.

Coding Instructions

Record the number of days during the 7-day look-back period (or since admission/entry or reentry if less than 7 days) that the resident received any type of medication, antigen, vaccine, etc., by subcutaneous, intramuscular, or intradermal injection.

*Insulin injections **are** counted in this item as well as in Item N0350.*

- Count the number of days that the resident received any type of injection (subcutaneous, intramuscular, or intradermal) while a resident of the nursing home.
- Record the number of days that any type of injection (subcutaneous, intramuscular, or intradermal) was received in Item N0300.

N0300: Injections (cont.)

Coding Tips and Special Populations

- For subcutaneous pumps, code only the number of days that the resident actually required a subcutaneous injection to restart the pump.

- If an antigen or vaccination is provided on one day, and another vaccine is provided on the next day, the number of days the resident received injections would be **coded as 2 days.**

- If two injections were administered on the same day, the number of days the resident received injections would be **coded as 1 day.**

Examples

1. During the 7-day look-back period, Mr. T. received an influenza shot on Monday, a PPD test (for tuberculosis) on Tuesday, and a Vitamin B_{12} injection on Wednesday.

    Coding: N0300 would be **coded 3.**
    Rationale: The resident received injections on 3 separate days during the 7-day look-back period.

2. During the 7-day look-back period, Miss C. received both an influenza shot and her vitamin B_{12} injection on Thursday.

    Coding: N0300 would be **coded 1.**
    Rationale: The resident received injections on one day during the 7-day look-back period.

N0350: Insulin

N0350. Insulin	
Enter Days ☐	A. **Insulin injections - Record the number of days that insulin injections** were received during the last 7 days or since admission/entry or reentry if less than 7 days
Enter Days ☐	B. **Orders for insulin - Record the number of days the physician (or authorized assistant or practitioner) changed the resident's insulin orders** during the last 7 days or since admission/entry or reentry if less than 7 days

Item Rationale

Health-related Quality of Life

- Insulin is a medication used to treat diabetes mellitus (DM).

- Individualized meal plans should be created with the resident's input to ensure appropriate meal intake. Residents are more likely to be compliant with their DM diet if they have input related to food choices.

N0350: Insulin (cont.)

Planning for Care

- Orders for insulin may have to change depending on the resident's condition (e.g., fever or other illness) and/or laboratory results.

- Ensure that dosage and time of injections take into account meals, activity, etc., based on individualized resident assessment.

- Monitor for adverse effects of insulin injections (e.g., hypoglycemia).

- Monitor HbA1c and blood glucose levels to ensure appropriate amounts of insulin are being administered.

Steps for Assessment

1. Review the resident's medication administration records for the 7-day look-back period (or since admission/entry or reentry if less than 7 days).
2. Determine if the resident received insulin injections during the look-back period.
3. Determine if the physician (or nurse practitioner, physician assistant, or clinical nurse specialist if allowable under state licensure laws) changed the resident's insulin orders during the look-back period.
4. Count the number of days insulin injections were received and/or insulin orders changed.

Coding Instructions for N0350A

- Enter in Item N0350A, the number of days during the 7-day look-back period (or since admission/entry or reentry if less than 7 days) that insulin injections were received.

Coding Instructions for N0350B

- Enter in Item N0350B, the number of days during the 7-day look-back period (or since admission/entry or reentry if less than 7 days) that the physician (nurse practitioner, physician assistant, or clinical nurse specialist if allowable under state licensure laws) changed the resident's insulin orders.

Coding Tips and Special Populations

- For sliding scale orders:
  - A sliding scale dosage schedule that is written to cover different dosages depending on lab values **does not** count as an order change simply because a different dose is administered based on the sliding scale guidelines.
  - If the sliding scale order is new, discontinued, or is the first sliding scale order for the resident, these days **can** be counted and coded.
- For subcutaneous insulin pumps, code only the number of days that the resident actually required a subcutaneous injection to restart the pump.

N0410: Medications Received

N0410. Medications Received

Indicate the number of DAYS the resident received the following medications during the last 7 days or since admission/entry or reentry if less than 7 days. Enter "0" if medication was not received by the resident during the last 7 days

Enter Days	
☐	A. Antipsychotic
Enter Days ☐	B. Antianxiety
Enter Days ☐	C. Antidepressant
Enter Days ☐	D. Hypnotic
Enter Days ☐	E. Anticoagulant (warfarin, heparin, or low-molecular weight heparin)
Enter Days ☐	F. Antibiotic
Enter Days ☐	G. Diuretic

Item Rationale

Health-related Quality of Life

- Medications are an integral part of the care provided to residents of nursing homes. They are administered to try to achieve various outcomes, such as curing an illness, diagnosing a disease or condition, arresting or slowing a disease's progress, reducing or eliminating symptoms, or preventing a disease or symptom.

- Residents taking medications in these medication categories and pharmacologic classes are at risk of side effects that can adversely affect health, safety, and quality of life.

- While assuring that only those medications required to treat the resident's assessed condition are being used, it is important to assess the need to reduce these medications wherever possible and ensure that the medication is the most effective for the resident's assessed condition.

- As part of all medication management, it is important for the interdisciplinary team to consider non-pharmacological approaches. Educating the nursing home staff and providers about non-pharmacological approaches in addition to and/or in conjunction with the use of medication may minimize the need for medications or reduce the dose and duration of those medications.

> **DEFINITIONS**
>
> **ADVERSE CONSEQUENCE**
> An unpleasant symptom or event that is caused by or associated with a medication, impairment or decline in an individual's physical condition, mental, functional or psychosocial status. It may include various types of adverse drug reactions (ADR) and interactions (e.g., medication-medication, medication-food, and medication-disease).
>
> **NON-PHARMACOLOGICAL INTERVENTION**
> Approaches that do not involve the use of medication to address a medical condition.

N0410: Medications Received (cont.)

Planning for Care

- The indications for initiating, withdrawing, or withholding medication(s), as well as the use of non-pharmacological interventions, are determined by assessing the resident's underlying condition, current signs and symptoms, and preferences and goals for treatment. This includes, where possible, the identification of the underlying cause(s), since a diagnosis alone may not warrant treatment with medication.

- Target symptoms and goals for use of these medications should be established for each resident. Progress toward meeting the goals should be evaluated routinely.

- Possible adverse effects of these medications should be well understood by nursing staff. Educate nursing home staff to be observant for these adverse effects.

- Implement systematic monitoring of each resident taking any of these medications to identify adverse consequences early.

Steps for Assessment

1. Review the resident's medical record for documentation that any of these medications were received by the resident during the 7-day look-back period (or since admission/entry or reentry if less than 7 days).
2. Review documentation from other health care settings where the resident may have received any of these medications while a resident of the nursing home (e.g., valium given in the emergency room).

Coding Instructions

- **N0410A, Antipsychotic:** Record the number of days an antipsychotic medication was received by the resident at any time during the 7-day look-back period (or since admission/entry or reentry if less than 7 days)

- **N0410B, Antianxiety:** Record the number of days an anxiolytic medication was received by the resident at any time during the 7-day look-back period (or since admission/entry or reentry if less than 7 days).

- **N0410C, Antidepressant:** Record the number of days an antidepressant medication was received by the resident at any time during the 7-day look-back period (or since admission/entry or reentry if less than 7 days).

DEFINITIONS

DOSE

The total amount/strength/ concentration of a medication given at one time or over a period of time. The individual dose is the amount/strength/ concentration received at each administration. The amount received over a 24-hour period may be referred to as the "daily dose."

MONITORING

The ongoing collection and analysis of information (such as observations and diagnostic test results) and comparison to baseline and current data in order to ascertain the individual's response to treatment and care, including progress or lack of progress toward a goal. Monitoring can detect any improvements, complications or adverse consequences of the condition or of the treatments; and support decisions about adding, modifying, continuing, or discontinuing, any interventions.

N0410: Medications Received (cont.)

- **N0410D, Hypnotic:** Record the number of days a hypnotic medication was received by the resident at any time during the 7-day look-back period (or since admission/entry or reentry if less than 7 days).

- **N0410E, Anticoagulant (e.g., warfarin, heparin, or low- molecular weight heparin):** Record the number of days an anticoagulant medication was received by the resident at any time during the 7-day look-back period (or since admission/entry or reentry if less than 7 days). Do not code antiplatelet medications such as aspirin/extended release, dipyridamole, or clopidogrel here.

- **N0410F, Antibiotic:** Record the number of days an antibiotic medication was received by the resident at any time during the 7-day look-back period (or since admission/entry or reentry if less than 7 days).

- **N0410G, Diuretic:** Record the number of days a diuretic medication was received by the resident at any time during the 7-day look-back period (or since admission/entry or reentry if less than 7 days).

Coding Tips and Special Populations

> **DEFINITION**
>
> **SLEEP HYGIENE**
> Practices, habits and environmental factors that promote and/or improve sleep patterns.

- Code medications in Item N0410 according to the medication's therapeutic category and/or pharmacological classification, not how it is used. For example, although oxazepam may be prescribed for use as a hypnotic, it is categorized as an antianxiety medication. Therefore, in this section, it would be coded as an antianxiety medication and not as a hypnotic.

- Include any of these medications given to the resident by any route (e.g., PO, IM, or IV) in any setting (e.g., at the nursing home, in a hospital emergency room) while a resident of the nursing home.

- Code a medication even if it was given only once during the look-back period.

- Count long-acting medications, such as fluphenazine decanoate or haloperidol decanoate, that are given every few weeks or monthly **only** if they are given during the 7-day look-back period (or since admission/entry or reentry if less than 7 days).

- Combination medications should be coded in all categories/pharmacologic classes that constitute the combination. For example, if the resident receives a single tablet that combines an antipsychotic and an antidepressant, then both antipsychotic and antidepressant categories should be coded.

- Over-the-counter sleeping medications are not coded as hypnotics, as they are not categorized as hypnotic medications.

- When residents are having difficulty sleeping, nursing home staff should explore non-pharmacological interventions (e.g., sleep hygiene approaches that individualize the sleep and wake times to accommodate the person's wishes and prior customary routine) to try to improve sleep prior to initiating pharmacologic interventions. If residents are currently on sleep-enhancing medications, nursing home staff can try non-pharmacologic interventions to help reduce the need for these medications or eliminate them.

N0410: Medications Received (cont.)

- Many psychoactive medications increase confusion, sedation, and falls. For those residents who are already at risk for these conditions, nursing home staff should develop plans of care that address these risks.

- Adverse drug reaction (ADR) is a form of adverse consequence. It may be either a secondary effect of a medication that is usually undesirable and different from the therapeutic effect of the medication or any response to a medication that is noxious and unintended and occurs in doses for prophylaxis, diagnosis, or treatment. The term "side effect" is often used interchangeably with ADR; however, side effects are but one of five ADR categories, the others being hypersensitivity, idiosyncratic response, toxic reactions, and adverse medication interactions. A side effect is an expected, well-known reaction that occurs with a predictable frequency and may or may not constitute an adverse consequence.

- Doses of psychoactive medications differ in acute and long-term treatment. Doses should always be the lowest possible to achieve the desired therapeutic effects and be deemed necessary to maintain or improve the resident's function, well-being, safety, and quality of life. Duration of treatment should also be in accordance with pertinent literature, including clinical practice guidelines.

- Since medication issues continue to evolve and new medications are being approved regularly, it is important to refer to a current authoritative source for detailed medication information, such as indications and precautions, dosage, monitoring, or adverse consequences.

- During the first year in which a resident on a psychoactive medication is admitted, or after the nursing home has initiated such medication, nursing home staff should attempt to taper the medication or perform gradual dose reduction (GDR) as long as it is not medically contraindicated. Information on GDR and tapering of medications can be found in the **State Operations Manual, Appendix PP, Guidance to Surveyors for Long Term Care Facilities** (the **State Operations Manual** can be found at http://www.cms.gov/Manuals/IOM/list.asp).

- Prior to discontinuing a psychoactive medication, residents may need a GDR or tapering to avoid withdrawal syndrome (e.g., for medications such as selective serotonin reuptake inhibitors [SSRIs], tricyclic antidepressants [TCAs], etc.).

> **DEFINITION**
>
> **GRADUAL DOSE REDUCTION (GDR)** Step-wise tapering of a dose to determine whether or not symptoms, conditions, or risks can be managed by a lower dose or whether or not the dose or medication can be discontinued.

> **DEFINITION**
>
> **MEDICATION INTERACTION**
>
> The impact of medication or other substance (such as nutritional supplements including herbal products, food, or substances used in diagnostic studies) upon another medication. The interactions may alter absorption, distribution, metabolism, or elimination. These interactions may decrease the effectiveness of the medication or increase the potential for adverse consequences.

N0410: Medications Received (cont.)

- Residents who are on antidepressants should be closely monitored for worsening of depression and/or suicidal ideation/behavior, especially during initiation or change of dosage in therapy. Stopping antidepressants abruptly puts one at higher risk of suicidal ideation and behavior.

- Anticoagulants must be monitored with dosage frequency determined by clinical circumstances, duration of use, and stability of monitoring results (e.g., Prothrombin Time [PT]/International Normalization Ratio [INR]).

  — Multiple medication interactions exist with use of anticoagulants (information on common medication-medication interactions can be found in the **State Operations Manual, Appendix PP, Guidance to Surveyors for Long Term Care Facilities** [the **State Operations Manual** can be found at http://www.cms.gov/Manuals/IOM/list.asp]), which may

    o significantly increase PT/INR results to levels associated with life-threatening bleeding, or

    o decrease PT/INR results to ineffective levels, or increase or decrease the serum concentration of the interacting medication.

- Herbal and alternative medicine products are considered to be dietary supplements by the Food and Drug Administration (FDA). These products are not regulated by the FDA (e.g., they are not reviewed for safety and effectiveness like medications) and their composition is not standardized (e.g., the composition varies among manufacturers). Therefore, they should not be counted as medications (e.g. chamomile, valerian root). Keep in mind that, for clinical purposes, it is important to document a resident's intake of such herbal and alternative medicine products elsewhere in the medical record and to monitor their potential effects as they can interact with medications the resident is currently taking. For more information consult the FDA website http://www.fda.gov/food/dietarysupplements/consumerinformation/ucm110567.htm.

Example

1. The Medication Administration Record for Mrs. P. reflects the following:

- Risperidone 0.5 mg PO BID PRN: Received once a day on Monday, Wednesday, and Thursday.

- Lorazepam 1 mg PO QAM: Received every day.

- Temazepam 15 mg PO QHS PRN: Received at bedtime on Tuesday and Wednesday only.

  Coding: Medications in N0410, would be checked as follows: **A. Antipsychotic,** resperidone is an antipsychotic medication, **B. Antianxiety,** lorazepam is an antianxiety medication, and **D. Hypnotic,** temazepam is a hypnotic medication. Please note: if a resident is receiving medications in all three categories simultaneously there must be a clear clinical indication for the use of these medications. Administration of these types of medications, particularly in this combination, could be interpreted as chemically restraining the resident. Adequate documentation is essential in justifying their use.

N0410: Medications Received (cont.)

Additional information on psychoactive medications can be found in the **Diagnostic and Statistical Manual of Mental Disorders, Fourth Edition (DSM-IV)** (or subsequent editions) (http://www.psychiatryonline.com/resourceTOC.aspx?resourceID=1), and the **State Operations Manual, Appendix PP, Guidance to Surveyors for Long Term Care Facilities** [the **State Operations Manual** can be found at (http://www.cms.gov/Manuals/IOM/list.asp)].

Additional information on medications can be found in:

The Orange Book, http://www.fda.gov/cder/ob/default.htm

The National Drug Code Directory, http://www.fda.gov/cder/ndc/database/Default.htm

SECTION O: SPECIAL TREATMENTS, PROCEDURES, AND PROGRAMS

Intent: The intent of the items in this section is to identify any special treatments, procedures, and programs that the resident received during the specified time periods.

O0100: Special Treatments, Procedures, and Programs

Facilities may code treatments, programs and procedures that the resident performed themselves independently or after set-up by facility staff. Do not code services that were provided solely in conjunction with a surgical procedure or diagnostic procedure, such as IV medications or ventilators. Surgical procedures include routine pre- and post-operative procedures.

O0100. Special Treatments, Procedures, and Programs Check all of the following treatments, procedures, and programs that were performed during the last **14 days**	1. While NOT a Resident	2. While a Resident
1. **While NOT a Resident** Performed *while NOT a resident* of this facility and within the *last 14 days*. Only check column 1 if resident entered (admission or reentry) IN THE LAST 14 DAYS. If resident last entered 14 or more days ago, leave column 1 blank 2. **While a Resident** Performed *while a resident* of this facility and within the *last 14 days*	↓ Check all that apply ↓	
Cancer Treatments		
A. Chemotherapy	☐	☐
B. Radiation	☐	☐
Respiratory Treatments		
C. Oxygen therapy	☐	☐
D. Suctioning	☐	☐
E. Tracheostomy care	☐	☐
F. Ventilator or respirator	☐	☐
G. BiPAP/CPAP	☐	☐
Other		
H. IV medications	☐	☐
I. Transfusions	☐	☐
J. Dialysis	☐	☐
K. Hospice care	☐	☐
L. Respite care		☐
M. Isolation or quarantine for active infectious disease (does not include standard body/fluid precautions)	☐	☐
None of the Above		
Z. None of the above	☐	☐

Item Rationale

Health-related Quality of Life

- The treatments, procedures, and programs listed in Item O0100, Special Treatments, Procedures, and Programs, can have a profound effect on an individual's health status, self-image, dignity, and quality of life.

O0100: Special Treatments, Procedures, and Programs (cont.)

Planning for Care

- Reevaluation of special treatments and procedures the resident received or performed, or programs that the resident was involved in during the 14-day look-back period is important to ensure the continued appropriateness of the treatments, procedures, or programs.

- Residents who perform any of the treatments, programs, and/or procedures below should be educated by the facility on the proper performance of these tasks, safety and use of any equipment needed, and be monitored for appropriate use and continued ability to perform these tasks.

Steps for Assessment

1. Review the resident's medical record to determine whether or not the resident received or performed any of the treatments, procedures, or programs within the last 14 days.

Coding Instructions for Column 1

Check all treatments, procedures, and programs received or performed by the resident **prior** to admission/entry or reentry to the facility and within the 14-day look-back period. Leave Column 1 blank if the resident was admitted/entered or reentered the facility more than 14 days ago. If no items apply in the last 14 days, **check Z, none of the above**.

Coding Instructions for Column 2

Check all treatments, procedures, and programs received or performed by the resident **after** admission/entry or reentry to the facility and within the 14-day look-back period.

Coding Tips

- Facilities may code treatments, programs and procedures that the resident performed themselves independently or after set-up by facility staff. Do not code services that were provided solely in conjunction with a surgical procedure or diagnostic procedure, such as IV medications or ventilators. Surgical procedures include routine pre- and post-operative procedures.

- **O0100A, Chemotherapy**

Code any type of chemotherapy agent administered as an antineoplastic given by any route in this item. Each drug should be evaluated to determine its reason for use before coding it here. The drugs coded here are those actually used for cancer treatment. For example, megestrol acetate is classified in the **Physician's Desk Reference (PDR)** as an antineoplastic drug. One of its side effects is appetite stimulation and weight gain. If megestrol acetate is being given only for appetite stimulation, do **not** code it as chemotherapy in this item, as the resident is not receiving the medication for chemotherapy purposes in this situation. IV's, IV medication, and blood transfusions administered during chemotherapy are **not** recorded under items K0510A (Parenteral/IV), O0100H (IV Medications), or O01001 (Transfusions).

- **O0100B, Radiation**

Code intermittent radiation therapy, as well as radiation administered via radiation implant in this item.

O0100: Special Treatments, Procedures, and Programs (cont.)

- ## O0100C, Oxygen therapy

Code continuous or intermittent oxygen administered via mask, cannula, etc., delivered to a resident to relieve hypoxia in this item. Code oxygen used in Bi-level Positive Airway Pressure/Continuous Positive Airway Pressure (BiPAP/CPAP) here. Do not code hyperbaric oxygen for wound therapy in this item. This item may be coded if the resident places or removes his/her own oxygen mask, cannula.

- ## O0100D, Suctioning

Code only tracheal and/or nasopharyngeal suctioning in this item. Do not code oral suctioning here. This item may be coded if the resident performs his/her own tracheal and/or nasopharyngeal suctioning.

- ## O0100E, Tracheostomy care

Code cleansing of the tracheostomy and/or cannula in this item. This item may be coded if the resident performs his/her own tracheostomy care.

- ## O0100F, Ventilator or respirator

Code any type of electrically or pneumatically powered closed-system mechanical ventilator support devices that ensure adequate ventilation in the resident who is, or who may become, unable to support his or her own respiration in this item. A resident who is being weaned off of a respirator or ventilator in the last 14 days should also be coded here. Do not code this item when the ventilator or respirator is used only as a substitute for BiPAP or CPAP.

- ## O0100G, BiPAP/CPAP

Code any type of CPAP or BiPAP respiratory support devices that prevent the airways from closing by delivering slightly pressurized air through a mask continuously or via electronic cycling throughout the breathing cycle. The BiPAP/CPAP mask enables the individual to support his or her own respiration by providing enough pressure when the individual inhales to keep his or her airways open, unlike ventilators that "breathe" for the individual. If a ventilator or respirator is being used as a substitute for BiPAP/CPAP, code here. This item may be coded if the resident places or removes his/her own BiPAP/CPAP mask.

- ## O0100H, IV medications

Code any drug or biological given by intravenous push, epidural pump, or drip through a central or peripheral port in this item. Do **not** code flushes to keep an IV access port patent, or IV fluids without medication here. Epidural, intrathecal, and baclofen pumps may be coded here, as they are similar to IV medications in that they must be monitored frequently and they involve continuous administration of a substance. Subcutaneous pumps are **not** coded in this item. Do **not** include IV medications of any kind that were administered during dialysis or chemotherapy. Dextrose 50% and/or Lactated Ringers given IV are not considered medications, and should not be coded here. To determine what products are considered medications or for more information consult the FDA website:

- The Orange Book, http://www.fda.gov/cder/ob/default.htm
- The National Drug Code Directory, http://www.fda.gov/cder/ndc/database/Default.htm

O0100: Special Treatments, Procedures, and Programs (cont.)

- **O0100I, Transfusions**

Code transfusions of blood or any blood products (e.g., platelets, synthetic blood products), which are administered directly into the bloodstream in this item. Do **not** include transfusions that were administered during dialysis or chemotherapy.

- **O0100J, Dialysis**

Code peritoneal or renal dialysis that occurs at the nursing home or at another facility in this item. Record treatments of hemofiltration, Slow Continuous Ultrafiltration (SCUF), Continuous Arteriovenous Hemofiltration (CAVH), and Continuous Ambulatory Peritoneal Dialysis (CAPD) in this item. IVs, IV medication, and blood transfusions administered during dialysis are considered part of the dialysis procedure and are **not** to be coded under items K0510A (Parenteral/IV), O0100H (IV medications), or O0100I (transfusions). This item may be coded if the resident performs his/her own dialysis.

- **O0100K, Hospice care**

Code residents identified as being in a hospice program for terminally ill persons where an array of services is provided for the palliation and management of terminal illness and related conditions. The hospice must be licensed by the state as a hospice provider and/or certified under the Medicare program as a hospice provider.

- **O0100L, Respite care**

Code only when the resident's care program involves a short-term stay in the facility for the purpose of providing relief to a primary home-based caregiver(s) in this item.

- **O0100M, Isolation for active infectious disease (does not include standard precautions)**

Code only when the resident requires transmission-based precautions and single room isolation (alone in a separate room) because of active infection (i.e., symptomatic and/or have a positive test and are in the contagious stage) with highly transmissible or epidemiologically significant pathogens that have been acquired by physical contact or airborne or droplet transmission. Do not code this item if the resident only has a history of infectious disease (e.g., s/p MRSA or s/p C-Diff - no active symptoms). Do not code this item if the precautions are standard precautions, because these types of precautions apply to everyone. Standard precautions include hand hygiene compliance, glove use, and additionally may include masks, eye protection, and gowns. Examples of when the isolation criterion would not apply include urinary tract infections, encapsulated pneumonia, and wound infections.

Code for "single room isolation" only when all of the following conditions are met:

1. The resident has active infection with highly transmissible or epidemiologically significant pathogens that have been acquired by physical contact or airborne or droplet transmission.
2. Precautions are over and above standard precautions. That is, transmission-based precautions (contact, droplet, and/or airborne) must be in effect.
3. The resident is in a room alone because of active infection and cannot have a roommate. This means that the resident must be in the room alone and not cohorted with a roommate regardless of whether the roommate has a similar active infection that requires isolation.

O0100: Special Treatments, Procedures, and Programs (cont.)

4. The resident must remain in his/her room. This requires that all services be brought to the resident (e.g. rehabilitation, activities, dining, etc.).

The following resources are being provided to help the facility interdisciplinary team determine the best method to contain and/or prevent the spread of infectious disease based on the type of infection and clinical presentation of the resident related to the specific communicable disease. The CDC guidelines also outline isolation precautions and go into detail regarding the different types of Transmission-Based Precautions (Contact, Droplet, and Airborne).

- 2007 Guideline for Isolation Precautions: Preventing Transmission of Infectious Agents in Healthcare Settings http://www.cdc.gov/hicpac/2007IP/2007isolationPrecautions.html

- SHEA/APIC Guideline: Infection Prevention and Control in the Long Term Care Facility http://www.apic.org/Resource_/TinyMceFileManager/Practice_Guidance/id_APIC-SHEA_GuidelineforICinLTCFs.pdf

As the CDC guideline notes, there are psychosocial risks associated with such restriction, and it has been recommended that psychosocial needs be balanced with infection control needs in the long-term care setting.

If a facility transports a resident who meets the criteria for single room isolation to another healthcare setting to receive medically needed services (e.g. dialysis, chemotherapy, blood transfusions, etc.) which the facility does not or cannot provide, they should follow CDC guidelines for transport of patients with communicable disease, and may still code O0100M for single room isolation since it is still being maintained while the resident is in the facility.

Finally, when coding for isolation, the facility should review the resident's status and determine if the criteria for a Significant Change of Status Assessment (SCSA) is met based on the effect the infection has on the resident's function and plan of care. The definition and criteria of "significant change of status" is found in Chapter 2, page 20. Regardless of whether the resident meets the criteria for an SCSA, a modification of the resident's plan of care will likely need to be completed.

- **O0100Z, None of the above**

Code if none of the above treatments, procedures, or programs were received or performed by the resident.

O0250: Influenza Vaccine

O0250. Influenza Vaccine - Refer to current version of RAI manual for current flu season and reporting period	
Enter Code ☐	**A.** Did the **resident receive the Influenza vaccine in this facility** for this year's Influenza season? 　0. **No →** Skip to O0250C, If Influenza vaccine not received, state reason 　1. **Yes →** Continue to O0250B, Date vaccine received
	B. Date vaccine received → Complete date and skip to O0300A, Is the resident's Pneumococcal vaccination up to date? ☐☐ – ☐☐ – ☐☐☐☐ 　Month　　　Day　　　Year
Enter Code ☐	**C. If Influenza vaccine not received, state reason:** 　1. **Resident not in facility** during this year's flu season 　2. **Received outside of this facility** 　3. **Not eligible** - medical contraindication 　4. **Offered and declined** 　5. **Not offered** 　6. **Inability to obtain vaccine** due to a declared shortage 　9. **None of the above**

O0250: Influenza Vaccine (cont.)

Item Rationale

Health-related Quality of Life

- When infected with influenza, older adults and persons with underlying health problems are at increased risk for complications and are more likely than the general population to require hospitalization.

- An institutional Influenza A outbreak can result in up to 60 percent of the population becoming ill, with 25 percent of those affected developing complications severe enough to result in hospitalization or death.

- Influenza-associated mortality results not only from pneumonia, but also from subsequent events arising from cardiovascular, cerebrovascular, and other chronic or immunocompromising diseases that can be exacerbated by influenza.

Planning for Care

- Influenza vaccines have been proven effective in preventing hospitalizations.

- Determining the rate of vaccination and causes for non-vaccination assists nursing homes in reaching the Healthy People 2020 (http://www.healthypeople.gov/2020/topicsobjectives2020/overview.aspx?topicid=23) national goal of 90 percent immunization among nursing home residents.

Steps for Assessment

1. Review the resident's medical record to determine whether an influenza vaccine was received in the facility for this year's influenza season. If vaccination status is unknown, proceed to the next step.

2. Ask the resident if he or she received an influenza vaccine outside of the facility for this year's Influenza season. If vaccination status is still unknown, proceed to the next step.

3. If the resident is unable to answer, then ask the same question of the responsible party/legal guardian and/or primary care physician. If vaccination status is still unknown, proceed to the next step.

4. If vaccination status cannot be determined, administer the vaccine to the resident according to standards of clinical practice.

Coding Instructions for O0250A, Did the Resident Receive the Influenza Vaccine in This Facility for This Year's Influenza Season?

- **Code 0, no:** if the resident **did NOT receive the influenza vaccine in this facility** during this year's influenza season. Proceed to **If influenza vaccine not received, state reason** (O0250C).

- **Code 1, yes:** if the resident **did receive the influenza vaccine in this facility** during this year's influenza season. Continue to **Date Vaccine Received** (O0250B).

O0250: Influenza Vaccine (cont.)

Coding Instructions for O0250B, Date Vaccine Received

- Enter date vaccine received. Do not leave any boxes blank. If the month contains only a single digit, fill in the first box of the month with a "0". For example, January 7, 2012 should be entered as 01-07-2012. If the day only contains a single digit, then fill the first box of the day with the "0". For example, May 6, 2012 should be entered as 05-06-2012. A full 8 character date is required. If the date is unknown or the information is not available, a single dash needs to be entered in the first box.

Coding Instructions for O0250C, If Influenza Vaccine Not Received, State Reason

If the resident has not received the influenza vaccine for this year's influenza season (i.e., 0250A=0), code the reason from the following list:

- **Code 1, Resident not in facility during this year's influenza season:** resident not in the facility during this year's influenza season.
- **Code 2, Received outside of this facility:** includes influenza vaccinations administered in any other setting (e.g., physician office, health fair, grocery store, hospital, fire station) during this year's influenza season.
- **Code 3, Not eligible—medical contraindication:** if influenza vaccine not received due to medical contraindications, including allergic reaction to eggs or other vaccine component(s), a physician order not to immunize, or an acute febrile illness is present. However, the resident should be vaccinated if contraindications end.
- **Code 4, Offered and declined:** resident or responsible party/legal guardian has been informed of what is being offered and chooses not to accept the influenza vaccine.
- **Code 5, Not offered:** resident or responsible party/legal guardian not offered the influenza vaccine.
- **Code 6, Inability to obtain vaccine due to a declared shortage:** influenza vaccine unavailable at the facility due to declared influenza vaccine shortage. However, the resident should be vaccinated once the facility receives the vaccine. The annual supply of inactivated influenza vaccine and the timing of its distribution cannot be guaranteed in any year.
- **Code 9, None of the above:** if none of the listed reasons describe why the influenza vaccine was not administered. This code is also used if the answer is unknown.

Coding Tips and Special Populations

- The influenza season varies annually. Information about current influenza season can be obtained by accessing the CDC Seasonal Influenza (Flu) website. This website provides information on influenza activity and has an interactive map that shows geographic spread of influenza: http://www.cdc.gov/flu/weekly/fluactivitysurv.htm, http://www.cdc.gov/flu/weekly/usmap.htm. Facilities can also contact their local health department website for their local influenza surveillance information. The influenza season ends when influenza is no longer active in your geographic area.
- Once the influenza vaccination has been administered to a resident for the current influenza season, this value is carried forward until the new influenza season begins.

O0250: Influenza Vaccine (cont.)

Examples

1. Mrs. J. received the influenza vaccine in the facility during this year's influenza season, on January 7, 2010.

   Coding: O0250A would be **coded 1, yes**; O0250B would be **coded 01-07-2010**, and O0250C would be skipped.

   Rationale: Mrs. J. received the vaccine in the facility on January 7, 2010, during this year's influenza season.

2. Mr. R. did not receive the influenza vaccine in the facility during this year's influenza season due to his known allergy to egg protein.

   Coding: O0250A would be **coded 0, no**; O0250B is skipped, and O0250C would be **coded 3, not eligible-medical contraindication.**

   Rationale: Allergies to egg protein is a medical contraindication to receiving the influenza vaccine, therefore, Mr. R did not receive the vaccine.

3. Resident Mrs. T. received the influenza vaccine at her doctor's office during this year's Influenza season. Her doctor provided documentation of Mrs. T.'s receipt of the vaccine to the facility to place in Mrs. T.'s medical record. He also provided documentation that Mrs. T. was explained the benefits and risks for the vaccine prior to administration.

   Coding: O0250A would be **coded 0, no**; and O0250C would be **coded 2, received outside of this facility.**

   Rationale: Mrs. T. received the influenza vaccine at her doctor's office during this year's Influenza season.

4. Mr. K. wanted to receive the influenza vaccine if it arrived prior to his scheduled discharge October 5th. Mr. K. was discharged prior to the facility receiving their annual shipment of influenza vaccine, and therefore, Mr. K. did not receive the influenza vaccine in the facility. Mr. K. was encouraged to receive the influenza vaccine at his next scheduled physician visit.

   Coding: O0250A would be **coded 0, no**; O0250B is skipped, and O0250C would be **coded 9, none of the above.**

   Rationale: Mr. K. was unable to receive the influenza vaccine in the facility due to the fact that the facility did not receive its shipment of influenza vaccine until after his discharge. None of the codes in O0250C, **Influenza vaccine not received, state reason**, are applicable.

O0300: Pneumococcal Vaccine

O0300. Pneumococcal Vaccine	
Enter Code ☐	**A. Is the resident's Pneumococcal vaccination up to date?** 0. **No** → Continue to O0300B, If Pneumococcal vaccine not received, state reason 1. **Yes** → Skip to O0400, Therapies
Enter Code ☐	**B. If Pneumococcal vaccine not received, state reason:** 1. **Not eligible** - medical contraindication 2. **Offered and declined** 3. **Not offered**

Item Rationale

Health-related Quality of Life

- Pneumococcal disease accounts for more deaths than any other vaccine-preventable bacterial disease.

- Case fatality rates for pneumococcal bacteremia are approximately 20%; however, they can be as high as 60% in the elderly (CDC, 2009).

Planning for Care

- Early detection of outbreaks is essential to control outbreaks of pneumococcal disease in long-term care facilities.

- Conditions that increase the risk of invasive pneumococcal disease include: decreased immune function, damaged or no spleen, chronic diseases of the heart, lungs, liver and kidneys. Other risk factors include smoking and cerebrospinal fluid (CSF) leak (CDC, 2009).

- Determining the rate of pneumococcal vaccination and causes for non-vaccination assists nursing homes in reaching the Healthy People 2020 (http://www.healthypeople.gov/2020/topicsobjectives2020/overview.aspx?topicid=23) national goal of 90% immunization among nursing home residents.

Steps for Assessment

1. Determine whether or not the resident should receive the vaccine.

   - All adults 65 years of age or older should receive the pneumococcal vaccine. However, certain person should be vaccinated before the age of 65, which include but are not limited to the following:

     — Immunocompromised persons 2 years of age and older who are at increased risk of pneumococcal disease should be vaccinated. This group includes those with the risk factors listed under **Planning for Care,** as well as Hodgkin's disease, leukemia, lymphoma, multiple myeloma, nephrotic syndrome, cochlear implant, or those who have had organ transplants and are on immunosuppressive protocols. Those on chemotherapy who are immunosuppressed, or those taking high-dose corticosteriods (14 days or longer) should also be vaccinated.

     — Individuals 2 years of age or older with asymptomatic or symptomatic HIV should be vaccinated.

O0300: Pneumococcal Vaccine (cont.)

— Individuals living in environments or social settings (e.g., nursing homes and other long-term care facilities) with an identified increased risk of invasive pneumococcal disease or its complications should be considered for vaccination populations.

— If vaccination status is unknown or the resident/family is uncertain whether or not the vaccine was received, the resident should be vaccinated.

- Pneumococcal vaccine is given once in a lifetime, with certain exceptions. Revaccination is recommended for the following:

— Individuals 2 years of age or older who are at highest risk for serious pneumococcal infection and for those who are likely to have a rapid decline in pneumococcal antibody levels. Those at highest risk include individuals with asplenia (functional or anatomic), sickle-cell disease, HIV infections or AIDS, cancer, leukemia, lymphoma, Hodgkin disease, multiple myeloma, generalized malignancy, chronic renal failure, nephrotic syndrome, or other conditions associated with immunosuppression (e.g., organ or bone marrow transplant, medication regimens that lower immunity (such as chemotherapy or long-term steroids).

— Persons 65 years or older should be administered a second dose of pneumococcal vaccine if they received the first dose of vaccine more than 5 years earlier and were less than 65 years old at the time of the first dose.

- If the resident has had a severe allergic reaction to vaccine components or following a prior dose of the vaccine, they should not be vaccinated.

If the resident has a moderate to severe acute illness, he or she should not be vaccinated until his or her condition improves. However, someone with a minor illness (e.g., a cold) should be vaccinated since minor illnesses are not a contraindication to receiving the vaccine.

[Centers for Disease Control and Prevention. (2009, May). *The Pink Book: Chapters: Epidemiology and Prevention of Vaccine Preventable Diseases (11th ed.)*. Retrieved from http://www.cdc.gov/vaccines/pubs/pinkbook/index.html#chapters]

Note: Please refer to the algorithm below for pneumococcal vaccine administration ONLY.

O0300: Pneumococcal Vaccine (cont.)

<u>Figure 1</u> Adopted from the CDC Recommendations and Reports, Prevention of Pneumococcal Disease: Recommendations of the Advisory Committee on Immunization Practices (ACIP) Recommended Adult Immunization Schedule --- United States. (2009, January 9). *MMWR, 57(53),*Q-1-Q-4.

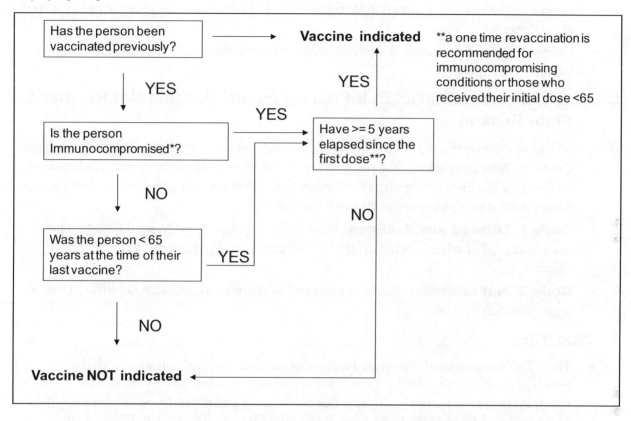

2. Review the resident's medical record and interview resident or responsible party/legal guardian and/or primary care physician to determine pneumococcal vaccination status, using the following steps:

    - Review the resident's medical record to determine whether a pneumococcal vaccine has been received. If vaccination status is unknown, proceed to the next step.

    - Ask the resident if he/she received a pneumococcal vaccine. If vaccination status is still unknown, proceed to the next step.

    - If the resident is unable to answer, ask the same question of a responsible party/legal guardian and/or primary care physician. If vaccination status is still unknown, proceed to the next step.

    - If vaccination status cannot be determined, administer the appropriate vaccine to the resident, according to the standards of clinical practice.

O0300: Pneumococcal Vaccine (cont.)

Coding Instructions O0300A, Is the Resident's Pneumococcal Vaccination Up to Date?

- **Code 0, no:** if the resident's pneumococcal vaccination status is not up to date or cannot be determined. Proceed to item O0300B, **If Pneumococcal vaccine not received, state reason**.

- **Code 1, yes:** if the resident's pneumococcal vaccination status is up to date. Skip to O0400, **Therapies**.

Coding Instructions O0300B, If Pneumococcal Vaccine Not Received, State Reason

If the resident has not received a pneumococcal vaccine, code the reason from the following list:

- **Code 1, Not eligible:** if the resident is not eligible due to medical contraindications, including a life-threatening allergic reaction to the pneumococcal vaccine or any vaccine component(s) or a physician order not to immunize.

- **Code 2, Offered and declined:** resident or responsible party/legal guardian has been informed of what is being offered and chooses not to accept the pneumococcal vaccine.

- **Code 3, Not offered:** resident or responsible party/legal guardian not offered the pneumococcal vaccine.

Coding Tips

- The CDC has evaluated inactivated influenza vaccine co-administration with the pneumococcal vaccine systematically among adults. It is safe to give these two vaccinations simultaneously. If the influenza vaccine and pneumococcal vaccine will be given to the resident at the same time, they should be administered at different sites (CDC, 2009). If the resident has had both upper extremities amputated or intramuscular injections are contraindicated in the upper extremities, administer the vaccine(s) according to clinical standards of care.

Examples

1. Mr. L., who is 72 years old, received the pneumococcal vaccine at his physician's office last year.

    Coding: O0300A would be **coded 1, yes**; skip to O0400, **Therapies**.

    Rationale: Mr. L is over 65 years old and received the pneumococcal vaccine in his physician's office last year at age 71.

O0300: Pneumococcal Vaccine (cont.)

2. Mrs. B, who is 95 years old, has never received a pneumococcal vaccine. Her physician has an order stating that she is NOT to be immunized.

    Coding: O0300A would be **coded 0, no**; and O0300B would be **coded 1, not eligible.**

    Rationale: Mrs. B. has never received the pneumococcal vaccine, therefore, her vaccine is not up to date. Her physician has written an order for her not to receive a pneumococcal vaccine, thus she is not eligible for the vaccine.

3. Mrs. A. received the pneumococcal vaccine at age 62 when she was hospitalized for a broken hip. She is now 78 and is being admitted to the nursing home for rehabilitation. Her covering physician offered the pneumococcal vaccine to her during his last visit in the nursing home, which she accepted. The facility administered the pneumococcal vaccine to Mrs. A.

    Coding: O0300A would be **coded 1, yes**; skip to O0400, **Therapies.**

    Rationale: Mrs. A. received the pneumococcal vaccine prior to the age of 65. Guidelines suggest that she should be revaccinated since she is over the age of 65 <u>and</u> 5 years have passed since her original vaccination. Mrs. A received the pneumococcal vaccine in the facility.

4. Mr. T. received the pneumococcal vaccine at age 62 when he was living in a congregate care community. He is now 65 years old and is being admitted to the nursing home for chemotherapy and respite care.

    Coding: O0300A would be **coded 1, yes**; skip to O0400, **Therapies**.

    Rationale: Mr. T. received his first dose of pneumococcal vaccine prior to the age of 65 due to him residing in congregate care at the age of 62. Even though Mr. T. is now immunocompromised, less than 5 years have lapsed since he originally received the vaccine. He would be considered up to date with his vaccination.

O0400: Therapies

O0400. Therapies

A. Speech-Language Pathology and Audiology Services

Enter Number of Minutes

1. **Individual minutes** - record the total number of minutes this therapy was administered to the resident **individually** in the last 7 days

Enter Number of Minutes

2. **Concurrent minutes -** record the total number of minutes this therapy was administered to the resident **concurrently with one other resident** in the last 7 days

Enter Number of Minutes

3. **Group minutes -** record the total number of minutes this therapy was administered to the resident as **part of a group of residents** in the last 7 days

If the sum of individual, concurrent, and group minutes is zero, → skip to O0400A5, Therapy start date

Enter Number of Days

4. **Days** - record the **number of days** this therapy was administered for **at least 15 minutes** a day in the last 7 days

5. **Therapy start date** - record the date the most recent therapy regimen (since the most recent entry) started

   Month — Day — Year

6. **Therapy end date** - record the date the most recent therapy regimen (since the most recent entry) ended - enter dashes if therapy is ongoing

   Month — Day — Year

B. Occupational Therapy

Enter Number of Minutes

1. **Individual minutes** - record the total number of minutes this therapy was administered to the resident **individually** in the last 7 days

Enter Number of Minutes

2. **Concurrent minutes -** record the total number of minutes this therapy was administered to the resident **concurrently with one other resident** in the last 7 days

Enter Number of Minutes

3. **Group minutes -** record the total number of minutes this therapy was administered to the resident as **part of a group of residents** in the last 7 days

If the sum of individual, concurrent, and group minutes is zero, → skip to O0400B5, Therapy start date

Enter Number of Days

4. **Days** - record the **number of days** this therapy was administered for **at least 15 minutes** a day in the last 7 days

5. **Therapy start date** - record the date the most recent therapy regimen (since the most recent entry) started

   Month — Day — Year

6. **Therapy end date** - record the date the most recent therapy regimen (since the most recent entry) ended - enter dashes if therapy is ongoing

   Month — Day — Year

C. Physical Therapy

Enter Number of Minutes

1. **Individual minutes** - record the total number of minutes this therapy was administered to the resident **individually** in the last 7 days

Enter Number of Minutes

2. **Concurrent minutes -** record the total number of minutes this therapy was administered to the resident **concurrently with one other resident** in the last 7 days

Enter Number of Minutes

3. **Group minutes -** record the total number of minutes this therapy was administered to the resident as **part of a group of residents** in the last 7 days

If the sum of individual, concurrent, and group minutes is zero, → skip to O0400C5, Therapy start date

Enter Number of Days

4. **Days** - record the **number of days** this therapy was administered for **at least 15 minutes** a day in the last 7 days

5. **Therapy start date** - record the date the most recent therapy regimen (since the most recent entry) started

   Month — Day — Year

6. **Therapy end date** - record the date the most recent therapy regimen (since the most recent entry) ended - enter dashes if therapy is ongoing

   Month — Day — Year

O0400 continued on next page

O0400: Therapies (cont.)

	O0400. Therapies - Continued
	D. Respiratory Therapy
Enter Number of Minutes ☐☐☐☐	**1. Total minutes** - record the total number of minutes this therapy was administered to the resident in the last 7 days If zero, → skip to O0400E, Psychological Therapy
Enter Number of Days ☐	**2. Days** - record the **number of days** this therapy was administered for **at least 15 minutes** a day in the last 7 days
	E. Psychological Therapy (by any licensed mental health professional)
Enter Number of Minutes ☐☐☐☐	**1. Total minutes** - record the total number of minutes this therapy was administered to the resident in the last 7 days If zero, → skip to O0400F, Recreational Therapy
Enter Number of Days ☐	**2. Days** - record the **number of days** this therapy was administered for **at least 15 minutes** a day in the last 7 days
	F. Recreational Therapy (includes recreational and music therapy)
Enter Number of Minutes ☐☐☐☐	**1. Total minutes** - record the total number of minutes this therapy was administered to the resident in the last 7 days If zero, → skip to O0450, Resumption of Therapy
Enter Number of Days ☐	**2. Days** - record the **number of days** this therapy was administered for **at least 15 minutes** a day in the last 7 days

Item Rationale

Health-related Quality of Life

- Maintaining as much independence as possible in activities of daily living, mobility, and communication is critically important to most people. Functional decline can lead to depression, withdrawal, social isolation, breathing problems, and complications of immobility, such as incontinence and pressure ulcers, which contribute to diminished quality of life. The qualified therapist, in conjunction with the physician and nursing administration, is responsible for determining the necessity for, and the frequency and duration of, the therapy services provided to residents.

- Rehabilitation (i.e., via Speech-Language Pathology Services and Occupational and Physical Therapies) and respiratory, psychological, and recreational therapy can help residents to attain or maintain their highest level of well-being and improve their quality of life.

Planning for Care

- Code only medically necessary therapies that occurred after admission/readmission to the nursing home that were (1) ordered by a physician (physician's assistant, nurse practitioner, and/or clinical nurse specialist) based on a qualified therapist's assessment (i.e., one who meets Medicare requirements or, in some instances, under such a person's direct supervision) and treatment plan, (2) documented in the resident's medical record, and (3) care planned and periodically evaluated to ensure that the resident receives needed therapies and that current treatment plans are effective. Therapy treatment may occur either inside or outside of the facility.

- **For definitions of the types of therapies listed in this section, please refer to the Glossary in Appendix A.**

O0400: Therapies (cont.)

Steps for Assessment

1. Review the resident's medical record (e.g., rehabilitation therapy evaluation and treatment records, recreation therapy notes, mental health professional progress notes), and consult with each of the qualified care providers to collect the information required for this item.

Coding Instructions for Speech-Language Pathology and Audiology Services and Occupational and Physical Therapies

- **Individual minutes**—Enter the total number of minutes of therapy that were provided on an individual basis in the last 7 days. **Enter 0** if none were provided. Individual services are provided by one therapist or assistant to one resident at a time.

- **Concurrent minutes**—Enter the total number of minutes of therapy that were provided on a concurrent basis in the last 7 days. **Enter 0** if none were provided. Concurrent therapy is defined as the treatment of 2 residents at the same time, when the residents are not performing the same or similar activities, regardless of payer source, both of whom must be in line-of-sight of the treating therapist or assistant for Medicare Part A. When a Part A resident receives therapy that meets this definition, it is defined as concurrent therapy for the Part A resident regardless of the payer source for the second resident. For Part B, residents may not be treated concurrently: a therapist may treat one resident at a time, and the minutes during the day when the resident is treated individually are added, even if the therapist provides that treatment intermittently (first to one resident and then to another). For all other payers, follow Medicare Part A instructions.

- **Group minutes**—Enter the total number of minutes of therapy that were provided in a group in the last 7 days. **Enter 0** if none were provided. Group therapy is defined for Part A as the treatment of 4 residents, regardless of payer source, who are performing the same or similar activities, and are supervised by a therapist or an assistant who is not supervising any other individuals. For Medicare Part B, treatment of two patients (or more), regardless of payer source, at the same time is documented as group treatment. For all other payers, follow Medicare Part A instructions.

- **Days**—Enter the number of days therapy services were provided in the last 7 days. A day of therapy is defined as skilled treatment for 15 minutes or more during the day. Use total minutes of therapy provided (individual plus concurrent plus group), without any adjustment, to determine if the day is counted. For example, if the resident received 20 minutes of concurrent therapy, the day requirement is considered met. **Enter 0** if therapy was provided but for less than 15 minutes every day for the last 7 days. If the total number of minutes (individual plus concurrent plus group) during the last 7 days is 0, skip this item and leave blank.

- **Therapy Start Date**—Record the date the most recent therapy regimen (since the most recent entry/reentry) started. This is the date the initial therapy evaluation is conducted regardless if treatment was rendered or not or the date of resumption (O0450B) on the resident's EOT OMRA, in cases where the resident discontinued and then resumed therapy.

O0400: Therapies (cont.)

- **Therapy End Date**—Record the date the most recent therapy regimen (since the most recent entry) ended. This is the last date the resident <u>received</u> skilled therapy treatment. Enter dashes if therapy is ongoing.

Coding Instructions for Respiratory, Psychological, and Recreational Therapies

- **Total Minutes**—Enter the actual number of minutes therapy services were provided in the last 7 days. **Enter 0** if none were provided.

- **Days**—Enter the number of days therapy services were provided in the last 7 days. A day of therapy is defined as treatment for 15 minutes or more in the day.

   Enter 0 if therapy was provided but for less than 15 minutes every day for the last 7 days. If the total number of minutes during the last 7 days is 0, skip this item and leave blank.

Coding Tips and Special Populations

- **Therapy Start Date:**
   1. Look at the date at A1600.
   2. Determine whether the resident has had skilled rehabilitation therapy at any time from that date to the present date.
   3. If so, enter the date that the therapy regimen started; if there was more than one therapy regimen since the A1600 date, enter the start date of the most recent therapy regimen.

- Psychological Therapy is provided by any licensed mental health professional, such as psychiatrists, psychologists, clinical social workers, and clinical nurse specialists in mental health as allowable under applicable state laws. Psychiatric technicians are not considered to be licensed mental health professionals and their services may not be counted in this item.

Minutes of therapy

- Includes only therapies that were provided once the individual is actually living/being cared for at the long-term care facility. Do **NOT** include therapies that occurred while the person was an inpatient at a hospital or recuperative/rehabilitation center or other long-term care facility, or a recipient of home care or community-based services.

- If a resident returns from a hospital stay, an initial evaluation must be performed after entry to the facility, and only those therapies that occurred since admission/reentry to the facility and after the initial evaluation shall be counted.

- The therapist's time spent on documentation or on initial evaluation is not included.

- The therapist's time spent on subsequent reevaluations, conducted as part of the treatment process, should be counted.

O0400: Therapies (cont.)

- Family education when the resident is present is counted and must be documented in the resident's record.

- Only skilled therapy time (i.e., requires the skills, knowledge and judgment of a qualified therapist and all the requirements for skilled therapy are met) shall be recorded on the MDS. In some instances, the time during which a resident received a treatment modality includes partly skilled and partly unskilled time; only time that is skilled may be recorded on the MDS. Therapist time during a portion of a treatment that is non-skilled; during a non-therapeutic rest period; or during a treatment that does not meet the therapy mode definitions may not be included.

- The time required to adjust equipment or otherwise prepare the treatment area for skilled rehabilitation service is the set-up time and is to be included in the count of minutes of therapy delivered to the resident. Set-up may be performed by the therapist, therapy assistant, or therapy aide.

- Set-up time shall be recorded under the mode for which the resident receives initial treatment when he/she receives more than one mode of therapy per visit.
  — Code as individual minutes when the resident receives only individual therapy or individual therapy followed by another mode(s);
  — Code as concurrent minutes when the resident receives only concurrent therapy or concurrent therapy followed by another mode(s); and
  — Code as group minutes when the resident receives only group therapy or group therapy followed by another mode(s).

- For Speech-Language Pathology Services (SLP) and Physical (PT) and Occupational Therapies (OT) include only skilled therapy services. Skilled therapy services **must** meet **all** of the following conditions (Refer to Medicare Benefit Policy Manual, Chapters 8 and 15, for detailed requirements and policies):
  — for Part A, services must be ordered by a physician. For Part B the plan of care must be certified by a physician following the therapy evaluation;
  — the services must be directly and specifically related to an active written treatment plan that is approved by the physician after any needed consultation with the qualified therapist and is based on an initial evaluation performed by a qualified therapist prior to the start of therapy services in the facility;
  — the services must be of a level of complexity and sophistication, or the condition of the resident must be of a nature that requires the judgment, knowledge, and skills of a therapist;
  — the services must be provided with the expectation, based on the assessment of the resident's restoration potential made by the physician, that the condition of the patient will improve materially in a reasonable and generally predictable period of time, or the services must be necessary for the establishment of a safe and effective maintenance program;
  — the services must be considered under accepted standards of medical practice to be specific and effective treatment for the resident's condition; and,

O0400: Therapies (cont.)

- — the services must be reasonable and necessary for the treatment of the resident's condition; this includes the requirement that the amount, frequency, and duration of the services must be reasonable and they must be furnished by qualified personnel.

- Include services provided by a qualified occupational/physical therapy assistant who is employed by (or under contract with) the long-term care facility only if he or she is under the direction of a qualified occupational/physical therapist. Medicare does not recognize speech-language pathology assistants; therefore, services provided by these individuals are not to be coded on the MDS.

- For purposes of the MDS, when the payer for therapy services is not Medicare Part B, follow the definitions and coding for Medicare Part A.

- Record the actual minutes of therapy. **Do not round therapy minutes (e.g., reporting) to the nearest 5th minute**. The conversion of units to minutes or minutes to units is not appropriate. Please note that therapy logs are not an MDS requirement but reflect a standard clinical practice expected of all therapy professionals. These therapy logs may be used to verify the provision of therapy services in accordance with the plan of care and to validate information reported on the MDS assessment.

- When therapy is provided staff need to document the different modes of therapy and set up minutes that are being included on the MDS. It is important to keep records of time included for each. When submitting a part B claim, minutes reported on the MDS may not match the time reported on a claim. For example, therapy aide set-up time is recorded on the MDS when it precedes skilled therapy; however, the therapy aide set-up time is not included for billing purposes on a therapy Part B claim.

- For purposes of the MDS, providers should record services for respiratory, psychological, and recreational therapies (Item O0400D, E, and F) when the following criteria are met:

  - — the physician orders the therapy;
  - — the physician's order includes a statement of frequency, duration, and scope of treatment;
  - — the services must be directly and specifically related to an active written treatment plan that is based on an initial evaluation performed by qualified personnel (See Glossary in Appendix A for definitions of respiratory, psychological and recreational therapies);
  - — the services are required and provided by qualified personnel (See Glossary in Appendix A for definitions of respiratory, psychological and recreational therapies);
  - — the services must be reasonable and necessary for treatment of the resident's condition.

Non-Skilled Services

- Services provided at the request of the resident or family that are not medically necessary (sometimes referred to as family-funded services) shall **not** be counted in item O0400 **Therapies**, even when performed by a therapist or an assistant.

- Nursing homes may elect to have licensed professionals perform repetitive exercises and other maintenance treatments or to supervise aides performing these maintenance services.

O0400: Therapies (cont.)

In these situations, the services shall **not** be coded as therapy in item O0400 **Minutes**, since the specific interventions would be considered restorative nursing care when performed by nurses or aides. Services provided by therapists, licensed or not, that are not specifically listed in this manual or on the MDS item set shall **not** be coded as therapy in Item 0400. These services should be documented in the resident's medical record.

- Once the qualified therapist has designed a maintenance program and discharged the resident from a rehabilitation (i.e., skilled) therapy program, the services performed by the therapist and the assistant are **not** to be reported in item O0400A, B, or C **Therapies** The services may be reported on the MDS assessment in item O0500 **Restorative Nursing Care**, provided the requirements for restorative nursing program are met.

- Services provided by therapy aides are **not** skilled services (see therapy aide section below).

- When a resident refuses to participate in therapy, it is important for care planning purposes to identify why the resident is refusing therapy. However, the time spent investigating the refusal or trying to persuade the resident to participate in treatment is not a skilled service and shall not be included in the therapy minutes.

Co-treatment

For Part A:

When two clinicians (therapists or therapy assistants), each from a different discipline, treat one resident at the same time with different treatments, both disciplines may code the treatment session in full. All policies regarding mode, modalities and student supervision must be followed as well as all other federal, state, practice and facility policies. For example, if two therapists (from different disciplines) were conducting a group treatment session, the group must be comprised of four participants who were doing the same or similar activities in each discipline. The decision to co-treat should be made on a case by case basis and the need for co-treatment should be well documented for each patient. Because co-treatment is appropriate for specific clinical circumstances and would not be suitable for all residents, its use should be limited.

For Part B:

Therapists, or therapy assistants, working together as a "team" to treat one or more patients **cannot** each bill separately for the same or different service provided at the same time to the same patient.

CPT codes are used for billing the services of one therapist or therapy assistant. The therapist cannot bill for his/her services and those of another therapist or a therapy assistant, when both provide the same or different services, at the same time, to the same patient(s). Where a physical and occupational therapist both provide services to one patient at the same time, only one therapist can bill for the entire service or the PT and OT can divide the service units. For example, a PT and an OT work together for 30 minutes with one patient on transfer activities. The PT and OT could each bill one unit of 97530. Alternatively, the 2 units of 97530 could be billed by either the PT or the OT, but not both.

O0400: Therapies (cont.)

Similarly, if two therapy assistants provide services to the same patient at the same time, only the service of one therapy assistant can be billed by the supervising therapist or the service units can be split between the two therapy assistants and billed by the supervising therapist(s).

Therapy Aides and Students

Therapy Aides

Therapy Aides cannot provide skilled services. Only the time a therapy aide spends on set-up preceding skilled therapy may be coded on the MDS (e.g., set up the treatment area for wound therapy) and should be coded under the appropriate mode for the skilled therapy (individual, concurrent, or group) in O0400. The therapy aide must be under direct supervision of the therapist or assistant (i.e., the therapist/assistant must be in the facility and immediately available).

Therapy Students

Medicare Part A—Therapy students are not required to be in line-of-sight of the professional supervising therapist/assistant (**Federal Register**, August 8, 2011). Within individual facilities, supervising therapists/assistants must make the determination as to whether or not a student is ready to treat patients without line-of-sight supervision. Additionally all state and professional practice guidelines for student supervision must be followed.

Time may be coded on the MDS when the therapist provides skilled services and direction to a student who is participating in the provision of therapy. All time that the student spends with patients should be documented.

- Medicare Part B—The following criteria must be met in order for services provided by a student to be billed by the long-term care facility:
  — The qualified professional is present and in the room for the entire session. The student participates in the delivery of services when the qualified practitioner is directing the service, making the skilled judgment, and is responsible for the assessment and treatment.
  — The practitioner is not engaged in treating another patient or doing other tasks at the same time.
  — The qualified professional is the person responsible for the services and, as such, signs all documentation. (A student may, of course, also sign but it is not necessary because the Part B payment is for the clinician's service, not for the student's services.)
  — Physical therapy assistants and occupational therapy assistants are not precluded from serving as clinical instructors for therapy assistant students while providing services within their scope of work and performed under the direction and supervision of a qualified physical or occupational therapist.

O0400: Therapies (cont.)

Modes of Therapy

A resident may receive therapy via different modes during the same day or even treatment session. When developing the plan of care, the therapist and assistant must determine which mode(s) of therapy and the amount of time the resident receives for each mode and code the MDS appropriately. The therapist and assistant should document the reason a specific mode of therapy was chosen as well as anticipated goals for that mode of therapy. For any therapy that does not meet one of the therapy mode definitions below, those minutes may not be counted on the MDS. (Please also see the section on group therapy for limited exceptions related to group size.) The therapy mode definitions must always be followed and apply regardless of when the therapy is provided in relationship to all assessment windows (i.e., applies whether or not the resident is in a look back period for an MDS assessment).

Individual Therapy

The treatment of one resident at a time. The resident is receiving the therapist's or the assistant's full attention. Treatment of a resident individually at intermittent times during the day is individual treatment, and the minutes of individual treatment are added for the daily count. For example, the speech-language pathologist treats the resident individually during breakfast for 8 minutes and again at lunch for 13 minutes. The total of individual time for this day would be 21 minutes.

When a therapy student is involved with the treatment of a resident, the minutes may be coded as individual therapy when only one resident is being treated by the therapy student and supervising therapist/assistant (Medicare A and Medicare B). The supervising therapist/assistant shall not be engaged in any other activity or treatment when the resident is receiving therapy under Medicare B. However, for those residents whose stay is covered under Medicare A, the supervising therapist/assistant shall not be treating or supervising other individuals **and** he/she is able to immediately intervene/assist the student as needed.

Example:

- A speech therapy graduate student treats Mr. A for 30 minutes. Mr. A.'s therapy is covered under the Medicare Part A benefit. The supervising speech-language pathologist is not treating any patients at this time but is not in the room with the student or Mr. A. Mr. A.'s therapy may be coded as 30 minutes of individual therapy on the MDS .

Concurrent Therapy

Medicare Part A

The treatment of 2 residents, who are not performing the same or similar activities, at the same time, <u>regardless of payer source</u>, both of whom must be in line-of-sight of the treating therapist or assistant.

- NOTE: The minutes being coded on the MDS are unadjusted minutes, meaning, the minutes are coded in the MDS as the full time spent in therapy; however, the software grouper will allocate the minutes appropriately. In the case of concurrent therapy, the minutes will be divided by 2.

O0400: Therapies (cont.)

When a therapy student is involved with the treatment, and one of the following occurs, the minutes may be coded as concurrent therapy:

- The therapy student is treating one resident and the supervising therapist/assistant is treating another resident, and both residents are in line of sight of the therapist/assistant or student providing their therapy.; or

- The therapy student is treating 2 residents, <u>regardless of payer source,</u> both of whom are in line-of-sight of the therapy student, and the therapist is not treating any residents and not supervising other individuals; or

- The therapy student is not treating any residents and the supervising therapist/assistant is treating 2 residents at the same time, regardless of payer source, both of whom are in line-of-sight.

Medicare Part B

- The treatment of two or more residents who may or may not be performing the same or similar activity, regardless of payer source, at the same time is documented as group treatment

Examples:

- A physical therapist provides therapies that are not the same or similar, to Mrs. Q and Mrs. R at the same time, for 30 minutes. Mrs. Q's stay is covered under the Medicare SNF PPS Part A benefit. Mrs. R. is paying privately for therapy. Based on the information above, the therapist would code each individual's MDS for this day of treatment as follows:

  — Mrs. Q. received concurrent therapy for 30 minutes.

  — Mrs. R received concurrent therapy for 30 minutes.

- A physical therapist provides therapies that are not the same or similar, to Mrs. S. and Mrs. T. at the same time, for 30 minutes. Mrs. S.'s stay is covered under the Medicare SNF PPS Part A benefit. Mr. T.'s therapy is covered under Medicare Part B. Based on the information above, the therapist would code each individual's MDS for this day of treatment as follows:

  — Mrs. S. received concurrent therapy for 30 minutes.

  — Mr. T. received group therapy (Medicare Part B definition) for 30 minutes. (Please refer to the Medicare Benefit Policy Manual, Chapter 15, and the Medicare Claims Processing Manual, Chapter 5, for coverage and billing requirements under the Medicare Part B benefit.)

- An Occupational Therapist provides therapy to Mr. K. for 60 minutes. An occupational therapy graduate student who is supervised by the occupational therapist, is treating Mr. R. at the same time for the same 60 minutes but Mr. K. and Mr. R. are not doing the same or similar activities. Both Mr. K. and Mr. R's stays are covered under the Medicare Part A benefit. Based on the information above, the therapist would code each individual's MDS for this day of treatment as follows:

  — Mr. K. received concurrent therapy for 60 minutes.

  — Mr. R. received concurrent therapy for 60 minutes.

O0400: Therapies (cont.)

Group Therapy

Medicare Part A

The treatment of 4 residents, regardless of payer source, who are performing the same or similar activities, and are supervised by a therapist or assistant who is not supervising any other individuals.

- NOTE: The minutes being coded on the MDS are unadjusted minutes, meaning, the minutes are coded in the MDS as the full time spent in therapy; however, the software grouper will allocate the minutes appropriately. In the case of group therapy, the minutes will be divided by 4.

When a therapy student is involved with group therapy treatment, and one of the following occurs, the minutes may be coded as group therapy:

- The therapy student is providing the group treatment and the supervising therapist/assistant is not treating any residents and is not supervising other individuals (students or residents); or
- The supervising therapist/assistant is providing the group treatment and the therapy student is not providing treatment to any resident. In this case, the student is simply assisting the supervising therapist.

Medicare Part B

The treatment of 2 or more individuals simultaneously, regardless of payer source, who may or may not be performing the same activity.

- When a therapy student is involved with group therapy treatment, and one of the following occurs, the minutes may be coded as group therapy:
- The therapy student is providing group treatment and the supervising therapist/assistant is not engaged in any other activity or treatment; or
- The supervising therapist/assistant is providing group treatment and the therapy student is not providing treatment to any resident.

Examples:

- A Physical Therapist provides similar therapies to Mr. W, Mr. X, Mrs. Y. and Mr. Z. at the same time, for 30 minutes. Mr. W. and Mr. X.'s stays are covered under the Medicare SNF PPS Part A benefit. Mrs. Y.'s therapy is covered under Medicare Part B, and Mr. Z has private insurance paying for therapy. Based on the information above, the therapist would code each individual's MDS for this day of treatment as follows:
  — Mr W. received group therapy for 30 minutes.
  — Mr. X. received group therapy for 30 minutes.
  — Mrs. Y. received group therapy for 30 minutes. (Please refer to the Medicare Benefit Policy Manual, Chapter 15, and the Medicare Claims Processing Manual, Chapter 5, for coverage and billing requirements under the Medicare Part B benefit.)
  — Mr. Z. received group therapy for 30 minutes.

O0400: Therapies (cont.)

- Mrs. V, whose stay is covered by SNF PPS Part A benefit, begins therapy in an individual session. After 13 minutes the therapist begins working with Mr. S., whose therapy is covered by Medicare Part B, while Mrs. V. continues with her skilled intervention and is in line-of-sight of the treating therapist. The therapist provides treatment during the same time period to Mrs. V. and Mr. S. for 24 minutes who are not performing the same or similar activities, at which time Mrs. V.'s therapy session ends. The therapist continues to treat Mr. S. individually for 10 minutes. Based on the information above, the therapist would code each individual's MDS for this day of treatment as follows:

  — Mrs. V. received individual therapy for 13 minutes and concurrent therapy for 24.

  — Mr. S. received group therapy (Medicare Part B definition) for 24 minutes and individual therapy for 10 minutes. (Please refer to the **Medicare Benefit Policy Manual**, Chapter 15, and the **Medicare Claims Processing Manual**, Chapter 5, for coverage and billing requirements under the Medicare Part B benefit.)

- Mr. A. and Mr. B., whose stays are covered by Medicare Part A, begin working with a physical therapist on two different therapy interventions. After 30 minutes, Mr. A. and Mr. B are joined by Mr. T. and Mr. E., whose stays are also covered by Medicare Part A., and the therapist begins working with all of them on the same therapy goals as part of a group session. After 15 minutes in this group session, Mr. A. becomes ill and is forced to leave the group, while the therapist continues working with the remaining group members for an additional 15 minutes. Based on the information above, the therapist would code each individual's MDS for this day of treatment as follows:

  — Mr. A. received concurrent therapy for 30 minutes and group therapy for 15 minutes.

  — Mr. B. received concurrent therapy for 30 minutes and group therapy for 30 minutes.

  — Mr. T. received group therapy for 30 minutes.

  — Mr. E. received group therapy for 30 minutes.

Therapy Modalities

Only skilled therapy time (i.e., require the skills, knowledge and judgment of a qualified therapist and all the requirements for skilled therapy are met, see page O-17) shall be recorded on the MDS. In some instances, the time a resident receives certain modalities is partly skilled and partly unskilled time; only the time that is skilled may be recorded on the MDS. For example, a resident is receiving TENS (transcutaneous electrical nerve stimulation) for pain management. The portion of the treatment that is skilled, such as proper electrode placement, establishing proper pulse frequency and duration, and determining appropriate stimulation mode, shall be recorded on the MDS. In other instances, some modalities only meet the requirements of skilled therapy in certain situations. For example, the application of a hot pack is often not a skilled intervention. However, when the resident's condition is complicated and the skills, knowledge, and judgment of the therapist are required for treatment, then those minutes associated with skilled therapy time may be recorded on the MDS. The use and rationale for all therapy modalities, whether skilled or unskilled should always be documented as part of the patient's plan of care.

O0400: Therapies (cont.)

Dates of Therapy

A resident may have more than one regimen of therapy treatment during an episode of a stay. When this situation occurs the Therapy Start Date for the most recent episode of treatment for the particular therapy (SLP, PT, or OT) should be coded. When a resident's episode of treatment for a given type of therapy extends beyond the ARD (i.e., therapy is ongoing), enter dashes in the appropriate Therapy End Date. Therapy is considered to be ongoing if:

- The resident was discharged and therapy was planned to continue had the resident remained in the facility, or
- The resident's SNF benefit exhausted and therapy continued to be provided, or
- The resident's payer source changed and therapy continued to be provided.

For example, Mr. N. was admitted to the nursing home following a fall that resulted in a hip fracture in November 2011. Occupational and Physical therapy started December 3, 2011. His physical therapy ended January 27, 2012 and occupational therapy ended January 29, 2012. Later on during his stay at the nursing home, due to the progressive nature of his Parkinson's disease, he was referred to SLP and OT February 10, 2012 (he remained in the facility the entire time). The speech-language pathologist evaluated him on that day and the occupational therapist evaluated him the next day. The ARD for Mr. N.'s MDS assessment is February 28, 2012. Coding values for his MDS are:

- Item O0400A5 (SLP start date) is 02102012,
- O0400A6 (SLP end date) is dash filled,
- O0400B5 (OT start date) is 02112012,
- O0400B6 (OT end date) is dash filled,
- O0400C5 (PT start date) is 12032011, and
- O0400C6 (PT end date) is 01272012.

NOTE: When an EOT-R is completed, the Therapy Start Date (O0400A5, O0400B5, and O0400C5) on the next assessment is the same as the Resumption of Therapy Date (O0450B) on the EOT-R. If therapy is ongoing, the Therapy End Date (O0400A6, O0400B6, and O0400C6) would be filled out with dashes.

General Coding Example:

Following a stroke, Mrs. F. was admitted to the skilled nursing facility in stable condition for rehabilitation therapy on 10/06/11 under Part A skilled nursing facility coverage. She had slurred speech, difficulty swallowing, severe weakness in both her right upper and lower extremities, and a Stage III pressure ulcer on her left lateral malleolus. She was referred to SLP, OT, and PT with the long-term goal of returning home with her daughter and son-in-law. Her initial SLP evaluation was performed on 10/06/11, the PT initial evaluation on 10/07/11, and the OT initial evaluation on 10/09/11. She was also referred to recreational therapy and respiratory therapy. The interdisciplinary team determined that 10/19/11 was an appropriate ARD for her Medicare-required 14-day MDS. During the look-back period she received the following:

O0400: Therapies (cont.)

- Speech-language pathology services that were provided over the 7-day look-back period. Individual dysphagia treatments; Monday-Friday for 30 minute sessions each day.
- Cognitive training; Monday and Thursday for 35 minute concurrent therapy sessions and Tuesday, Wednesday and Friday 25 minute group sessions.
- Individual speech techniques; Tuesday and Thursday for 20-minute sessions each day.

  Coding:

  O0400A1 would be **coded 190**; O0400A2 would be **coded 70**; O0400A3 would be **coded 75**; O0400A4 would bc **coded 5**; O0400A5 would be **coded 10062011**; and O0400A6 would be **coded with dashes**.

  Rationale:

  Individual minutes totaled 190 over the 7-day look-back period [(30 × 5) + (20 × 2) = 190]; concurrent minutes totaled 70 over the 7-day look-back period (35 × 2 = 70); and group minutes totaled 75 over the 7-day look-back period (25 × 3 = 75). Therapy was provided 5 out of the 7 days of the look-back period. Date speech-language pathology services began was 10-06-2011, and dashes were used as the therapy end date value because the therapy was ongoing.

Occupational therapy services that were provided over the 7-day look-back period:

- Individual sitting balance activities; Monday and Wednesday for 30-minute co-treatment sessions with PT each day (OT and PT each code the session as 30 minutes for each discipline).
- Individual wheelchair seating and positioning; Monday, Wednesday, and Friday for the following times: 23 minutes, 18 minutes, and 12 minutes.
- Balance/coordination activities; Tuesday-Friday for 20 minutes each day in group sessions.

  Coding:

  O0400B1 would be **coded 113**, O0400B2 would be **coded 0**, O0400B3 would be **coded 80**, O0400B4 would be **coded 5**, O0400B5 would be **coded 10092011**, and O0400B6 would be **coded with dashes**.

  Rationale:

  Individual minutes totaled 113 over the 7-day look-back period [(30 × 2) + 23 + 18 + 12 = 113]; concurrent minutes totaled 0 over the 7-day look-back period (0 × 0 = 0); and group minutes totaled 80 over the 7-day look-back period (20 × 4 = 80). Therapy was provided 5 out of the 7 days of the look-back period. Date occupational therapy services began was 10-09-2011and dashes were used as the therapy end date value because the therapy was ongoing.

Physical therapy services that were provided over the 7-day look-back period:

- Individual wound debridement followed by application of routine wound dressing; Monday the session lasted 22 minutes, 5 minutes of which were for the application of the dressing. On Thursday the session lasted 27 minutes, 6 minutes of which were for the

O0400: Therapies (cont.)

application of the dressing. For each session the therapy aide spent 7 minutes preparing the debridement area (set-up time) for needed therapy supplies and equipment for the therapist to conduct wound debridement.

- Individual sitting balance activities; on Monday and Wednesday for 30-minute co-treatment sessions with OT (OT and PT each code the session as 30 minutes for each discipline).

- Individual bed positioning and bed mobility training; Monday-Friday for 35 minutes each day.

- Concurrent therapeutic exercises; Monday-Friday for 20 minutes each day.

Coding:
O0400C1 would be **coded 287,** O0400C2 would be **coded 100,** O0400C3 would be **coded 0,** O0400C4 would be **coded 5,** O0400C5 would be **coded 10072011,** and O0400C6 would be **coded with dashes.**

Rationale:
Individual minutes totaled 287 over the 7-day look-back period $[(30 \times 2) + (35 \times 5) + (22 - 5) + 7 + (27 - 6) + 7 = 287]$; concurrent minutes totaled 100 over the 7-day look-back period $(20 \times 5 = 100)$; and group minutes totaled 0 over the 7-day look-back period $(0 \times 0 = 0)$. Therapy was provided 5 out of the 7 days of the look-back period. Date physical therapy services began was 10-07-2011, and dashes were used as the therapy end date value because the therapy was ongoing.

Respiratory therapy services that were provided over the 7-day look-back period:

Respiratory therapy services; Sunday-Thursday for 10 minutes each day.

Coding:
O0400D1 would be **coded 50,** O0400D2 would be **coded 0.**

Rationale:
Total minutes were 50 over the 7-day look-back period $(10 \times 5 = 50)$. Although a total of 50 minutes of respiratory therapy services were provided over the 7-day look-back period, there were not any days that respiratory therapy was provided for 15 minutes or more. Therefore, O0400D equals **zero days.**

Psychological therapy services that were provided over the 7-day look-back period:

Psychological therapy services were not provided at all over the 7-day look-back period.

Coding:
O0400E1 would be **coded 0,** O0400E2 would be **left blank.**

Rationale:
There were no minutes or days of psychological therapy services provided over the 7-day look-back period.

Recreational therapy services that were provided over the 7-day look-back period:

Recreational therapy services; Tuesday, Wednesday, and Friday for 30-minute sessions each day.

O0400: Therapies (cont.)

Coding:
O0400F1 would be **coded 90**, O0400F2 would be **coded 3**.

Rationale:
Total minutes were 90 over the 7-day look-back period ($30 \times 3 = 90$). Sessions provided were longer than 15 minutes each day, therefore each day recreational therapy was performed can be counted.

O0400. Therapies	
A. Speech-Language Pathology and Audiology Services	

Enter Number of Minutes: `1` `9` `0`

1. **Individual minutes** - record the total number of minutes this therapy was administered to the resident **individually** in the last 7 days

Enter Number of Minutes: `7` `0`

2. **Concurrent minutes** - record the total number of minutes this therapy was administered to the resident **concurrently with one other resident** in the last 7 days

Enter Number of Minutes: `7` `5`

3. **Group minutes** - record the total number of minutes this therapy was administered to the resident as **part of a group of residents** in the last 7 days

If the sum of individual, concurrent, and group minutes is zero, → skip to O0400A5, Therapy start date

Enter Number of Days: `5`

4. **Days** - record the **number of days** this therapy was administered for **at least 15 minutes** a day in the last 7 days

5. **Therapy start date** - record the date the most recent therapy regimen (since the most recent entry) started

`1` `0` – `0` `6` – `2` `0` `1` `1`
Month   Day   Year

6. **Therapy end date** - record the date the most recent therapy regimen (since the most recent entry) ended - enter dashes if therapy is ongoing

`-` `-` – `-` `-` – `-` `-` `-` `-`
Month   Day   Year

B. Occupational Therapy

Enter Number of Minutes: `1` `1` `3`

1. **Individual minutes** - record the total number of minutes this therapy was administered to the resident **individually** in the last 7 days

Enter Number of Minutes: `0`

2. **Concurrent minutes** - record the total number of minutes this therapy was administered to the resident **concurrently with one other resident** in the last 7 days

Enter Number of Minutes: `8` `0`

3. **Group minutes** - record the total number of minutes this therapy was administered to the resident as **part of a group of residents** in the last 7 days

If the sum of individual, concurrent, and group minutes is zero, → skip to O0400B5, Therapy start date

Enter Number of Days: `5`

4. **Days** - record the **number of days** this therapy was administered for **at least 15 minutes** a day in the last 7 days

5. **Therapy start date** - record the date the most recent therapy regimen (since the most recent entry) started

`1` `0` – `0` `9` – `2` `0` `1` `1`
Month   Day   Year

6. **Therapy end date** - record the date the most recent therapy regimen (since the most recent entry) ended - enter dashes if therapy is ongoing

`-` `-` – `-` `-` – `-` `-` `-` `-`
Month   Day   Year

O0400 continued on next page

O0400: Therapies (cont.)

	O0400. Therapies - Continued
	C. Physical Therapy
Enter Number of Minutes `2` `8` `7`	1. **Individual minutes** - record the total number of minutes this therapy was administered to the resident **individually** in the last 7 days
Enter Number of Minutes `1` `0` `0`	2. **Concurrent minutes** - record the total number of minutes this therapy was administered to the resident **concurrently with one other resident** in the last 7 days
Enter Number of Minutes `0`	3. **Group minutes** - record the total number of minutes this therapy was administered to the resident as **part of a group of residents** in the last 7 days
	If the sum of individual, concurrent, and group minutes is zero, → skip to O0400C5, Therapy start date
Enter Number of Days `5`	4. **Days** - record the **number of days** this therapy was administered for **at least 15 minutes** a day in the last 7 days
	5. **Therapy start date** - record the date the most recent therapy regimen (since the most recent entry) started 6. **Therapy end date** - record the date the most recent therapy regimen (since the most recent entry) ended - enter dashes if therapy is ongoing
	`1` `0` – `0` `7` – `2` `0` `1` `1` `-` `-` – `-` `-` – `-` `-` `-` `-` Month Day Year Month Day Year
	D. Respiratory Therapy
Enter Number of Minutes `5` `0`	1. **Total minutes** - record the total number of minutes this therapy was administered to the resident in the last 7 days If zero, → skip to O0400E, Psychological Therapy
Enter Number of Days `0`	2. **Days** - record the **number of days** this therapy was administered for **at least 15 minutes** a day in the last 7 days
	E. Psychological Therapy (by any licensed mental health professional)
Enter Number of Minutes `0`	1. **Total minutes** - record the total number of minutes this therapy was administered to the resident in the last 7 days If zero, → skip to O0400F, Recreational Therapy
Enter Number of Days ` `	2. **Days** - record the **number of days** this therapy was administered for **at least 15 minutes** a day in the last 7 days
	F. Recreational Therapy (includes recreational and music therapy)
Enter Number of Minutes `9` `0`	1. **Total minutes** - record the total number of minutes this therapy was administered to the resident in the last 7 days If zero, → skip to O0450, Resumption of Therapy
Enter Number of Days `3`	2. **Days** - record the **number of days** this therapy was administered for **at least 15 minutes** a day in the last 7 days

O0450: Resumption of Therapy

	O0450. Resumption of Therapy - Complete only if A0310C = 2 or 3 and A0310F = 99
Enter Code ` `	A. **Has a previous rehabilitation therapy regimen (speech, occupational, and/or physical therapy) ended, as reported on this End of Therapy OMRA, and has this regimen now resumed at exactly the same level for each discipline?** 0. **No** → Skip to O0500, Restorative Nursing Programs 1. **Yes**
	B. **Date on which therapy regimen resumed:** `  ` – `  ` – `    ` Month Day Year

Item Rationale

In cases where therapy resumes after the EOT OMRA is performed and the resumption of therapy date is no more than 5 consecutive calendar days after the last day of therapy provided,

O0450: Resumption of Therapy (cont.)

and the therapy services have resumed at the same RUG-IV classification level that had been in effect prior to the EOT OMRA, an End of Therapy OMRA with Resumption (EOT-R) may be completed. The EOT-R reduces the number of assessments that need to be completed and reduces the number of interview items residents must answer.

Coding Instructions:

When an EOT OMRA has been performed, determine whether therapy will resume. If it will, determine whether therapy will resume no more than five consecutive calendar days after the last day of therapy was provided AND whether the therapy services will resume at the same level for each discipline, if **no, skip to O0500**, Restorative Nursing Programs. If Yes, **code item O0450A as 1**. Determine when therapy will resume and code item **O0450B with the date** that therapy will resume. For example:

- Mrs. A. who was in RVL did not receive therapy on Saturday and Sunday because the facility did not provide weekend services and she missed therapy on Monday because of a doctor's appointment. She resumed therapy on Tuesday, November 13, 2011. The IDT determined that her RUG-IV therapy classification level did not change as she had not had any significant clinical changes during the lapsed therapy days. When the EOT was filled out, item **O0450 A was coded as 1** because therapy was resuming within 5 days from the last day of therapy and it was resuming at the same RUG-IV classification level. Item **O0450B was coded as 11132011** because therapy resumed on November 13, 2011.

NOTE: If the EOT OMRA has not been accepted in the QIES ASAP when therapy resumes, code the EOT-R items (O0450A and O0450B) on the assessment and submit the record. If the EOT OMRA without the EOT-R items have been accepted into the QIES ASAP system, then submit a modification request for that EOT OMRA with the only changes being the completion of the Resumption of Therapy items (O0450A and O0450B) and check X0900E to indicate that the reason for modification is the addition of the Resumption of Therapy date.

NOTE: When an EOT-R is completed, the Therapy start date (O0400A5, O0400B5, and O0400C5) on the next PPS assessment is the date of the Resumption of therapy on the EOT-R (O0450B). If therapy is ongoing, the Therapy end date (O0400A6, O0400B6, and O0400C6) would be filled out with dashes.

O0500: Restorative Nursing Programs

O0500. Restorative Nursing Programs	
Record the **number of days** each of the following restorative programs was performed (for at least 15 minutes a day) in the last 7 calendar days (enter 0 if none or less than 15 minutes daily)	
Number of Days	Technique
☐	A. Range of motion (passive)
☐	B. Range of motion (active)
☐	C. Splint or brace assistance
Number of Days	Training and Skill Practice In:
☐	D. Bed mobility
☐	E. Transfer
☐	F. Walking
☐	G. Dressing and/or grooming
☐	H. Eating and/or swallowing
☐	I. Amputation/prostheses care
☐	J. Communication

Item Rationale

Health-related Quality of Life

- Maintaining independence in activities of daily living and mobility is critically important to most people.
- Functional decline can lead to depression, withdrawal, social isolation, and complications of immobility, such as incontinence and pressure ulcers.

Planning for Care

- Restorative nursing program refers to nursing interventions that promote the resident's ability to adapt and adjust to living as independently and safely as possible. This concept actively focuses on achieving and maintaining optimal physical, mental, and psychosocial functioning.
- A resident may be started on a restorative nursing program when he or she is admitted to the facility with restorative needs, but is not a candidate for formalized rehabilitation therapy, or when restorative needs arise during the course of a longer-term stay, or in conjunction with formalized rehabilitation therapy. Generally, restorative nursing programs are initiated when a resident is discharged from formalized physical, occupational, or speech rehabilitation therapy.

Steps for Assessment

1. Review the restorative nursing program notes and/or flow sheets in the medical record.
2. For the 7-day look-back period, enter the number of days on which the technique, training or skill practice was performed for a total of at least 15 minutes during the 24-hour period.
3. The following criteria for restorative nursing programs must be met in order to code O0500:

O0500: Restorative Nursing Programs (cont.)

- Measureable objective and interventions must be documented in the care plan and in the medical record. If a restorative nursing program is in place when a care plan is being revised, it is appropriate to reassess progress, goals, and duration/frequency as part of the care planning process. Good clinical practice would indicate that the results of this reassessment should be documented in the resident's medical record.

- Evidence of periodic evaluation by the licensed nurse must be present in the resident's medical record. When not contraindicated by state practice act provisions, a progress note written by the restorative aide and countersigned by a licensed nurse is sufficient to document the restorative nursing program once the purpose and objectives of treatment have been established.

- Nursing assistants/aides must be trained in the techniques that promote resident involvement in the activity.

- A registered nurse or a licensed practical (vocational) nurse must supervise the activities in a restorative nursing program. Sometimes, under licensed nurse supervision, other staff and volunteers will be assigned to work with specific residents. Restorative nursing does not require a physician's order. Nursing homes may elect to have licensed rehabilitation professionals perform repetitive exercises and other maintenance treatments or to supervise aides performing these maintenance services. In these situations, the services may not be coded as therapy in item O0400, Therapies, because the specific interventions are considered restorative nursing services. The therapist's time actually providing the maintenance service can be included when counting restorative nursing minutes. Although therapists may participate, members of the nursing staff are still responsible for overall coordination and supervision of restorative nursing programs.

- This category does not include groups with more than four residents per supervising helper or caregiver.

Coding Instructions

- This item does not include procedures or techniques carried out by or under the direction of qualified therapists, as identified in **Speech-Language Pathology and Audiology Services** item O0400A, **Occupational Therapy** item O0400B, and **Physical Therapy** O0400C.

- The time provided for items O0500A-J must be coded separately, in time blocks of 15 minutes or more. For example, to check **Technique—Range of Motion [Passive]** item O0500A, 15 or more minutes of passive range of motion (PROM) must have been provided during a 24-hour period in the last 7 days. The 15 minutes of time in a day may be totaled across 24 hours (e.g., 10 minutes on the day shift plus 5 minutes on the evening shift). However, 15-minute time increments cannot be obtained by combining 5 minutes of **Technique—Range of Motion [Passive]** item O0500A, 5 minutes of **Technique— Range of Motion [Active]** item O0500B, and 5 minutes of **Splint or Brace Assistance** item O0500C, over 2 days in the last 7 days.

- Review for each activity throughout the 24-hour period. **Enter 0**, if none.

O0500: Restorative Nursing Programs (cont.)

Technique

Activities provided by restorative nursing staff.

- **O0500A, Range of Motion (Passive)**

  Code provision of passive movements in order to maintain flexibility and useful motion in the joints of the body. These exercises must be individualized to the resident's needs, planned, monitored, evaluated and documented in the resident's medical record.

- **O0500B, Range of Motion (Active)**

  Code exercises performed by the resident, with cueing, supervision, or physical assist by staff that are individualized to the resident's needs, planned, monitored, evaluated, and documented in the resident's medical record. Include active ROM and active-assisted ROM.

- **O0500C, Splint or Brace Assistance**

  Code provision of (1) verbal and physical guidance and direction that teaches the resident how to apply, manipulate, and care for a brace or splint; or (2) a scheduled program of applying and removing a splint or brace. These sessions are individualized to the resident's needs, planned, monitored, evaluated, and documented in the resident's medical record.

Training and Skill Practice

Activities including repetition, physical or verbal cueing, and/or task segmentation provided by any staff member under the supervision of a licensed nurse.

- **O0500D, Bed Mobility**

  Code activities provided to improve or maintain the resident's self-performance in moving to and from a lying position, turning side to side and positioning himself or herself in bed. These activities are individualized to the resident's needs, planned, monitored, evaluated, and documented in the resident's medical record.

- **O0500E, Transfer**

  Code activities provided to improve or maintain the resident's self-performance in moving between surfaces or planes either with or without assistive devices. These activities are individualized to the resident's needs, planned, monitored, evaluated, and documented in the resident's medical record.

- **O0500F, Walking**

  Code activities provided to improve or maintain the resident's self-performance in walking, with or without assistive devices. These activities are individualized to the resident's needs, planned, monitored, evaluated, and documented in the resident's medical record.

O0500: Restorative Nursing Programs (cont.)

- **O0500G, Dressing and/or Grooming**

  Code activities provided to improve or maintain the resident's self-performance in dressing and undressing, bathing and washing, and performing other personal hygiene tasks. These activities are individualized to the resident's needs, planned, monitored, evaluated, and documented in the resident's medical record.

- **O0500H, Eating and/or Swallowing**

  Code activities provided to improve or maintain the resident's self-performance in feeding oneself food and fluids, or activities used to improve or maintain the resident's ability to ingest nutrition and hydration by mouth. These activities are individualized to the resident's needs, planned, monitored, evaluated, and documented in the resident's medical record.

- **O0500I, Amputation/ Prosthesis Care**

  Code activities provided to improve or maintain the resident's self-performance in putting on and removing a prosthesis, caring for the prosthesis, and providing appropriate hygiene at the site where the prosthesis attaches to the body (e.g., leg stump or eye socket). Dentures are not considered to be prostheses for coding this item. These activities are individualized to the resident's needs, planned, monitored, evaluated, and documented in the resident's medical record.

- **O0500J, Communication**

  Code activities provided to improve or maintain the resident's self-performance in functional communication skills or assisting the resident in using residual communication skills and adaptive devices. These activities are individualized to the resident's needs, planned, monitored, evaluated, and documented in the resident's medical record.

Coding Tips and Special Populations

- For range of motion (passive): the caregiver moves the body part around a fixed point or joint through the resident's available range of motion. The resident provides no assistance.

- For range of motion (active): any participation by the resident in the ROM activity should be coded here.

- For both active and passive range of motion: movement by a resident that is incidental to dressing, bathing, etc., does not count as part of a formal restorative nursing program. For inclusion in this section, active or passive range of motion must be a component of an individualized program that is planned, monitored evaluated, and documented in the resident's medical record. Range of motion should be delivered by staff who are trained in the procedures.

- For splint or brace assistance: assess the resident's skin and circulation under the device, and reposition the limb in correct alignment.

- The use of continuous passive motion (CPM) devices in a restorative nursing program is coded when the following criteria are met: (1) ordered by a physician, (2) nursing staff

O0500: Restorative Nursing Programs (cont.)

have been trained in technique (e.g., properly aligning resident's limb in device, adjusting available range of motion), and (3) monitoring of the device. Nursing staff should document the application of the device and the effects on the resident. Do not include the time the resident is receiving treatment in the device. Include only the actual time staff were engaged in applying and monitoring the device.

- Remember that persons with dementia learn skills best through repetition that occurs multiple times per day.

- Grooming programs, including programs to help residents learn to apply make-up, may be considered restorative nursing programs when conducted by a member of the activity staff. These grooming programs would need to be individualized to the resident's needs, planned, monitored, evaluated, and documented in the resident's medical record.

Examples

1. Mr. V. has lost range of motion in his right arm, wrist, and hand due to a cerebrovascular accident (CVA) experienced several years ago. He has moderate to severe loss of cognitive decision-making skills and memory. To avoid further ROM loss and contractures to his right arm, the occupational therapist fabricated a right resting hand splint and instructions for its application and removal. The nursing coordinator developed instructions for providing passive range of motion exercises to his right arm, wrist, and hand three times per day. The nurse's aides and Mr. V.'s wife have been instructed in how and when to apply and remove the hand splint and how to do the passive ROM exercises. These plans are documented in Mr. V.'s care plan. The total amount of time involved each day in removing and applying the hand splint and completing the ROM exercises is 30 minutes (15 minutes to perform ROM exercises and 15 minutes to apply/remove the splint). The nurse's aides report that there is less resistance in Mr. V.'s affected extremity when bathing and dressing him.

    Coding: Both **Splint or Brace Assistance** item (O0500C), and **Range of Motion (Passive)** item (O0500A), would be **coded 7.**

    Rationale: Because this was the number of days these restorative nursing techniques were provided.

2. Mrs. R.'s right shoulder ROM has decreased slightly over the past week. Upon examination and X-ray, her physician diagnosed her with right shoulder impingement syndrome. Mrs. R. was given exercises to perform on a daily basis to help improve her right shoulder ROM. After initial training in these exercises by the physical therapist, Mrs. R. and the nursing staff were provided with instructions on how to cue and sometimes actively assist Mrs. R. when she cannot make the full ROM required by the exercises on her own. Her exercises are to be performed for 15 minutes, two times per day at change of shift in the morning and afternoon. This information is documented in Mrs. R.'s medical record. The nursing staff cued and sometimes actively assisted Mrs. R. two times daily over the past 7 days.

    Coding: **Range of motion (active)** item (O0500B), would be **coded 7.**

    Rationale: Because this was the number of days restorative nursing training and skill practice for active ROM were provided.

O0500: Restorative Nursing Programs (cont.)

3. Mrs. K. was admitted to the nursing facility 7 days ago following repair to a fractured hip. Physical therapy was delayed due to complications and a weakened condition. Upon admission, she had difficulty moving herself in bed and required total assistance for transfers. To prevent further deterioration and increase her independence, the nursing staff implemented a plan on the second day following admission to teach her how to move herself in bed and transfer from bed to chair using a trapeze, the bed rails, and a transfer board. The plan was documented in Mrs. K.'s medical record and communicated to all staff at the change of shift. The charge nurse documented in the nurse's notes that in the 5 days Mrs. K. has been receiving training and skill practice for bed mobility for 20 minutes a day and transferring for 25 minutes a day, her endurance and strength have improved, and she requires only extensive assistance for transferring. Each day the amount of time to provide this nursing restorative intervention has been decreasing, so that for the past 5 days, the average time is 45 minutes.

    Coding: Both **Bed Mobility** item (O0500D), **Transfer** item (O0500E), would be **coded 5.**

    Rationale: Because this was the number of days that restorative nursing training and skill practice for bed mobility and transfer were provided.

4. Mrs. D. is receiving training and skill practice in walking using a quad cane. Together, Mrs. D. and the nursing staff have set progressive walking distance goals. The nursing staff has received instruction on how to provide Mrs. D. with the instruction and guidance she needs to achieve the goals. She has three scheduled times each day where she learns how to walk with her quad cane. Each teaching and practice episode for walking, supervised by a nursing assistant, takes approximately 15 minutes.

    Coding: **Walking** item (O0500F), would be **coded 7.**

    Rationale: Because this was the number of days that restorative nursing skill and practice training for walking was provided.

5. Mrs. J. had a CVA less than a year ago resulting in left-sided hemiplegia. Mrs. J. has a strong desire to participate in her own care. Although she cannot dress herself independently, she is capable of participating in this activity of daily living. Mrs. J.'s overall care plan goal is to maximize her independence in ADLs. A plan, documented on the care plan, has been developed to assist Mrs. J. in how to maintain the ability to put on and take off her blouse with no physical assistance from the staff. All of her blouses have been adapted for front closure with velcro. The nursing assistants have been instructed in how to verbally guide Mrs. J. as she puts on and takes off her blouse to enhance her efficiency and maintain her level of function. It takes approximately 20 minutes per day for Mrs. J. to complete this task (dressing and undressing).

    Coding: **Dressing or Grooming** item (O0500G), would be **coded 7.**

    Rationale: Because this was the number of days that restorative nursing training and skill practice for dressing and grooming were provided.

O0500: Restorative Nursing Programs (cont.)

6. Mr. W.'s cognitive status has been deteriorating progressively over the past several months. Despite deliberate nursing restoration, attempts to promote his independence in feeding himself, he will not eat unless he is fed.

    Coding: Eating and/or Swallowing item (O0500H), would be **coded 0.**

    Rationale: Because restorative nursing skill and practice training for eating and/or swallowing were not provided over the last 7 days.

7. Mrs. E. has Amyotrophic Lateral Sclerosis. She no longer has the ability to speak or even to nod her head "yes" or "no." Her cognitive skills remain intact, she can spell, and she can move her eyes in all directions. The speech-language pathologist taught both Mrs. E. and the nursing staff to use a communication board so that Mrs. E. could communicate with staff. The communication board has been in use over the past 2 weeks and has proven very successful. The nursing staff, volunteers, and family members are reminded by a sign over Mrs. E.'s bed that they are to provide her with the board to enable her to communicate with them. This is also documented in Mrs. E.'s care plan. Because the teaching and practice using the communication board had been completed 2 weeks ago and Mrs. E. is able to use the board to communicate successfully, she no longer receives skill and practice training in communication.

    Coding: Communication item (O0500J), would be **coded 0.**

    Rationale: Because the resident has mastered the skill of communication, restorative nursing skill and practice training for communication was no longer needed or provided over the last 7 days.

O0600: Physician Examinations

O0600. Physician Examinations	
Enter Days	Over the last 14 days, **on how many days did the physician (or authorized assistant or practitioner) examine the resident?**

Item Rationale

Health-related Quality of Life

-   Health status that requires frequent physician examinations can adversely affect an individual's sense of well-being and functional status and can limit social activities.

Planning for Care

-   Frequency of physician examinations can be an indication of medical complexity and stability of the resident's health status.

O0600: Physician Examinations (cont.)

Steps for Assessment

1. Review the physician progress notes for evidence of examinations of the resident by the physician or other authorized practitioners.

Coding Instructions

- Record the **number of days** that physician progress notes reflect that a physician examined the resident (or since admission if less than 14 days ago).

Coding Tips and Special Populations

- Includes medical doctors, doctors of osteopathy, podiatrists, dentists, and authorized physician assistants, nurse practitioners, or clinical nurse specialists working in collaboration with the physician as allowable by state law.

- Examination (partial or full) can occur in the facility or in the physician's office. Included in this item are telehealth visits as long as the requirements are met for physician/practitioner type as defined above and whether it qualifies as a telehealth billable visit. For eligibility requirements and additional information about Medicare telehealth services refer to:

  — Chapter 15 of the *Medicare Benefit Policy Manual* (Pub. 100-2) and Chapter 12 of the *Medicare Claims Processing Manual* (Pub. 100-4) may be accessed at: http://www.cms.gov/Regulations-and-Guidance/Guidance/Manuals/Internet-Only-Manuals-IOMs.html.

- Do not include physician examinations that occurred prior to admission or readmission to the facility (e.g., during the resident's acute care stay).

- Do not include physician examinations that occurred during an emergency room visit or hospital observation stay.

- If a resident is evaluated by a physician off-site (e.g., while undergoing dialysis or radiation therapy), it can be coded as a physician examination as long as documentation of the physician's evaluation is included in the medical record. The physician's evaluation can include partial or complete examination of the resident, monitoring the resident for response to the treatment, or adjusting the treatment as a result of the examination.

- The licensed psychological therapy by a Psychologist (PhD) should be recorded in O0400E, **Psychological Therapy**.

- Does not include visits made by Medicine Men.

O0700: Physician Orders

O0700. Physician Orders	
Enter Days [ ][ ]	Over the last 14 days, **on how many days did the physician (or authorized assistant or practitioner) change the resident's orders?**

Item Rationale

Health-related Quality of Life

- Health status that requires frequent physician order changes can adversely affect an individual's sense of well-being and functional status and can limit social activities.

Planning for Care

- Frequency of physician order changes can be an indication of medical complexity and stability of the resident's health status.

Steps for Assessment

1. Review the physician order sheets in the medical record.
2. Determine the number of days during the 14-day look-back period that a physician changed the resident's orders.

Coding Instructions

- Enter the **number of days** during 14-day look-back period (or since admission, if less than 14 days ago) in which a physician changed the resident's orders.

Coding Tips and Special Populations

- Includes orders written by medical doctors, doctors of osteopathy, podiatrists, dentists, and physician assistants, nurse practitioners, or clinical nurse specialists working in collaboration with the physician as allowable by state law.
- Includes written, telephone, fax, or consultation orders for new or altered treatment. Does **not** include standard admission orders, return admission orders, renewal orders, or clarifying orders without changes. Orders written on the day of admission as a result for an unexpected change/deterioration in condition or injury are considered as new or altered treatment orders and should be counted as a day with order changes.
- The prohibition against counting standard admission or readmission orders applies regardless of whether or not the orders are given at one time or are received at different times on the date of admission or readmission.
- Do not count orders prior to the date of admission or re-entry.
- A sliding scale dosage schedule that is written to cover different dosages depending on lab values, does **not** count as an order change simply because a different dose is administered based on the sliding scale guidelines.

O0700: Physician Orders (cont.)

- When a PRN (as needed) order was already on file, the potential need for the service had already been identified. Notification of the physician that the PRN order was activated does **not** constitute a new or changed order and may **not** be counted when coding this item.

- A Medicare Certification/Recertification is a renewal of an existing order and should **not** be included when coding this item.

- If a resident has multiple physicians (e.g., surgeon, cardiologist, internal medicine), and they all visit and write orders on the same day, the MDS must be coded as 1 day during which a physician visited, and 1 day in which orders were changed.

- Orders requesting a consultation by another physician may be counted. However, the order must be reasonable (e.g., for a new or altered treatment).

- An order written on the last day of the MDS observation period for a consultation planned 3-6 months in the future should be carefully reviewed.

- Orders written to increase the resident's RUG classification and facility payment are **not** acceptable.

- Orders for transfer of care to another physician may **not** be counted.

- Do **not** count orders written by a pharmacist.

SECTION P: RESTRAINTS

Intent: The intent of this section is to record the frequency over the 7-day look-back period that the resident was restrained by any of the listed devices at any time during the day or night. Assessors will evaluate whether or not a device meets the definition of a physical restraint and code only the devices that meet the definition in the appropriate categories of Item P0100.

CMS is committed to reducing unnecessary physical restraints in nursing homes and ensuring that residents are free of physical restraints unless deemed necessary and appropriate as permitted by regulation. Proper interpretation of the physical restraint definition is necessary to understand if nursing homes are accurately assessing manual methods or physical or mechanical devices, materials or equipment as physical restraints and meeting the federal requirement for restraint use (see Centers for Medicare & Medicaid Services. [2007, June 22]. Memorandum to State Survey Agency Directors from CMS Director, Survey and Certification Group: Clarification of Terms Used in the Definition of Physical Restraints as Applied to the Requirements for Long Term Care Facilities. Retrieved December 18, 2012, from http://www.cms.gov/Medicare/Provider-Enrollment-and-Certification/SurveyCertificationGenInfo/downloads/SCLetter07-22.pdf).

Are Restraints Prohibited by CMS?

> **DEFINITIONS**
>
> **PHYSICAL RESTRAINTS**
> Any manual method or physical or mechanical device, material or equipment attached or adjacent to the resident's body that the individual cannot remove easily, which restricts freedom of movement or normal access to one's body (State Operations Manual, Appendix PP).

Federal regulations and CMS guidelines do not prohibit use of physical restraints in nursing homes, except when they are imposed for discipline or convenience and are not required to treat the resident's medical symptoms. The regulation specifically states, "The resident has the right to be free from any physical or chemical restraints imposed for the purposes of discipline or convenience and not required to treat the resident's medical symptoms" (42 CFR 483.13(a)). Research and standards of practice show that physical restraints have many negative side effects and risks that far outweigh any benefit from their use.

Prior to using any physical restraint, the nursing home must assess the resident to properly identify the resident's needs and the medical symptom(s) that the restraint is being employed to address. If a physical restraint is needed to treat the resident's medical symptom, the nursing home is responsible for assessing the appropriateness of that restraint. When the decision is made to use a physical restraint, CMS encourages, to the extent possible, gradual restraint reduction because there are many negative outcomes associated with restraint use.

While a restraint-free environment is not a federal requirement, the use of physical restraints should be the exception, not the rule.

P0100: Physical Restraints

P0100. Physical Restraints		
Physical restraints are any manual method or physical or mechanical device, material or equipment attached or adjacent to the resident's body that the individual cannot remove easily which restricts freedom of movement or normal access to one's body		
	↓ Enter Codes in Boxes	
		Used in Bed
	☐	A. Bed rail
	☐	B. Trunk restraint
	☐	C. Limb restraint
Coding:	☐	D. Other
0. **Not used**		**Used in Chair or Out of Bed**
1. **Used less than daily**	☐	E. Trunk restraint
2. **Used daily**	☐	F. Limb restraint
	☐	G. Chair prevents rising
	☐	H. Other

Item Rationale

Health-related Quality of Life

- Although the requirements describe the narrow instances when physical restraints may be used, growing evidence supports that physical restraints have a limited role in medical care. Physical restraints limit mobility and increase the risk for a number of adverse outcomes, such as functional decline, agitation, diminished sense of dignity, depression, and pressure ulcers.

- Residents who are cognitively impaired are at a higher risk of entrapment and injury or death caused by physical restraints. It is vital that physical restraints used on this population be carefully considered and monitored. In many cases, the risk of using the physical restraint may be greater than the risk of it not being used.

- The risk of restraint-related injury and death is significant when physical restraints are used.

Planning for Care

- When the use of physical restraints is considered, thorough assessment of problems to be addressed by restraint use is necessary to determine reversible causes and contributing factors and to identify alternative methods of treating non-reversible issues.

- When the interdisciplinary team determines that the use of physical restraints is the appropriate course of action, and there is a signed physician order that gives the medical symptom supporting the use of the restraint, the least restrictive manual method or physical or mechanical device, material or equipment that will meet the resident's needs must be selected.

- Care planning must focus on preventing the adverse effects of physical restraint use.

P0100: Physical Restraints (cont.)

Steps for Assessment

1. Review the resident's medical record (e.g., physician orders, nurses' notes, nursing assistant documentation) to determine if physical restraints were used during the 7-day look-back period.

2. Consult the nursing staff to determine the resident's cognitive and physical status/limitations.

3. Considering the physical restraint definition as well as the clarifications listed below, observe the resident to determine the effect the restraint has on the resident's normal function. Do not focus on the type, intent, or reason behind its use.

4. Evaluate whether the resident can easily and voluntarily remove any manual method or physical or mechanical device, material, or equipment attached or adjacent to his or her body. If the resident cannot easily and voluntarily do this, continue with the assessment to determine whether or not the manual method or physical or mechanical device, material or equipment restrict freedom of movement or restrict the resident's access to his or her own body.

5. Any manual method or physical or mechanical device, material or equipment should be classified as a restraint only when it meets the criteria of the physical restraint definition. This can only be determined on a case-by-case basis by individually assessing each and every manual method or physical or mechanical device, material or equipment (whether or not it is listed specifically on the MDS) attached or adjacent to the resident's body, and the effect it has on the resident.

6. Determine if the manual method or physical or mechanical device, material, or equipment meets the definition of a physical restraint as clarified below. Remember, the decision about coding any manual method or physical or mechanical device, material, equipment as a restraint depends on the effect it has on the resident.

7. Any manual method or physical or mechanical device, material, or equipment that meets the definition of a physical restraint must have:

   - physician documentation of a medical symptom that supports the use of the restraint,

   - a physician's order for the type of restraint and parameters of use, and

   - a care plan and a process in place for systematic and gradual restraint reduction (and/or elimination, if possible), as appropriate.

Clarifications

- **"Remove easily"** means that the manual method or physical or mechanical device, material, or equipment can be removed intentionally by the resident in the same manner as it was applied by the staff (e.g., side rails are put down or not climbed over, buckles are intentionally unbuckled, ties or knots are intentionally untied), considering the resident's physical condition and ability to accomplish his or her objective (e.g., transfer to a chair, get to the bathroom in time).

- **"Freedom of movement"** means any change in place or position for the body or any part of the body that the person is physically able to control or access.

P0100: Physical Restraints (cont.)

- **"Medical symptoms/diagnoses"** are defined as an indication or characteristic of a physical or psychological condition. Objective findings derived from clinical evaluation of the resident's subjective symptoms and medical diagnoses should be considered when determining the presence of medical symptom(s) that might support restraint use. **The resident's subjective symptoms may not be used as the sole basis for using a restraint. In addition, the resident's medical symptoms/diagnoses should not be viewed in isolation; rather, the medical symptoms identified should become the context in which to determine the most appropriate method of treatment related to the resident's condition, circumstances, and environment, and not a way to justify restraint use.**

- The identification of medical symptoms should assist the nursing home in determining if the specific medical symptom can be improved or addressed by using other, less restrictive interventions. The nursing home should perform all due diligence and document this process to ensure that they have exhausted alternative treatments and less restrictive measures before a physical restraint is employed to treat the medical symptom, protect the resident's safety, help the resident attain or maintain his or her highest level of physical or psychological well-being and support the resident's goals, wishes, independence, and self-direction.

- **Physical restraints as an intervention do not treat the underlying causes of medical symptoms. Therefore, as with other interventions, physical restraints should not be used without also seeking to identify and address the physical or psychological condition causing the medical symptom.**

- Physical restraints may be used, if warranted, as a temporary symptomatic intervention while the actual cause of the medical symptom is being evaluated and managed. Additionally, physical restraints may be used as a symptomatic intervention when they are immediately necessary to prevent a resident from injuring himself/herself or others and/or to prevent the resident from interfering with life-sustaining treatment when no other less restrictive or less risky interventions exist.

- Therefore, a clear link must exist between physical restraint use and how it benefits the resident by addressing the specific medical symptom. If it is determined, after thorough evaluation and attempts at using alternative treatments and less restrictive methods, that a physical restraint must still be employed, the medical symptoms that support the use of the restraint must be documented in the resident's medical record, ongoing assessments, and care plans. There also must be a physician's order reflecting the use of the physical restraint and the specific medical symptom being treated by its use. The physician's order alone is not sufficient to employ the use of a physical restraint. CMS will hold the nursing home ultimately accountable for the appropriateness of that determination.

P0100: Physical Restraints (cont.)

Coding Instructions

Identify all physical restraints that were used at any time (day or night) during the 7-day look-back period.

After determining whether or not an item listed in (P0100) is a physical restraint and was used during the 7-day look-back period, code the frequency of use:

- **Code 0, not used:** if the item was not used during the 7-day look-back **or** it was used but did not meet the definition.
- **Code 1, used less than daily:** if the item met the definition and was used less than daily.
- **Code 2, used daily:** if the item met the definition and was used on a daily basis during the look-back period.

Coding Tips and Special Populations

- Any manual method or physical or mechanical device, material or equipment, that does not fit into the listed categories but that meets the definition of a physical restraint, and has not been excluded from this section, should be coded in items P0100D or P0100H, Other. These devices, although not coded on the MDS, must be assessed, care-planned, monitored, and evaluated.

- In classifying any manual method or physical or mechanical device, material or equipment as a physical restraint, the assessor must consider the effect it has on the resident, not the purpose or intent of its use. It is possible that a manual method or physical or mechanical device, material or equipment may improve a resident's mobility but also have the effect of physically restraining him or her.

- Exclude from this section items that are typically used in the provision of medical care, such as catheters, drainage tubes, casts, traction, leg, arm, neck, or back braces, abdominal binders, and bandages that are serving in their usual capacity to meet medical need(s).

- **Bed rails** include any combination of partial or full rails (e.g., one-side half-rail, one-side full rail, two-sided half-rails or quarter-rails, rails along the side of the bed that block three-quarters to the whole length of the mattress from top to bottom, etc.). Include in this category enclosed bed systems.

  — *Bed rails used as positioning devices.* If the use of bed rails (quarter-, half- or three-quarter, one or both, etc.) meet the definition of a physical restraint even though they may improve the resident's mobility in bed, the nursing home must code their use as a restraint at P0100A.

  — *Bed rails used with residents who are immobile.* If the resident is immobile and cannot voluntarily get out of bed because of a physical limitation or because proper assistive devices were not present, the bed rails do not meet the definition of a physical restraint.

  For residents who have no voluntary movement, the staff need to determine if there is an appropriate use of bed rails. Bed rails may create a visual barrier and deter

P0100: Physical Restraints (cont.)

physical contact from others. Some residents have no ability to carry out voluntary movements, yet they exhibit involuntary movements. Involuntary movements, resident weight, and gravity's effects may lead to the resident's body shifting toward the edge of the bed. When bed rails are used in these cases, the resident could be at risk for entrapment. For this type of resident, clinical evaluation of alternatives (e.g., a concave mattress to keep the resident from going over the edge of the bed), coupled with frequent monitoring of the resident's position, should be considered. While the bed rails may not constitute a physical restraint, they may affect the resident's quality of life and create an accident hazard.

- **Trunk restraints** include any manual method or physical or mechanical device, material or equipment attached or adjacent to the resident's body that the resident cannot easily remove such as, but not limited to, vest or waist restraints or belts used in a wheelchair that either restricts freedom of movement or access to his or her body

- **Limb restraints** include any manual method or physical or mechanical device, material or equipment that the resident cannot easily remove, that restricts movement of any part of an upper extremity (i.e., hand, arm, wrist) or lower extremity (i.e., foot, leg) that either restricts freedom of movement or access to his or her own body. Hand mitts/mittens are included in this category.

- **Trunk or limb restraints**, if used in both bed and chair, should be marked in both sections.

- **Chairs that prevent rising** include any type of chair with a locked lap board, that places the resident in a recumbent position that restricts rising, chairs that are soft and low to the floor, chairs that have a cushion placed in the seat that prohibit the resident from rising, geriatric chairs, and enclosed-frame wheeled walkers.

  — For residents who have the ability to transfer from other chairs, but cannot transfer from a geriatric chair, the geriatric chair would be considered a restraint to that individual, and should be coded as P0100G–Chair Prevents Rising.

  — For residents who have no ability to transfer independently, the geriatric chair does not meet the definition of a restraint, and should not be coded at P0100G–Chair Prevents Rising.

  — Geriatric chairs used for residents who are immobile. For residents who have no voluntary or involuntary movement, the geriatric chair does not meet the definition of a restraint.

  — Enclosed-frame wheeled walkers, with or without a posterior seat, and other devices like it should not automatically be classified as a physical restraint. These types of walkers are only classified as a physical restraint if the resident cannot exit the walker via opening a gate, bar, strap, latch, removing a tray, etc. When deemed a physical restraint, these walkers should be coded at P0100G–Chair Prevents Rising.

- **Restraints used in emergency situations.** If the resident needs emergency care, physical restraints may be used for brief periods to permit medical treatment to proceed, unless the

P0100: Physical Restraints (cont.)

resident or legal representative has previously made a valid refusal of the treatment in question. The resident's right to participate in care planning and the right to refuse treatment are addressed at 42 CFR §§483.10(b)(4) and 483.20(k)(2)(ii) respectively. The use of physical restraints in this instance should be limited to preventing the resident from interfering with life-sustaining procedures only and not for routine care.

— A resident who is injuring himself/herself or is threatening physical harm to others may be physically restrained in an emergency to safeguard the resident and others. A resident whose unanticipated violent or aggressive behavior places him/her or others in imminent danger does not have the right to refuse the use of physical restraints, as long as those restraints are used as a last resort to protect the safety of the resident or others and use is limited to the immediate episode.

Additional Information

- **Restraint reduction/elimination.** It is further expected, for residents whose care plan indicates the need for physical restraints, that the nursing home engages in a systematic and gradual process towards reducing (or eliminating, if possible) the restraints (e.g., gradually increasing the time for ambulation and strengthening activities). This systematic process also applies to recently-admitted residents for whom physical restraints were used in the previous setting.

- **Restraints as a fall prevention approach.** Although physical restraints have been traditionally used as a fall prevention approach, they have major drawbacks and can contribute to serious injuries. Falls do not constitute self-injurious behavior nor a medical symptom supporting the use of physical restraints. There is no evidence that the use of physical restraints, including but not limited to side rails, will prevent, reduce, or eliminate falls. In fact, in some instances, reducing the use of physical restraints may actually decrease the risk of falling. Additionally, falls that occur while a person is physically restrained often result in more severe injuries.

- **Request for restraints.** While a resident, family member, legal representative, or surrogate may request use of a physical restraint, the nursing home is responsible for evaluating the appropriateness of that request, just as they would for any medical treatment. As with other medical treatments, such as the use of prescription drugs, a resident, family member, legal representative, or surrogate has the right to refuse treatment, but not to demand its use when it is not deemed medically necessary.

According to 42 CFR 483.13(a), "The resident has the right to be free from any physical or chemical restraints imposed for the purposes of discipline or convenience and not required to treat the resident's medical symptoms." CMS expects that no resident will be physically restrained for discipline or convenience. Prior to employing any physical restraint, the nursing home must perform a prescribed resident assessment to properly identify the resident's needs and the medical symptom the physical restraint is being employed to address. The guidelines in the State Operations Manual (SOM) state, "...the legal surrogate or representative cannot give permission to use restraints for the sake of discipline or staff convenience or when the restraint is not necessary to treat the resident's medical symptoms. That is, the facility may not use restraints in violation of regulation

P0100: Physical Restraints (cont.)

solely based on a resident, legal surrogate or representative's request or approval." The SOM goes on to state, "While Federal regulations affirm the resident's right to participate in care planning and to refuse treatment, the regulations do not create the right for a resident, legal surrogate or representative to demand that the facility use specific medical interventions or treatment that the facility deems inappropriate. Statutory requirements hold the facility ultimately accountable for the resident's care and safety, including clinical decisions."

SECTION Q: PARTICIPATION IN ASSESSMENT AND GOAL SETTING

Intent: The items in this section are intended to record the participation and expectations of the resident, family members, or significant other(s) in the assessment, and to understand the resident's overall goals. Discharge planning follow-up is already a regulatory requirement (CFR 483.20 (i) (3)). Section Q of the MDS uses a person-centered approach and to insure that all individuals have the opportunity to learn about home and community based services and have an opportunity to receive long term care in the least restrictive setting possible. Interviewing the resident or designated individuals places the resident or their family at the center of decision-making.

Q0100: Participation in Assessment

Q0100. Participation in Assessment	
Enter Code [ ]	A. Resident participated in assessment 　　0. No 　　1. Yes
Enter Code [ ]	B. Family or significant other participated in assessment 　　0. No 　　1. Yes 　　9. No family or significant other available
Enter Code [ ]	C. Guardian or legally authorized representative participated in assessment 　　0. No 　　1. Yes 　　9. No guardian or legally authorized representative available

Item Rationale

Health-related Quality of Life

- Residents who actively participate in the assessment process and in developing their care plan through interview and conversation often experience improved quality of life and higher quality care based on their needs, goals, and priorities.

Planning for Care

- Each care plan should be individualized and resident-driven. Whenever possible, the resident should be actively involved-except in unusual circumstances such as if the individual is unable to understand the proceedings or is comatose. Involving the resident in all assessment interviews and care planning meetings is also important to address dignity and self-determination survey and certification requirements (CFR §483.15 Quality of Life).

> **DEFINITIONS**
>
> **RESIDENT'S PARTICIPATION IN ASSESSMENT**
>
> The resident actively engages in interviews and conversations to meaningfully contribute to the completion of the MDS 3.0. Interdisciplinary team members should engage the resident during assessment in order to determine the resident's expectations and perspective during assessment.

Q0100: Participation in Assessment (cont.)

- During the care planning meetings, he or she should be made comfortable and verbal communication should be directly with him or her.

- Residents should be asked about inviting family members, significant others, and/or guardian/legally authorized representatives to participate, and if they desire that they be involved in the assessment process.

- If the individual resident is unable to understand the process, his or her family member, significant other, and/or guardian/legally authorized representative, who represents the individual, should be invited to attend the assessment process whenever possible.

- When the resident is unable to participate in the assessment process, a family member or significant other, and/or guardian or legally authorized representatives can provide information about the resident's needs, goals, and priorities.

Steps for Assessment

1. Review the medical record for documentation that the resident, family member and/or significant other, and guardian or legally authorized representative participated in the assessment process.

2. Ask the resident, the family member or significant other (when applicable), and the guardian or legally authorized representative (when applicable) if he or she actively participated in the assessment process.

3. Ask staff members who completed the assessment whether or not the resident, family or significant other, or guardian or legally authorized representative participated in the assessment process.

> **DEFINITIONS**
>
> **FAMILY OR SIGNIFICANT OTHER**
> A spousal, kinship (e.g., sibling, child, parent, nephew), or in-law relationship; a partner, housemate, primary community caregiver or close friend. Significant other does not, however, include staff at the nursing home.
>
> **GUARDIAN/LEGALLY AUTHORIZED REPRESENTATIVE**
> A person who is authorized, under applicable law, to make decisions for the resident, including giving and withholding consent for medical treatment.

Coding Instructions for Q0100A, Resident Participated in Assessment

Record the participation of the resident in the assessment process.

- **Code 0, No:** if the resident did not actively participate in the assessment process.

- **Code 1, Yes:** if the resident actively and meaningfully participated in the assessment process.

Coding Instructions for Q0100B, Family or Significant Other Participated in Assessment

Record the participation of the family or significant other in the assessment process.

- **Code 0, No:** if the family or significant other did not participate in the assessment process.

Q0100: Participation in Assessment (cont.)

- **Code 1, Yes:** if the family or significant other(s) did participate in the assessment process.
- **Code 9, No family or significant other available:** None of the above—resident has no family or significant other.

Coding Instructions for Q0100C, Guardian or Legally Authorized Representative Participated in Assessment

Record the participation of the guardian or legally authorized representative in the assessment process.

- **Code 0, No:** if guardian or legally authorized representative did not participate in the assessment process.
- **Code 1, Yes:** if guardian or legally authorized representative did participate in the assessment process.
- **Code 9, No guardian or legally authorized representative available:** None of the above -- resident has no guardian or legally authorized representative.

Coding Tips

- While family, significant others, or, if necessary, the guardian or legally authorized representative can be involved, the response selected must reflect the resident's perspective if he or she is able to express it.

- Significant other does not include nursing home staff.

- No family or significant other available means the individual resident has no family or significant other, not that they were not consulted.

Q0300: Resident's Overall Expectation

Complete only when A0310E=1. (First assessment on admission/entry or reentry).

Q0300. Resident's Overall Expectation	
Complete only if A0310E = 1	
Enter Code ☐	**A. Select one for resident's overall goal established during assessment process** 1. Expects to be **discharged to the community** 2. Expects to **remain in this facility** 3. Expects to be **discharged to another facility/institution** 9. **Unknown or uncertain**
Enter Code ☐	**B. Indicate information source for Q0300A** 1. **Resident** 2. If not resident, then **family or significant other** 3. If not resident, family, or significant other, then **guardian or legally authorized representative** 9. **Unknown or uncertain**

Q0300: Resident's Overall Expectation (cont.)

Item Rationale

This item identifies the resident's general expectations and goals for nursing home stay. The resident should be asked about his or her own expectations regarding return to the community and goals for care. The resident may not be aware of the option of returning to the community and that services and supports may be available in the community to meet long-term care needs. Additional assessment information may be needed to determine whether the resident requires additional community services and supports.

Some residents have very clear and directed expectations that will change little prior to discharge. Other residents may be unsure or may be experiencing an evolution in their thinking as their clinical condition changes or stabilizes.

Health-related Quality of Life

- Unless the resident's goals for care are understood, his or her needs, goals, and priorities are not likely to be met.

Planning for Care

- The resident's goals should be the basis for care planning.

DEFINITIONS
DISCHARGE To release from nursing home care. Can be to home, another community setting, or healthcare setting.

Steps for Assessment

1. Ask the resident about his or her overall expectations to be sure that he or she has participated in the assessment process and has a better understanding of his or her current situation and the implications of alternative choices.

2. Ask the resident to consider his or her current health status, expectations regarding improvement or worsening, social supports and opportunities to obtain services and supports in the community.

3. If goals have not already been stated directly by the resident and documented since admission, ask the resident directly about what his or her expectation is regarding the outcome of this nursing home admission and expectations about returning to the community.

4. The resident's stated goals should be recorded here. The goals for the resident, as described by the family, significant other, guardian, or legally authorized representative may also be recorded in the clinical record.

5. Because of a temporary (e.g., delirium) or permanent (e.g., profound dementia) condition, some residents may be unable to provide a clear response. If the resident is unable to communicate his or her preference either verbally or nonverbally, the information can be obtained from the family or significant other, as designated by the individual. If family or the significant other is not available, the information should be obtained from the guardian or legally authorized representative.

Q0300: Resident's Overall Expectation (cont.)

6. Encourage the involvement of family or significant others in the discussion, if the resident consents. While family, significant others, or the guardian or legally authorized representative can be involved if the resident is uncertain about his or her goals, the response selected must reflect the resident's perspective if he or she is able to express it.

7. In some guardianship situations, the decision-making authority regarding the individual's care is vested in the guardian. But this should not create a presumption that the individual resident is not able to comprehend and communicate their wishes.

Coding Instructions for Q0300A, Resident's Overall Goals Established during Assessment Process

Record the resident's expectations as expressed by him or her. It is important to document his or her expectations.

- **Code 1, Expects to be discharged to the community:** if the resident indicates an expectation to return home, to assisted living, or to another community setting.

- **Code 2, Expects to remain in this facility:** if the resident indicates that he or she expects to remain in the nursing home.

- **Code 3, Expects to be discharged to another facility/institution:** if the resident expects to be discharged to another nursing home, rehabilitation facility, or another institution.

- **Code 9, Unknown or uncertain:** if the resident is uncertain or if the resident is not able to participate in the discussion or indicate a goal, and family, significant other, or guardian or legally authorized representative do not exist or are not available to participate in the discussion.

Coding Tips

- This item is individualized and resident-driven rather than what the nursing home staff judge to be in the best interest of the resident. This item focuses on exploring the resident's expectations; not whether or not the staff considers them to be realistic.

- Q0300A, Code 1 "Expects to be discharged to the community" may include newly admitted Medicare SNF residents with a facility arranged discharge plan or non-Medicare and Medicaid residents with adequate supports already in place that would not require referral to a local contact agency (LCA). It may also include residents who ask to talk to someone about the possibility of leaving this facility and returning to live and receive services in the community (Q0500B, Code 1).

- Avoid trying to guess what the resident might identify as a goal or to judge the resident's goal. Do not infer a response based on a specific advance directive, e.g., "do not resuscitate" (DNR).

- The resident should be provided options, as well as, access to information that allows him or her to make the decision and to be supported in directing his or her care planning.

Q0300: Resident's Overall Expectation (cont.)

- If the resident is unable to communicate his or her preference either verbally or nonverbally, or has been legally determined incompetent, the information can be obtained from the family or significant other, as designated by the individual. Families, significant others or legal guardians should be consulted as part of the assessment.

Coding Instructions for Q0300B, Indicate Information Source for Q0300A

- **Code 1, Resident:** if the resident is the source for completing this item.

- **Code 2, If not resident, then family or significant other:** if the resident is unable to respond and a family member or significant other is the source for completing this item.

- **Code 3, If not resident, family or significant other, then guardian or legally authorized representative:** if the guardian or legally authorized representative is the source for completing this item because the resident is unable to respond and a family member or significant other is not available to respond.

- **Code 9, Unknown or uncertain (none of the above):** if the resident cannot respond and the family or significant other, or guardian or legally authorized representative does not exist or cannot be contacted or is unable to respond (Q0300A= 9).

Examples

1. Mrs. F. is a 55-year-old married woman who had a cerebrovascular accident (CVA, also known as stroke) 2 weeks ago. She was admitted to the nursing home 1 week ago for rehabilitation, specifically for transfer, gait training, and wheelchair mobility training. Mrs. F. is extremely motivated to return home. Her husband is supportive and has been busy adapting their home to promote her independence. Her goal is to return home once she has completed rehabilitation.

    Coding: Q0300A would be **coded 1, Expects to be discharged to the community**.
    Q0300B would be **coded 1, Resident**.
    Rationale: Mrs. F. has clear expectations and a goal to return home.

2. Mr. W. is a 73-year-old man who has severe heart failure and renal dysfunction. He also has a new diagnosis of metastatic colorectal cancer and was readmitted to the nursing home after a prolonged hospitalization for lower gastrointestinal (GI) bleeding. He relies on nursing staff for all activities of daily living (ADLs). He indicates that he is "strongly optimistic" about his future and only wants to think "positive thoughts" about what is going to happen and needs to believe that he will return home.

    Coding: Q0300A would be **coded 1, Expects to be discharged to the community**.
    Q0300B would be **coded 1, Resident**.

Q0300: Resident's Overall Expectation (cont.)

Rationale: Mr. W has a clear goal to return home. Even if the staff believe this is unlikely based on available social supports and past nursing home residence, this item should be coded based on the resident's expressed goals.

3. Ms. T. is a 93-year-old woman with chronic renal failure, oxygen dependent chronic obstructive pulmonary disease (COPD), severe osteoporosis, and moderate dementia. When queried about her care preferences, she is unable to voice consistent preferences for her own care, simply stating that "It's such a nice day. Now let's talk about it more." When her daughter is asked about goals for her mother's care, she states that "We know her time is coming. The most important thing now is for her to be comfortable. Because of monetary constraints, the level of care that she needs, and other work and family responsibilities we cannot adequately meet her needs at home. Other than treating simple things, what we really want most is for her to live out whatever time she has in comfort and for us to spend as much time as we can with her." The assessor confirms that the daughter wants care oriented toward making her mother comfortable in her final days and that the family does not have the capacity to provide all the care the resident needs.

    Coding: Q0300A would be **coded 2, Expects to remain in this facility**.
    Q0300B would be **coded 2, Family or significant other**.
    Rationale: Ms. T is not able to respond, but her daughter has clear expectations that her mother will remain in the nursing home where she will be made comfortable for her remaining days.

4. Mrs. G., an 84-year-old female with severe dementia, is admitted by her daughter for a 7-day period. Her daughter stated that she "just needs to have a break." Her mother has been wandering at times and has little interactive capacity. The daughter is planning to take her mother back home at the end of the week.

    Coding: Q0300A would be **coded 1, Expects to be discharged to the community**.
    Q0300B would be **coded 2, Family or significant other**.
    Rationale: Mrs. G. is not able to respond but her daughter has clear expectations that her mother will return home at the end of the 7-day respite visit.

5. Mrs. C. is a 72-year-old woman who had been living alone and was admitted to the nursing home for rehabilitation after a severe fall. Upon admission, she was diagnosed with moderate dementia and was unable to voice consistent preferences for her own care. She has no living relatives and no significant other who is willing to participate in her care decisions. The court appointed a legal guardian to oversee her care. Community-based services, including assisted living and other residential care situations, were discussed with the guardian. The guardian decided that it is in Mrs. C.'s best interest that she be discharged to a nursing home that has a specialized dementia care unit once rehabilitation was complete.

    Coding: Q0300A would be **coded 3, Expects to be discharged to another facility/institution**.
    Q0300B would be **coded 3, Guardian or legally authorized representative**.

Q0300: Resident's Overall Expectation (cont.)

Rationale: Mrs. C. is not able to respond and has no family or significant other available to participate in her care decisions. A court-appointed legal guardian determined that it is in Mrs. C.'s best interest to be discharged to a nursing home that could provide dementia care once rehabilitation was complete.

6. Ms. K. is a 40-year-old with cerebral palsy and a learning disability. She lived in a group home 5 years ago, but after a hospitalization for pneumonia she was admitted to the nursing home for respiratory therapy. Although her group home bed is no longer available, she is now medically stable and there is no medical reason why she could not transition back to the community. Ms. K. states she wants to return to the group home. Her legal guardian agrees that she should return to the community to a small group home.

> **Coding:** Q0300A would be **coded 1, Expects to be discharged to the community (small group homes are considered to be community setting).**
> Q0300B would be **coded 1, Resident**

Rationale: Ms. K. understands and is able to respond and says she would like to go back to the group home. Her expression of choice should be recorded. When the legal guardian, with legal decision-making authority under state law, was told that Ms. K. is medically stable and would like to go back to the community, she confirmed that it is in Ms. K.'s best interest to be transferred to a group home. This information should also be recorded in the individual's clinical record. (If Ms. K had not been able to communicate her choice and the guardian made the decision, Q0300B would have been coded 3.)

Q0400: Discharge Plan

Q0400. Discharge Plan	
Enter Code	**A. Is active discharge planning already occurring for the resident to return to the community?** 0. **No** 1. **Yes** → Skip to Q0600, Referral

Item Rationale

Health-related Quality of Life

- Returning home or to a non-institutional setting can be very important to a resident's health and quality of life.

- For residents who have been in the facility for a long time, it is important to discuss with them their interest in talking with local contact agency (LCA) experts about returning to the community. There are improved community resources and supports that may benefit these residents and allow them to return to a community setting.

- Being discharged from the nursing home without adequate discharge planning occurring (planning and implementation of a plan before discharge) could result in the resident's decline and increase the chances for rehospitalization and aftercare, so a thorough examination of the options with the resident and local community experts is imperative.

Q0400: Discharge Plan (cont.)

Planning for Care

- Many nursing home residents may be able to return to the community if they are provided appropriate assistance and referral to community resources.

- Important progress has been made so that individuals have more choices, care options, and available supports to meet care preferences and needs in the least restrictive setting possible. This progress resulted from the 1999 U. S. Supreme Court decision in Olmstead v. L.C., which states that residents needing long term services and supports have a right to receive services in the least restrictive and most integrated setting.

- The care plan should include the name and contact information of a primary care provider chosen by the resident, family, significant other, guardian or legally authorized representative, arrangements for the durable medical equipment (if needed), formal and informal supports that will be available, the persons and provider(s) in the community who will meet the resident's needs, and the place the resident is going to be living.

- Each situation is unique to the resident, his/her family, and/or guardian/legally authorized representative. A referral to the Local Contact Agency (LCA) may be appropriate for many individuals, who could be maintained in the community homes of their choice for long periods of time, depending on the residential setting and support services available. For example, a referral to the LCA may be appropriate for some individuals with Alzheimer's disease. There are many individuals with this condition being maintained in their own homes for long periods of time, depending on the residential setting and support services available. The interdisciplinary should not assume that any particular resident is unable to be discharged. A successful transition will depend on the services, settings, and sometimes family support services that are available.

- Discharge instructions should include at a minimum:
  — the individuals preferences and needs for care and supports;
    o personal identification and contact information, including Advance Directives;
    o provider contact information of primary care physician, pharmacy, and community care agency including personal care services (if applicable) etc.;
    o brief medical history;
    o current medications, treatments, therapies, and allergies;
    o arrangements for durable medical equipment;
    o arrangements for housing;
    o arrangements for transportation to follow-up appointments; and
    o contact information at the nursing home if a problem arises during discharge
  — A follow-up appointment with the designated primary care provider in the community and other specialists (as appropriate).
  — Medication education.

Q0400: Discharge Plan (cont.)

— Prevention and disease management education, focusing especially on warning symptoms for when to call the doctor.

— Who to call in case of an emergency or if symptoms of decline occur.

— Nursing facility procedures and discharge planning for subacute and rehabilitation community discharges are most often well-defined and efficient.

— Section Q has broadened the scope of the traditional boundary of discharge planning for sub-acute residents to encompass long stay residents. In addition to home health and other medical services, discharge planning may include expanded resources such as assistance with locating housing, transportation, employment if desired, and social engagement opportunities.

   o   Asking the resident and family about whether they want to talk to someone about a return to the community gives the resident voice and respects his or her wishes. This step in no way guarantees discharge but provides an opportunity for the resident to interact with LCA experts.

   o   The NF is responsible for making referrals to the LCAs under the process that the State has set up. The LCA is responsible for contacting referred residents and assisting with transition services planning. They should work closely together. The LCA is the entity that does the community support planning, (e.g. housing, home modification, setting up a household, transportation, community inclusion planning, etc.). A referral to the LCA may come from the nursing facility by phone, by e-mails or by a state's on-line/website or by other state-approved processes. In most cases, further screening and consultation with the resident, their family and the interdisciplinary team by the nursing home social worker or staff member would likely be an important step in the referral determination process.

   o   Each NH needs to develop relationships with their LCAs to work with them to contact the resident and their family, guardian or significant others concerning a potential return to the community. A thorough review of medical, psychological, functional, and financial information is necessary in order to assess what each individual resident needs and whether or not there are sufficient community resources and finances to support a transition to the community.

   o   Enriched transition resources including housing, in-home caretaking services and meals, home modifications, etc. are now more readily available. Resource availability and eligibility coverage varies across States and local communities.

   o   Should a planned relocation not occur, it might create stress and disappointment for the resident and family that will require support and nursing home care planning interventions.

• Involve community mental health resources (as appropriate) to ensure that the resident has support and active coping skills that will help him or her to readjust to community living.

Q0400: Discharge Plan (cont.)

- Use teach-back methods to ensure that the resident understands all of the factors associated with his or her discharge.

- For additional guidance, see CMS' **Planning for Your Discharge: A checklist for patients and caregivers preparing to leave a hospital, nursing home, or other health care setting**. Available at http://www.medicare.gov/Publications/Pubs/pdf/11376.pdf

Steps for Assessment

1. A review should be conducted of the care plan, the medical record, and clinician progress notes, including but not limited to nursing, physician, social services, and therapy to consider the resident's discharge planning needs.

2. If the resident is unable to communicate his or her preference either verbally or nonverbally, or has been legally determined incompetent, the information can be obtained from the family or significant other or guardian, as designated by the individual.

3. If a nursing facility has a discharge planning and referral and resource process for short stay residents that includes arranging for home health services, durable medical equipment, medical services, and appointments, etc., and the capability to address a resident's needs and arrange for that resident to discharge back to the community, a referral to the LCA may not be necessary. Additionally, some non-Medicare and Medicaid residents may have resources, informal and formal supports, and finances already in place that would not require referral to a local contact agency (LCA) to access them.

4. Record the resident's expectations as expressed/communicated, whether you assess that they are realistic or not realistic.

5. If the resident's discharge needs cannot be met by the nursing facility, an evaluation of the community living situation to evaluate whether it can meet the resident's needs should be conducted by the LCA, along with other community providers who will be providing the transition and other community based services to determine the need for assistive/adaptive devices, medical supplies, and equipment and other services.

6. The resident, his or her interdisciplinary team, and LCA (when a referral has been made to a local contact agency) should determine the services and assistance that the resident will need post discharge (e.g., homemaker, meal preparation, ADL assistance, transportation, prescription assistance).

7. Eligibility for financial assistance through various funding sources (e.g., private funds, family assistance, Medicaid, long-term care insurance) should be considered prior to discharge to identify the options available to the individual (e.g., home, assisted living, board and care, or group homes, etc.).

8. A determination of family involvement, capability and support after discharge should also be made.

Q0400: Discharge Plan (cont.)

Coding Instructions for Q0400A, Is Active Discharge planning already occurring for the Resident to Return to the Community?

- **Code 0, No:** if there is not active discharge planning already occurring for the resident to return to the community.

- **Code 1, Yes:** if there is active discharge planning already occurring for the resident to return to the community; skip to **Referral** item (Q0600).

Q0490: Resident's Preference to Avoid Being Asked Question Q0500B

For Quarterly, Correction to Quarterly, and Not-OBRA Assessments. (A0310A=02, 06, 99)

Q0490. Resident's Preference to Avoid Being Asked Question Q0500B
Complete only if A0310A = 02, 06, or 99
Enter Code ☐	Does the resident's clinical record document a request that this question be asked only on comprehensive assessments? 0. **No** 1. **Yes** → Skip to Q0600, Referral 8. **Information not available**

Item Rationale

This item directs a check of the resident's clinical record to determine if the resident and/or family, etc. have indicated on a previous OBRA comprehensive assessment (A0310A = 01, 03, 04 or 05) that they do not want to be asked question Q0500B until their next comprehensive assessment. Some residents and their families do not want to be asked about their preference for returning to the community and would rather not be asked about it. Item Q0550 allows them to opt-out of being asked question Q0500B on quarterly (non-comprehensive) assessments. If there is a notation in the clinical record that the resident does not want to be asked again, and this is a quarterly assessment, then skip to item Q0600, **Referral**.

Note: Let the resident know that they can change their mind at any time and should be referred to the LCA if they voice their request, regardless of schedule of MDS assessment(s).

If this is a comprehensive assessment, do not skip to item Q0600, continue to item Q0500B.

Coding Instructions for Q0490, Does the resident's clinical record document a request that this question be asked only on comprehensive assessments?

- **Code 0, No:** if there is no notation in the resident's clinical record that he or she does not want to be asked Question Q0500B again.

Q0490: Resident's Preference to Avoid Being Asked Question Q0500B (cont.)

- **Code 1, Yes:** if there is a notation in the resident's clinical record to not ask Question Q0500B again, except on comprehensive assessments.

Unless this is a comprehensive assessment (A0310A=01, 03, 04, 05), skip to item Q0600, **Referral.** If this is a comprehensive assessment, proceed to the next item Q0500B.

- **Code 8, Information not available:** if there is no information available in the resident's clinical record or prior MDS 3.0 assessment.

Coding Tips

- Carefully review the resident's clinical record, including prior MDS 3.0 assessments, to determine if the resident or other respondent has previously responded No to item Q0550.

If this is a comprehensive assessment, proceed to item Q0500B, regardless of the previous responses to item Q0550A.

Examples

1. Ms. G is a 45-year old woman, 300 pounds, who is cognitively intact. She has CHF and shortness of breath requiring oxygen at all times. Ms. G also requires 2 person assistance with bathing and transfers to the commode. She was admitted to the nursing home 3 years ago after her daughter who was caring for her passed away. The nursing home social worker discussed options in which she could be cared for in the community but Ms. G refused to consider leaving the nursing home. During the review of her clinical record, the assessor found that on her last MDS assessment, Ms. G stated that she did not want to be asked again about returning to community living, that she has friends in the nursing facility and really likes the activities.

    Coding: Q0490 would be **coded 1, Yes, skip to Q0600; because this is a quarterly assessment.**

    If this is a comprehensive assessment, then proceed to the next item Q0500B.

    Rationale: On her last MDS 3.0 assessment, Ms. G indicates her preference to not want to be asked again about returning to community living (No on Q0550A).

2. Mrs. R is an 82-year-old widowed woman with advanced Alzheimer's disease. She has resided at the nursing home for 4½ years and her family requests that she not be interviewed because she becomes agitated and upset and cannot be cared for by family members or in the community. The resident is not able to be interviewed.

    Coding: Q0490 would be **coded 1, Yes, skip to Q0600;**

    Unless this is a comprehensive assessment, then proceed to the next item Q0500B.

    Rationale: Mrs. R is not able to be interviewed. Her family requests that she opt out of the return to the community question because she becomes agitated.

Q0500: Return to Community

For Admission, Quarterly, and Annual Assessments.

Q0500. Return to Community	
Enter Code ☐	**B. Ask the resident** (or family or significant other if resident is unable to respond): **"Do you want to talk to someone about the possibility of leaving this facility and returning to live and receive services in the community?"** 0. **No** 1. **Yes** 9. **Unknown or uncertain**

Item Rationale

The goal of follow-up action is to initiate and maintain collaboration between the nursing home and the local contact agency to support the resident's expressed interest in being transitioned to community living. This includes the nursing home supporting the resident in achieving his or her highest level of functioning and the local contact agency providing informed choices for community living and assisting the resident in transitioning to community living. The underlying intention of the return to the community item is to insure that all individuals have the opportunity to learn about home and community based services and have an opportunity to receive long term services and supports in the least restrictive setting. CMS has found that in many cases individuals requiring long term services, and/or their families, are unaware of community based services and supports that could adequately support individuals in community living situations.

Health-related Quality of Life

- Returning home or to a non-institutional setting can be very important to the resident's health and quality of life.
- This item identifies the resident's desire to speak with someone about returning to community living. Based on the Americans with Disabilities Act and the 1999 U.S. Supreme Court decision in **Olmstead v. L.C.,** residents needing long-term care services have a right to receive services in the least restrictive and most integrated setting.
- Item Q0500B requires that the resident be asked the question directly and formalizes the opportunity for the resident to be informed of and consider his or her options to return to community living. This ensures that the resident's desire to learn about the possibility of returning to the community will be obtained and appropriate follow-up measures will be taken.
- The goal is to obtain the informed choice and preferences expressed by the resident and to provide information about available community supports and services.

Planning for Care

- Many nursing home residents may be able to return to the community if they are provided appropriate assistance to facilitate care in a non-institutional setting.

Q0500: Return to Community (cont.)

Steps for Assessment: Interview Instructions

1. At the initial admission assessment and in subsequent follow-up assessments (as applicable), make the resident comfortable by assuring him or her that this is a routine question that is asked of all residents.

2. Ask the resident if he or she would like to speak with someone about the possibility of returning to live in the community. Inform the resident that answering yes to this item signals the resident's request for more information and will initiate a contact by someone with more information about supports available for living in the community. A successful transition will depend on the resident's preferences and choices and the services, settings, and sometimes family supports that are available. In many cases individuals requiring long term care services, and/or their families, are unaware of community based services and supports that could adequately support individuals in community living situations. Answering yes does not commit the resident to leave the nursing home at a specific time; nor does it ensure that the resident will be able to move back to the community. Answering no is also not a permanent commitment. Also inform the resident that he or she can change his or her decision (i.e., whether or not he or she wants to speak with someone) at any time.

3. Explain that this item is meant to provide the opportunity for the resident to get information and explore the possibility of different settings for receiving ongoing care. A viable and workable discharge plan requires that the nursing home social worker or staff talk with the resident before making a referral to a local contact agency to explore topics such as: what returning to the community means, i.e., a variety of settings based on preferences and needs; the arrangements and planning that the NF/SNF can make; and obtaining family or legal guardian input. This step will help the resident clarify their discharge goals and identify important information for the LCA or, in some instances may indicate that the resident does not want to be referred to the LCA at this time. Also explain that the resident can change his/her mind at any time.

4. If the resident is unable to communicate his or her preference either verbally or nonverbally, the information can then be obtained from family or a significant other, as designated by the individual. If family or significant others are not available, a guardian or legally authorized representative, if one exists, can provide the information.

5. Ask the resident if he or she wants information about different kinds of supports that may be available for community living. Responding yes will be a way for the individual—and his or her family, significant other, or guardian or legally authorized representative—to obtain additional information about services and supports that would be available to support community living.

Coding Instructions for Q0500B, Ask the resident (or family or significant other or guardian or legally authorized representative if resident is unable to understand or respond): "Do you want to talk to someone about the possibility of leaving this facility and returning to live and receive services in the community?"

Q0500: Return to Community (cont.)

- **Code 0, No:** if the resident (or family or significant other, or guardian or legally authorized representative) states that he or she does not want to talk to someone about the possibility of returning to the community.

- **Code 1, Yes:** if the resident (or family or significant other, or guardian or legally authorized representative) states that he or she does want to talk to someone about the possibility of returning to the community.

- **Code 9, Unknown or uncertain:** if the resident cannot <u>understand or</u> respond and the family or significant other is not available to respond on the resident's behalf and a guardian or legally authorized representative is not available or has not been appointed by the court.

Coding Tips

- A "yes" response to item Q0500B will trigger follow-up care planning and contact with the designated local contact agency about the resident's request within approximately 10 business days of a yes response being given. This code is intended to initiate contact with the local agency for follow-up as the resident desires.

- Follow-up is expected in a "reasonable" amount of time and 10 business days is a recommendation and not a requirement. The level and type of response needed by an individual is determined on a resident-by-resident basis. Some States may determine that the LCAs can make an initial telephone contact to identify the resident's needs and/or set up the face-to-face visit/appointment. However, it is expected that most residents will have a face to face visit. In some States, an initial meeting is set up with the resident, facility staff, and LCA together to talk with the resident about their needs and community care options.

- Some residents will have a very clear expectation and some may change their expectations over time. Residents may also be unsure or unaware of the opportunities available to them for community living with services and supports. Talking with the resident regarding discharge goals and plans before referral to the LCA is a critical step. It is important to clarify the resident's discharge needs and expectations, determine what the SNF/NF usually provides and can arrange, and obtain information about transition barriers or challenges based on family, financial, guardian, cognition, assuring health and safety, and/or intensive 24- hour care issues, etc.

- The SNF/NF should not assume that the resident cannot transition out of the SNF/NF due to their level of care needs. The SNF/NF can talk with the LCA to see what is available that does not require family support.

- Current return to community questions may upset residents who cannot understand what the question means and result in them being agitated or saddened by being asked the question. If the level of cognitive impairment is such that the resident does not understand Q0500, a family member, significant other guardian and/or legally appointed decision-maker for that individual could be asked the question.

Q0500: Return to Community (cont.)

Examples

1. Mr. B. is an 82-year-old male with COPD. He was referred to the nursing home by his physician for end-of-life palliative care. He responded, "I'm afraid I can't" to item Q0500B. The assessor should ask follow-up questions to understand why Mr. B. is afraid and explain that obtaining more information may help overcome some of his fears. He should also be informed that someone from a local agency is available to provide him with more information about receiving services and supports in the community. At the close of this discussion, Mr. B. says that he would like more information on community supports.

    Coding: Q0500B would be **coded 1, Yes**.

    Rationale: Coding Q0500B as yes should trigger a visit by the nursing home social worker (or facility social worker) to assess fears and concerns, with any additional follow-up care planning that is needed and to initiate contact with the designated local agency within approximately 10 business days.

2. Ms. C. is a 45-year-old woman with cerebral palsy and a learning disability who has been living in the Hope Nursing Home for the past 20 years. She once lived in a group home but became ill and required hospitalization for pneumonia. After recovering in the hospital, Ms. C. was sent to the nursing home because she now required regular chest physical therapy and was told that she could no longer live in her previous group home because her needs were more intensive. No one had asked her about returning to the community until now. When administered the MDS assessment, she responded yes to item Q0500B.

    Coding: Q0500B would be **coded 1, Yes**.

    Rationale: Ms. C.'s discussions with staff in the nursing home should result in a visit by the nursing home social worker or discharge planner. Her response should be noted in her care plan, and care planning should be initiated to assess her preferences and needs for possible transition to the community. Nursing home staff should contact the designated local contact agency within approximately 10 business days for them to initiate discussions with Ms. C. about returning to community living.

3. Mr. D. is a 65-year-old man with a severe heart condition and interstitial pulmonary fibrosis. At the last quarterly assessment, Mr. D. had been asked about returning to the community and his response was no. He also responds no to item Q0500B. The assessor should ask why he responded no. Depending on the response, follow-up questions could include, "Is it that you think you cannot get the care you need in the community? Do you have a home to return to? Do you have any family or friends to assist you in any way?" Mr. D. responds no to the follow-up questions and does not want to offer any more information or talk about it.

    Coding: Q0500B would be **coded 0, No**.

    Rationale:. During this assessment, he was asked about returning to the community and he responded no.

Q0550: Resident's Preference to Avoid Being Asked Question Q0500B again

Q0550. Resident's Preference to Avoid Being Asked Question Q0500B Again	
Enter Code ☐	**A. Does the resident** (or family or significant other or guardian, if resident is unable to respond) **want to be asked about returning to the community on all assessments?** (Rather than only on comprehensive assessments.) 0. **No** - then document in resident's clinical record and ask again only on the next comprehensive assessment 1. **Yes** 8. **Information not available**
Enter Code ☐	**B. Indicate information source for Q0550A** 1. **Resident** 2. If not resident, then **family or significant other** 3. If not resident, family or significant other, then **guardian or legally authorized representative** 8. **No information source available**

Item Rationale

Some individuals, such as those with cognitive impairments, mental illness, or end-stage life conditions, may be upset by asking them if they want to return to the community. CMS pilot tested Q0500 language and determined that respondents would be less likely to be upset by being asked if they want to talk to someone about returning to the community if they were given the opportunity to opt-out of being asked the question every quarter. The intent of the item is to achieve a better balance between giving residents a voice and a choice about the services they receive, while being sensitive to those individuals who may be unable to voice their preferences or be upset by being asked question Q0500B in the assessment process.

Coding Instructions for Q0550A, Does the resident, (or family or significant other or guardian, if resident is unable to respond) want to be asked about returning to the community on all assessments (rather than being asked yearly only on comprehensive assessments)?

- **Code 0, No:** if the resident (or family or significant other, or guardian or legally authorized representative) states that he or she does not want to be asked again on quarterly assessments about returning to the community. Then document in resident's clinical record and ask question Q0500B again only on the next comprehensive assessment.

- **Code 1, Yes:** if the resident (or family or significant other, or guardian or legally authorized representative) states that he or she does want to be asked the return to community question Q0500B on all assessments.

- **Code 9, Information not available:** if the resident cannot respond and the family or significant other is not available to respond on the resident's behalf and a guardian or legally authorized representative is not available or has not been appointed by the court.

Q0550: Resident's Preference to Avoid Being Asked Question Q0500B again (cont.)

Coding Instructions for Q0550B, Indicate information source for Q0550A

- **Code 1, Resident:** if resident responded to Q0550A.
- **Code 2, If not resident, then family or significant other.**
- **Code 3, If not resident, family or significant other, then guardian or legally authorized representative.**
- **Code 8, No information source available:** if the resident cannot respond and the family or significant other is not available to respond on the resident's behalf and a guardian or legally authorized representative is not available or has not been appointed by the court.

Example

1. Ms. W is an 81 year old woman who was admitted after a fall that broke her hip, wrist and collar bone. Her recovery is slow and her family visits regularly. Her apartment is awaiting her and she hopes within the next 4-6 months to be discharged home. She and her family requests that discharge planning occur when she can transfer and provide more self-care.

   Coding: Q0550A would be **coded 1, Yes.**

   Q0550B would be **coded 1, Resident.**

   Rationale: Ms. W. needs longer term restorative nursing care to recover from her falls before she can return home. She has some elderly family members who will provide caregiver support. She will likely need community supports and the social worker will consult with LCA staff to consider community services and supports in advance of her discharge.

Q0600: Referral

Q0600. Referral	
Enter Code ☐	Has a referral been made to the Local Contact Agency? (Document reasons in resident's clinical record) 0. **No** - referral not needed 1. **No** - referral is or may be needed (For more information see Appendix C, Care Area Assessment Resources #20) 2. **Yes** - referral made

Item Rationale

Health-related Quality of Life

- Returning home or to a non-institutional setting can be very important to the resident's health and quality of life.

Q0600: Referral (cont.)

Planning for Care

- Some nursing home residents may be able to return to the community if they are provided appropriate assistance and referral to appropriate community resources to facilitate care in a non-institutional setting.

Steps for Assessment: Interview Instructions

1. If Item Q0400A is coded 1, yes, then complete this item.
2. If Item Q0490B is coded 1, yes, then complete this item,
3. If Item Q0500B is coded 1, yes, then complete this item.

Coding Instructions

> **DEFINITIONS**
>
> **DESIGNATED LOCAL CONTACT AGENCY**
>
> Each state has community contact agencies that can provide individuals with information about community living options and available supports and services.
>
> These local contact agencies may be a single entry point agency, an Aging and Disability Resource Center (ADRC), an Area Agency on Aging (AAA), a Center for Independent Living (CIL), or other state designated entities.

- **Code 0, No - referral not needed;** determination has been made by the resident (or family or significant other, or guardian or legally authorized representative) and the care planning team that the designated local contact agency does not need to be contacted. If the resident's discharge planning has been completely developed by the nursing home staff, and there are no additional needs that the SNF/NF cannot arrange for, then there is no need for a LCA referral. Or, if resident or family, etc. responded no to Q0500B.

- **Code 1, No - referral is or may be needed;** determination has been made by the resident (or family or significant other, or guardian or legally authorized representative) that the designated local contact agency needs to be contacted but the referral has not been initiated at this time. If the resident has asked to talk to someone about available community services and supports and a referral is not made at this time, care planning and progress notes should indicate the status of discharge planning and why a referral was not initiated.

- **Code 2, Yes - referral made;** if referral was made to the local contact agency. For example, the resident responded yes to Q0500B. The facility care planning team was notified and initiated contact with the local contact agency.

  Section Q Point of Contact list for Local Contact Agencies:
  http://www.medicaid.gov/Medicaid-CHIP-Program-Information/By-Topics/Long-Term-Services-and-Support/Balancing/Money-Follows-the-Person.html

Q0600: Referral (cont.)

Coding Tips

- State Medicaid Agencies have designated Local Contact Agencies and a State point of contact (POC) to coordinate efforts to implement Section Q and designate LCAs for their State's skilled nursing facilities and nursing facilities. These local contact agencies may be single entry point agencies, Aging and Disability Resource Centers, Money Follows the Person programs, Area Agencies on Aging, Independent Living Centers, or other entities the State may designate.
- Several resources are available at the Return to Community web site at: http://www.cms.gov/CommunityServices/10_CommunityLivingInitiative.asp#TopOfPage.
  - The State-by-State list of Local Contact Agencies and POC Section Q Coordinator Information
  - MDS 3.0 Section Q Implementation Solutions contains Section Q questions and answers that can help States with implementation issues.
  - The Section Q Pilot Test Results report describes the results of user testing of the new items in Section Q.
- Resource availability and eligibility coverage varies across States and local communities and may present barriers to allowing some resident's return to their community. The nursing home and local agency staff members should guard against raising the resident and their family members' expectations of what can occur until more information is obtained.
- Close collaboration between the nursing facility and the local contact agency is needed to evaluate the resident's medical needs, finances and available community transition resources.
- The LCA can provide information to the SNF/NF on the available community living situations, and options for community based supports and services including the levels and scope of what is possible.
- The local contact agency team must explore community care options/supports and conduct appropriate care planning to determine if transitions back to the community is possible.
- Resident support and interventions by the nursing home staff may be necessary if the LCA transition is not successful because of unanticipated changes to the resident's medical condition, insufficient financial resources, problems with caregiving supports, community resource gaps, etc. preventing discharge to the community.
- When Q0600 is answered 1, No, a care area trigger requires a return to community care area assessment (CAA) and CAA 20 provides a step-by-step process for the facility to use in order to provide the resident an opportunity to discuss returning to the community.

Q0600: Referral (cont.)

Examples

1. Mr. S. is a 48-year-old man who suffered a stroke, resulting in paralysis below the waist. He is responsible for his 8-year old son, who now stays with his grandmother. At the last quarterly assessment, Mr. S. had been asked about returning to the community and his response was "Yes" to item Q0500B and he reports no contact from the LCA. Mr. S. is more hopeful he can return home as he becomes stronger in rehabilitation. He wants a location to be able to remain active in his son's school and use accessible public transportation when he finds employment. He is worried whether he can afford or find accessible housing with wheelchair accessible sinks, cabinets, countertops and appliances.

   Coding: Q0500B would be **coded 1, Yes**
   Q0600 would be **coded 2, Yes**.

   Rationale: The social worker or discharge planner would make a referral to the designated local contact agency for their area and Q0600 would be coded as 2, yes.

2. Ms. V. is an 82-year-old female with right sided paralysis, mild dementia, diabetes and was admitted by the family because of safety concerns because of falls and difficulties cooking and proper nutrition. She said yes to Q0500B. She needs to continue her rehabilitation therapy and regain her strength and ability to transfer. The social worker plans to talk to the resident and her family to determine whether a referral to the LCA is needed for Ms. V.

   Coding: Q0600 would be **coded 1, No**.

   Rationale: Ms. V indicated that she wanted to have an opportunity to talk to someone about return to community. The nursing home staff will focus on her therapies and talk to her and her family to obtain more information for discharge planning. Q0600 would be coded as no- "referral is or may be needed." The Care Area Assessment #20 is triggered and it will be used to guide the follow-up process. Because a referral was not made at this time, care planning and progress notes should indicate the status of discharge planning and why a referral was not initiated to the designated local contact agency.

SECTION S IS RESERVED FOR ADDITIONAL STATE-DEFINED ITEMS. THERE IS NO SECTION S IN THE FEDERAL MDS VERSION 3.0 ITEM SET. YOUR STATE MAY CHOOSE TO DESIGNATE A SECTION S.

SECTION V: CARE AREA ASSESSMENT (CAA) SUMMARY

Intent: The MDS does not constitute a comprehensive assessment. Rather, it is a preliminary assessment to identify potential resident problems, strengths, and preferences. Care Areas are triggered by MDS item responses that indicate the need for additional assessment based on problem identification, known as "triggered care areas," which form a critical link between the MDS and decisions about care planning.

There are 20 CAAs in Version 3.0 of the RAI, which includes the addition of "Pain" and "Return to the Community Referral." These CAAs cover the majority of care areas known to be problematic for nursing home residents. The Care Area Assessment (CAA) process provides guidance on how to focus on key issues identified during a comprehensive MDS assessment and directs facility staff and health professionals to evaluate triggered care areas.

The interdisciplinary team (IDT) then identifies relevant assessment information regarding the resident's status. After obtaining input from the resident, the resident's family, significant other, guardian, or legally authorized representative, the IDT decides whether or not to develop a care plan for triggered care areas. Chapter 4 of this manual provides detailed instructions on the CAA process and development of an individualized care plan.

Whereas the MDS identifies actual or potential problem areas, the CAA process provides for further assessment of the triggered areas by guiding staff to look for causal or confounding factors, some of which may be reversible. It is important that the CAA documentation include the causal or unique risk factors for decline or lack of improvement. The plan of care then addresses these factors, with the goal of promoting the resident's highest practicable level of functioning: (1) improvement where possible, or (2) maintenance and prevention of avoidable declines. Documentation should support your decision making regarding whether to proceed with a care plan for a triggered CAA and the type(s) of care plan interventions that are appropriate for a particular resident. Documentation may appear anywhere in the clinical record, e.g., progress notes, consults, flowsheets, etc.

V0100: Items From the Most Recent Prior OBRA or PPS Assessment

V0100. Items From the Most Recent Prior OBRA or Scheduled PPS Assessment	
Complete only if A0310E = 0 and if the following is true for the **prior assessment**: A0310A = 01- 06 or A0310B = 01- 06	
Enter Code ☐☐	**A. Prior Assessment Federal OBRA Reason for Assessment** (A0310A value from prior assessment) 01. **Admission** assessment (required by day 14) 02. **Quarterly** review assessment 03. **Annual** assessment 04. **Significant change in status** assessment 05. **Significant correction** to **prior comprehensive** assessment 06. **Significant correction** to **prior quarterly** assessment 99. None of the above
Enter Code ☐☐	**B. Prior Assessment PPS Reason for Assessment** (A0310B value from prior assessment) 01. **5-day** scheduled assessment 02. **14-day** scheduled assessment 03. **30-day** scheduled assessment 04. **60-day** scheduled assessment 05. **90-day** scheduled assessment 06. **Readmission/return** assessment 07. **Unscheduled assessment used for PPS** (OMRA, significant or clinical change, or significant correction assessment) 99. None of the above
	C. Prior Assessment Reference Date (A2300 value from prior assessment) ☐☐ – ☐☐ – ☐☐☐☐ Month Day Year
Enter Score ☐☐	**D. Prior Assessment Brief Interview for Mental Status (BIMS) Summary Score** (C0500 value from prior assessment)
Enter Score ☐☐	**E. Prior Assessment Resident Mood Interview (PHQ-9©) Total Severity Score** (D0300 value from prior assessment)
Enter Score ☐☐	**F. Prior Assessment Staff Assessment of Resident Mood (PHQ-9-OV) Total Severity Score** (D0600 value from prior assessment)

Item Rationale

The items in V0100 are used to determine whether to trigger several of the CAAs that compare a resident's current status with their prior status. The values of these items are derived from a prior OBRA or scheduled PPS assessment that was performed since the most recent admission of any kind (i.e., since the most recent entry or reentry), if one is available. Items V0100A, B, C, D, E and F are skipped on the first assessment (OBRA or PPS) following the most recent admission of any kind (i.e., when A0310E = 1, Yes). Complete these items only if a prior assessment has been completed since the most recent admission of any kind to the facility (i.e., when A0310E = 0, No) and if the prior assessment is an OBRA or a scheduled PPS assessment. If such an assessment is available, the values of V0100A, B, C, D, E, and F should be copied from the corresponding items on that prior assessment.

Coding Instructions for V0100A, Prior Assessment Federal OBRA Reason for Assessment (A0310A Value from Prior Assessment)

- Record in V0100A the value for A0310A (Federal OBRA Reason for Assessment) from the most recent prior OBRA or scheduled PPS assessment, if one is available (see "Item Rationale", above, for details). One of the available values (01 through 06 or 99) must be selected.

V0100: Items From the Most Recent Prior OBRA or PPS Assessment (cont.)

Coding Instructions for V0100B, Prior Assessment PPS Reason for Assessment (A0310B Value from Prior Assessment)

- Record in V0100B the value for A0310B (PPS Assessment) from the most recent prior OBRA or scheduled PPS assessment, if one is available (see "Item Rationale", above, for details). One of the available values (01 through 07 or 99) must be selected.

  Note: The values for V0100A and V0100B cannot both be 99, indicating that the prior assessment is neither an OBRA nor a PPS assessment. If the value of V0100A is 99 (None of the above), then the value for V0100B must be 01 through 07, indicating a PPS assessment. If the value of V0100B is 99 (None of the above), then the value for V0100A must be 01 through 06, indicating an OBRA assessment.

Coding Instructions for V0100C, Prior Assessment Reference Date (A2300 Value from Prior Assessment)

- Record in V0100C the value of A2300 (Assessment Reference Date) from the most recent prior OBRA or scheduled PPS assessment, if one is available (see "Item Rationale", above, for details).

Coding Instructions for V0100D, Prior Assessment Brief Interview for Mental Status (BIMS) Summary Score (C0500 Value from Prior Assessment)

- Record in V0100D, the value for C0500 Mental Status (BIMS) Summary Score from the most recent prior OBRA or scheduled PPS assessment, if one is available (see "Item Rationale", above, for details).This item will be compared with the corresponding item on the current assessment to evaluate resident improvement or decline in the Delirium care area.

Coding Instructions for V0100E, Prior Assessment Resident Mood Interview (PHQ-9©) Total Severity Score (D0300 Value from Prior Assessment)

- Record in V0100E the value of D0300 (Resident Mood Interview [PHQ-9©] Total Severity Score) from the most recent prior OBRA or scheduled PPS assessment, if one is available (see "Item Rationale," above, for details). This item will be compared with the corresponding item on the current assessment to evaluate resident decline in the Mood State care area.

Coding Instructions for V0100F, Prior Assessment Staff Assessment of Resident Mood (PHQ-9-OV©) Total Severity Score (D0600 Value from Prior Assessment)

- Record in V0100F the value for item D0600 (Staff Assessment of Resident Mood [PHQ-9-OV©] Total Severity Score) from the most recent prior OBRA or scheduled PPS assessment, if one is available (see "Item Rationale", above, for details). This item will be compared with the corresponding item on the current assessment to evaluate resident decline in the Mood State care area.

V0200: CAAs and Care Planning

V0200. CAAs and Care Planning

1. Check column A if Care Area is triggered.
2. For each triggered Care Area, indicate whether a new care plan, care plan revision, or continuation of current care plan is necessary to address the problem(s) identified in your assessment of the care area. The Care Planning Decision column must be completed within 7 days of completing the RAI (MDS and CAA(s)). Check column B if the triggered care area is addressed in the care plan.
3. Indicate in the Location and Date of CAA Documentation column where information related to the CAA can be found. CAA documentation should include information on the complicating factors, risks, and any referrals for this resident for this care area.

A. CAA Results

Care Area	A. Care Area Triggered	B. Care Planning Decision	Location and Date of CAA documentation
	↓ Check all that apply ↓		
01. Delirium	☐	☐	
02. Cognitive Loss/Dementia	☐	☐	
03. Visual Function	☐	☐	
04. Communication	☐	☐	
05. ADL Functional/Rehabilitation Potential	☐	☐	
06. Urinary Incontinence and Indwelling Catheter	☐	☐	
07. Psychosocial Well-Being	☐	☐	
08. Mood State	☐	☐	
09. Behavioral Symptoms	☐	☐	
10. Activities	☐	☐	
11. Falls	☐	☐	
12. Nutritional Status	☐	☐	
13. Feeding Tube	☐	☐	
14. Dehydration/Fluid Maintenance	☐	☐	
15. Dental Care	☐	☐	
16. Pressure Ulcer	☐	☐	
17. Psychotropic Drug Use	☐	☐	
18. Physical Restraints	☐	☐	
19. Pain	☐	☐	
20. Return to Community Referral	☐	☐	

B. Signature of RN Coordinator for CAA Process and Date Signed

1. Signature

2. Date

☐☐ – ☐☐ – ☐☐☐☐
Month — Day — Year

C. Signature of Person Completing Care Plan Decision and Date Signed

1. Signature

2. Date

☐☐ – ☐☐ – ☐☐☐☐
Month — Day — Year

V0200: CAAs and Care Planning (cont.)

Item Rationale

- Items V0200A 01 through 20 document which triggered care areas require further assessment, decision as to whether or not a triggered care area is addressed in the resident care plan, and the location and date of CAA documentation. The CAA Summary documents the interdisciplinary team's and the resident, resident's family or representative's final decision(s) on which triggered care areas will be addressed in the care plan.

Coding Instructions for V0200A, CAAs

- Facility staff are to use the RAI triggering mechanism to determine which care areas require review and additional assessment. The triggered care areas are checked in Column A "Care Area Triggered" in the CAAs section. For each triggered care area, use the CAA process and current standard of practice, evidence-based or expert-endorsed clinical guidelines and resources to conduct further assessment of the care area. Document relevant assessment information regarding the resident's status. Chapter 4 of this manual provides detailed instructions on the CAA process, care planning, and documentation.

- For each triggered care area, Column B "Care Planning Decision" is checked to indicate that a new care plan, care plan revision, or continuation of the current care plan is necessary to address the issue(s) identified in the assessment of that care area. The "Care Planning Decision" column must be completed within 7 days of completing the RAI, as indicated by the date in V0200C2, which is the date that the care planning decision(s) were completed and that the resident's care plan was completed. For each triggered care area, indicate the date and location of the CAA documentation in the "Location and Date of CAA Documentation" column. Chapter 4 of this manual provides detailed instructions on the CAA process, care planning, and documentation.

Coding Instructions for V0200B, Signature of RN Coordinator for CAA Process and Date Signed

V0200B1, Signature

- Signature of the RN coordinating the CAA process.

V0200B2, Date

- Date that the RN coordinating the CAA process certifies that the CAAs have been completed. The CAA review must be completed no later than the 14th day of admission (admission date + 13 calendar days) for an Admission assessment and within 14 days of the Assessment Reference Date (A2300) for an Annual assessment, Significant Change in Status Assessment, or a Significant Correction to Prior Comprehensive Assessment. This date is considered the date of completion for the RAI.

V0200: CAAs and Care Planning (cont.)

Coding Instructions for V0200C, Signature of Person Completing Care Plan Decision and Date Signed

V0200C1, Signature

- Signature of the staff person facilitating the care planning decision-making. Person signing does not have to be an RN.

V0200C2, Date

- The date on which a staff member completes the Care Planning Decision column (V0200A, Column B), which is done after the care plan is completed. The care plan must be completed within 7 days of the completion of the comprehensive assessment (MDS and CAAs), as indicated by the date in V0200B2.

- Following completion of the MDS,CAAs (V0200A, Columns A and B) and the care plan, the MDS 3.0 comprehensive assessment record must be transmitted to the QIES Assessment Submission and Processing (ASAP) system within 14 days of the V0200C2 date.

Clarifications:

- The signatures at V0200B1 and V0200C1 can be provided by the same person, if the person actually completed both functions. However, it is not a requirement that the same person complete both functions.

- If a resident is discharged prior to the completion of Section V, a comprehensive assessment may be in progress when a resident is discharged. Although the resident has been discharged, the facility may complete and submit the assessment. **The following guidelines apply to completing a <u>comprehensive assessment</u>* when the resident has been discharged**:

  1. Complete all required MDS items from Section A through Section Z and indicate the date of completion in Z0500B. Encode and verify these items.

  2. Complete the care area triggering process by checking all triggered care areas in V0200A, Column A.

  3. Sign and enter the date the CAAs were completed at V0200B1 and V0200B2.

  4. Dash fill all of the "Care Planning Decision" items in V0200A, Column B, which indicates that the decisions are unknown.

  5. Sign and enter the date that care planning decisions were completed at V0200C1 and V0200C2. Use the same date used in V0200B2.

  6. Submit the record.

  *Please see Chapter 2 for additional detailed instructions regarding options for when residents are discharged prior to completion of the RAI.

SECTION X: CORRECTION REQUEST

Intent: The purpose of Section X is to identify an MDS record to be modified or inactivated. The following items identify the existing assessment record that is in error. Section X is only completed if Item A0050, Type of Record, is coded a 2 (Modify existing record) or a 3 (Inactivate existing record). In Section X, the facility must reproduce the information EXACTLY as it appeared on the existing erroneous record, even if the information is incorrect. This information is necessary to locate the existing record in the National MDS Database.

A modification request is used to correct a QIES ASAP record containing incorrect MDS item values due to:

- transcription errors,
- data entry errors,
- software product errors,
- item coding errors, and/or
- other error requiring modification

The modification request record contains correct values for all MDS items (not just the values previously in error), including the Section X items. The corrected record will replace the prior erroneous record in the QIES ASAP database.

In some cases, an incorrect MDS record requires a completely new assessment of the resident in addition to a modification request for that incorrect record. Please refer to Chapter 5 of this manual, Submission and Correction of the MDS Assessments, to determine if a new assessment is required in addition to a modification request.

An inactivation request is used to move an existing record in the QIES ASAP database from the active file to an archive (history file) so that it will not be used for reporting purposes. Inactivations should be used when the event did not occur (e.g., a discharge was submitted when the resident was not discharged). The inactivation request only includes Item A0050 and the Section X items. All other MDS sections are skipped.

The modification and inactivation processes are automated and neither completely removes the prior erroneous record from the QIES ASAP database. The erroneous record is archived in a history file. In certain cases, it is necessary to delete a record and not retain any information about the record in the QIES ASAP database. This requires a request from the facility to the facility's state agency to manually delete all traces of a record from the QIES ASAP database. The policy and procedures for a Manual Correction/Deletion Request are provided in Chapter 5 of this manual.

A Manual Deletion Request is required **only** in the following three cases:

1. **Item A0410 Submission Requirement is incorrect.** Submission of MDS assessment records to the QIES ASAP system constitutes a release of private information and must conform to privacy laws. Only records required by the State and/or the Federal governments may be stored in the QIES ASAP database. If a record has been submitted with the incorrect Submission Requirement value in Item A0410, then that record must be manually deleted and, in some cases, a new record with a corrected A0410 value submitted. Item A0410 cannot be corrected by modification or inactivation. See Chapter 5 of this manual for details.

2. **Inappropriate submission of a test record as a production record.** Removal of a test record from the QIES ASAP database requires manual deletion. Otherwise information for a "bogus" resident will be retained in the database and this resident will appear on some reports to the facility.

3. **Record was submitted for the wrong facility.** If a QIES ASAP record was submitted for an incorrect facility, the record must be removed manually and then a new record for the correct facility must be submitted to the **QIES ASAP database. Manual deletion of the record for the wrong facility** is necessary to ensure that the resident is not associated with that facility and does not appear on reports to that facility.

X0150: Type of Provider

X0150. Type of Provider	
Enter Code	Type of provider 1. Nursing home (SNF/NF) 2. Swing Bed

Coding Instructions for X0150, **Type of Provider**

This item contains the type of provider identified from the prior erroneous record to be modified/inactivated.

- **Code 1, Nursing home (SNF/NF):** if the facility is a Nursing home (SNF/NF).
- **Code 2, Swing Bed:** if the facility is a Swing Bed facility.

X0200: Name of Resident

These items contain the resident's name from the prior erroneous record to be modified/inactivated.

X0200. Name of Resident on existing record to be modified/inactivated
A. First name:
C. Last name:

Coding Instructions for X0200A, **First Name**

- Enter the first name of the resident exactly as submitted for item A0500A "Legal Name of Resident—First Name" on the prior erroneous record to be modified/inactivated. Start entry with the leftmost box. If the first name was left blank on the prior record, leave X0200A blank.
- Note that the first name in X0200A does not have to match the current value of A0500A on a modification request. The entries may be different if the modification is correcting the first name.

X0200: Name of Resident (cont.)

Coding Instructions for X0200C, Last Name

- Enter the last name of the resident exactly as submitted for item A0500C "Legal Name of Resident— Last Name" on the prior erroneous record to be modified/inactivated. Start entry with the leftmost box. The last name in X0200C cannot be blank.

- Note that the last name in X0200C does not have to match the current value of A0500C on a modification request. The entries may be different if the modification is correcting the last name.

X0300: Gender

X0300. Gender on existing record to be modified/inactivated	
Enter Code [ ]	1. Male 2. Female

Coding Instructions for X0300, Gender

- Enter the gender code 1 "Male," 2 "Female," or – (dash value indicating unable to determine) exactly as submitted for item A0800 "Gender" on the prior erroneous record to be modified/inactivated.

- Although a dash (indicating unable to determine) is no longer an acceptable value in A0800, a dash must be used in X0300 on a modification or inactivation request to locate a record if a dash was previously entered in A0800 on the original record.

- Note that the gender in X0300 does not have to match the current value of A0800 on a modification request. The entries may be different if the modification is correcting the gender.

X0400: Birth Date

X0400. Birth Date on existing record to be modified/inactivated
[ ][ ] – [ ][ ] – [ ][ ][ ][ ] Month   Day   Year

Coding Instructions for X0400, Birth Date

- Fill in the boxes with the birth date exactly as submitted for item A0900 "Birth Date" on the prior erroneous record to be modified/inactivated. If the month or day contains only a single digit, fill in the first box with a 0 For example, January 2, 1918, should be entered as:

0	1		0	2		1	9	1	8

If the birth date in MDS item A0900 on the prior record was a partial date, with day of the month unknown and the day of the month boxes were left blank, then the day of the month boxes must be blank in X0400. If the birth date in MDS item A0900 on the prior record was a partial date with both month and day of the month unknown and the month and day of the month boxes were left blank, then the month and day of the month boxes must be blank in X0400.

- Note that the birth date in X0400 does not have to match the current value of A0900 on a modification request. The entries may be different if the modification is correcting the birth date.

X0500: Social Security Number

X0500. Social Security Number on existing record to be modified/inactivated

☐☐☐ - ☐☐ - ☐☐☐☐

Coding Instructions for X0500, Social Security Number

- Fill in the boxes with the Social Security number exactly as submitted for item A0600 "Social Security and Medicare numbers" on the prior erroneous record to be modified/inactivated. If the Social Security number was unknown or unavailable and left blank on the prior record, leave X0500 blank.
- Note that the Social Security number in X0500 does not have to match the current value of A0600 on a modification request. The entries may be different if the modification is correcting the Social Security number.

X0600: Type of Assessment/Tracking

These items contain the reasons for assessment/tracking from the prior erroneous record to be modified/inactivated.

X0600. Type of Assessment on existing record to be modified/inactivated

Enter Code	A. Federal OBRA Reason for Assessment 01. **Admission** assessment (required by day 14) 02. **Quarterly** review assessment 03. **Annual** assessment 04. **Significant change in status** assessment 05. **Significant correction** to **prior comprehensive** assessment 06. **Significant correction** to **prior quarterly** assessment 99. **None of the above**
Enter Code	B. PPS Assessment **PPS Scheduled Assessments for a Medicare Part A Stay** 01. **5-day** scheduled assessment 02. **14-day** scheduled assessment 03. **30-day** scheduled assessment 04. **60-day** scheduled assessment 05. **90-day** scheduled assessment 06. **Readmission/return** assessment **PPS Unscheduled Assessments for a Medicare Part A Stay** 07. **Unscheduled assessment used for PPS** (OMRA, significant or clinical change, or significant correction assessment) **Not PPS Assessment** 99. **None of the above**
Enter Code	C. PPS Other Medicare Required Assessment - OMRA 0. **No** 1. **Start of therapy** assessment 2. **End of therapy** assessment 3. **Both Start and End of therapy** assessment 4. **Change of therapy** assessment
Enter Code	D. Is this a Swing Bed clinical change assessment? Complete only if X0150 = 2 0. **No** 1. **Yes**
Enter Code	F. Entry/discharge reporting 01. **Entry** tracking record 10. **Discharge** assessment-**return not anticipated** 11. **Discharge** assessment-**return anticipated** 12. **Death in facility** tracking record 99. **None of the above**

X0600: Type of Assessment/Tracking (cont.)

Coding Instructions for X0600A, Federal OBRA Reason for Assessment

- Fill in the boxes with the Federal OBRA reason for assessment/tracking code exactly as submitted for item A0310A "Federal OBRA Reason for Assessment" on the prior erroneous record to be modified/inactivated.
- Note that the Federal OBRA reason for assessment/tracking code in X0600A must match the current value of A0310A on a modification request.
- If item A0310A was incorrect on an assessment that we previously submitted and accepted by the ASAP system, then the original assessment must be inactivated and a new record with a new date must be submitted.

Coding Instructions for X0600B, PPS Assessment

- Fill in the boxes with the PPS assessment type code exactly as submitted for item A0310B "PPS Assessment" on the prior erroneous record to be modified/inactivated.
- Note that the PPS assessment code in X0600B must match the current value of A0310B on a modification request.
- If item A0310B was incorrect on an assessment that we previously submitted and accepted by the ASAP system, then the original assessment must be inactivated and a new record with a new date must be submitted.

Coding Instructions for X0600C, PPS Other Medicare Required Assessment—OMRA

- Fill in the boxes with the PPS OMRA code exactly as submitted for item A0310C "PPS—OMRA" on the prior erroneous record to be modified/inactivated.
- Note that the PPS OMRA code in X0600C must match the current value of A0310C on a modification request.
- If item A0310C was incorrect on an assessment that we previously submitted and accepted by the ASAP system, then the original assessment must be inactivated and a new record with a new date must be submitted.

Coding Instructions for X0600D, Is this a Swing Bed clinical change assessment? (Complete only if X0150=2)

- Enter the code exactly as submitted for item A0310D "Is this a Swing Bed clinical change assessment?" on the prior erroneous record to be modified/inactivated.
- **Code 0, no:** if the assessment submitted was not coded as a swing bed clinical change assessment.
- **Code 1, yes:** if the assessment submitted was coded as a swing bed clinical change assessment.

X0600: Type of Assessment/Tracking (cont.)

- Note that the code in X0600D must match the current value of A0310D on a modification request.

- If item A0310D was incorrect on an assessment that we previously submitted and accepted by the ASAP system, then the original assessment must be inactivated and a new record with a new date must be submitted.

Coding Instructions for X0600F, Entry/discharge reporting

- Enter the number corresponding to the entry/discharge code exactly as submitted for item A0310F "Entry/discharge reporting" on the prior erroneous record to be modified/inactivated.

    01. Entry tracking record

    10. Discharge assessment-return not anticipated

    11. Discharge assessment-return anticipated

    12. Death in facility tracking record

    99. None of the above

- Note that the Entry/discharge code in X0600F must match the current value of A0310F on a modification request.

- If item A0310F was incorrect on an assessment that we previously submitted and accepted by the ASAP system, then the original assessment must be inactivated and a new record with a new date must be submitted.

X0700: Date on Existing Record to Be Modified/Inactivated – Complete one only

The item that is completed in this section is the event date for the prior erroneous record to be modified/inactivated. The event date is the assessment reference date for an assessment record, the discharge date for a discharge record, or the entry date for an entry record. In the QIES ASAP system, this date is often referred to as the "target date." Enter only one (1) date in X0700.

X0700. Date on existing record to be modified/inactivated - **Complete one only**
A. Assessment Reference Date - Complete only if X0600F = 99 ☐☐ - ☐☐ - ☐☐☐☐ Month   Day   Year
B. Discharge Date - Complete only if X0600F = 10, 11, or 12 ☐☐ - ☐☐ - ☐☐☐☐ Month   Day   Year
C. Entry Date - Complete only if X0600F = 01 ☐☐ - ☐☐ - ☐☐☐☐ Month   Day   Year

X0700: Date on Existing Record to Be Modified/Inactivated (cont.)

Coding Instructions for X0700A, Assessment Reference Date— Complete Only if X0600F = 99

- If the prior erroneous record to be modified/inactivated is an OBRA assessment or a PPS assessment, where X0600F = 99, enter the assessment reference date here exactly as submitted in item A2300 "Assessment Reference Date" on the prior record.
- Note that the assessment reference date in X0700A must match the current value of A2300 on a modification request.

Coding Instructions for X0700B, Discharge Date—Complete Only If X0600F = 10, 11, or 12

- If the prior erroneous record to be modified/inactivated is a discharge record (indicated by X0600F = 10, 11, or 12), enter the discharge date here exactly as submitted for item A2000 "Discharge Date" on the prior record. If the prior erroneous record was a discharge combined with an OBRA or PPS assessment, then that prior record will contain both a completed assessment reference date (A2300) and discharge date (A2000) and these two dates will be identical. If such a record is being modified or inactivated, enter the prior discharge date in X0700B and leave the prior assessment reference date in X0700A blank.
- Note that the discharge date in X0700B must match the current value of A2000 on a modification request.

Coding Instructions for X0700C, Entry Date—Complete Only If X0600F = 01

- If the prior erroneous record to be modified/inactivated is an entry record (indicated by X0600F = 01), enter the entry date here exactly as submitted for item A1600 "Entry Date [date of admission/reentry into the facility]" on the prior record.
- Note that the entry date in X0700C must match the current value of A1600 on a modification request.

X0800: Correction Attestation Section

The items in this section indicate the number of times the QIES ASAP database record has been corrected, the reason for the current modification/inactivation request, the person attesting to the modification/inactivation request, and the date of the attestation.

This item may be populated automatically by the nursing home's date entry software, however, if it is not, the nursing home should enter this information.

Correction Attestation Section - Complete this section to explain and attest to the modification/inactivation request
X0800. Correction Number
Enter Number [ ] [ ] Enter the number of correction requests to modify/inactivate the existing record, including the present one

X0800: Correction Attestation Section (cont.)

Coding Instructions for X0800, Correction Number

- Enter the total number of correction requests to modify/inactivate the QIES ASAP record that is in error. Include the present modification/inactivation request in this number.
- For the first correction request (modification/inactivation) for an MDS record, code a value of 01 (zero-one); for the second correction request, code a value of 02 (zero-two); etc. With each succeeding request, X0800 is incremented by one. For values between one and nine, a leading zero should be used in the first box. For example, enter "01" into the two boxes for X0800.
- This item identifies the total number of correction requests following the original assessment or tracking record, including the present request. Note that Item X0800 is used to track successive correction requests in the QIES ASAP database.

X0900: Reasons for Modification

The items in this section indicate the possible reasons for the modification request of the record in the QIES ASAP database. Check all that apply. These items should only be completed when A0050 = 2, indicating a modification request. If A0050 = 3, indicating an inactivation request, these items should be skipped.

X0900. Reasons for Modification - Complete only if Type of Record is to modify a record in error (A0050 = 2)
↓ Check all that apply
☐ A. Transcription error
☐ B. Data entry error
☐ C. Software product error
☐ D. Item coding error
☐ E. End of Therapy - Resumption (EOT-R) date
☐ Z. Other error requiring modification If "Other" checked, please specify: _____

Coding Instructions for X0900A, Transcription Error

- Check the box if any errors in the prior QIES ASAP record were caused by data transcription errors.
- A transcription error includes any error made recording MDS assessment or tracking form information from other sources. An example is transposing the digits for the resident's weight (e.g., recording "191" rather than the correct weight of "119" that appears in the medical record).

Coding Instructions for X0900B, Data Entry Error

- Check the box if any errors in the prior QIES ASAP record were caused by data entry errors.
- A data entry error includes any error made while encoding MDS assessment or tracking form information into the facility's computer system. An example is an error where the response to the individual minutes of physical therapy O0400C1 is incorrectly encoded as "3000" minutes rather than the correct number of "0030" minutes.

X0900: Reasons for Modification (cont.)

Coding Instructions for X0900C, Software Product Error

- Check the box if any errors in the prior QIES ASAP record were caused by software product errors.
- A software product error includes any error created by the encoding software, such as storing an item in the wrong format (e.g., storing weight as "020" instead of "200").

Coding Instructions for X0900D, Item Coding Error

- Check the box if any errors in the prior QIES ASAP record were caused by item coding errors.
- An item coding error includes any error made coding an MDS item (for exceptions when certain items may not be modified see Chapter 5), such as choosing an incorrect code for the Activities of Daily Living (ADL) bed mobility self-performance item G0110A1 (e.g., choosing a code of "4" for a resident who requires limited assistance and should be coded as "2"). Item coding errors may result when an assessor makes an incorrect judgment or misunderstands the RAI coding instructions.

Coding Instructions for X0900E, End of Therapy-Resumption (EOT-R) date

- Check the box if the End of Therapy-Resumption (EOT-R) date (item O0450B) has been added with the modified record (i.e., the provider has determined that the EOT-R policy was applicable after submitting the original EOT record not indicating a resumption of therapy date in item O0450B).
- Do not check this box if the modification is correcting the End of Therapy Resumption date (item O0450B) in a previous EOT-R assessment. In this case, the reason for modification is an item Coding Error and box X0900D should be checked.

Coding Instructions for X0900Z, Other Error Requiring Modification

- Check the box if any errors in the prior QIES ASAP record were caused by other types of errors not included in Items X0900A through X0900E.
- Such an error includes any other type of error that causes a QIES ASAP record to require modification under the Correction Policy. An example would be when a record is prematurely submitted prior to final completion of editing and review. Facility staff should describe the "other error" in the space provided with the item.

X1050: Reasons for Inactivation

The items in this section indicate the possible reasons for the inactivation request. Check all that apply. These items should only be completed when A0050 = 3, indicating an inactivation request. If A0050 = 2, indicating a modification request, these items should be skipped.

X1050. Reasons for Inactivation - Complete only if Type of Record is to inactivate a record in error (A0050 = 3)
↓ Check all that apply
☐ A. Event did not occur
☐ Z. Other error requiring inactivation / If "Other" checked, please specify: _____

X1050: Reasons for Inactivation (cont.)

Coding Instructions for X1050A, Event Did Not Occur

- Check the box if the prior QIES ASAP record does not represent an event that actually occurred.
- An example would be a discharge record submitted for a resident, but there was no actual discharge. There was **no event**.

Coding Instructions for X1050Z, Other Reason Requiring Inactivation

- Check the box if any errors in the prior QIES ASAP record were caused by other types of errors not included in Item X1050A.
- Facility staff should describe the "other error" in the space provided with the item.

X1100: RN Assessment Coordinator Attestation of Completion

The items in this section identify the RN coordinator attesting to the correction request and the date of the attestation.

Coding Instructions for X1100A, Attesting Individual's First Name

- Enter the first name of the facility staff member attesting to the completion of the corrected information. Start entry with the leftmost box.

Coding Instructions for X1100B, Attesting Individual's Last Name

- Enter the last name of the facility staff member attesting to the completion of the corrected information. Start entry with the leftmost box.

Coding Instructions for X1100C, Attesting Individual's Title

- Enter the title of the facility staff member attesting to the completion of the corrected information on the line provided.

X1100: RN Assessment Coordinator Attestation of Completion (cont.)

Coding Instructions for X1100D, **Signature**

- The attesting individual must sign the correction request here, certifying the completion of the corrected information. The entire correction request should be completed and signed within 14 days of detecting an error in a QIES ASAP record. The correction request, including the signature of the attesting facility staff, must be kept with the modified or inactivated MDS record and retained in the resident's medical record or electronic medical record.

Coding Instructions for X1100E, **Attestation Date**

- Enter the date the attesting facility staff member attested to the completion of the corrected information.
- Do not leave any boxes blank. For a one-digit month or day, place a zero in the first box. For example, January 2, 2011, should be entered as:

0	1		0	2		2	0	1	1

Coding Tip for X1100, **RN Assessment Coordinator Attestation of Completion**

- If an inactivation is being completed, Z0400 must also be completed.

SECTION Z: ASSESSMENT ADMINISTRATION

Intent: The intent of the items in this section is to provide billing information and signatures of persons completing the assessment.

Z0100: Medicare Part A Billing

Z0100. Medicare Part A Billing	
Enter Code	**A. Medicare Part A HIPPS code** (RUG group followed by assessment type indicator):
	B. RUG version code:
	C. Is this a Medicare Short Stay assessment? 0. No 1. Yes

Item Rationale

- Used to capture the Resource Utilization Group (RUG) followed by Health Insurance Prospective Payment System (HIPPS) modifier based on type of assessment.

Coding Instructions for Z0100A, **Medicare Part A HIPPS Code**

- Typically the software data entry product will calculate this value.
- The HIPPS code is a Skilled Nursing Facility (SNF) Part A billing code and is composed of a five-position code representing the RUG group code, plus a two-position assessment type indicator. For information on HIPPS, access: http://www.cms.gov/ProspMedicareFeeSvcPmtGen/02_HIPPSCodes.asp#TopOfPage.
- If the value for Z0100A is not automatically calculated by the software data entry product, enter the HIPPS code in the spaces provided (see Chapter 6 of this manual, Medicare Skilled Nursing Home Prospective Payment System, for a step-by-step worksheet for manually determining the RUG code and a table that defines the assessment type indicator).
- Note that the RUG included in this HIPPS code takes into account all MDS items used in the RUG logic and is the "normal" group since the classification considers the rehabilitation therapy received. This classification uses all reported speech/language pathology and auditory services, occupational therapy, and physical therapy values in Item O0400 (Therapies).
- This HIPPS code is usually used for Medicare SNF Part A billing by the provider.
- Left-justify the 5-character HIPPS code. The extra two spaces are supplied for future use, if necessary.

> **DEFINITIONS**
>
> **MEDICARE-COVERED STAY**
>
> Skilled Nursing Facility stays billable to Medicare Part A. Does not include stays billable to Medicare Advantage HMO plans.

> **DEFINITIONS**
>
> **HIPPS CODE**
>
> Health Insurance Prospective Payment System code is comprised of the RUG category calculated by the assessment followed by an indicator of the type of assessment that was completed.

Z0100: Medicare Part A Billing (cont.)

Coding Instructions for Z0100B, RUG Version Code

- Typically the software data entry product will calculate this value.

- If the value for Z0100B is not automatically calculated by the software data entry product, enter the RUG version code in the spaces provided. This is the version code appropriate to the RUG included in the Medicare Part A HIPPS code in Item Z0100A.

- With MDS 3.0 implementation on October 1, 2010, the initial Medicare RUG-IV Version Code is "1.0066".

Coding Instructions for Z0100C, Is This a Medicare Short Stay Assessment?

- **Code 0, No:** if this is not a Medicare Short Stay Assessment.
- **Code 1, Yes:** if this is a Medicare Short Stay Assessment.

Coding Tip

- The CMS standard RUG-IV grouper automatically determines whether or not this is a Medicare Short Stay Assessment. MDS software typically makes this determination automatically. If the value for Z0100C is not automatically calculated by the software data entry product, use the definition found in Chapter 6 to determine the correct response.

> **DEFINITIONS**
>
> **MEDICARE SHORT STAY ASSESSMENT** is a Start of Therapy Other Medicare Required Assessment (OMRA) and is used for a short Medicare Part A stay that was not long enough to allow a complete rehabilitation therapy regimen to be established. This type of assessment allows an alternative Medicare Short Stay assessment RUG rehabilitation therapy classification as described in Chapter 6, Medicare Skilled Nursing Home Prospective Payment System.

Z0150: Medicare Part A Non-Therapy Billing

Z0150. Medicare Part A Non-Therapy Billing
A. Medicare Part A non-therapy HIPPS code (RUG group followed by assessment type indicator):
B. RUG version code:

Item Rationale

Used to capture the Resource Utilization Group non-therapy (RUG) followed by Health Insurance Prospective Payment System (HIPPS) modifier based on type of assessment. The non- therapy RUG is the code obtained when all rehabilitation therapy is ignored and will be limited to the Extensive Services, Special Care High, Special Care Low, Clinically Complex, Behavior and Cognitive Performance, and the Physical Function codes.

Z0150: Medicare Part A Non-Therapy Billing (cont.)

Coding Instructions for Z0150A, Medicare Part A Non-therapy HIPPS Code

- Typically the software data entry product will calculate this value.
- The HIPPS code is a SNF Part A billing code and is comprised of a five-position code representing the RUG code, plus a two-position assessment type indicator. For information on HIPPS, access http://www.cms.gov/ProspMedicareFeeSvcPmtGen/02_HIPPSCodes.asp#TopOfPage.
- If the value for Z0150A is not automatically calculated by the software data entry product, enter the HIPPS code in the spaces provided (see Chapter 6 of this manual, Medicare Skilled Nursing Home Prospective Payment System, for a step-by-step worksheet for manually determining the RUG-IV group and a table that defines assessment type indicator). Note that the RUG included in this HIPPS code is the "non- therapy" group and classification ignores the rehabilitation therapy received. This classification ignores all reported speech/language pathology and auditory services, occupational therapy, and physical therapy values in Item O0400 (Therapies).
- In some instances, this non-therapy HIPPS code may be required for Medicare SNF Part A billing by the provider.
- Left-justify the 5-character HIPPS code. The extra two spaces are supplied for future use, if necessary.

Coding Instructions for Z0150B, RUG Version Code

- Typically the software data entry product will calculate this value.
- If the value for Z0150B is not automatically calculated by the software data entry product, enter the RUG version code in the spaces provided. This is the version code appropriate to the RUG included in the Medicare Part A non-therapy HIPPS code in Item Z0150A.
- With MDS 3.0 implementation on October 1, 2010, the initial Medicare RUG-IV Version Code is "1.0066".

Z0200: State Medicaid Billing (if required by the state)

Z0200. State Medicaid Billing (if required by the state)
A. RUG Case Mix group:
B. RUG version code:

Item Rationale

- Used to capture the payment code in states that employ the MDS for Medicaid case-mix reimbursement.

Z0200: State Medicaid Billing (cont.)

Coding Instructions for Z0200A, RUG Case Mix Group

- If the state has selected a standard RUG model, this item will usually be populated automatically by the software data entry product. Otherwise, enter the case-mix code calculated based on the MDS assessment.

Coding Instructions for Z0200B, RUG Version Code

- If the state has selected a standard RUG model, this item will usually be populated automatically by the software data entry product. Otherwise, enter the case mix version code in the spaces provided. This is the version code appropriate to the code in Item Z0200A.

Z0250: Alternate State Medicaid Billing (if required by state)

Z0250. Alternate State Medicaid Billing (if required by the state)
A. RUG Case Mix group:
B. RUG version code:

Item Rationale

- Used to capture an alternate payment group in states that employ the MDS for Medicaid case-mix reimbursement. States may want to capture a second payment group for Medicaid purposes to allow evaluation of the fiscal impact of changing to a new payment model or to allow blended payment between two models during a transition period.

Coding Instructions for Z0250A, RUG Case Mix Group

- If the state has selected a standard RUG model, this item will usually be populated automatically by the software data entry product. Otherwise, enter the case-mix code calculated based on the MDS assessment.

Coding Instructions for Z0250B, RUG Version Code

- If the state has selected a standard RUG model, this item will usually be populated automatically by the software data entry product. Otherwise, enter the case mix version code in the spaces provided. This is the version code appropriate to the code in Item Z0250A.

Z0300: Insurance Billing

Z0300. Insurance Billing
A. RUG billing code:
⬚⬚⬚⬚⬚⬚⬚⬚⬚⬚
B. RUG billing version:
⬚⬚⬚⬚⬚⬚⬚⬚⬚⬚

Item Rationale

- Allows providers and vendors to capture case-mix codes required by other payers (e.g. private insurance or the Department of Veterans Affairs).

Coding Instructions for Z0300A, RUG billing code

- If the other payer has selected a standard RUG model, this item may be populated automatically by the software data entry product. Otherwise, enter the billing code in the space provided. This code is for use by other payment systems such as private insurance or the Department of Veterans Affairs.

Coding Instructions for Z0300B, RUG billing version

- If the other payor has selected a standard RUG model, this item may be populated automatically by the software data entry product. Otherwise, enter an appropriate billing version in the spaces provided. This is the billing version appropriate to the billing code in Item Z0300A.

Z0400: Signatures of Persons Completing the Assessment or Entry/Death Reporting

Z0400. Signature of Persons Completing the Assessment or Entry/Death Reporting

I certify that the accompanying information accurately reflects resident assessment information for this resident and that I collected or coordinated collection of this information on the dates specified. To the best of my knowledge, this information was collected in accordance with applicable Medicare and Medicaid requirements. I understand that this information is used as a basis for ensuring that residents receive appropriate and quality care, and as a basis for payment from federal funds. I further understand that payment of such federal funds and continued participation in the government-funded health care programs is conditioned on the accuracy and truthfulness of this information, and that I may be personally subject to or may subject my organization to substantial criminal, civil, and/or administrative penalties for submitting false information. I also certify that I am authorized to submit this information by this facility on its behalf.

Signature	Title	Sections	Date Section Completed
A.			
B.			
C.			
D.			
E.			
F.			
G.			
H.			
I.			
J.			
K.			
L.			

Item Rationale

- To obtain the signature of all persons who completed any part of the MDS. Legally, it is an attestation of accuracy with the primary responsibility for its accuracy with the person selecting the MDS item response. Each person completing a section or portion of a section of the MDS is required to sign the Attestation Statement.

- The importance of accurately completing and submitting the MDS cannot be over-emphasized. The MDS is the basis for:

  — the development of an individualized care plan;

  — the Medicare Prospective Payment System

  — Medicaid reimbursement programs

  — quality monitoring activities, such as the quality indicator/quality measure reports

  — the data-driven survey and certification process

  — the quality measures used for public reporting

  — research and policy development.

Z0400: Signatures of Persons Completing the Assessment (cont.)

Coding Instructions

- All staff who completed any part of the MDS must enter their signatures, titles, sections or portion(s) of section(s) they completed, and the date completed.

- If a staff member cannot sign Z0400 on the same day that he or she completed a section or portion of a section, when the staff member signs, use the date the item originally was completed.

- Read the Attestation Statement carefully. You are certifying that the information you entered on the MDS, to the best of your knowledge, most accurately reflects the resident's status. Penalties may be applied for submitting false information.

Coding Tips and Special Populations

- Two or more staff members can complete items within the same section of the MDS. When filling in the information for Z0400, any staff member who has completed a sub- set of item within a section should identify which item(s) he/she completed within that section.
- Nursing homes may use electronic signatures for medical record documentation, including the MDS, when permitted to do so by state and local law and when authorized by the nursing home's policy. Nursing homes must have written policies in place that meet any and all state and federal privacy and security requirements to ensure proper security measures to protect the use of an electronic signature by anyone other than the person to whom the electronic signature belongs.

- Although the use of electronic signatures for the MDS does not require that the entire record be maintained electronically, most facilities have the option to maintain a resident's record by computer rather than hard copy.

- Whenever copies of the MDS are printed and dates are automatically encoded, be sure to note that it is a "copy" document and not the original.

Z0500: Signature of RN Assessment Coordinator Verifying Assessment Completion

Z0500. Signature of RN Assessment Coordinator Verifying Assessment Completion	
A. Signature:	B. Date RN Assessment Coordinator signed assessment as complete: ☐☐ – ☐☐ – ☐☐☐☐ Month Day Year

Item Rationale

- Federal regulation requires the RN assessment coordinator to sign and thereby certify that the assessment is complete.

Z0500: Signature of RN Assessment Coordinator Verifying Assessment Completion (cont.)

Steps for Assessment

1. Verify that all items on this assessment or tracking record are complete.
2. Verify that Item Z0400 (Signature of Persons Completing the Assessment) contains attestation for all MDS sections.

Coding Instructions

- For Z0500B, use the actual date that the MDS was completed, reviewed, and signed as complete by the RN assessment coordinator. This date will generally be later than the date(s) at Z0400, which documents when portions of the assessment information were completed by assessment team members.
- If for some reason the MDS cannot be signed by the RN assessment coordinator on the date it is completed, the RN assessment coordinator should use the actual date that it is signed.

Coding Tips

- The RN assessment coordinator is not certifying the accuracy of portions of the assessment that were completed by other health professionals.
- Nursing homes may use electronic signatures for medical record documentation, including the MDS, when permitted to do so by state and local law and when authorized by the nursing home's policy. Nursing homes must have written policies in place that meet any and all state and federal privacy and security requirements to ensure proper security measures to protect the use of an electronic signature by anyone other than the person to whom the electronic signature belongs.
- Although the use of electronic signatures for the MDS does not require that the entire record be maintained electronically, most facilities have the option to maintain a resident's record by computer rather than hard copy.
- Whenever copies of the MDS are printed and dates are automatically encoded, be sure to note that it is a "copy" document and not the original.

CHAPTER 4:   CARE AREA ASSESSMENT (CAA) PROCESS AND CARE PLANNING

4.1   Background and Rationale

The Omnibus Budget Reconciliation Act of 1987 (OBRA 1987) mandated that nursing facilities provide necessary care and services to help each resident attain or maintain the highest practicable well-being. Facilities must ensure that residents improve when possible and do not deteriorate unless the resident's clinical condition demonstrates that the decline was unavoidable.

Regulations require facilities to complete, at a minimum and at regular intervals, a comprehensive, standardized assessment of each resident's functional capacity and needs, in relation to a number of specified areas (e.g., customary routine, vision, and continence). The results of the assessment, which must accurately reflect the resident's status and needs, are to be used to develop, review, and revise each resident's comprehensive plan of care.

This chapter provides information about the Care Area Assessments (CAAs), Care Area Triggers (CATs), and the process for care plan development for nursing home residents.

4.2   Overview of the Resident Assessment Instrument (RAI) and Care Area Assessments (CAAs)

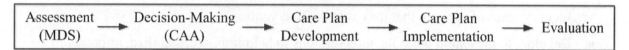

Assessment (MDS) → Decision-Making (CAA) → Care Plan Development → Care Plan Implementation → Evaluation

As discussed in Chapter 1, the updated Resident Assessment Instrument (RAI) consists of three basic components: 1) the Minimum Data Set (MDS) Version 3.0, 2) the Care Area Assessment (CAA) process, and 3) the RAI Utilization Guidelines. The RAI-related processes help staff identify key information about residents as a basis for identifying resident-specific issues and objectives. In accordance with 42 CFR 483.20(k) the facility must develop a comprehensive care plan for each resident that includes measurable objectives and timetables to meet a resident's medical, nursing, and mental and psychosocial needs that are identified in the comprehensive assessment. The services that are to be furnished to attain or maintain the resident's highest practicable physical, mental, and psychosocial well-being and any services that would otherwise be required but are not provided due to the resident's exercise of rights including the right to refuse treatment.

The MDS is a starting point. The Minimum Data Set (MDS) is a standardized instrument used to assess nursing home residents. It is a collection of basic physical (e.g., medical conditions, mood, and vision), functional (e.g., activities of daily living, behavior), and psychosocial (e.g., preferences, goals, and interests) information about residents. For example, assessing a resident's orientation and recall helps staff complete portions of the MDS that relate to cognition (Section C), and weighing a resident and identifying his or her food intake helps staff complete portions of the MDS related to nutritional status (Section K). When it is completed, the MDS provides a foundation for a more thorough assessment and the development of an individualized care plan. The MDS 3.0 manual explains in detail how to complete the MDS.

The information in the MDS constitutes the core of the required State-specified Resident Assessment Instrument (RAI). Based on assessing the resident, the MDS identifies actual or potential areas of concern. The remainder of the RAI process supports the efforts of nursing home staff, health professionals, and practitioners to further assess these triggered areas of concern in order to identify, to the extent possible, whether the findings represent a problem or risk requiring further intervention, as well as the causes and risk factors related to the triggered care area under assessment. These conclusions then provide the basis for developing an individualized care plan for each resident.

The CAA process framework. The CAA process provides a framework for guiding the review of triggered areas, and clarification of a resident's functional status and related causes of impairments. It also provides a basis for additional assessment of potential issues, including related risk factors. The assessment of the causes and contributing factors gives the interdisciplinary team (IDT) additional information to help them develop a comprehensive plan of care.

When implemented properly, the CAA process should help staff:

- Consider each resident as a whole, with unique characteristics and strengths that affect his or her capacity to function;

- Identify areas of concern that may warrant interventions;

- Develop, to the extent possible, interventions to help improve, stabilize, or prevent decline in physical, functional, and psychosocial well-being, in the context of the resident's condition, choices, and preferences for interventions; and

- Address the need and desire for other important considerations, such as advanced care planning and palliative care; e.g., symptom relief and pain management.

4.3   What Are the Care Area Assessments (CAAs)?

The completed MDS must be analyzed and combined with other relevant information to develop an individualized care plan. To help nursing facilities apply assessment data collected on the MDS, Care Area Assessments (CAAs) are triggered responses to items coded on the MDS specific to a resident's possible problems, needs or strengths. Specific "CAT logic" for each care area is identified under section 4.10 (The Twenty Care Areas). The CAAs reflect conditions, symptoms, and other areas of concern that are common in nursing home residents and are commonly identified or suggested by MDS findings. Interpreting and addressing the care areas identified by the CATs is the basis of the Care Area Assessment process, and can help provide additional information for the development of an individualized care plan.

Table 1. Care Area Assessments in the Resident Assessment Instrument, Version 3.0

1. Delirium	2. Cognitive Loss/Dementia
3. Visual Function	4. Communication
5. Activity of Daily Living (ADL) Functional / Rehabilitation Potential	6. Urinary Incontinence and Indwelling Catheter
7. Psychosocial Well-Being	8. Mood State
9. Behavioral Symptoms	10. Activities
11. Falls	12. Nutritional Status
13. Feeding Tubes	14. Dehydration/Fluid Maintenance
15. Dental Care	16. Pressure Ulcer
17. Psychotropic Medication Use	18. Physical Restraints
19. Pain	20. Return to Community Referral

The CAA process does not mandate any specific tool for completing the further assessment of the triggered areas, nor does it provide any specific guidance on how to understand or interpret the triggered areas. Instead, facilities are instructed to identify and use tools that are current and grounded in current clinical standards of practice, such as evidence-based or expert-endorsed research, clinical practice guidelines, and resources. When applying these evidence-based resources to practice, the use of sound clinical problem solving and decision making (often called "critical thinking") skills is imperative.

By statute, the RAI must be completed within 14 days of admission. As an integral part of the RAI, CAAs must be completed and documented within the same time frame. While a workup cannot always be completed within 14 days, it is expected that nursing homes will assess resident needs, plan care and implement interventions in a timely manner.

CAAs are not required for Medicare PPS assessments. They are required only for OBRA comprehensive assessments (Admission, Annual, Significant Change in Status, or Significant Correction of a Prior Comprehensive). However, when a Medicare PPS assessment is combined with an OBRA comprehensive assessment, the CAAs must be completed in order to meet the requirements of the OBRA comprehensive assessment.

4.4 What Does the CAA Process Involve?

Facilities use the findings from the comprehensive assessment to develop an individualized care plan to meet each resident's needs (42 CFR 483.20(b)). The CAA process discussed in this manual refers to identifying and clarifying areas of concern that are triggered based on how specific MDS items are coded on the MDS. The process focuses on evaluating these triggered care areas using the CAAs, but does not provide exact detail on how to select pertinent interventions for care planning. Interventions must be individualized and based on applying effective problem solving and decision making approaches to all of the information available for each resident.

Care Area Triggers (CATs) identify conditions that may require further evaluation because they may have an impact on specific issues and/or conditions, or the risk of issues and/or conditions for the resident. Each triggered item must be assessed further through the use of the CAA process to facilitate care plan decision making, but it may or may not represent a condition that should or will be addressed in the care plan. The significance and causes of any given trigger may vary for different residents or in different situations for the same resident. Different CATs may have common causes, or various items associated with several CATs may be connected.

CATs provide a "flag" for the IDT members, indicating that the triggered care area needs to be assessed more completely prior to making care planning decisions. Further assessment of a triggered care area may identify causes, risk factors, and complications associated with the care area condition. The plan of care then addresses these factors with the goal of promoting the resident's highest practicable level of functioning: (1) improvement where possible or (2) maintenance and prevention of avoidable declines.

A risk factor increases the chances of having a negative outcome or complication. For example, impaired bed mobility may increase the risk of getting a pressure ulcer. In this example, impaired bed mobility is the risk factor, unrelieved pressure is the effect of the compromised bed mobility, and the potential pressure ulcer is the complication.

A care area issue/condition (e.g., falls) may result from a single underlying cause (e.g., administration of a new medication that causes dizziness) or from a combination of multiple factors (e.g., new medication, resident forgot walker, bed too high or too low, etc.). There can also be a single cause of multiple triggers and impairments. For example, hypothyroidism is an example of a common, potentially reversible medical condition that can have diverse physical, functional, and psychosocial complications. Thus, if a resident has hypothyroidism, it is possible that the MDS might trigger any or several of the following CAAs depending on whether or not the hypothyroidism is controlled, there is an acute exacerbation, etc.: Delirium (#1), Cognitive Loss/Dementia (#2), Visual Function (#3), Communication (#4), ADL Functional/Rehabilitation (#5), Urinary Incontinence (#6), Psychosocial Well-Being (#7), Mood State (#8), Behavior Symptoms (#9), Activities (#10), Falls (#11), Nutritional Status (#12), Dehydration (#14), Psychotropic Medication Use (#17), and Pain (#19). Even if the MDS does not trigger a particular care area, the facility can use the CAA process and resources at any time to further assess the resident.

Recognizing the connection among these symptoms and treating the underlying cause(s) to the extent possible, can help address complications and improve the resident's outcome. Conversely, failing to recognize the links and instead trying to address the triggers or MDS findings in isolation may have little if any benefit for the resident with hypothyroidism or other complex or mixed causes of impaired behavior, cognition, and mood.

For example, it is necessary to assess a resident's orientation and recall in order to complete portions of the MDS that relate to cognitive patterns (Section C) and to obtain a resident's weight and identify his or her food intake in order to complete MDS items related to nutritional status (Section K). A positive finding in Section C may trigger one or several CAAs, including Delirium (#1), Cognitive Loss/Dementia (#2), and ADL Functional/Rehabilitation Potential (#5).

Additional evaluation is then required to identify whether the resident has delirium, dementia, or both; how current symptoms and patterns compare to their usual or previous baseline, whether potentially reversible causes are present, what else might be needed to identify underlying causes (including medical diagnoses and history), and what symptomatic and cause-specific interventions are appropriate for the resident. If the Nutritional Status (#12) CAA also triggered, due to weight loss and the resident being found to have delirium, then it is possible that both findings could have a common cause (e.g., an infection or medication side effects), that delirium resulted in impaired nutritional status, or that impaired nutritional status led to delirium, or still other possibilities. Thus, identifying the sequence of events is essential to understanding causes and choosing appropriate interventions.

The RAI is not intended to provide diagnostic advice, nor is it intended to specify which triggered areas may be related to one another or and how those problems relate to underlying causes. It is up to the IDT, including the resident's physician, to determine these connections and underlying causes as they assess the triggered care areas and any other areas pertinent to the individual resident.

Not all triggers identify deficits or problems. Some triggers indicate areas of resident strengths, and can suggest possible approaches to improve a resident's functioning or minimize decline. For example, MDS item responses indicate the "resident believes he or she is capable of increased independence in at least some ADLs" (Item G0900A) may focus the assessment and care plan on functional areas most important to the resident or on the area with the greatest potential for improvement.

In addition to identifying causes and risk factors that contribute to the resident's care area issues or conditions, the CAA process may help the IDT:

- Identify and address associated causes and effects;

- Determine whether and how multiple triggered conditions are related;

- Identify a need to obtain additional medical, functional, psychosocial, financial, or other information about a resident's condition that may be obtained from sources such as the resident, the resident's family or other responsible party, the attending physician, direct care staff, rehabilitative staff, or that requires laboratory and diagnostic tests;

- Identify whether and how a triggered condition actually affects the resident's function and quality of life, or whether the resident is at particular risk of developing the conditions;

- Review the resident's situation with a health care practitioner (e.g., attending physician, medical director, or nurse practitioner), to try to identify links among causes and between causes and consequences, and to identify pertinent tests, consultations, and interventions;

- Determine whether a resident could potentially benefit from rehabilitative interventions;

- Begin to develop an individualized care plan with measurable objectives and timetables to meet a resident's medical, functional, mental and psychosocial needs as identified through the comprehensive assessment.

4.5   Other Considerations Regarding Use of the CAAs

Assigning responsibility for completing the MDS and CAAs. Per the OBRA statute, the resident's assessment must be conducted or coordinated by a registered nurse (RN) with the appropriate participation of health professionals. It is common practice for facilities to assign specific MDS items or portion(s) of items (and subsequently CAAs associated with those items) to those of various disciplines (e.g., the dietitian completes the Nutritional Status and Feeding Tube CAAs, if triggered). The proper assessment and management of CAAs that are triggered for a given resident may involve aspects of diagnosis and treatment selection that exceed the scope of training or practice of any one discipline involved in the care (for example, identifying specific medical conditions or medication side effects that cause anorexia leading to a resident's weight loss). It is the facility's responsibility to obtain the input that is needed for clinical decision making (e.g., identifying causes and selecting interventions) that is consistent with relevant clinical standards of practice. For example, a physician may need to get a more detailed history or perform a physical examination in order to establish or confirm a diagnosis and/or related complications.

Identifying policies and practices related to the assessment and care planning processes. Under the OBRA regulations, 42 CFR 483.75(i) identifies the medical director as being responsible for overseeing the " implementation of resident care policies" in each facility, "and the coordination of medical care in the facility." Therefore, it is recommended that the facility's IDT members collaborate with the medical director to identify current evidence-based or expert-endorsed resources and standards of practice that they will use for the expanded assessments and analyses that may be needed to adequately address triggered areas. The facility should be able to provide surveyors the resources that they have used upon request as part of the survey review process.[1]

CAA documentation. CAA documentation helps to explain the basis for the care plan by showing how the IDT determined that the underlying causes, contributing factors, and risk factors were related to the care area condition for a specific resident; for example, the documentation should indicate the basis for these decisions, why the finding(s) require(s) an intervention, and the rationale(s) for selecting specific interventions. Based on the review of the comprehensive assessment, the IDT and the resident and/or the resident's representative determine the areas that require care plan intervention(s) and develop, revise, or continue the individualized care plan.

- Relevant documentation for each triggered CAA describes: causes and contributing factors;

- The nature of the issue or condition (may include presence or lack of objective data and subjective complaints). In other words, what exactly is the issue/problem for this resident and why is it a problem;

- Complications affecting or caused by the care area for this resident;

- Risk factors related to the presence of the condition that affects the staff's decision to proceed to care planning;

---

[1]   In Appendix C, CMS has provided CAA resources that facilities may choose to use but that are neither mandatory nor endorsed by the government. Please note that Appendix C does not provide an all-inclusive list.

- Factors that must be considered in developing individualized care plan interventions, including the decision to care plan or not to care plan various findings for the individual resident;

- The need for additional evaluation by the attending physician and other health professionals, as appropriate;

- The resource(s), or assessment tool(s) used for decision-making, and conclusions that arose from performing the CAA;

- Completion of Section V (CAA Summary; see Chapter 3 for coding instructions) of the MDS.

Written documentation of the CAA findings and decision making process may appear anywhere in a resident's record; for example, in discipline-specific flow sheets, progress notes, the care plan summary notes, a CAA summary narrative, etc. Nursing homes should use a format that provides the information as outlined in this manual and the State Operations Manual (SOM). If it is not clear that a facility's documentation provides this information, surveyors may ask facility staff to provide such evidence.

Use the "Location and Date of CAA Documentation" column on the CAA Summary (Section V of the MDS 3.0) to note where the CAA information and decision making documentation can be found in the resident's record. Also indicate in the column "Care Planning Decision" whether the triggered care area is addressed in the care plan.

4.6   When Is the RAI Not Enough?

Federal requirements support a nursing home's ongoing responsibility to assess residents. The Quality of Care regulation requires that "each resident must receive and the facility must provide the necessary care and services to attain or maintain the highest practicable physical, mental, and psychosocial well-being, in accordance with the comprehensive assessment and plan of care" (42 CFR 483.25 [F 309]).

Services provided or arranged by the nursing home must also meet professional standards of quality. Per 42 CFR 483.75(b), the facility must operate and provide services in compliance with all applicable Federal, State, and local laws, regulations, and codes, and with accepted professional standards and principles that apply to professionals providing services in such a facility. Furthermore, surveyor guidance within OBRA (e.g., F314 42 CFR 483.25(c) Pressure Sores and F329 42 CFR 483.25(l) Unnecessary Medications) identifies additional elements of assessment and care related to specific issues and/or conditions that are consistent with professional standards.

Therefore, facilities are responsible for assessing and addressing all care issues that are relevant to individual residents, regardless of whether or not they are covered by the RAI (42 CFR 483.20(b)), including monitoring each resident's condition and responding with appropriate interventions.

Limitations of the RAI-related instruments. The RAI provides tools related to assessment including substantial detail for completing the MDS, how CATs are triggered, and a framework for the CAA process. However, the process of completing the MDS and related portions of the

RAI does not constitute the entire assessment that may be needed to address issues and manage the care of individual residents.

Neither the MDS nor the remainder of the RAI includes all of the steps, relevant factors, analyses, or conclusions needed for clinical problem solving and decision making for the care of nursing home residents. By themselves, neither the MDS nor the CAA process provide sufficient information to determine if the findings from the MDS are problematic or merely incidental, or if there are multiple causes of a single trigger or multiple triggers related to one or several causes. Although a detailed history is often essential to correctly identify and address causes of symptoms, the RAI was not designed to capture a history (chronology) of a resident's symptoms and impairments. Thus, it can potentially be misleading or problematic to care plan individual MDS findings or CAAs without any additional thought or investigation.

- The MDS may not trigger every relevant issue
- Not all triggers are clinically significant
- The MDS is not a diagnostic tool or treatment selection guide
- The MDS does not identify causation or history of problems

Although facilities have the latitude to choose approaches to the CAA process, compliance with various OBRA requirements can be enhanced by using additional relevant clinical problem solving and decision making processes to analyze and address MDS findings and CAAs. Table 2 provides a framework for a more complete approach to clinical problem solving and decision making essential to the appropriate care of individuals with multiple and/or complex illnesses and impairments.

4.7 The RAI and Care Planning

As required at 42 CFR 483.25, the comprehensive care plan is an interdisciplinary communication tool. It must include measurable objectives and time frames and must describe the services that are to be furnished to attain or maintain the resident's highest practicable physical, mental, and psychosocial well-being. The care plan must be reviewed and revised periodically, and the services provided or arranged must be consistent with each resident's written plan of care. Refer to 42 CFR 483.20(d), which notes that a nursing home must maintain all resident assessments completed within the previous 15 months in the resident's active record and use the results of the assessments to develop, review, and revise the resident's comprehensive plan of care. Regulatory requirements related to care planning in nursing homes are located at 42 CFR 483.20(k)(1) and (2) and are specified in the interpretive guidelines (F tags) in Appendix PP of the State Operations Manual (SOM). The SOM can be found at: http://www.cms.gov/Manuals/IOM/list.asp.

Good assessment is the starting point for good clinical problem solving and decision making and ultimately for the creation of a sound care plan. The CAAs provide a link between the MDS and care planning. The care plan should be revised on an ongoing basis to reflect changes in the resident and the care that the resident is receiving (see.42 CFR 483.20(k), Comprehensive Care Plans). This Chapter does not specify a care plan structure or format.

Table 2. Clinical Problem Solving and Decision Making Process Steps and Objectives

Process Step / Objectives *	Key Tasks **
Recognition / Assessment *Gather essential information about the individual*	– Identify and collect information that is needed to identify an individual's conditions that enables proper definition of their conditions, strengths, needs, risks, problems, and prognosis – Obtain a personal and medical history – Perform a physical assessment
Problem definition *Define the individual's problems, risks, and issues*	– Identify any current consequences and complications of the individual's situation, underlying condition and illnesses, etc. – Clearly state the individual's issues and physical, functional, and psychosocial strengths, problems, needs, deficits, and concerns – Define significant risk factors
Diagnosis / Cause-and-effect analysis *Identify physical, functional, and psychosocial causes of risks, problems, and other issues, and relate to one another and to their consequences*	– Identify causes of, and factors contributing to, the individual's current dysfunctions, disabilities, impairments, and risks – Identify pertinent evaluations and diagnostic tests – Identify how existing symptoms, signs, diagnoses, test results, dysfunctions, impairments, disabilities, and other findings relate to one another – Identify how addressing those causes is likely to affect consequences
Identifying goals and objectives of care *Clarify purpose of providing care and of specific interventions, and the criteria that will be used to determine whether the objectives are being met*	– Clarify prognosis – Define overall goals for the individual – Identify criteria for meeting goals
Selecting interventions / planning care *Identify and implement interventions and treatments to address the individual's physical, functional, and psychosocial needs, concerns, problems, and risks*	– Identify specific symptomatic and cause-specific interventions (physical, functional, and psychosocial) – Identify how current and proposed treatments and services are expected to address causes, consequences, and risk factors, and help attain overall goals for the individual – Define anticipated benefits and risks of various interventions – Clarify how specific treatments and services will be evaluated for their effectiveness and possible adverse consequences
Monitoring of progress *Review individual's progress towards goals and modify approaches as needed*	– Identify the individual's response to interventions and treatments – Identify factors that are affecting progress towards achieving goals – Define or refine the prognosis – Define or refine when to stop or modify interventions – Review effectiveness and adverse consequences related to treatments – Adjust interventions as needed – Identify when care objectives have been achieved sufficiently to allow for discharge, transfer, or change in level of care

* Refers to key steps in the care delivery process, related to clinical problem solving and decision making
** Refers to key tasks at each step in the care delivery process

The care plan is driven not only by identified resident issues and/or conditions but also by a resident's unique characteristics, strengths, and needs. A care plan that is based on a thorough assessment, effective clinical decision making, and is compatible with current standards of clinical practice can provide a strong basis for optimal approaches to quality of care and quality of life needs of individual residents. A well developed and executed assessment and care plan:

- Looks at each resident as a whole human being with unique characteristics and strengths;

- Views the resident in distinct functional areas for the purpose of gaining knowledge about the resident's functional status (MDS);

- Gives the IDT a common understanding of the resident;

- Re-groups the information gathered to identify possible issues and/or conditions that the resident may have (i.e., triggers);

- Provides additional clarity of potential issues and/or conditions by looking at possible causes and risks (CAA process);

- Develops and implements an interdisciplinary care plan based on the assessment information gathered throughout the RAI process, with necessary monitoring and follow-up;

- Reflects the resident/resident representative input and goals for health care;

- Provides information regarding how the causes and risks associated with issues and/or conditions can be addressed to provide for a resident's highest practicable level of well-being (care planning);

- Re-evaluates the resident's status at prescribed intervals (i.e., quarterly, annually, or if a significant change in status occurs) using the RAI and then modifies the individualized care plan as appropriate and necessary.

Following the decision to address a triggered condition on the care plan, key staff or the IDT should subsequently:

- Review and revise the current care plan, as needed; and

- Communicate with the resident or his/her family or representative regarding the resident, care plans, and their wishes.

The overall care plan should be oriented towards:

1. Preventing avoidable declines in functioning or functional levels or otherwise clarifying why another goal takes precedence (e.g., palliative approaches in end of life situation).

2. Managing risk factors to the extent possible or indicating the limits of such interventions.

3. Addressing ways to try to preserve and build upon resident strengths.

4. Applying current standards of practice in the care planning process.

5. Evaluating treatment of measurable objectives, timetables and outcomes of care.

6. Respecting the resident's right to decline treatment.

7. Offering alternative treatments, as applicable.

8. Using an appropriate interdisciplinary approach to care plan development to improve the resident's functional abilities.

9. Involving resident, resident's family and other resident representatives as appropriate.

10. Assessing and planning for care to meet the resident's medical, nursing, mental and psychosocial needs.

11. Involving the direct care staff with the care planning process relating to the resident's expected outcomes.

12. Addressing additional care planning areas that are relevant to meeting the resident's needs in the long-term care setting.

4.8   CAA Tips and Clarifications

Care planning is a process that has several steps that may occur at the same time or in sequence. The following key steps and considerations may help the IDT develop the care plan after completing the comprehensive assessment:

1) Care Plan goals should be measurable. The IDT may agree on intermediate goal(s) that will lead to outcome objectives. Intermediate goal(s) and objectives must be pertinent to the resident's condition and situation (i.e., not just automatically applied without regard for their individual relevance), measurable, and have a time frame for completion or evaluation.

2) Care plan goal statements should include: The **subject (first or third person)**, the **verb**, the **modifiers**, the **time frame, and the goal(s)**.

EXAMPLE:

Subject	Verb	Modifiers	Time frame	Goal
Mr. Jones **OR** I	will walk	fifty feet daily with the help of one nursing assistant	the next 30 days	in order to maintain continence and eat in the dining area

3) A separate care plan is not necessarily required for each area that triggers a CAA. Since a single trigger can have multiple causes and contributing factors and multiple items can have a common cause or related risk factors, it is acceptable and may sometimes be more appropriate to address multiple issues within a single care plan segment or to cross reference related interventions from several care plan segments. For example, if impaired ADL function, mood state, falls and altered nutritional status are all determined to be caused by an infection and medication-related adverse consequences, it may be appropriate to have a single care plan that addresses these issues in relation to the common causes.

4) The RN coordinator is required to sign and date the Care Area Assessment (CAA) Summary after all triggered CAAs have been reviewed to certify completion of the comprehensive assessment (CAAs Completion Date, V0200B2). Facilities have 7 days after completing the RAI assessment to develop or revise the resident's care plan. Facilities should use the date at V0200B2 to determine the date at V0200C2 by which the care plan must be completed (V0200B2 + 7 days).

5) The 7-day requirement for completion or modification of the care plan applies to the Admission, SCSA, SCPA, and/or Annual RAI assessments. A new care plan does

not need to be developed after each SCSA, SCPA, or Annual reassessment. Instead, the nursing home may revise an existing care plan using the results of the latest comprehensive assessment. Facilities should also evaluate the appropriateness of the care plan at all times including after Quarterly assessments, modifying as needed.

6) If the RAI (MDS and CAAs) is not completed until the last possible date (the end of calendar day 14 of the stay), many of the appropriate care area issues, risk factors, or conditions may have already been identified, causes may have been considered, and a preliminary care plan and related interventions may have been initiated. A complete care plan is required no later than 7 days after the RAI is completed.

7) Review of the CAAs after completing the MDS may raise questions about the need to modify or continue services. Conditions that originally triggered the CAA may no longer be present because they resolved, or consideration of alternative causes may be necessary because the initial approach to an issue, risk, or condition did not work or was not fully implemented.

8) On the Annual assessment, if a resident triggers the same CAA(s) that triggered on the last comprehensive assessment, the CAA should be reviewed again. Even if the CAA is triggered for the same reason (no difference in MDS responses), there may be a new or changed related event identified during CAA review that might call for a revision to the resident's plan of care. The IDT with the input of the resident, family or resident's representative determines when a problem or potential problem needs to be addressed in the care plan.

9) The RN Coordinator for the CAA process (V0200B1) does not need to be the same RN as the RN Assessment Coordinator who verifies completion of the MDS assessment (Z0500). The date entered in V0200B2 on the CAA Summary is the date on which the RN Coordinator for the CAA process verified completion of the CAAs, which includes assessment of each triggered care area and completion of the location and date of the CAA assessment documentation section. See Chapter 2 for detailed instructions on the RAI completion schedule.

10) The Signature of Person Completing Care Plan Decision (V0200C1) can be that of any person(s) who facilitates the care plan decision making. It is an interdisciplinary process. The date entered in V0200C2 is the day the RN certifies that the CAAs have been completed and the day V0200C1 is signed.

4.9 Using the Care Area Assessment (CAA) Resources

Based on the preceding discussions in this Chapter, the following summarizes the steps involved in the CAA process, for those facilities that choose to use the CAA resources in this manual.

Please note: **Because MDS 3.0 trigger logic is complex, please refer to the CAT Logic tables within each CAA description (Section 4.10) for detailed information on triggers.**

Step 1: Identification of Triggered CAAs. After completing the MDS, identify triggered care areas. Many facilities will use automated systems to trigger CAAs. The resulting set of triggered CAAs generated by the software program should be matched against the trigger definitions to make sure that triggered CAAs have been correctly identified. CMS has developed test files for facility validation of a software program's triggering logic. Generally, software vendors use these test files to test their systems, but the nursing home is responsible for ensuring that the software is triggering correctly.

It is prudent to consider whether or not the software has triggered relevant CAAs for individual residents. For example, did the software miss some CAAs you thought should have been triggered? Do some of the CAAs seem to be missing and are there other CAAs triggered that you did not expect?

For nursing homes that do not use an automated system, the CAT logic will provide the information necessary to manually identify triggered CAAs. The CAT logic is found within the CAT logic tables of each care area's description in section 4.10. These tables provide the MDS items that trigger the 20 (twenty) care areas. Facilities are not required to use this information or to maintain it in the resident's clinical record. Rather, the information is a resource that may be used by the IDT members to determine which CAAs are triggered from a completed MDS.

To identify the triggered CAAs manually using the CAT logic tables in section 4.10:

1. Compare the completed MDS with the CAT logic tables to determine which CAAs have been triggered for review.
2. The CAT logic table will list the MDS item numbers and specific codes that will trigger the particular CAA. To identify a triggered CAA, match the resident's MDS item responses with the MDS item number(s) and code(s) for each care area as listed in the CAT logic tables within section 4.10. If a particular item response matches a code in the CAT logic table for a particular care area, read through the logic statement and qualifiers (i.e., 'IF', 'AND', and 'OR') for that particular care area to determine if that care area is triggered. This means that further assessment using the CAA process is required for that particular care area.
3. Note which CAAs are triggered by particular MDS items. If desired, circle or highlight the trigger indicator or the title of the column.
4. Continue through the CAT logic tables for each of the 20 (twenty) care areas matching recorded MDS item responses with trigger indicators until all triggered CAAs have been identified.
5. When the CAT logic review is completed, document on the CAA Summary which CAAs were triggered by checking the boxes in the column titled "Care Area Triggered."

Step 2: Analysis of Triggered CAAs. Review a triggered CAA by doing an in-depth, resident-specific assessment of the triggered condition in terms of the potential need for care plan interventions. While reviewing the CAA, consider what MDS items caused the CAA to be triggered. This is also an opportunity to consider any issues and/or conditions that may contribute to the triggered condition, but are not necessarily captured in MDS data. Review of CAAs helps staff to decide if care plan intervention is necessary, and what types of intervention may be appropriate.

Using the results of the assessment can help the interdisciplinary team (IDT) and the resident and/or resident's representative to identify areas of concern that:

*   Warrant intervention;

- Affect the resident's capacity to help identify and implement interventions to improve, stabilize, or maintain current level of function to the extent possible, based upon the resident's condition and choices and preferences for interventions;

- Can help to minimize the onset or progression of impairments and disabilities; and

- Can help to address the need and desire for other specialized services (e.g. palliative care, including symptom relief and pain management).

Use the information gathered thus far to make a clear issue or problem statement. An issue or problem is different from a finding (e.g., a single piece of information from the MDS or a test result). The chief complaint (e.g., the resident has a headache, is vomiting, or is not participating in activities) is not the same thing as an issue or problem statement that clearly identifies the situation. Trying to care plan a chief complaint may lead to inappropriate, irrelevant, or problematic interventions.

Example:

Chief Complaint: New onset of falls

Problem Statement: Resident currently falling 2-3 times per week. Falls are preceded by lightheadedness. Most falls occurred after she stood up and started walking; a few falls occurred while attempting to stand up from a sitting or lying position.

It is clear that the problem statement reflects assessment findings from which the investigation may continue and relevant conclusions drawn.

While the CAAs can help the IDT identify conditions or findings that could potentially be a problem or risk for the resident, additional thought is needed to define these issues and determine whether and to what extent the care area issue and/or condition is a problem or issue needing an intervention (assessment, testing, treatment, etc.) or simply a minor or inconsequential finding that does not need additional care planning. For example, a resident may exhibit sadness without being depressed or may appear to be underweight despite having a stable nutritional status consistent with their past history. The IDT should identify and document the functional and behavioral implications of identified problematic issues/conditions, limitations, improvement possibilities, and so forth (e.g., how the condition is a problem for the resident; how the condition limits or impairs the resident's ability to complete activities of daily living; or how the condition affects the resident's well-being in some way).

Identify links among triggers and their causes. CMS does not require that each care area triggered be care planned separately. The IDT may find during their discussions that several problematic issues and/or conditions have a related cause, or they might identify that those issues and/or conditions stand alone and are unrelated. Goals and approaches for each problematic issue and/or condition may overlap, and consequently the IDT may decide to address the problematic issues and/or conditions collectively in the care plan.

For example, behavior, mood, cognition, communication, and psychosocial well-being typically have common risk factors and common or closely related causes of related impairments. Thus, the following CATs naturally coexist and could be combined, assessed through the CAA process, and care planned together as a starting point for any resident: Delirium (CAA #1), Cognitive

Loss/Dementia (CAA #2), Communication (CAA #4), Psychosocial Well-Being (CAA #7), Mood State (CAA #8) Behavioral Symptoms (CAA #9), and Psychotropic Drug Use (CAA #17).

Usually, illnesses and impairments happen in sequence (i.e., one thing leads to another, which leads to another, and so on). The symptom or trigger often represents only the most recent or most apparent finding in a series of complications or related impairments. Thus, a detailed history is often essential to identifying causes and selecting the most beneficial interventions, e.g., the sequence over time of how the resident developed incontinence, pain, or anorexia. While the MDS presents diverse information about residents, and the CAAs cover various implications and complications, neither one is designed to give a detailed or chronological medical, psychosocial, or personal history. For example, knowing that the Behavioral Symptoms CAA (#9) is triggered and that the resident also has a diagnosis of UTI is not enough information to know whether the diagnosis of UTI is old or new, whether there is any link between the behavioral issue and the UTI, and whether there are other conditions such as kidney stones or bladder obstruction that might be causing or predisposing the resident to a UTI.

It is the facility's responsibility to refer to sources as needed to help with clinical problem solving and decision making that is consistent with professional standards of practice. It is often necessary to involve the attending physician to identify specific underlying causes of problems, including multiple causes of a single problem or multiple problems or complications related to one or more underlying causes.

Steps 3 and 4: Decision Making and CAA Documentation. The care plan is driven not only by identified resident issues and/or conditions but also by a resident's unique characteristics, strengths, and needs. The resident, family, or resident's representative should be an integral part of the team care planning process. A care plan that is based on a thorough assessment, effective clinical decision making, and is compatible with professional standards of practice should support optimal approaches to addressing quality of care and quality of life needs of individual residents.

Key components of the care plan may include, but are not limited to the following:

*   Specific interventions, including those that address common causes of multiple issues

*   Additional follow-up and clarification

*   Items needing additional assessment, testing, and review with the practitioner

*   Items that may require additional monitoring but do not require other interventions

Staff who have participated in the assessment and who have provided pertinent information about the resident's status for triggered care areas should be a part of the IDT that develops the resident's care plan. In order to provide continuity of care for the resident and good communication with all persons involved in the resident's care, information from the assessment that led the team to their care planning decision should be clearly documented. **See Table 2. Clinical Problem Solving and Decision Making Process Steps and Objectives.**

Documentation related to CAAs should include the items previously discussed in Section 4.5.

4.10 The Twenty Care Areas

NOTE: Each of the following descriptions of the Twenty Care Areas includes a table listing the Care Area Trigger (CAT) logical specifications. For those MDS items that require a numerical response, the logical specifications will reference the numerical response that triggered the Care Area. For those MDS items that require a check mark response (e.g. H0100, J0800, K0510, etc.), the logical specifications will reference this response in numerical form when the check box response is one that triggers a Care Area. Therefore, in the tables below, when a check mark has been placed in a check box item on the MDS and triggers a Care Area, the logical specifications will reference a value of "1." Example: "H0100A=1" means that a check mark has been placed in the check box item H0100A. Similarly, the Care Area logical specifications will reference a value of "0" (zero) to indicate that a check box item is not checked. Example: "I4800=0" means that a check mark has not been placed in the check box item I4800.

1. Delirium

Delirium is acute brain failure caused by medical conditions, which presents with psychiatric symptoms, acute confusion, and fluctuations in levels of consciousness. It is a serious condition that can be caused by medical issues/conditions such as medication-related adverse consequences, infections, or dehydration. It can easily be mistaken for the onset or progression of dementia, particularly in individuals with more advanced pre-existing dementia.

Unlike dementia, delirium typically has a rapid onset (hours to days). Typical signs include fluctuating states of consciousness; disorientation; decreased environmental awareness and behavioral changes; difficulty paying attention; fluctuating behavior or cognitive function throughout the day; restlessness; sleepiness periodically during the day; rambling, nonsensical speech; and altered perceptions, such as misinterpretations (illusions), seeing or feeling things that are not there (hallucinations), or a fixed false belief (delusions).

Delirium CAT Logic Table

Triggering Conditions (any of the following):

1. Worsening mental status is indicated by the BIMS summary score having a non-missing value of 00 to 15 on both the current non-admission comprehensive assessment (A0310A = 03, 04 or 05) and the prior assessment, and the summary score on the current non-admission assessment being less than the prior assessment as indicated by:

$$(A0310A = 03, 04, OR\ 05)\ AND$$

$$((C0500 >= 0)\ AND\ (C0500 <= 15))\ AND$$

$$((V0100D >= 0)\ AND\ (V0100D <= 15))\ AND$$

$$(C0500 < V0100D)$$

2. Acute mental status change is indicated on the current comprehensive assessment as follows:

$$C1600 = 1$$

Delirium is never a part of normal aging, and it is associated with high mortality and morbidity unless it is recognized and treated appropriately. Staff who are closely involved with residents should report promptly any new onset or worsening of cognitive impairment and the other aforementioned symptoms in that resident.

When this CAA is triggered, nursing home staff should follow their facility's chosen protocol or policy for performing the CAA. This CAA is triggered if the resident is exhibiting a worsening or an acute change in mental status.

The information gleaned from the assessment should be used to identify and address the underlying clinical issue(s) and/or condition(s), as well as to identify related underlying causes and contributing and/or risk factors. The next step is to develop an individualized care plan based directly on these conclusions. The focus of the care plan should be to address the underlying clinical issues/conditions identified through this assessment process (e.g., treating infections, addressing dehydration, identifying and treating hypo- or hyperthyroidism, relieving pain and depression, managing medications, and promoting adaptation and a comfortable environment for the resident to function. Other simple preventive measures that can be applied in all settings include addressing hearing and visual impairments to the extent possible (e.g., with the use of glasses and hearing aids) and minimizing the use of indwelling urinary catheters.

2. Cognitive Loss/Dementia

Cognitive prerequisites for an independent life include the ability to remember recent events and the ability to make safe daily decisions. Although the aging process may be associated with mild impairment, decline in cognition is often the result of other factors such as delirium, another mental health issue and/or condition, a stroke, and/or dementia. Dementia is not a specific condition but a syndrome that may be linked to several causes. According to the *Diagnostic and Statistical Manual, Fourth Edition, Text Revision* (DSM-IV-TR), the dementia syndrome is defined by the presence of three criteria: a short-term memory issue and/or condition and trouble with at least one cognitive function (e.g., abstract thought, judgment, orientation, language, behavior) and these troubles have an impact on the performance of activities of daily living. The cognitive loss/dementia CAA focuses on declining or worsening cognitive abilities that threaten personal independence and increase the risk for long-term nursing home placement or impair the potential for return to the community.

When this CAA is triggered, nursing home staff should follow their facility's chosen protocol or policy for performing the CAA. This CAA is triggered when a resident has evidence of cognitive loss.

Cognitive Loss/Dementia CAT Logic Table

Triggering Conditions (any of the following):

1. BIMS summary score is less than 13 as indicated by:

   C0500 >= 00 AND C0500 < 13

2. BIMS summary score has a missing value and there is a problem with short-term memory as indicated by:

   (C0500 = 99, -, OR ^) AND

   (C0700 = 1)

3. BIMS summary score has a missing value and there is a problem with long-term memory as indicated by:

   (C0500 = 99, -, OR ^) AND

   (C0800 = 1)

4. BIMS summary score has missing value of 99 or – and at least some difficulty making decisions regarding tasks of daily life as indicated by:

   (C0500 = 99, -, OR ^) AND

   (C1000 >= 1 AND C1000 <= 3)

5. BIMS, staff assessment or clinical record suggests presence of inattention, disorganized thinking, altered level of consciousness or psychomotor retardation as indicated by:

   (C1300A = 1 OR C1300A = 2) OR

   (C1300B = 1 OR C1300B = 2) OR

   (C1300C = 1 OR C1300C = 2) OR

   (C1300D = 1 OR C1300D = 2)

6. Presence of any behavioral symptom (verbal, physical or other) as indicated by:

   (E0200A >= 1 AND E0200A <= 3) OR

   (E0200B >= 1 AND E0200B <= 3) OR

   (E0200C >= 1 AND E0200C <= 3)

7. Rejection of care occurred at least 1 day in the past 7 days as indicated by:

   E0800 >= 1 AND E0800 <= 3

8. Wandering occurred at least 1 day in the past 7 days as indicated by:

   E0900 >= 1 AND E0900 <= 3

The information gleaned from the assessment should be used to evaluate the situation, to identify and address (where possible) the underlying cause(s) of cognitive loss/dementia, as well as to identify any related possible contributing and/or risk factors. The next step is to develop an individualized care plan based directly on these conclusions. It is important to define the nature of the impairment, e.g., identify whether the cognitive issue and/or condition is new or a worsening or change in existing cognitive impairment—characteristics of potentially reversible delirium—or whether it indicates a long-term, largely irreversible cognitive loss. If the issue and/or condition is apparently not related to reversible causes, assessment should focus on the details of the cognitive issue/condition (i.e., forgetfulness and/or impulsivity and/or behavior issues/conditions, etc.) and risk factors for the resident presented by the cognitive loss, to facilitate care planning specific to the resident's needs, issues and/or conditions, and strengths. The focus of the care plan should be to optimize remaining function by addressing underlying issues identified through this assessment process, such as relieving pain, optimizing medication use, ensuring optimal sensory input (e.g., with the use of glasses and hearing aids), and promoting as much social and functional independence as possible while maintaining health and safety.

3. Visual Function

The aging process leads to a decline in visual acuity, for example, a decreased ability to focus on close objects or to see small print, a reduced capacity to adjust to changes in light and dark and diminished ability to discriminate colors. The safety and quality consequences of vision loss are wide ranging and can seriously affect physical safety, self-image, and participation in social, personal, self-care, and rehabilitation activities.

When this CAA is triggered, nursing home staff should follow their facility's chosen protocol or policy for performing the CAA. This CAA is triggered when a resident has a diagnosis of glaucoma, macular degeneration or cataracts or B1000 is coded 1-4.

Visual Function CAT Logic Table

Triggering Conditions (any of the following):

1. Cataracts, glaucoma, or macular degeneration on the current assessment as indicated by:

$$I6500 = 1$$

2. Vision item has a value of 1 through 4 indicating vision problems on the current assessment as indicated by:

$$B1000 >= 1 \text{ AND } B1000 <= 4$$

The information gleaned from the assessment should be used to identify and address the underlying cause(s) of the resident's declining visual acuity, identifying residents who have treatable conditions that place them at risk of permanent blindness (e.g., glaucoma, diabetes, retinal hemorrhage) and those who have impaired vision whose quality of life could be improved through use of appropriate visual appliances, as well as to determine any possibly related contributing and/or risk factors. The next step is to develop an individualized care plan based directly on these conclusions. The focus of the care plan should be to prevent decline when possible and to enhance vision to the extent possible when reversal of visual impairment is not possible, as well as to address any underlying clinical issues and/or conditions identified through the CAA or subsequent assessment process. This might include treating infections and glaucoma or providing appropriate glasses or other visual appliances to improve visual acuity, quality of life, and safety.

4. Communication

Normal communication involves related activities, including expressive communication (making oneself understood to others, both verbally and via non-verbal exchange) and receptive communication (comprehending or understanding the verbal, written, or visual communication of others). Typical expressive issues and/or conditions include disruptions in language, speech, and voice production. Typical receptive communication issues and/or conditions include changes or difficulties in hearing, speech discrimination, vocabulary comprehension, and reading and interpreting facial expressions. While many conditions can affect how a person expresses and comprehends information, the communication CAA focuses on the interplay between the person's communication status and his or her cognitive skills for everyday decision making.

When this CAA is triggered, nursing home staff should follow their facility's chosen protocol or policy for performing the CAA. This CAA is triggered when a resident's ability to hear, to express ideas and wants, or to understand verbal content may be impaired.

Communication CAT Logic Table

Triggering Conditions (any of the following):

1. Hearing item has a value of 1 through 3 indicating hearing problems on the current assessment as indicated by:

$$B0200 >= 1 \text{ AND } B0200 <= 3$$

1. Impaired ability to make self understood through verbal and non-verbal expression of ideas/wants as indicated by:

$$B0700 >= 1 \text{ AND } B0700 <= 3$$

2. Impaired ability to understand others through verbal content as indicated by:

$$B0800 >= 1 \text{ AND } B0800 <= 3$$

The information gleaned from the assessment should be used to evaluate the characteristics of the problematic issue/condition and the underlying cause(s), the success of any attempted remedial actions, the person's ability to compensate with nonverbal strategies (e.g., the ability to visually follow non-verbal signs and signals), and the willingness and ability of caregivers to ensure effective communication. The assessment should also help to identify any related possible contributing and/or risk factors. The next step is to develop an individualized care plan based directly on these conclusions. The focus of the care plan should be to address any underlying issues/conditions and causes, as well as verbal and nonverbal strategies, in order to help the resident improve quality of life, health, and safety. In the presence of reduced language skills, both caregivers and the resident can strive to expand their nonverbal communication skills, for example, touch, facial expressions, eye contact, hand movements, tone of voice, and posture.

5. ADL Functional/Rehabilitation Potential

The ADL Functional/Rehabilitation CAA addresses the resident's self-sufficiency in performing basic activities of daily living, including dressing, personal hygiene, walking, transferring, toilet use, bed mobility, and eating. Nursing home staff should identify and address, to the extent possible, any issues or conditions that may impair function or impede efforts to improve that function. The resident's potential for improved functioning should also be clarified before rehabilitation is attempted.

When this CAA is triggered, nursing home staff should follow their facility's chosen protocol or policy for performing the CAA. This CAA is triggered when a resident requires assistance to improve performance or to prevent avoidable functional decline.

The information gleaned from the assessment should be used to identify the resident's actual functional deficits and risk factors, as well as to identify any possible contributing and/or risk factors related to the functional issues/conditions. The next step is to develop an individualized care plan based directly on these conclusions. The focus of the care plan should be to address the underlying cause or causes, improving or maintaining function when possible, and preventing additional decline when improvement is not possible. An ongoing assessment is critical to identify and address risk factors that can lead to functional decline.

ADL Functional/Rehabilitation Potential CAT Logic Table

Triggering Conditions (any of the following):

1. Cognitive skills for daily decision making has a value of 0 through 2 or BIMS summary score is 5 or greater, while ADL assistance for bed mobility was needed as indicated by:

(G0110A1 >= 1 AND G0110A1 <= 4) AND

((C1000 >= 0 AND C1000 <= 2) OR

(C0500 >= 5 AND C0500 <= 15))

2. Cognitive skills for daily decision making has a value of 0 through 2 or BIMS summary score is 5 or greater, while ADL assistance for transfer between surfaces (excluding to/from bath/toilets) was needed as indicated by:

(G0110B1 >= 1 AND G0110B1 <= 4) AND

((C1000 >= 0 AND C1000 <= 2) OR

(C0500 >= 5 AND C0500 <= 15))

3. Cognitive skills for daily decision making has a value of 0 through 2 or BIMS summary score is 5 or greater, while ADL assistance for walking in his/her room was needed as indicated by:

(G0110C1 >= 1 AND G0110C1 <= 4) AND

((C1000 >= 0 AND C1000 <= 2) OR

(C0500 >= 5 AND C0500 <= 15))

4. Cognitive skills for daily decision making has a value of 0 through 2 or BIMS summary score is 5 or greater, while ADL assistance for walking in corridor was needed as indicated by:

$$(G0110D1 >= 1 \text{ AND } G0110D1 <= 4) \text{ AND}$$
$$((C1000 >= 0 \text{ AND } C1000 <= 2) \text{ OR}$$
$$(C0500 >= 5 \text{ AND } C0500 <= 15))$$

5. Cognitive skills for daily decision making has a value of 0 through 2 or BIMS summary score is 5 or greater, while ADL assistance for locomotion on unit (including with wheel chair, if applicable) was needed as indicated by:

$$(G0110E1 >= 1 \text{ AND } G0110E1 <= 4) \text{ AND}$$
$$((C1000 >= 0 \text{ AND } C1000 <= 2) \text{ OR}$$
$$(C0500 >= 5 \text{ AND } C0500 <= 15))$$

6. Cognitive skills for daily decision making has a value of 0 through 2 or BIMS summary score is 5 or greater, while ADL assistance for locomotion off unit (including with wheel chair, if applicable) was needed as indicated by:

$$(G0110F1 >= 1 \text{ AND } G0110F1 <= 4) \text{ AND}$$
$$((C1000 >= 0 \text{ AND } C1000 <= 2) \text{ OR}$$
$$(C0500 >= 5 \text{ AND } C0500 <= 15))$$

7. Cognitive skills for daily decision making has a value of 0 through 2 or BIMS summary score is 5 or greater, while ADL assistance for dressing was needed as indicated by:

$$(G0110G1 >= 1 \text{ AND } G0110G1 <= 4) \text{ AND}$$
$$((C1000 >= 0 \text{ AND } C1000 <= 2) \text{ OR}$$
$$(C0500 >= 5 \text{ AND } C0500 <= 15))$$

8. Cognitive skills for daily decision making has a value of 0 through 2 or BIMS summary score is 5 or greater, while ADL assistance for eating was needed as indicated by:

$$(G0110H1 >= 1 \text{ AND } G0110H1 <= 4) \text{ AND}$$
$$((C1000 >= 0 \text{ AND } C1000 <= 2) \text{ OR}$$
$$(C0500 >= 5 \text{ AND } C0500 <= 15))$$

9. Cognitive skills for daily decision making has a value of 0 through 2 or BIMS summary score is 5 or greater, while ADL assistance for toilet use was needed as indicated by:

$$(G0110I1 >= 1 \text{ AND } G0110I1 <= 4) \text{ AND}$$
$$((C1000 >= 0 \text{ AND } C1000 <= 2) \text{ OR}$$
$$(C0500 >= 5 \text{ AND } C0500 <= 15))$$

10. Cognitive skills for daily decision making has a value of 0 through 2 or BIMS summary score is 5 or greater, while ADL assistance for grooming/personal hygiene was needed as indicated by:

$$(G0110J1 >= 1 \text{ AND } G0110J1 <= 4) \text{ AND}$$
$$((C1000 >= 0 \text{ AND } C1000 <= 2) \text{ OR}$$

$$(C0500 >= 5 \text{ AND } C0500 <= 15))$$

11. Cognitive skills for daily decision making has a value of 0 through 2 or BIMS summary score is 5 or greater, while ADL assistance for self-performance bathing (excluding washing of back and hair) has a value of 1 through 4 as indicated by:

$$(G0120A >= 1 \text{ AND } G0120A <= 4) \text{ AND}$$

$$((C1000 >= 0 \text{ AND } C1000 <= 2) \text{ OR}$$

$$(C0500 >= 5 \text{ AND } C0500 <= 15))$$

12. Cognitive skills for daily decision making has a value of 0 through 2 or BIMS summary score is 5 or greater, while balance during transition has a value of 1 or 2 for any item as indicated by:

$$((G0300A = 1 \text{ OR } G0300A = 2) \text{ OR}$$

$$(G0300B = 1 \text{ OR } G0300B = 2) \text{ OR}$$

$$(G0300C = 1 \text{ OR } G0300C = 2) \text{ OR}$$

$$(G0300D = 1 \text{ OR } G0300D = 2) \text{ OR}$$

$$(G0300E = 1 \text{ OR } G0300E = 2)) \text{ AND}$$

$$((C1000 >= 0 \text{ AND } C1000 <= 2) \text{ OR}$$

$$(C0500 >= 5 \text{ AND } C0500 <= 15))$$

13. Cognitive skills for daily decision making has a value of 0 through 2 or BIMS summary score is 5 or greater, while resident believes he/she is capable of increased independence as indicated by:

$$G0900A = 1 \text{ AND}$$

$$((C1000 >= 0 \text{ AND } C1000 <= 2) \text{ OR}$$

$$(C0500 >= 5 \text{ AND } C0500 <= 15))$$

14. Cognitive skills for daily decision making has a value of 0 through 2 or BIMS summary score is 5 or greater, while direct care staff believe resident is capable of increased independence as indicated by:

$$G0900B = 1 \text{ AND}$$

$$((C1000 >= 0 \text{ AND } C1000 <= 2) \text{ OR}$$

$$(C0500 >= 5 \text{ AND } C0500 <= 15))$$

6. Urinary Incontinence and Indwelling Catheter

Urinary incontinence is the involuntary loss or leakage of urine or the inability to urinate in a socially acceptable manner. There are several types of urinary incontinence (e.g., functional, overflow, stress, and urge) and the individual resident may experience more than one type at a time (mixed incontinence).

Although aging affects the urinary tract and increases the potential for urinary incontinence, urinary incontinence itself is not a normal part of aging. Urinary incontinence can be a risk factor for various complications, including skin rashes, falls, and social isolation. Often, it is at least partially correctable. Incontinence may affect a resident's psychological well-being and social interactions. Incontinence also may lead to the potentially troubling use of indwelling catheters, which can increase the risk of life threatening infections.

This CAA is triggered if the resident is incontinent of urine or uses a urinary catheter. When this CAA is triggered, nursing home staff should follow their facility's chosen protocol or policy for performing the CAA.

Urinary Incontinence and Indwelling Catheter CAT Logic Table

Triggering Conditions (any of the following):

1. ADL assistance for toileting was needed as indicated by:

    (G0110I1 >= 2 AND G0110I1 <= 4)

2. Resident requires a indwelling catheter as indicated by:

    H0100A = 1

3. Resident requires an external catheter as indicated by:

    H0100B = 1

4. Resident requires intermittent catheterization as indicated by:

    H0100D = 1

5. Urinary incontinence has a value of 1 through 3 as indicated by:

    H0300 >= 1 AND H0300 <= 3

6. Resident has moisture associated skin damage as indicated by:

    M1040H = 1

Successful management will depend on accurately identifying the underlying cause(s) of the incontinence or the reason for the indwelling catheter. Some of the causes can be successfully treated to reduce or eliminate incontinence episodes or the reason for catheter use. Even when incontinence cannot be reduced or resolved, effective incontinence management strategies can prevent complications related to incontinence. Because of the risk of substantial complications with the use of indwelling urinary catheters, they should be used for appropriate indications and when no other viable options exist. The assessment should include consideration of the risks and benefits of an indwelling (suprapubic or urethral) catheter, the potential for removal of the catheter, and consideration of complications resulting from the use of an indwelling catheter (e.g., urethral erosion, pain, discomfort, and bleeding). The next step is to develop an individualized care plan based directly on these conclusions.

7. Psychosocial Well-Being

Involvement in social relationships is a vital aspect of life, with most adults having meaningful relationships with family, friends, and neighbors. When these relationships are challenged, it can cloud other aspects of life. Decreases in a person's social relationships may affect psychological well-being and have an impact on mood, behavior, and physical activity. Similarly, declines in physical functioning or cognition or a new onset or worsening of pain or other health or mental health issues/conditions may affect both social relationships and mood. Psychosocial well-being may also be negatively impacted when a person has significant life changes such as the death of a loved one. Thus, other contributing factors also must be considered as a part of this assessment.

When this CAA is triggered, nursing home staff should follow their facility's chosen protocol or policy for performing the CAA. This CAA is triggered when a resident exhibits minimal interest in social involvement.

Psychosocial Well-Being CAT Logic Table

Triggering Conditions (any of the following):

1. Resident mood interview indicates the presence of little interest or pleasure in doing things as indicated by:

    D0200A1 = 1

2. Staff assessment of resident mood indicates the presence of little interest or pleasure in doing things as indicated by:

    D0500A1 = 1

3. Interview for activity preference item "How important is it to you to do your favorite activities?" has a value of 3 or 4 as indicated by:

    F0500F = 3 OR F0500F = 4

4. Staff assessment of daily and activity preferences did not indicate that resident prefers participating in favorite activities:

    F0800Q = 0

5. Physical behavioral symptoms directed toward others has a value of 1 through 3 and neither dementia nor Alzheimer's disease is present as indicated by:

    (E0200A >= 1 AND E0200A <= 3) AND

    (I4800 = 0 OR I4800 = -) AND

    (I4200 = 0 OR I4200 = -)

6. Verbal behavioral symptoms directed toward others has a value of 1 through 3 and neither dementia nor Alzheimer's disease is present as indicated by:

    (E0200B >=1 AND E0200B <= 3) AND

    (I4800 = 0 OR I4800 = -) AND

    (I4200 = 0 OR I4200 = -)

7. Any six items for interview for activity preferences has the value of 4 and resident is primary respondent for daily and activity preferences as indicated by:

    (Any 6 of F0500A through F0500H = 4) AND

    (F0600 = 1)

The information gleaned from the assessment should be used to identify whether their minimal involvement is typical or customary for that person or a possible indication of a problem. If it is problematic, then address the underlying cause(s) of the resident's minimal social involvement and factors associated with reduced social relationships and engagement, as well as to identify any related possible contributing and/or risk factors. The next step is to develop an individualized care plan based directly on these conclusions. The focus of the care plan should be to address the underlying cause or causes in order to stimulate and facilitate social engagement.

8. Mood State

Sadness and anxiety are normal human emotions, and fluctuations in mood are also normal. But mood states (which reflect more enduring patterns of emotions) may become as extreme or overwhelming as to impair personal and psychosocial function. Mood disorders such as depression reflect a problematic extreme and should not be confused with normal sadness or mood fluctuation.

The mood section of the MDS screens for—but is not intended to definitively diagnose—any mood disorder, including depression. Mood disorders may be expressed by sad mood, feelings of emptiness, anxiety, or uneasiness. They may also result in a wide range of bodily complaints and dysfunctions, including weight loss, tearfulness, agitation, aches, and pains. However, because none of these symptoms is specific for a mood disorder, diagnosis of mood disorders requires additional assessment and confirmation of findings. In addition, other problems (e.g., lethargy, fatigue, weakness, or apathy) with different causes, which require a very different approach, can be easily confused with depression.

When this CAA is triggered, nursing home staff should follow their facility's chosen protocol or policy for performing the CAA. This CAA is triggered if the Resident Mood Interview, Staff Assessment of Mood, or certain other specific issues indicate a mood issue and/or condition may be present.

Mood State CAT Logic Table

Triggering Conditions (any of the following):

1. Resident has had thoughts he/she would be better off dead, or thoughts of hurting him/herself as indicated by:

D0200I1 = 1

2. Staff assessment of resident mood suggests resident states life isn't worth living, wishes for death, or attempts to harm self as indicated by:

D0500I1 = 1

3. The resident mood interview total severity score has a non-missing value (0 to 27) on both the current non-admission comprehensive assessment (A0310A = 03, 04, or 05) and the prior assessment, and the resident interview summary score on the current non-admission comprehensive assessment (D0300) is greater than the prior assessment (V0100E) as indicated by:

((A0310A = 03) OR (A0310A = 04) OR (A0310A = 05)) AND

$$((D0300 >= 00) \text{ AND } (D0300 <= 27)) \text{ AND}$$
$$((V0100E >= 00) \text{ AND } (V0100E <= 27)) \text{ AND}$$
$$(D0300 > V0100E)$$

4. The resident mood interview is not successfully completed (missing value on D0300), the staff assessment of resident mood has a non-missing value (0 to 30) on both the current non-admission comprehensive assessment (A0310A = 03, 04, or 05) and the prior assessment, and the staff assessment current total severity score on the current non-admission comprehensive assessment (D0600) is greater than the prior assessment (V0100F) as indicated by:

$$((A0310A = 03) \text{ OR } (A0310A = 04) \text{ OR } (A0310A = 05)) \text{ AND}$$
$$((D0300 < 00) \text{ OR } (D0300 > 27)) \text{ AND}$$
$$((D0600 >= 00) \text{ AND } (D0600 <= 30)) \text{ AND}$$
$$((V0100F >= 00) \text{ AND } (V0100F <= 30)) \text{ AND}$$
$$(D0600 > V0100F)$$

5. The resident mood interview is successfully completed and the current total severity score has a value of 10 through 27 as indicated by:

$$D0300 >= 10 \text{ AND } D0300 <= 27$$

6. The staff assessment of resident mood is recorded and the current total severity score has a value of 10 through 30 as indicated by:

$$D0600 >= 10 \text{ AND } D0600 <= 30$$

The information gleaned from the assessment should be used as a starting point to assess further in order to confirm a mood disorder and get enough detail of the situation to consider whether treatment is warranted. If a mood disorder is confirmed, the individualized care plan should, in part, focus on identifying and addressing underlying causes, to the extent possible.

9. Behavioral Symptoms

In the world at large, human behavior varies widely and is often dysfunctional and problematic. While behavior may sometimes be related to or caused by illness, behavior itself is only a symptom and not a disease. The MDS only identifies certain behaviors, but is not intended to determine the significance of behaviors, including whether they are problematic and need an intervention.

Therefore, it is essential to assess behavior symptoms carefully and in detail in order to determine whether, and why, behavior is problematic and to identify underlying causes. The behavior CAA focuses on potentially problematic behaviors in the following areas: wandering (e.g., moving with no rational purpose, seemingly being oblivious to needs or safety), verbal abuse (e.g., threatening, screaming at, or cursing others), physical abuse (e.g., hitting, shoving, kicking, scratching, or sexually abusing others), other behavioral symptoms not directed at others (e.g., making disruptive sounds or noises, screaming out, smearing or throwing food or feces, hoarding, rummaging through other's belongings), inappropriate public sexual behavior or public disrobing, and rejection of care (e.g., verbal or physical resistance to taking medications, taking injections, completing a variety of activities of daily living or eating). Understanding the nature of the issue/condition and addressing the underlying causes have the potential to improve the quality of the resident's life and the quality of the lives of those with whom the resident interacts.

When this CAA is triggered, nursing home staff should follow their facility's chosen protocol or policy for performing the CAA. This CAA is triggered when the resident is identified as exhibiting certain troubling behavioral symptoms.

Behavioral Symptoms CAT Logic Table

Triggering Conditions (any of the following):

1. Rejection of care has a value of 1 through 3 indicating resident has rejected evaluation or care necessary to achieve his/her goals for health and well-being as indicated by:

$$E0800 >= 1 \text{ AND } E0800 <= 3$$

2. Wandering has a value of 1 through 3 as indicated by:

$$E0900 >= 1 \text{ AND } E0900 <= 3$$

3. Change in behavior indicates behavior, care rejection or wandering has gotten worse since prior assessment as indicated by:

$$E1100 = 2$$

4. Presence of at least one behavioral symptom as indicated by:

$$E0300 = 1$$

The information gleaned from the assessment should be used to determine why the resident's behavioral symptoms are problematic in contrast to a variant of normal, whether and to what extent the behavior places the resident or others at risk for harm, and any related contributing and/or risk factors. The next step is to develop an individualized care plan based directly on these conclusions. The focus of the care plan should be to address the underlying cause or causes, reduce the frequency of truly problematic behaviors, and minimize any resultant harm.

10. Activities

The capabilities of residents vary, especially as abilities and expectations change, illness intervenes, opportunities become less frequent, and/or extended social relationships become less common. The purpose of the activities CAA is to identify strategies to help residents become more involved in relevant activities, including those that have interested and stimulated them in the past and/or new or modified ones that are consistent with their current functional and cognitive capabilities.

When this CAA is triggered, nursing home staff should follow their facility's chosen protocol or policy for performing the CAA. This CAA is triggered when the resident may have evidence of decreased involvement in social activities.

Activities CAT Logic Table

Triggering Conditions (any of the following):

1. Resident has little interest or pleasure in doing things as indicated by:

    D0200A1 = 1

2. Staff assessment of resident mood suggests resident states little interest or pleasure in doing things as indicated by:

    D0500A1 = 1

3. Any 6 items for interview for activity preferences has the value of 4 (not important at all) or 5 (important, but cannot do or no choice) as indicated by:

    Any 6 of F0500A through F0500H = 4 or 5

4. Any 6 items for staff assessment of activity preference item L through T are not checked as indicated by:

    Any 6 of F0800L through F0800T = 0

The information gleaned from the assessment should be used to identify residents who have either withdrawn from recreational activities or who are uneasy entering into activities and social relationships, to identify the resident's interests, and to identify any related possible contributing and/or risk factors. The next step is to develop an individualized care plan based directly on these conclusions. The care plan should focus on addressing the underlying cause(s) of activity limitations and the development or inclusion of activity programs tailored to the resident's interests and to his or her cognitive, physical/functional, and social abilities and improve quality of life.

11. Falls

A "fall" refers to unintentionally coming to rest on the ground, floor, or other lower level but not as a result of an external force (e.g., being pushed by another resident). A fall without injury is still a fall. Falls are a leading cause of morbidity and mortality among the elderly, including nursing home residents. Falls may indicate functional decline and/or the development of other serious conditions, such as delirium, adverse medication reactions, dehydration, and infections. A potential fall is an episode in which a resident lost his/her balance and would have fallen without staff intervention.

When this CAA is triggered, nursing home staff should follow their facility's chosen protocol or policy for performing the CAA. This CAA is triggered when the resident has had recent history of falls and balance problems.

Falls CAT Logic Table

Triggering Conditions (any of the following):

1. Wandering occurs as indicated by a value of 1 through 3 as follows:

   E0900 >= 1 AND E0900 <= 3

2. Balance problems during transition indicated by a value of 1 or 2 for any item as follows:

   (G0300A = 1 OR G0300A = 2) OR

   (G0300B = 1 OR G0300B = 2) OR

   (G0300C = 1 OR G0300C = 2) OR

   (G0300D = 1 OR G0300D = 2) OR

   (G0300E = 1 OR G0300E = 2)

3. For OBRA admission assessment: fall history at admission indicates resident fell anytime in the last month prior to admission as indicated by:

   If A0310A = 01 AND J1700A = 1

4. For OBRA admission assessment: fall history at admission indicates resident fell anytime in the last 2 to 6 months prior to admission as indicated by:

   If A0310A = 01 AND J1700B = 1

5. Resident has fallen at least one time since admission or the prior assessment as indicated by:

   J1800 = 1

6. Resident received antianxiety medication on one or more of the last 7 days or since admission/entry or reentry as indicated by:

   N0410B>= 1 AND N0410B<=7

7. Resident received antidepressant medication on one or more of the last 7 days or since admission/entry or reentry as indicated by:

   N0410C> = 1 AND N0410C<=7

8. Trunk restraint used in bed as indicated by a value of 1 or 2 as follows:

   P0100B = 1 OR P0100B = 2

9. Trunk restraint used in chair or out of bed as indicated by a value of 1 or 2 as follows:

   P0100E = 1 OR P0100E = 2

The information gleaned from the assessment should be used to identify and address the underlying cause(s) of the resident's fall(s), as well as to identify any related possible causes and contributing and/or risk factors. The next step is to develop an individualized care plan based directly on these conclusions. The focus of the care plan should be to address the underlying cause(s) of the resident's fall(s), as well as the factors that place him or her at risk for falling.

12. Nutritional Status

Undernutrition is not a response to normal aging, but it can arise from many diverse causes, often acting together. It may cause or reflect acute or chronic illness, and it represents a risk factor for subsequent decline.

The Nutritional Status CAA process reflects the need for an in-depth analysis of residents with impaired nutrition and those who are at nutritional risk. This CAA triggers when a resident has or is at risk for a nutrition issue/condition. Some residents who are triggered for follow-up will already be significantly underweight and thus undernourished, while other residents will be at risk of undernutrition. This CAA may also trigger based on loss of appetite with little or no accompanying weight loss and despite the absence of obvious, outward signs of impaired nutrition.

Nutritional Status CAT Logic Table

Triggering Conditions (any of the following):

1. Dehydration is selected as a problem health condition as indicated by:

$$J1550C = 1$$

2. Body mass index (BMI) is too low or too high as indicated by:

$$BMI < 18.5000 \text{ OR } BMI > 24.9000$$

3. Any weight loss as indicated by a value of 1 or 2 as follows:

$$K0300 = 1 \text{ OR } K0300 = 2$$

4. Any planned or unplanned weight gain as indicated by a value of 1 or 2 as follows:

$$K0310 = 1 \text{ OR } K0310 = 2$$

5. Parenteral/IV feeding while NOT a resident or while a resident is used as nutritional approach as indicated by:

$$K0510A1 = 1 \text{ OR } K0510A2 = 1$$

6. Mechanically altered diet while NOT a resident or while a resident is used as nutritional approach as indicated by:

$$K0510C1 = 1 \text{ OR } K0510C2 = 1$$

7. Therapeutic diet while NOT a resident or while a resident is used as nutritional approach as indicated by:

$$K0510D1 = 1 \text{ OR } K0510D2 = 1$$

8. Resident has one or more unhealed pressure ulcer(s) at Stage 2 or higher, or one or more likely pressure ulcers that are unstageable at this time as indicated by:

$$((M0300B1 > 0 \text{ AND } M0300B1 <= 9) \text{ OR}$$
$$(M0300C1 > 0 \text{ AND } M0300C1 <= 9) \text{ OR}$$
$$(M0300D1 > 0 \text{ AND } M0300D1 <= 9) \text{ OR}$$
$$(M0300E1 > 0 \text{ AND } M0300E1 <= 9) \text{ OR}$$
$$(M0300F1 > 0 \text{ AND } M0300F1 <= 9) \text{ OR}$$
$$(M0300G1 > 0 \text{ AND } M0300G1 <= 9))$$

13. Feeding Tubes

This CAA focuses on the long-term (greater than 1 month) use of feeding tubes. It is important to balance the benefits and risks of feeding tubes in individual residents in deciding whether to make such an intervention a part of the plan of care. In some acute and longer term situations, feeding tubes may provide adequate nutrition that cannot be obtained by other means. In other circumstances, feeding tubes may not enhance survival or improve quality of life, e.g., in individuals with advanced dementia. Also, feeding tubes can be associated with diverse complications that may further impair quality of life or adversely impact survival. For example, tube feedings will not prevent aspiration of gastric contents or oral secretions and feeding tubes may irritate or perforate the stomach or intestines.

When this CAA is triggered, nursing home staff should follow their facility's chosen protocol or policy for performing the CAA. This CAA is triggered when the resident has a need for a feeding tube for nutrition.

Feeding Tubes CAT Logic Table

Triggering Conditions (any of the following):

1. Feeding tube while NOT a resident or while a resident is used as nutritional approach as indicated by:

$$K0510B1 = 1 \text{ OR } K0510B2 = 1$$

The information gleaned from the assessment should be used to identify and address the resident's status and underlying issues/conditions that necessitated the use of a feeding tube. In addition, the CAA information should be used to identify any related risk factors. The next step is to develop an individualized care plan based directly on these conclusions. The focus of the care plan should be to address the underlying cause(s), including any reversible issues and conditions that led to using a feeding tube.

14. Dehydration/Fluid Maintenance

Dehydration is a condition in which there is an imbalance of water and related electrolytes in the body. As a result, the body may become less able to maintain adequate blood pressure and electrolyte balance, deliver sufficient oxygen and nutrients to the cells, and rid itself of wastes. In older persons, diagnosing dehydration is accomplished primarily by a detailed history, laboratory testing (e.g., electrolytes, BUN, creatinine, serum osmolality, urinary sodium), and to a lesser degree by a physical examination. Abnormal vital signs, such as falling blood pressure and an increase in the pulse rate, may sometimes be meaningful symptoms of dehydration in the elderly.

When this CAA is triggered, nursing home staff should follow their facility's chosen protocol or policy for performing the CAA.

Dehydration/Fluid Maintenance CAT Logic Table

Triggering Conditions (any of the following):

1. Fever is selected as a problem health condition as indicated by:

$$J1550A = 1$$

2. Vomiting is selected as a problem health condition as indicated by:

$$J1550B = 1$$

3. Dehydration is selected as a problem health condition as indicated by:

$$J1550C = 1$$

4. Internal bleeding is selected as a problem health condition as indicated by:

$$J1550D = 1$$

5. Infection present as indicated by:

$$(I1700 = 1) \text{ OR}$$
$$(I2000 = 1) \text{ OR}$$
$$(I2100 = 1) \text{ OR}$$
$$(I2200 = 1) \text{ OR}$$
$$(I2300 = 1) \text{ OR}$$
$$(I2400 = 1) \text{ OR}$$
$$(I2500 = 1) \text{ OR}$$
$$((M1040A = 1))$$

6. Constipation present as indicated by:

$$H0600 = 1$$

7. Parenteral/IV feeding while NOT a resident or while a resident is used as nutritional approach as indicated by:

$$K0510A1 = 1 \text{ OR } K0510A2 = 1$$

8. Feeding tube while NOT a resident or while a resident is used as nutritional approach as indicated by:

$$K0510B1 = 1 \text{ OR } K0510B2 = 1$$

The information gleaned from the assessment should be used to identify whether the resident is dehydrated or at risk for dehydration, as well as to identify any related possible causes and contributing and/or risk factors. The next step is to develop an individualized care plan based directly on these conclusions. The focus of the care plan should be to prevent dehydration by addressing risk factors, to maintain or restore fluid and electrolyte balance, and to address the underlying cause or causes of any current dehydration.

15. Dental Care

The ability to chew food is important for adequate oral nutrition. Having clean and attractive teeth or dentures can promote a resident's positive self-image and personal appearance, thereby enhancing social interactions. Medical illnesses and medication-related adverse consequences may increase a resident's risk for related complications such as impaired nutrition and communication deficits. The dental care CAA addresses a resident's risk of oral disease, discomfort, and complications.

When this CAA is triggered, nursing home staff should follow their facility's chosen protocol or policy for performing the CAA. This CAA is triggered when a resident has indicators of an oral/dental issue and/or condition.

Dental Care CAT Logic Table

Triggering Conditions (any of the following):

1. Any dental problem indicated by:

$$(L0200A = 1) \text{ OR}$$

$$(L0200B = 1) \text{ OR}$$

$$(L0200C = 1) \text{ OR}$$

$$(L0200D = 1) \text{ OR}$$

$$(L0200E = 1) \text{ OR}$$

$$(L0200F = 1)$$

The information gleaned from the assessment should be used to identify the oral/dental issues and/or conditions and to identify any related possible causes and/or contributing risk factors. The next step is to develop an individualized care plan based directly on these conclusions. The focus of the care plan should be to address the underlying cause or causes of the resident's issues and/or conditions.

16. Pressure Ulcer

A pressure ulcer can be defined as a localized injury to the skin and/or underlying tissue, usually over a bony prominence, as a result of pressure or pressure in combination with shear and/or friction. Pressure ulcers can have serious consequences for the elderly and are costly and time consuming to treat. They are a common preventable and treatable condition among elderly people with restricted mobility.

When this CAA is triggered, nursing home staff should follow their facility's chosen protocol or policy for performing the CAA.

Pressure Ulcer CAT Logic Table

Triggering Conditions (any of the following):

1. ADL assistance for bed mobility was needed, or activity did not occur, or activity only occurred once or twice as indicated by:

$$(G0110A1 >= 1 \text{ AND } G0110A1 <= 4) \text{ OR}$$

$$(G0110A1 = 7 \text{ OR } G0110A1 = 8)$$

2. Frequent urinary incontinence as indicated by:

$$H0300 = 2 \text{ OR } H0300 = 3$$

3. Frequent bowel continence as indicated by:

$$H0400 = 2 \text{ OR } H0400 = 3$$

4. Weight loss in the absence of physician-prescribed regimen as indicated by:

$$K0300 = 2$$

5. Resident at risk for developing pressure ulcers as indicated by:

$$M0150 = 1$$

6. Resident has one or more unhealed pressure ulcer(s) at Stage 2 or higher, or one or more likely pressure ulcers that are unstageable at this time as indicated by:

$$((M0300B1 > 0 \text{ AND } M0300B1 <= 9) \text{ OR}$$

$$(M0300C1 > 0 \text{ AND } M0300C1 <= 9) \text{ OR}$$

$$(M0300D1 > 0 \text{ AND } M0300D1 <= 9) \text{ OR}$$

$$(M0300E1 > 0 \text{ AND } M0300E1 <= 9) \text{ OR}$$

$$(M0300F1 > 0 \text{ AND } M0300F1 <= 9) \text{ OR}$$

$$(M0300G1 > 0 \text{ AND } M0300G1 <= 9))$$

7. Resident has one or more unhealed pressure ulcer(s) at Stage 1 as indicated by:

$$M0300A > 0 \text{ AND } M0300A <= 9$$

8. Resident has one or more pressure ulcer(s) that has gotten worse since prior assessment as indicated by:

$$(M0800A > 0 \text{ AND } M0800A <= 9) \text{ OR}$$

$$(M0800B > 0 \text{ AND } M0800B <= 9) \text{ OR}$$

$$(M0800C > 0 \text{ AND } M0800C <= 9)$$

9. Trunk restraint used in bed has value of 1 or 2 as indicated by:

$$P0100B = 1 \text{ OR } P0100B = 2$$

10. Trunk restraint used in chair or out of bed has value of 1 or 2 as indicated by:

$$P0100E = 1 \text{ OR } P0100E = 2$$

The information gleaned from the assessment should be used to draw conclusions about the status of a resident's pressure ulcers(s) and to identify any related causes and/or contributing risk factors. The next step is to develop an individualized care plan based directly on these conclusions. If a pressure ulcer is not present, the goal is to prevent them by identifying the resident's risks and implementing preventive measures. If a pressure ulcer is present, the goal is to heal or close it.

17. Psychotropic Medication Use

Any medication, prescription or non-prescription, can have benefits and risks, depending on various factors (e.g., active medical conditions, coexisting medication regimen). However, psychotropic medications, prescribed primarily to affect cognition, mood, or behavior, are among the most frequently prescribed agents for elderly nursing home residents. While these medications can often be beneficial, they can also cause significant complications such as postural hypotension, extrapyramidal symptoms (e.g., akathisia, dystonia, tardive dyskinesia), and acute confusion (delirium).

When this CAA is triggered, nursing home staff should follow their facility's chosen protocol or policy for performing the CAA.

The information gleaned from the assessment should be used to draw conclusions about the appropriateness of the resident's medication, in consultation with the physician and the consultant pharmacist, and to identify any adverse consequences, as well as any related possible causes and/or contributing risk factors. The next step is to develop an individualized care plan based directly on these conclusions. Important goals of therapy include maximizing the resident's functional potential and well-being, while minimizing the hazards associated with medication side effects.

Psychotropic Medication Use CAT Logic Table

Triggering Conditions (any of the following):

1. Antipsychotic medication administered to resident on one or more of the last 7 days or since admission/entry or reentry as indicated by:

    N0410A>= 1 AND N0410A<=7

2. Antianxiety medication administered to resident on one or more of the last 7 days or since admission/entry or reentry as indicated by:

    N0410B>= 1 AND N0410B<=7

3. Antidepressant medication administered to resident on one or more of the last 7 days or since admission/entry or reentry as indicated by:

    N0410C>= 1 AND N0410C<=7

4. Hypnotic medication administered to resident on one or more of the last 7 days or since admission/entry or reentry as indicated by:

    N0410D>= 1 AND N0410D<=7

18. Physical Restraints

A physical restraint is defined as any manual method or physical or mechanical device, material, or equipment attached or adjacent to the resident's body that the individual cannot remove easily and that restricts freedom of movement or normal access to one's body. The important consideration is the effect of the device on the resident, and not the purpose for which the device was placed on the resident. This category also includes the use of passive restraints such as chairs that prevent rising.

Physical restraints are only rarely indicated, and at most, should be used only as a short-term, temporary intervention to treat a resident's medical symptoms. They should not be used for purposes of discipline or convenience. Before a resident is restrained, the facility must determine the presence of a specific medical symptom that would require the use of the restraint and how the use of the restraint would treat the medical symptom, protect the resident's safety, and assist the resident in attaining or maintaining his or her highest practicable level of physical and psychosocial well-being.

Restraints are often associated with negative physical and psychosocial outcomes (e.g., loss of muscle mass, contractures, lessened mobility and stamina, impaired balance, skin breakdown, constipation, and incontinence). Adverse psychosocial effects of restraint use may include a feeling of shame, hopelessness, and stigmatization as well as agitation.

The physical restraint CAA identifies residents who are physically restrained during the look-back period. When this CAA is triggered, nursing home staff should follow their facility's chosen protocol or policy for performing the CAA.

Physical Restraints CAT Logic Table

Triggering Conditions (any of the following):

1. Bed rail restraint used in bed has value of 1 or 2 as indicated by:

   P0100A = 1 OR P0100A = 2

2. Trunk restraint used in bed has value of 1 or 2 as indicated by:

   P0100B = 1 OR P0100B = 2

3. Limb restraint used in bed has value of 1 or 2 as indicated by:

   P0100C = 1 OR P0100C = 2

4. Other restraint used in bed has value of 1 or 2 as indicated by:

   P0100D = 1 OR P0100D = 2

5. Trunk restraint used in chair or out of bed has value of 1 or 2 as indicated by:

   P0100E = 1 OR P0100E = 2

6. Limb restraint used in chair or out of bed has value of 1 or 2 as indicated by:

   P0100F = 1 OR P0100F = 2

7. Chair restraint that prevents rising used in chair or out of bed has value of 1 or 2 as indicated by:

   P0100G = 1 OR P0100G = 2

8. Other restraint used in chair or out of bed has value of 1 or 2 as indicated by:

   P0100H = 1 OR P0100H = 2

The information gleaned from the assessment should be used to identify the specific reasons for and the appropriateness of the use of the restraint and any adverse consequences caused by or risks related to restraint use.

The focus of an individualized care plan based directly on these conclusions should be to address the underlying physical or psychological condition(s) that led to restraint use. By addressing underlying conditions and causes, the facility may eliminate the medical symptom that led to using restraints. In addition, a review of underlying needs, risks, or issues/conditions may help to identify other potential kinds of treatments. The ultimate goal is to eliminate restraint use by employing alternatives. When elimination of restraints is not possible, assessment must result in using the least restrictive device possible.

19. Pain

Pain is "an unpleasant sensory and emotional experience associated with actual or potential tissue damage." Pain can be affected by damage to various organ systems and tissues, for example, musculoskeletal (e.g., arthritis, fractures, injury from peripheral vascular disease, wounds), neurological (e.g., diabetic neuropathy, herpes zoster), and cancer. The presence of pain can also increase suffering in other areas, leading to an increased sense of helplessness, anxiety, depression, decreased activity, decreased appetite, and disrupted sleep.

As with all symptoms, pain symptoms are subjective and require a detailed history and additional physical examination, and sometimes additional testing, in order to clarify pain characteristics and causes and identify appropriate interventions. This investigation typically requires coordination between nursing staff and a health care practitioner.

When this CAA is triggered, nursing home staff should follow their facility's chosen protocol or policy for performing the CAA. This CAA is triggered when a resident has active symptoms of pain.

Pain CAT Logic Table

Triggering Conditions (any of the following):

1. Pain has made it hard for resident to sleep at night over the past 5 nights as indicated by:

$$J0500A = 1$$

2. Resident has limited day-to-day activity because of pain over past 5 days as indicated by:

$$J0500B = 1$$

3. Pain numeric intensity rating has a value from 7 to 10 as indicated by:

$$J0600A >= 07 \text{ AND } J0600A <= 10$$

4. Verbal descriptor of pain is severe or very severe as indicated by a value of 3 or 4 as as follows:

$$J0600B = 3 \text{ OR } J0600B = 4$$

5. Pain is frequent as indicated by a value of 1 or 2 and numeric pain intensity rating has a value of 4 through 10 or verbal descriptor of pain has a value of 2 through 4 as indicated by:

$$(J0400 = 1 \text{ OR } J0400 = 2) \text{ AND}$$

$$((J0600A >= 04 \text{ AND } J0600A <= 10) \text{ OR}$$

$$(J0600B >= 2 \text{ AND } J0600B <= 4))$$

6. Staff assessment reports resident indicates pain or possible pain in body language as indicated by:

$$(J0800A = 1) \text{ OR}$$

$$(J0800B = 1) \text{ OR}$$

$$(J0800C = 1) \text{ OR}$$

$$(J0800D = 1)$$

The information gleaned from the assessment should be used to identify the characteristics and possible causes, contributing factors, and risk factors related to the pain. The next step is to develop an individualized care plan based directly on these conclusions. The focus of the care plan should be to alleviate symptoms and, to the extent possible, address the underlying condition(s) that cause the pain.

Management of pain may include various interventions, including medications and other treatments that focus on improving the person's quality of life and ability to function. Therefore, it is important to tailor an individualized care plan related to pain to the characteristics, causes, and consequences of pain in the context of a resident's whole picture, including medical conditions, cognitive capabilities, goals, wishes, and personal and psychosocial function.

20. Return to Community Referral

All individuals have the right to choose the services they receive and the settings in which they receive those services. This right became law under the Americans with Disabilities Act (1990) and with further interpretation by the U.S. Supreme Court in the Olmstead vs. L.C. decision in 1999. This ruling stated that individuals have a right to receive care in the least restrictive (most integrated) setting and that governments (Federal and State) have a responsibility to enforce and support these choices.

An individual in a nursing home with adequate decision making capacity can choose to leave the facility and/or request to talk to someone about returning to the community at any time. The return to community referral portion of MDS 3.0 uses a person-centered approach to ensure that all individuals have the opportunity to learn about home and community based services and have an opportunity to receive long-term care in the last restrictive setting possible. The CAA associated with this portion of MDS 3.0 focuses on residents who want to talk to someone about returning to the community and promotes opening the discussion about the individual's preferences for settings for receipt of services.

Individual choices related to returning to community living will vary, e.g., returning to a former home or a different community home, or, the individual may choose to stay in the nursing home. The discharge assessment process requires nursing home staff to apply a systematic and objective protocol so that every individual has the opportunity to access meaningful information about community living options and community service alternatives, with the goal being to assist the individual in maintaining or achieving the highest level of functioning and integration possible. This includes ensuring that the individual or surrogate is fully informed and involved, identifying individual strengths, assessing risk factors, implementing a comprehensive plan of care, coordinating interdisciplinary care providers, fostering independent functioning, and using rehabilitation programs and community referrals.

When this CAA is triggered, nursing home staff should follow their facility's chosen protocol or policy for performing the CAA. This CAA is triggered when a resident expresses interest in returning to the community.

Return to Community Referral CAT Logic Table

Triggering Conditions (any of the following):

    1.   Referral is or may be needed but has not been made to local contact agency as indicated by:

$$Q0600 = 1$$

The information gleaned from the assessment should be used to assess the resident's situation and begin appropriate care planning, discharge planning, and other follow-up measures. The next step is to develop an individualized care plan based directly on these findings.

The goal of care planning is to initiate and maintain collaboration between the nursing facility and the local contact agency (LCA) to support the individual's expressed interest in being transitioned to community living. The nursing home staff is responsible for making referrals to the LCAs under the process that the State has established. The LCA is, in turn, responsible for contacting referred residents and assisting with transition services planning. This includes facility support for the individual in achieving his or her highest level of functioning and the involvement of the designated contact agency providing informed choices for community living. The LCA is the entity that does the necessary community support planning (e.g. housing, home modification, setting up a household, transportation, community inclusion planning, arranging of care support, etc.)This collaboration will enable the State-designated local contact agency to initiate communication by telephone or visit with the individual (and his or her family or significant others, if the individual so chooses) to talk about opportunities for returning to community living.

4.11 Reserved

CHAPTER 5: SUBMISSION AND CORRECTION OF THE MDS ASSESSMENTS

Nursing homes are required to submit Omnibus Budget Reconciliation Act required (OBRA) MDS records for all residents in Medicare- or Medicaid-certified beds regardless of the pay source. Skilled nursing facilities (SNFs) and hospitals with a swing bed agreement (swing beds) are required to transmit additional MDS assessments for all Medicare beneficiaries in a Part A stay reimbursable under the SNF Prospective Payment System (PPS).

5.1 Transmitting MDS Data

All Medicare and/or Medicaid-certified nursing homes and swing beds, or agents of those facilities, must transmit required MDS data records to CMS' Quality Improvement and Evaluation System (QIES) Assessment Submission and Processing (ASAP) system. Required MDS records are those assessments and tracking records that are mandated under OBRA and SNF PPS. Assessments that are completed for purposes other than OBRA and SNF PPS reasons are not to be submitted, e.g., private insurance, including but not limited to Medicare Advantage Plans. After completion of the required assessment and/or tracking records, each provider must create electronic transmission files that meet the requirements detailed in the current MDS 3.0 Data Submission Specifications available on the CMS MDS 3.0 web site at:

http://www.cms. gov/NursingHomeQualityInits/30_NHQIMDS30TechnicalInformation.asp

In addition, providers must be certain they are submitting MDS assessments under the appropriate authority. There must be a federal and/or state authority to submit MDS assessment data to the QIES ASAP system. The software used by providers should have a prompt for confirming the authority to submit each record.

The provider indicates the submission authority for a record in item A0410, Submission Requirement.

- Value = 1   Neither federal nor state required submission.
- Value = 2   State but not federal required submission (FOR NURSING HOMES ONLY).
- Value = 3   Federal required submission.

See Chapter 3 for details concerning the coding of item A0410, Submission Requirement. Note: CMS certified Swing Bed unit assessments are always Value 3, Federal required submission.

Providers must establish communication with the QIES ASAP system in order to submit a file. This is accomplished by using specialized communications software and hardware and the CMS wide area network. Details about these processes are available on the QIES Technical Support Office web site at: https://www.qtso.com.

Once communication is established with the QIES ASAP system, the provider can access the CMS MDS Welcome Page in the MDS system. This site allows providers to submit MDS assessment data and access various information sources such as Bulletins and Questions and Answers. The *Minimum Data Set (MDS) 3.0 Provider User's Guide* provides more detailed information about the MDS system. It is available on the QTSO MDS 3.0 web site at https://www.qtso.com/mds30.html.

When the transmission file is received by the QIES ASAP system, the system performs a series of validation edits to evaluate whether or not the data submitted meet the required standards. MDS records are edited to verify that clinical responses are within valid ranges and are consistent, dates are reasonable, and records are in the proper order with regard to records that were previously accepted by the QIES ASAP system for the same resident. The provider is notified of the results of this evaluation by error and warning messages on a Final Validation Report. All error and warning messages are detailed and explained in the *Minimum Data Set (MDS) 3.0 Provider User's Guide*.

5.2 Timeliness Criteria

In accordance with the requirements at 42 CFR §483.20(f)(1), (f)(2), and (f)(3), long-term care facilities participating in the Medicare and Medicaid programs must meet the following conditions:

- **Completion Timing:**
  - For all non-admission OBRA and PPS assessments, the MDS Completion Date (Z0500B) must be no later than 14 days after the Assessment Reference Date (ARD) (A2300).
  - For the Admission assessment, the MDS Completion Date (Z0500B) must be no later than 13 days after the Assessment Reference Date (ARD) (A2300).
  - For the Admission assessment, the Care Area Assessment (CAA) Completion Date (V0200B2) must be no more than 13 days after the Entry Date (A1600).
  - For the Annual assessment, the CAA Completion Date (V0200B2) must be no later than 14 days after the ARD (A2300).
  - For the other comprehensive MDS assessments, Significant Change in Status Assessment and Significant Correction to Prior Comprehensive Assessment, the CAA Completion Date (V0200B2) must be no later than 14 days from the ARD (A2300) and no later than 14 days from the determination date of the significant change in status or the significant error, respectively.
  - For Entry and Death in Facility tracking records, the MDS Completion Date (Z0500B) must be no later than 7 days from the Event Date (A1600 for an entry record; A2000 for a death-in-facility record).
- **State Requirements:** Many states have established additional MDS requirements for Medicaid payment and/or quality monitoring purposes. For information on state requirements, contact your State RAI Coordinator. (See Appendix B for a list of state RAI coordinators.)
- **Encoding Data:** Within 7 days after completing a resident's MDS assessment or tracking information, the provider should encode the MDS data (i.e., enter the information into the facility MDS software). The encoding requirements are as follows:

— For a comprehensive assessment (Admission, Annual, Significant Change in Status, and Significant Correction to Prior Comprehensive), encoding must occur within 7 days after the Care Plan Completion Date (V0200C2 + 7 days).

— For a Quarterly, Significant Correction to Prior Quarterly, Discharge, or PPS assessment, encoding must occur within 7 days after the MDS Completion Date (Z0500B + 7 days).

— For a tracking record, encoding should occur within 7 days of the Event Date (A1600 + 7 days for Entry records and A2000 + 7 days for Death in Facility records).

- **Submission Format:** For submission, the MDS data must be in record and file formats that conform to standard record layouts and data dictionaries, and pass standardized edits defined by CMS and the State. Each MDS record must be a separate file in a required XML format. The submission file is a compressed ZIP file that may contain multiple XML files. See the MDS 3.0 Data Submission Specifications on the CMS MDS 3.0 web site for details concerning file and record formats, XML structure, and ZIP files.

- **Transmitting Data:** Submission files are transmitted to the QIES ASAP system using the CMS wide area network. Providers must transmit all sections of the MDS 3.0 required for their State-specific instrument, including the Care Area Assessment Summary (Section V) and all tracking or correction information. Transmission requirements apply to all MDS 3.0 records used to meet both Federal and state requirements. Care plans are not required to be transmitted.

  — **Assessment Transmission:** Comprehensive assessments must be transmitted electronically within 14 days of the Care Plan Completion Date (V0200C2 + 14 days). All other MDS assessments must be submitted within 14 days of the MDS Completion Date (Z0500B + 14 days).

  — **Tracking Information Transmission:** For Entry and Death in Facility tracking records, information must be transmitted within 14 days of the Event Date (A1600 + 14 days for Entry records and A2000 + 14 days for Death in Facility records).

Submission Time Frame for MDS Records

Type of Assessment/Tracking	Primary Reason (A0310A)	Secondary Reason (A0310B)	Entry/Discharge Reporting (A0310F)	Final Completion or Event Date	Submit By
Admission Assessment	01	All values	10, 11, 99	V0200C2	V0200C2 + 14
Annual Assessment	03	All values	10, 11, 99	V0200C2	V0200C2 + 14
Sign. Change in Status Assessment	04	All values	10, 11, 99	V0200C2	V0200C2 + 14
Sign. Correction to Prior Comprehensive Assessment.	05	All values	10, 11, 99	V0200C2	V0200C2 + 14
Quarterly Review Assessment.	02	All values	10, 11, 99	Z0500B	Z0500B +14
Sign. Correction Prior Quarterly Assessment.	06	All values	10, 11, 99	Z0500B	Z0500B + 14

(continued)

Submission Time Frame for MDS Records (continued)

Type of Assessment/Tracking	Primary Reason (A0310A)	Secondary Reason (A0310B)	Entry/Discharge Reporting (A0310F)	Final Completion or Event Date	Submit By
PPS Assessment	99	01 through 07	10, 11, 99	Z0500B	Z0500B + 14
Discharge Assessment	All values	All values	10 or 11	Z0500B	Z0500B + 14
Death in Facility Tracking	99	99	12	A2000	A2000 + 14
Entry Tracking	99	99	1	A1600	A1600 + 14
Correction Request (Modification or Inactivation)	N/A	N/A	N/A	X1100E	X1100E + 14

Table Legend:

Item	Description
V0200C2	Care Plan Completion Date: Date of the signature of the person completing the care planning decision on the Care Area Assessment (CAA) Summary sheet (Section V), indicating which Care Areas are addressed in the care plan. This is the date of care plan completion.
Z0500B	MDS Assessment Completion Date: Date of the RN assessment coordinator's signature, indicating that the MDS assessment is complete.
A2000	Date of discharge or death
A1600	Date of entry
X1100E	Date of the RN coordinator's signature on the Correction Request (Section X) certifying completion of the correction request information and the corrected assessment or tracking information.

- **Assessment Schedule:** An OBRA assessment (comprehensive or quarterly) is due every quarter unless the resident is no longer in the facility. There should be no more than 92 days between OBRA assessments. An OBRA comprehensive assessment is due every year unless the resident is no longer in the facility. There should be no more than 366 days between comprehensive assessments. PPS assessments follow their own schedule. See Chapter 6 for details.

5.3 Validation Edits

The QIES ASAP system has validation edits designed to monitor the timeliness and accuracy of MDS record submissions. If transmitted MDS records do not meet the edit requirements, the system will provide error and warning messages on the provider's Final Validation Report.

Initial Submission Feedback. For each file submitted, the submitter will receive confirmation that the file was received for processing and editing by the MDS system. This confirmation information includes the file submission number as well as the date and time the file was received for processing.

Validation and Editing Process. Each time a user accesses the QIES ASAP system and transmits an MDS file, the QIES ASAP system performs three types of validation:

1. **Fatal File Errors.** If the file structure is unacceptable (e.g., it is not a ZIP file), the records in the ZIP file cannot be extracted, or the file cannot be read, then the file will be rejected. The Submitter Final Validation Report will list the Fatal File Errors. Files that are rejected must be corrected and resubmitted.

2. **Fatal Record Errors.** If the file structure is acceptable, then each MDS record in the file is validated individually for Fatal Record Errors. These errors include, but are not limited to:

   - Out of range responses (e.g., the valid codes for the item are 1, 2, 3, and 4 and the submitted value is a 6).
   - Inconsistent relationships between items. One example is a skip pattern violation. The resident is coded as comatose (B0100 = 1) but the Brief Interview for Mental Status is conducted (C0100 = 1). Another example is an inconsistent date pattern, such as the resident's Birth Date (Item A0900) is later than the Entry Date (Item A1600).

   Fatal Record Errors result in rejection of individual records by the QIES ASAP system. The provider is informed of Fatal Record Errors on the Final Validation Report. Rejected records must be corrected and resubmitted.

3. **Non-Fatal Errors (Warnings).** The record is also validated for Non-Fatal Errors. Non-Fatal Errors include, but are not limited to, missing or questionable data of a non-critical nature or item consistency errors of a non-critical nature. Examples are timing errors. Timing errors for a Quarterly assessment include (a) the submission date is more than 14 days after the MDS assessment completion date (Z0500B) or (b) the assessment completion is more than 14 days after the ARD (A2300). Another example is a record sequencing error, where an Entry record (A0310F = 01) is submitted after a Quarterly assessment record (A0310A = 02) with no intervening discharge record (A0310F = 10, 11 or 12). Any Non-Fatal Errors are reported to the provider in the Final Validation Report as warnings. The provider must evaluate each warning to identify necessary corrective actions.

Storage to the QIES ASAP System. If there are any Fatal Record Errors, the record will be rejected and not stored in the QIES ASAP system. If there are no Fatal Record Errors, the record is loaded into the QIES ASAP system, even if the record has Non-Fatal Errors (Warnings).

Detailed information on the validation edits and the error and warning messages is available in the MDS 3.0 Data Submission Specifications on the CMS MDS 3.0 web site and in Section 5 of the *Minimum Data Set (MDS) 3.0 Provider User's Guide* on the QTSO MDS 3.0 web site.

5.4 Additional Medicare Submission Requirements that Impact Billing Under the SNF PPS

As stated in CFR §413.343(a) and (b), providers reimbursed under the SNF PPS "are required to submit the resident assessment data described at §483.20…. in the manner necessary to administer the payment rate methodology described in §413.337." This provision includes the frequency, scope, and number of assessments required in accordance with the methodology described in CFR §413.337(c) related to the adjustment of the Federal rates for case mix. SNFs must submit assessments according to a standard schedule. This schedule must include performance of resident assessments in specified windows near the 5th, 14th, 30th, 60th, and 90th days of the Medicare Part A stay.

HIPPS Codes: Health Insurance Prospective Payment System (HIPPS) codes are billing codes used when submitting Medicare Part A SNF payment claims to the Part A/Part B Medicare Administrative Contractor (A/B MAC). The HIPPS code consists of five positions. The first three positions represent the Resource Utilization Group-IV (RUG-IV) case mix code for the SNF resident, and the last two positions are an Assessment Indicator (AI) code indicating which type of assessment was completed. Standard "grouper" logic and software for RUG-IV and the AI code are provided by CMS on the MDS 3.0 web site.

The standard grouper uses MDS 3.0 items to determine both the RUG-IV group and the AI code. It is anticipated that MDS 3.0 software used by the provider will incorporate the standard grouper to automatically calculate the RUG-IV group and AI code. Detailed logic for determining the RUG-IV group and AI code is provided in Chapter 6.

The HIPPS codes to be used for Medicare Part A SNF claims are included on the MDS. There are two different HIPPS codes.

1. The Medicare Part A HIPPS code (Item Z0100A) is most often used on the claim. The RUG version code in Item Z0100B documents which version of RUG-IV was used to determine the RUG-IV group in the Medicare Part A HIPPS code.
2. The Medicare non-therapy Part A HIPPS code (Item Z0150A) is used when the provider is required to bill the non-therapy HIPPS. An example when the non-therapy HIPPS is to be billed is when the resident has been receiving rehabilitation therapy (physical therapy, occupational therapy, and/or speech-language pathology services), all rehabilitation therapy ends, and the resident continues on Part A (see Chapter 6 for details, including other instances when this HIPPS code is used for billing purposes). The RUG version code in Item Z0150B documents which version of RUG-IV was used to determine the RUG-IV group in the Medicare non-therapy Part A HIPPS code.

There is also a Medicare Short Stay indicator (Item Z0100C) on the MDS. For a qualifying Medicare short stay, the RUG-IV grouper uses alternative rehabilitation classification logic when there has been insufficient time to establish a full rehabilitation regime. The standard grouper uses MDS 3.0 items to determine the Medicare short stay indicator. See Chapter 6 for details.

Both HIPPS codes (Z0100A and Z0150A), the RUG version codes (Z0100B and Z0150B), and the Medicare Short Stay indicator (Z0100C) must be submitted to the QIES ASAP system on all Medicare PPS assessment records (indicated by A0310B= 01, 02, 03, 04, 05, 06, or 07). All of these values are validated by the QIES ASAP system. The Final Validation Report will indicate if any of these items is in error and the correct value for an incorrect item. Note that an error in one of these items is usually a non-fatal warning and the record will still be accepted in the QIES ASAP system. A record will receive a fatal error (-3804) if the record is a Start of Therapy (SOT) Other Medicare-Required Assessment (OMRA) (A0310C = 1 or 3) and the QIES ASAP system calculated value for the Medicare Part A HIPPS code (Z0100A) is not a group that begins with 'R', i.e., Rehabilitation Plus Extensive Services or Rehabilitation group.

The Medicare Part A SNF claim cannot be submitted until the corresponding MDS Medicare PPS assessment has been accepted in the QIES ASAP system. The claim must include the correct HIPPS code for the assessment. If the HIPPS code on the assessment was in error, then the correct HIPPS code from the Final Validation report must be used on the claim (warning error message -3616a).

5.5 MDS Correction Policy

Once completed, edited, and accepted into the QIES ASAP system, providers may not change a previously completed MDS assessment as the resident's status changes during the course of the resident's stay – the MDS must be accurate as of the ARD. Minor changes in the resident's status should be noted in the resident's record (e.g., in progress notes), in accordance with standards of clinical practice and documentation. Such monitoring and documentation is a part of the provider's responsibility to provide necessary care and services. A significant change in the resident's status warrants a new comprehensive assessment (see Chapter 2 for details).

It is important to remember that the electronic record submitted to and accepted into the QIES ASAP system is the legal assessment. Corrections made to the electronic record after QIES ASAP acceptance or to the paper copy maintained in the medical record are not recognized as proper corrections. It is the responsibility of the provider to ensure that any corrections made to a record are submitted to the QIES ASAP system in accordance with the MDS Correction Policy.

Several processes have been put into place to assure that the MDS data are accurate both at the provider and in the QIES ASAP system:

- If an error is discovered within 7 days of the completion of an MDS and before submission to the QIES ASAP system, the response may be corrected using standard editing procedures on the hard copy (cross out, enter correct response, initial and date) and/or correction of the MDS record in the facility's database. The resident's care plan should also be reviewed for any needed changes.

- Software used by the provider to encode the MDS must run all standard edits as defined in the data specifications released by CMS.

- Enhanced record rejection standards have been implemented in the QIES ASAP system.

- If an MDS record contains responses that are out of range, e.g., a 4 is entered when only 0-3 are allowable responses for an item, or item responses are inconsistent (e.g., a skip pattern is not observed), the record is rejected. Rejected records are not stored in the QIES ASAP database.

- If an error is discovered in a record that has been accepted by the QIES ASAP system, Modification or Inactivation procedures **must** be implemented by the provider to assure that the QIES ASAP system information is corrected.

- Clinical corrections must also be undertaken as necessary to assure that the resident is accurately assessed, the care plan is accurate, and the resident is receiving the necessary care. A Significant Change in Status Assessment (SCSA, Significant Correction to

Prior Quarterly (SCQA) or a Significant Correction to Prior Comprehensive (SCPA) may be needed as well as corrections to the information in the QIES ASAP system. An SCSA is required only if a change in the resident's clinical status occurred. An SCPA or SCQA is required when an uncorrected significant error is identified. See Chapter 2 for details.

The remaining sections of this chapter present the decision processes necessary to identify the proper correction steps. A flow chart is provided at the end of these sections that summarizes these decisions and correction steps.

5.6 Correcting Errors in MDS Records That Have Not Yet Been Accepted Into the QIES ASAP System

If an MDS assessment is found to have errors that incorrectly reflect the resident's status, then that assessment must be corrected. The correction process depends upon the type of error. MDS assessments that have not yet been accepted in the QIES ASAP system include records that have been submitted and rejected, production records that were inadvertently submitted as test records, or records that have not been submitted at all. These records can generally be corrected and retransmitted without any special correction procedures, since they were never accepted by the QIES ASAP system. The paper copy should be corrected according to standard procedures detailed below.

Errors Identified During the Encoding Period

Facilities have up to 7 days to encode (enter into the software) and edit an MDS assessment after the MDS has been completed. Changes may be made to the electronic record for any item during the encoding and editing period, provided the response refers to the same observation period. To make revisions to the paper copy, enter the correct response, draw a line through the previous response without obliterating it, and initial and date the corrected entry. This procedure is similar to how an entry in the medical record is corrected.

When the data are encoded into the provider's MDS system from paper, the provider is responsible for verifying that all responses in the computer file match the responses on the paper form. Any discrepancies must be corrected in the computer file during the 7-day encoding period.

In addition, the provider is responsible for running encoded MDS assessment data against CMS and State-specific edits that software vendors are responsible for building into MDS Version 3.0 computer systems. For each MDS item, the response must be within the required range and also be consistent with other item responses. During this 7-day encoding period that follows the completion of the MDS assessment, a provider may correct item responses to meet required edits. Only MDS assessments that meet all of the required edits are considered complete. For corrected items, the provider must use the same observation period as was used for the original item completion (i.e., the same ARD (A2300) and look-back period). Both the electronic and paper copies of the MDS must be corrected.

Errors Identified After the Encoding Period

Errors identified after the encoding and editing period must be corrected within 14 days after identifying the errors. If the record in error is an Entry tracking record, Death in Facility tracking record, Discharge assessment, or PPS assessment record (i.e., MDS Item A0310A = 99), then the record should be corrected and submitted to the QIES ASAP system. The correction process may be more complex if the record in error is an OBRA comprehensive or quarterly assessment record (i.e., Item A0310A = 01 through 06).

Significant versus Minor Errors in a Nursing Home OBRA Comprehensive or Quarterly Assessment Record. OBRA comprehensive and Quarterly assessment errors are classified as significant or minor errors. Errors that inaccurately reflect the resident's clinical status and/or result in an inappropriate plan of care are considered **significant errors**. All other errors related to the coding of MDS items are considered **minor errors**.

If the only errors in the OBRA comprehensive or Quarterly assessment are minor errors, then the only requirement is for the record to be corrected and submitted to the QIES ASAP system.

The correction process is more complicated for nursing home OBRA comprehensive or Quarterly assessments with *any significant errors* identified after the end of the 7-day encoding and editing period but before the records have been accepted into the QIES ASAP system. First, the nursing home must correct the original OBRA comprehensive or Quarterly assessment to reflect the resident's actual status as of the ARD for that original assessment and submit the record. Second, to insure an up-to-date view of the resident's status and an appropriate care plan, the nursing home must perform an additional new assessment, either a Significant Change in Status Assessment or Significant Correction to Prior Assessment with a current observation period and ARD. If correction of the error on the MDS revealed that the resident's status met the criteria for a Significant Change in Status Assessment, then a Significant Change in Status assessment is required. If the criteria for a Significant Change in Status Assessment are not met, then a Significant Correction to Prior Assessment is required. See Chapter 2 for details.

In summary, the nursing home must take the following actions for an OBRA comprehensive or Quarterly assessment that has *not* been submitted to the QIES ASAP system when it contains significant errors:

- Correct the errors in the original OBRA comprehensive or quarterly assessment.
- Submit the corrected assessment.
- Perform a *new* assessment – a Significant Change in Status Assessment or a Significant Correction to Prior Assessment and update the care plan as necessary.

If the assessment was performed for Medicare purposes only (A0310A = 99 and A0310B = 01 through 07) or for a discharge (A0310A = 99 and A0310F = 10 or 11), no Significant Change in Status Assessment or Significant Correction to Prior Assessment is required. The provider would determine if the Medicare-required or Discharge assessment should be modified or inactivated. Care Area Assessments (Section V) and updated care planning are not required with Medicare-only and Discharge assessments.

5.7 Correcting Errors in MDS Records That Have Been Accepted Into the QIES ASAP System

Facilities should correct any errors necessary to insure that the information in the QIES ASAP system accurately reflects the resident's identification, location, overall clinical status, or payment status. A correction can be submitted for any accepted record, regardless of the age of the original record. A record may be corrected even if subsequent records have been accepted for the resident.

Errors identified in QIES ASAP system records must be corrected within 14 days after identifying the errors. Inaccuracies can occur for a variety of reasons, such as transcription errors, data entry errors, software product errors, item coding errors or other errors. The following two processes have been established to correct MDS records (assessments, Entry tracking records or Death in Facility tracking records) that have been accepted into the QIES ASAP system:

- Modification
- Inactivation

A Modification request moves the inaccurate record into history in the QIES ASAP system and replaces it with the corrected record as the active record. An Inactivation request also moves the inaccurate record into history in the QIES ASAP system, but does not replace it with a new record. Both the Modification and Inactivation processes require the MDS Correction Request items to be completed in Section X of the MDS 3.0.

The MDS Correction Request items in Section X contain the minimum amount of information necessary to enable location of the erroneous MDS record previously submitted and accepted into the QIES ASAP system. Section X items are defined in the MDS 3.0 Data Submission Specifications posted on the CMS MDS 3.0 web site.

When a facility maintains the MDS electronically without the use of electronic signatures, a hard copy of the Correction Request items in Section X must be kept with the corrected paper copy of the MDS record in the clinical file to track the changes made with the modification. In addition, the facility would keep a hard copy of the Correction Request items (Section X) with an inactivated record. For details on electronic records, see Chapter 2, Section 2.4.

Modification Requests

A Modification Request should be used when an MDS record (assessment, Entry tracking record or Death in Facility tracking record) is in the QIES ASAP system, but the information in the record contains clinical or demographic errors.

The Modification Request is used to modify most MDS items, including:

- Target Date
  - Entry Date (Item A1600) on an Entry tracking record (Item A0310F = 1)
  - Discharge Date (Item A2000) on a Discharge/Death in Facility record (Item A0310F = 10, 11, 12),

— Assessment Reference Date (Item A2300) on an OBRA or PPS assessment.*
- Type of Assessment (Item A0310)**
- Clinical Items (Items B0100-V0200C)

*Note: The ARD (Item A2300) can be changed when the ARD on the assessment represents a data entry/typographical error. However, the ARD cannot be altered if it results in a change in the look back period and alters the actual assessment timeframe. Consider the following examples:

- When entering the assessment into the facility's software, the ARD, intended to be 02/12/2013, was inadvertently entered as 02/02/2013. The interdisciplinary team (IDT) completed the assessment based on the ARD of 2/12/2013 (that is, the seven day look back was 2/06/2012 through 2/12/2013. This would be an acceptable use of the modification process to modify the ARD (A2300) to reflect 02/12/2013.

- An assessment was completed by the team and entered into the software based on the ARD of 1/10/2013 (and seven day look back of 1/04/2013 through 1/10/2013). Three weeks later, the IDT determines that the date used represents a date that is not compliant with the PPS schedule and proposes changing the ARD to 1/07/2013. This would alter the look back period and result in a new assessment (rather than correcting a typographical error); this would not be an acceptable modification and shall not occur.

**Note: The Type of Assessment items (Item A0310) can only be modified when the Item Set Code (ISC) of that assessment does not change. In other words, if the Item Subset (full list can be found in Chapter 2, Section 2.5) would change, the modification cannot be done. Consider the following examples:

- A stand-alone Discharge assessment (ISC = ND) was completed and accepted into the ASAP system. The provider later (that is, after the day of discharge) determined that the assessment should have been a 30-day PPS assessment combined with a Discharge assessment (ISC = NP). This modification would not be allowed as the ISC for the Discharge assessment combined with the 30-day PPS is different than the stand-alone Discharge ISC. This is an example of a missing 30-day assessment.

- An Admission assessment (ISC = NC) was completed and accepted into the ASAP system. The provider intended to code the assessment as an Admission and a 5-day PPS assessment (ISC = NC). The modification process could be used in this case as the ISC would not change.

There are a few items for which the modification process shall not be used. These items require the following correction measures if an error is identified:

- An Inactivation of the existing record followed by submission of a new corrected record is required to correct an error of the Type of Provider (Item A0200)
- An MDS 3.0 Manual Assessment Correction/Deletion Request is required to correct:
  — Submission Requirement (Item A0410),
  — State-assigned facility submission ID (FAC_ID),
  — Production/test code (PRODN_TEST_CD).

See Section 5.8 for details on the MDS 3.0 Manual Assessment Correction/Deletion Request.

When an error is discovered (except for those items listed in the preceding paragraph and instances listed in Section 5.8) in an MDS 3.0 Entry tracking record, Death in Facility tracking record, Discharge assessment, or PPS assessment that is not an OBRA assessment (where Item A0310A = 99), the provider must take the following actions to correct the record:

1. Create a corrected record with all items included, not just the items in error.
2. Complete the required Correction Request Section X items and include with the corrected record. Item A0050 should have a value of 2, indicating a modification request.
3. Submit this modification request record.

If errors are discovered in a nursing home OBRA comprehensive or Quarterly assessment (Item A0310A = 01 through 06) in the QIES ASAP system, then the nursing home must determine if there are any significant errors. If the *only errors are minor errors*, the nursing home must take the following actions to correct the OBRA assessment:

1. Create a corrected record with all items included, not just the items in error.
2. Complete the required Correction Request Section X items and include with the corrected record. Item A0050 should have a value of 2, indicating a modification request.
3. Submit this modification request record.

When any *significant error* is discovered in an OBRA comprehensive or Quarterly assessment in the QIES ASAP system, the nursing home must take the following actions to correct the OBRA assessment:

1. Create a corrected record with all items included, not just the items in error.
2. Complete the required Correction Request Section X items and include with the corrected record. Item A0050 should have a value of 2, indicating a modification request.
3. Submit this modification request record.
4. Perform a *new* Significant Correction to Prior Assessment or Significant Change in Status Assessment and update the care plan as necessary.

A Significant Change in Status Assessment would be required only if correction of the MDS item(s) revealed that the resident met the criteria for a Significant Change in Status Assessment.

If criteria for Significant Change in Status Assessment were not met, then a Significant Correction to Prior Assessment is required.

When errors in an OBRA comprehensive or Quarterly assessment in the QIES ASAP system have been corrected in a more current OBRA comprehensive or Quarterly assessment (Item A0310A = 01through 06), the nursing home is not required to perform a new additional assessment (Significant Change in Status or Significant Correction to Prior assessment). In this situation, the nursing home has already updated the resident's status and care plan. However, the nursing home must use the Modification process to assure that the erroneous assessment residing in the QIES ASAP system is corrected.

Inactivation Requests

An Inactivation should be used when a record has been accepted into the QIES ASAP system but the corresponding event did not occur. For example, a Discharge assessment was submitted for a resident but there was no actual discharge. An Inactivation (Item A0050 = 3) **must** be completed when any of the following items are inaccurate:

- Type of Provider (Item A0200)

- Type of Assessment (A0310) **when the Item Subset would change had the MDS been modified**

- Entry Date (Item A1600) on an Entry tracking record (Item A0310F = 1) **when the look-back period and/or clinical assessment would change had the MDS been modified**

- Discharge Date (Item A2000) on a Discharge/Death in Facility record (Item A0310F = 10, 11, 12) **when the look-back period and/or clinical assessment would change had the MDS been modified**

- Assessment Reference Date (Item A2300) on an OBRA or PPS assessment **when the look-back period and/or clinical assessment would change had the MDS been modified**

When inactivating a record, the provider is required to submit an electronic Inactivation Request record. This record is an MDS record but only the Section X items and Item A0050 are completed. This is sufficient information to locate the record in the QIES ASAP system, inactivate the record and document the reason for inactivation.

For instances when the provider determines that the Type of Provider is incorrect, the provider must inactivate the record in the QIES ASAP system, then complete and submit a new MDS 3.0 record with the correct Type of Provider, ensuring that the clinical information is accurate.

Inactivations should be rare and are appropriate only under the narrow set of circumstances that indicate a record is invalid.

In such instances a new ARD date must be established based on MDS requirements, which is the date the error is determined or later, but not earlier. The new MDS 3.0 record being submitted to replace the inactivated record must include new signatures and dates for all items based on the look-back period established by the new ARD and according to established MDS assessment completion requirements.

5.8 Special Manual Record Correction Request

A few types of errors in a record in the QIES ASAP system cannot be corrected with an automated Modification or Inactivation request. These errors are:

1. The record is a test record inadvertently submitted as production.

2. The record has the wrong submission requirement in Item A0410.
3. The record has the wrong facility ID in the control Item FAC_ID.

In all of these cases, the facility must contact the State Agency to have the problems fixed. The State Agency will send the facility the MDS 3.0 Manual Assessment Correction/Deletion Request form. The facility is responsible for completing the form. The facility **must** submit the completed form to the State Agency via <u>certified mail</u> through the United States Postal Service (USPS). The State Agency **must** approve the provider's request and submit a signed form to the QIES Help Desk via <u>certified mail</u> through the USPS.

When a test record is in the QIES ASAP system, the problem must be manually evaluated in the QIES ASAP system and the QIES ASAP system appropriately corrected. A normal Inactivation request will not totally fix the problem, since it will leave the test record in a history file and may also leave information about a fictitious resident. Manual correction is necessary to completely remove the test record and associated information.

A QIES ASAP system record with an incorrect submission requirement in Item A0410 is a very serious problem. Submission of MDS assessment records to the QIES ASAP system constitutes a release of private information and must conform to privacy laws. Item A0410 is intended to allow appropriate privacy safeguards, controlling who can access the record and whether the record can even be accepted into the QIES ASAP system. A normal Modification or Inactivation request cannot be used to correct the A0410 value, since a copy of the record in error will remain in the QIES ASAP system history file with the wrong access control. Consider a record in the QIES ASAP system with an A0410 value of 3 (federal submission requirement) but there was actually no state or federal requirement for the record (A0410 should have been 1). The record should not be in the QIES ASAP system at all and manual correction is necessary to completely remove the record from the QIES ASAP system. Consider a record with an A0410 value of 3 (federal submission requirement) but the record is only required by the state (A0410 should have been 2). In this case there is both federal and state access to the record, but access should be limited to the state. Manual correction is necessary to correct A0410 and reset access control, without leaving a copy of the record with the wrong access in the QIES ASAP system history file.

If a QIES ASAP system record has the wrong main facility ID (control item FAC_ID), then the record must be removed without leaving any trace in the QIES ASAP system. The record also should be resubmitted with the correct FAC_ID value when indicated.

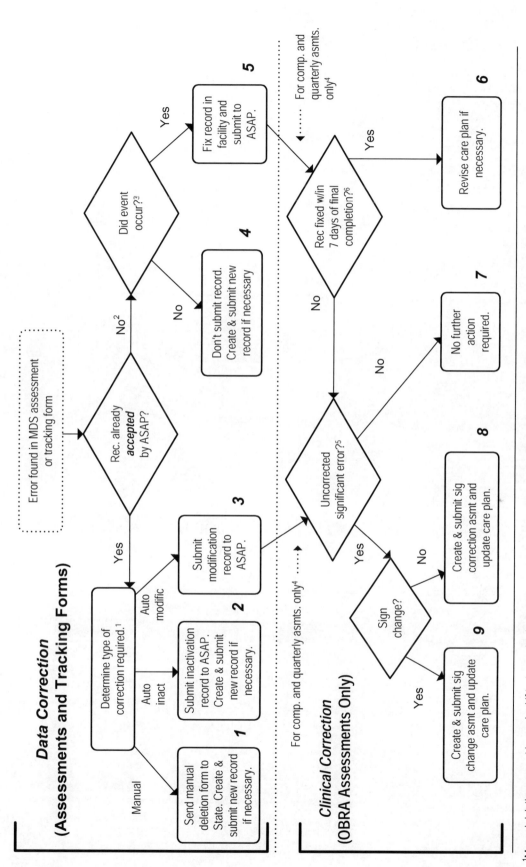

*Data Correction
(Assessments and Tracking Forms)*

Error found in MDS assessment or tracking form

Rec. already *accepted* by ASAP?

No[2]

Did event occur?[3]

Yes — Fix record in facility and submit to ASAP. **5**

No — Don't submit record. Create & submit new record if necessary **4**

Yes — Determine type of correction required.[1]

Manual — Send manual deletion form to State. Create & submit new record if necessary. **1**

Auto inact — Submit inactivation record to ASAP. Create & submit new record if necessary. **2**

Auto modific — Submit modification record to ASAP. **3**

For comp. and quarterly asmts. only[4]

Rec fixed w/in 7 days of final completion?[6]

Yes — Revise care plan if necessary. **6**

No

Uncorrected significant error?[5]

No — No further action required. **7**

Yes

Sign change?

No — Create & submit sig correction asmt and update care plan. **8**

Yes — Create & submit sig change asmt and update care plan. **9**

For comp. and quarterly asmts. only[4]

*Clinical Correction
(OBRA Assessments Only)*

[1]Manual deletion request is required if test record submitted as production record, if record contains incorrect FAC_ID, or if record was submitted with an incorrect submission requirement value (A0410), for example send in as federally required (A0410 = 3) but should have been state required (A0410 = 2). Otherwise, automated inactivation or modification required: (a) if event did not occur (see note #3 below), submit automated inactivation, (b) if event occurred, submit automated modification.
[2]Record has not been data entered, has not been submitted, or has been submitted and rejected by ASAP.
[3]The event occurred if the record reflects an actual entry or discharge or if an assessment was actually performed for the resident. If a record was created in error (e.g., a discharge was created for a resident who was not actually discharged), then the event did not occur.
[4]OBRA comprehensive assessments with A0310 A=01,03,04,05 and quarterly assessments with A0310B=02,06.
[5]The assessment contains a significant error which has not been corrected by a subsequent assessment.
[6]Final completion date is item V0200C2 for a comprehensive and Z0500B for all other assessments.

CHAPTER 6: MEDICARE SKILLED NURSING FACILITY PROSPECTIVE PAYMENT SYSTEM (SNF PPS)

6.1 Background

The Balanced Budget Act of 1997 included the implementation of a Medicare Prospective Payment System (PPS) for skilled nursing facilities (SNFs) and hospitals with a swing bed agreement, consolidated billing, and a number of related changes. The PPS system replaced the retrospective cost-based system for SNFs under Part A of the program (**Federal Register** Vol. 63, No. 91, May 12, 1998, Final Rule). Effective with cost reporting periods beginning on or after July 1, 2002, SNF-level services furnished in rural swing bed Hospitals are paid based on the SNF PPS instead of the previous, cost-related method (**Federal Register** Vol. 66, No. 147, July 31, 2001, Final Rule). However, the Medicare, Medicaid, and SCHIP Benefits Improvement and Protection Act of 2000 included an exemption of critical access hospital swing beds from the SNF PPS.

The SNF PPS is the culmination of substantial research efforts beginning as early as the 1970s that focus on the areas of nursing home payment and quality. In addition, it is based on a foundation of knowledge and work by a number of States that developed and implemented similar case mix payment methodologies for their Medicaid nursing home payment systems.

The current focus in the development of State and Federal payment systems for nursing home care is based on recognizing the differences among residents, particularly in the utilization of resources. Some residents require total assistance with their activities of daily living (ADLs) and have complex nursing care needs. Other residents may require less assistance with ADLs but may require rehabilitation or restorative nursing services. The recognition of these differences is the premise of a case mix system. Reimbursement levels differ based on the resource needs of the residents. Residents with heavy care needs require more staff resources and payment levels should be higher than for those residents with less intensive care needs. In a case mix adjusted payment system, the amount of reimbursement to the nursing home is based on the resource intensity of the resident as measured by items on the Minimum Data Set (MDS). Case mix reimbursement has become a widely adopted method for financing nursing home care. The case mix approach serves as the basis for the PPS for skilled nursing facilities and swing bed hospitals and is increasingly being used by States for Medicaid reimbursement for nursing homes.

6.2 Using the MDS in the Medicare Prospective Payment System

A key component of the Medicare SNF PPS is the case mix reimbursement methodology used to determine resident care needs. A number of nursing home case mix systems have been developed over the last 20 years. Since the early 1990s, however, the most widely adopted approach to case mix has been the Resource Utilization Groups (RUGs). This classification system uses information from the MDS assessment to classify SNF residents into a series of groups representing the residents' relative direct care resource requirements.

In 2005, the Centers for Medicare & Medicaid Services (CMS) initiated a national nursing home staff time measurement (STM) study, the Staff Time and Resource Intensity Verification (STRIVE) Project. The STRIVE project represents the first nationwide time study for nursing homes in the United States to be conducted since 1997, and the data collected has been used to update payment systems for Medicare SNFs and Medicaid nursing facilities (NFs). Based on this analysis, CMS has developed the RUG-IV classification system that incorporates the MDS 3.0 items.

Over half of the State Medicaid programs also use the MDS for their case mix payment systems. The RUG-IV system replaced the RUG-III for Medicare starting on October 1, 2010. However, State Medicaid agencies have the option to continue to use the RUG-III classification systems or adopt the RUG-IV system. CMS also provides the States alternative RUG-IV classification systems with 66, 57, or 48 groups with varying numbers of Rehabilitation groups (similar to the RUG-III 53, 44, and 34 groups). States have the option of selecting the system (RUG-III or RUG-IV) with the number of Rehabilitation groups that better suits their Medicaid long-term care population. State Medicaid programs always have the option to develop nursing home reimbursement systems that meet their specific program goals. The decision to implement a RUG-IV classification system for Medicaid is a State decision. Please contact your State Medicaid agency if you have questions about your State Medicaid reimbursement system.

The MDS assessment data is used to calculate the RUG-IV classification necessary for payment. The MDS contains extensive information on the resident's nursing and therapy needs, ADL impairments, cognitive status, behavioral problems, and medical diagnoses. This information is used to define RUG-IV groups that form a hierarchy from the greatest to the least resources used. Residents with more specialized nursing requirements, licensed therapies, greater ADL dependency, or other conditions will be assigned to higher groups in the RUG-IV hierarchy. Providing care to these residents is more costly and is reimbursed at a higher level.

6.3 Resource Utilization Groups Version IV (RUG-IV)

The RUG-IV classification system has eight major classification categories: Rehabilitation Plus Extensive Services, Rehabilitation, Extensive Services, Special Care High, Special Care Low, Clinically Complex, Behavioral Symptoms and Cognitive Performance Problems, and Reduced Physical Function (see Table 1). The categories, except for Extensive Services, are further divided by the intensity of the resident's ADL needs. The Special Care High, Special Care Low, and Clinically Complex categories are also divided by the presence of depression. Finally, the Behavioral Symptoms and Cognitive Performance Problems and the Reduced Physical Function categories are divided by the provision of restorative nursing services.

A calculation worksheet was developed in order to provide clinical staff with a better understanding of how the RUG-IV classification system works. The worksheet translates the standard software code into plain language to assist staff in understanding the logic behind the classification system. A copy of the calculation worksheet for the RUG-IV classification system for nursing homes can be found at the end of this section.

Table 1. Eight Major RUG-IV Classification Categories

Major RUG-IV Category	Characteristics Associated With Major RUG-IV Category
Rehabilitation Plus Extensive Services	Residents satisfying all of the following three conditions: • Having a minimum activity of daily living (ADL) dependency score of 2 or more. • Receiving physical therapy, occupational therapy, and/or speech-language pathology services while a resident. • While a resident, receiving complex clinical care and have needs involving tracheostomy care, ventilator/respirator, and/or infection isolation.
Rehabilitation	Residents receiving physical therapy, occupational therapy, and/or speech-language pathology services while a resident.
Extensive Services	Residents satisfying the following two conditions: • Having a minimum ADL dependency score of 2 or more. • While a resident, receiving complex clinical care and have needs involving: tracheostomy care, ventilator/respirator, and/or infection isolation.
Special Care High	Residents satisfying the following two conditions: • Having a minimum ADL dependency score of 2 or more. • Receiving complex clinical care or have serious medical conditions involving any one of the following: — comatose, — septicemia, — diabetes with insulin injections and insulin order changes, — quadriplegia with a higher minimum ADL dependence criterion (ADL score of 5 or more), — chronic obstructive pulmonary disease (COPD) with shortness of breath when lying flat, — fever with pneumonia, vomiting, weight loss, or tube feeding meeting intake requirement, — parenteral/IV feeding, or — respiratory therapy.

(continued)

Table 1. Eight Major RUG-IV Classification Categories (continued)

Major RUG-IV Category	Characteristics Associated With Major RUG-IV Category
Special Care Low	Residents satisfying the following two conditions: • Having a minimum ADL dependency score of 2 or more. • Receiving complex clinical care or have serious medical conditions involving any of the following: — cerebral palsy with ADL dependency score of 5 or more, — multiple sclerosis with ADL dependency score of 5 or more, — Parkinson's disease with ADL dependency score of 5 or more, — respiratory failure and oxygen therapy while a resident, — tube feeding meeting intake requirement, — ulcer treatment with two or more ulcers including venous ulcers, arterial ulcers or Stage II pressure ulcers, — ulcer treatment with any Stage III or IV pressure ulcer, — foot infections or wounds with application of dressing, — radiation therapy while a resident, or — dialysis while a resident.
Clinically Complex	Residents receiving complex clinical care or have conditions requiring skilled nursing management, interventions or treatments involving any of the following: • pneumonia, • hemiplegia with ADL dependency score of 5 or more, • surgical wounds or open lesions with treatment, • burns, • chemotherapy while a resident, • oxygen therapy while a resident, • IV medications while a resident, or • transfusions while a resident.

(continued)

Table 1. Eight Major RUG-IV Classification Categories (continued)

Major RUG-IV Category	Characteristics Associated With Major RUG-IV Category
Behavioral Symptoms and Cognitive Performance	Residents satisfying the following two conditions: • Having a maximum ADL dependency score of 5 or less. • Having behavioral or cognitive performance symptoms, involving any of the following: — difficulty in repeating words, temporal orientation, or recall (score on the Brief Interview for Mental Status <=9), — difficulty in making self understood, short term memory, or decision making (score on the Cognitive Performance Scale >=3), — hallucinations, — delusions, — physical behavioral symptoms toward others, — verbal behavioral symptoms toward others, — other behavioral symptoms, — rejection of care, or — wandering.
Reduced Physical Function	Residents whose needs are primarily for support with activities of daily living and general supervision.

6.4 Relationship between the Assessment and the Claim

The SNF PPS establishes a schedule of Medicare assessments. Each required Medicare assessment is used to support Medicare PPS reimbursement. There are scheduled PPS assessments performed around Day 5, Day 14, Day 30, Day 60, and Day 90 of a Medicare Part A stay (as defined in Chapter 2). These scheduled assessments establish per diem payment rates for associated standard payment periods. Unscheduled off-cycle assessments are performed under certain circumstances when required under the regulations (e.g., when the resident's condition changes). See Chapter 2 for greater detail on assessment types and requirements. These unscheduled assessments may impact the per diem payment rates for days within a standard payment period.

Numerous situations exist that impact the relationship between the assessment and the claim above and beyond the information provided in this chapter. It is the responsibility of the provider to ensure that claims submitted to Medicare are accurate and meet all Medicare requirements. For example, if resident's status does not meet the criteria for Medicare Part A SNF coverage, the provider is not to bill Medicare for any non-covered days. The assignment of a RUG is not an indication that the requirements for SNF Part A have been met. Once the resident no longer requires skilled services, the provider must not bill Medicare for days that are not covered. Therefore, the following information is not to be considered all inclusive and definitive. Refer to the **Medicare Claims Processing Manual**, Chapter 6, for detailed claims processing requirements and policies.

To verify that the Medicare bill accurately reflects the assessment information, two data items derived from the MDS assessment must be included on the Medicare claim:

Assessment Reference Date (ARD)

The ARD must be reported on the Medicare claim. CMS has developed internal mechanisms to link the assessment and billing records.

Health Insurance Prospective Payment System (HIPPS) Code

Each Medicare claim contains a five-position HIPPS code for the purpose of billing Part A covered days to the Part A/Part B Medicare Administrative Contractor (A/B MAC). The HIPPS code consists of the RUG-IV code and the Assessment Indicator (AI) as described below. CMS provides standard software and logic for HIPPS code calculation.

RUG-IV Group Code

The first three positions of the HIPPS code contain the RUG-IV group code to be billed for Medicare reimbursement. The RUG-IV group is calculated from the MDS assessment clinical data. See Section 6.6 for calculation details on each RUG group. CMS provides standard software, development tools, and logic for RUG-IV calculation. CMS software, or private software developed with the CMS tools, is used to encode and transmit the MDS assessment data and automatically calculates the RUG-IV group. CMS edits and validates the RUG-IV group code of transmitted MDS assessments. Skilled nursing facilities are not permitted to submit Medicare Part A claims until the assessments have been accepted into the CMS database, and they must use the RUG-IV code as validated by CMS when bills are filed, except in cases in which the facility must bill the default code (AAA). See Section 6.8 for details. The following RUG-IV group codes are used in the billing process:

Rehabilitation Plus Extensive Services:
RUX, RUL, RVX, RVL, RHX, RHL, RMX, RML, RLX
Rehabilitation:
RUA, RUB, RUC, RVA, RVB, RVC, RHA, RHB, RHC, RMA, RMB, RMC, RLA, RLB
Extensive Services:
ES3, ES2, ES1
Special Care High:
HE2, HE1, HD2, HD1, HC2, HC1, HB2, HB1
Special Care Low:
LE2, LE1, LD2, LD1, LC2, LC1, LB2, LB1
Clinically Complex:
CE2, CE1, CD2, CD1, CC2, CC1, CB2, CB1, CA2, CA1
Behavioral Symptoms and Cognitive Performance:
BB2, BB1, BA2, BA1

Reduced Physical Function:
PE2, PE1, PD2, PD1, PC2, PC1, PB2, PB1, PA2, PA1
Default:
AAA

There are two different Medicare HIPPS codes that may be recorded on the MDS 3.0 in Items Z0100A (Medicare Part A HIPPS code) and Z0150A (Medicare Part A non-therapy HIPPS code). The Medicare Part A HIPPS code may consist of any RUG-IV group code. The Medicare Part A non-therapy HIPPS code is restricted to the RUG-IV groups of Extensive Services and below. The HIPPS code included on the Medicare claim depends on the specific type of assessment involved.

The RUG codes in Items Z0100A and Z0150A are validated by CMS when the assessment is submitted. If the submitted RUG code is incorrect, the validation report will include a warning giving the correct code, and the facility must use the correct code in the HIPPS code on the bill.

The provider must ensure that all Medicare assessment requirements are met. When the provider fails to meet the Medicare assessment requirements, such as when the assessment is late (as evidenced by a late ARD), the provider may be required to bill the default code. In these situations, the provider is responsible to ensure that the default code and not the RUG group validated by CMS in Items Z0100A and Z01050A is billed for the applicable number of days. See Section 6.8 of this chapter for greater detail.

AI Code

The last two positions of the HIPPS code represent the Assessment Indicator (AI), identifying the assessment type. The AI coding system indicates the different types of assessments that define different PPS payment periods and is based on the coding of Item A0310. CMS provides standard software, development tools, and logic for AI code calculation. CMS software, or private software developed with the CMS tools, automatically calculates the AI code. The AI code is validated by CMS when the assessment is submitted. If the submitted AI code is incorrect on the assessment, the validation report will include a warning and provide the correct code. The facility is to use the correct AI code in the HIPPS code on the bill. The code consists of two digits, which are defined below. In situations when the provider is to bill the default code, such as a late assessment, the AI provided on the validation report is to be used along with the default code, AAA, on the Medicare claim. Refer to the **Medicare Claims Processing Manual**, Chapter 6, for detailed claims processing requirements and policies.

First AI Digit

The first digit of the AI code identifies scheduled PPS assessments that establish the RUG payment rate for the standard PPS scheduled payment periods. These assessments are PPS 5-day, 14-day, 30-day, 60-day, 90-day, and readmission/return. The Omnibus Budget Reconciliation Act (OBRA 1987) required assessments are also included, because they can be used under certain circumstances for payment (see Section 6.8). Table 2 displays the first AI code for each of the scheduled PPS assessment types and the standard payment period for each assessment type.

Table 2. Assessment Indicator First Digit Table

1st Digit Values	Assessment Type (abbreviation)	Standard* Scheduled Payment Period
0	Unscheduled PPS assessment (unsched)	Not applicable
1	PPS 5-day or readmission return (5d or readm)	Day 1 through 14
2	PPS 14-day (14d)	Day 15 through 30
3	PPS 30-day (30d)	Day 31 through 60
4	PPS 60-day (60d	Day 61 through 90
5	PPS 90-day (90d)	Day 91 through 100
6	OBRA assessment (not coded as a PPS assessment) **	Not applicable

* These are the payment periods that apply when only the scheduled Medicare-required assessments are performed. These are subject to change when unscheduled assessments used for PPS are performed, e.g., significant change in status, or when other requirements must be met.

**In some cases, such an assessment may be used for PPS if it is later determined that qualification for Part A coverage was present at the time of the assessment (see Missed Assessment, section 6.8). For these assessments A0310A will be 01 to 06 and A0310B will be 99.

Second AI Digit

The second digit of the AI code identifies unscheduled assessments used for PPS. Unscheduled PPS assessments are conducted in addition to the required standard scheduled PPS assessments and include the following OBRA unscheduled assessments: Significant Change in Status Assessment (SCSA) and Significant Correction to Comprehensive Assessment (SCPA), as well as the following PPS unscheduled assessments: Start of Therapy Other Medicare-required Assessment (OMRA), End of Therapy OMRA, Change of Therapy OMRA, and Swing Bed Clinical Change Assessment (CCA). Unscheduled assessments may be required at any time during the resident's Part A stay. They may be performed as separate assessments or combined with other assessments.

A stand-alone unscheduled assessment used for PPS will not establish the payment rate for a standard payment period. Rather a stand-alone unscheduled assessment will modify the payment rate for all or part of a standard payment period, but only when the rate for that standard period has been established by a prior PPS scheduled assessment. For example, if a PPS 14-day scheduled assessment has established the payment rate for the standard Day 15 to Day 30 payment period, then an SCSA with an ARD on Day 20 will modify the payment rate from the ARD (Day 20) to the end of the payment period (Day 30).

Special requirements apply when there are multiple assessments within one PPS scheduled assessment window. If an unscheduled PPS assessment (OMRA, SCSA, SCPA, or Swing Bed CCA) is required in the assessment window (including grace days) of a scheduled PPS assessment, and the ARD of the scheduled assessment is not set for a day that is prior to the ARD of the unscheduled assessment, then facilities must combine the scheduled and unscheduled assessments by setting the ARD of the scheduled assessment for the same day that the unscheduled assessment is required. In such cases, facilities should provide the proper response to the A0310 items to indicate which assessments are being combined, as completion of the combined assessment will be taken to fulfill the requirements for both the scheduled and unscheduled assessments. A scheduled PPS assessment cannot occur after an unscheduled assessment in the assessment window—the scheduled assessment must be combined with the unscheduled assessment using the appropriate ARD for the unscheduled assessment. The purpose of this policy is to minimize the number of assessments required for SNF PPS payment purposes and to ensure that the assessments used for payment provide the most accurate picture of the resident's clinical condition and service needs. More details about combining PPS assessments are provided in Chapter 2 of this manual and in Chapter 6, Section 30.3 of the Medicare Claims Processing Manual (CMS Pub. 100-04) available on the CMS web site.

Examples for combining PPS assessments are as follows:

- If the ARD for an SCSA is set for Day 13 (within the Day 13 to Day 18 window for the 14-Day assessment), then the 14-Day assessment cannot be later in the window. The 14-Day assessment must be combined with the SCSA with an ARD of Day 13. On this combined assessment, Item A0310B is set to 02 indicating the 14-Day assessment and Item A0310A is set to 04 indicating the SCSA.

- If the 14-Day assessment has an ARD of Day 15, then a Start of Therapy OMRA may occur later in the window (Day 16 to Day 18). If there are uncombined scheduled and unscheduled assessments in the assessment window, then the scheduled assessment must have the earliest ARD.

Different types of unscheduled assessments start modifying the payment rate on different dates.

- OBRA SCSA, OBRA SCPA, and Swing Bed CCA assessments begin modifying the payment rate on the ARD based on the Medicare RUG (Z0100A). The exception is when the ARD of the unscheduled assessment is a grace day of a scheduled PPS assessment. In that case, the Medicare RUG (Z0100A) calculated from the unscheduled assessment takes effect on the first day of the standard payment period for the scheduled assessment.

- A Start of Therapy OMRA Medicare RUG (item Z0100A) takes effect on the day therapy started.

- An End of Therapy OMRA Medicare Non-Therapy RUG (Z0150A) takes effect on the day after the last day of therapy provided.

- A Change of Therapy OMRA Medicare Therapy RUG (item Z0100A) takes effect on Day 1 of the Change of Therapy observation period (see Chapter 2 discussion of the Change in Therapy OMRA).

- In cases of an EOT-R when the therapy end date is in one payment period and the resumption date is in the next payment period, the facility should bill the non-therapy RUG given on the EOT OMRA beginning the day after the patient's last therapy session and begin billing the therapy RUG that was in effect prior to the EOT OMRA beginning on the day that therapy resumed (O0450B). If the resumption of therapy occurs after the next billing period has started, then this therapy RUG should be used until modified by a future scheduled or unscheduled assessment. For example, a resident misses therapy on Days 11, 12, and 13 and resumes therapy on Day 15. In this case the facility should bill the non-therapy RUG for Days 11, 12, 13, and 14 and on Day 15 the facility should bill the RUG that was in effect prior to the EOT.

Examples:

1. When rehabilitation therapy begins during the middle of a Medicare Part A stay, a Start of Therapy OMRA may optionally be performed with an ARD set for within 5 to 7 days after the earliest start of therapy date (items O0400A5, O0400B5, or O0400C5). The Start of Therapy OMRA changes the RUG payment rate previously established by a previous PPS assessment from the earliest start of therapy date through the end of the standard payment period. **Consider Example 1**.

   - EXAMPLE 1. The 14-Day assessment is performed with an ARD on Day 14. This assessment establishes the RUG payment for Days 15 through 30. Rehabilitation therapy starts on Day 18 and a Start of Therapy OMRA is performed with an ARD 6 days later on Day 24. The Start of Therapy OMRA will change the RUG payment starting on Day 18 until Day 30 (the end of the standard payment period).

2. The unscheduled Start of Therapy assessment changes the RUG payment rate for days prior to the ARD of that Start of Therapy assessment. Because of this policy, there are cases where a Start of Therapy OMRA can change the RUG payment rate for an entire standard payment period. **Consider Example 2**.

   - EXAMPLE 2. The scheduled 14-day assessment is performed with ARD on Day 14 of the stay. This 14-day assessment establishes the RUG payment rate for the standard Day 15 to Day 30 payment period. Rehabilitation therapy had started on Day 13. The facility opts to perform a Start of Therapy OMRA with ARD on Day 19 (6 days after the start of therapy). This Start of Therapy OMRA will change the RUG payment beginning with Day 13 through Day 30 (the end of the standard payment period). In this case, the HIPPS code from the Start of Therapy OMRA will be used for the entire Day 15 through Day 30 payment period and the 14-day assessment will not be used for billing. If the entire set of claims for the stay is reviewed, then there will be no HIPPS code with an Assessment Indictor code for the 14-day assessment. This does not present a SNF billing compliance problem. Examination of all the assessments and claims will indicate that a 14-day assessment was performed but that the Start of Therapy OMRA controlled the payment rate for the entire Day 15 to Day 30 payment period.

Example 2 also illustrates that there are cases where a single Start of Therapy OMRA can change the RUG payment rate in 2 separate payment periods. In Example 2, the Start of

Therapy OMRA changes the RUG payment rate for the last 2 days (Days 13 and 14) of the 5-Day assessment payment period and all of the days (Days 15 through 30) of the 14-Day assessment payment period.

3. When all rehabilitation therapy ends, an End of Therapy OMRA must be performed with an ARD set for within 1 to 3 days after the end of therapy, in order to establish a Medicare Non-Therapy RUG (Z0150A) for billing beginning with the day after therapy ended until the end of the current payment period. After the End of Therapy OMRA, a Medicare RUG in the Rehabilitation Plus Extensive or Rehabilitation groups should not be billed unless rehabilitation therapy starts again. **Example 3** presents the most common situation.

   - EXAMPLE 3. Rehabilitation therapy ends on Day 20 of a Medicare stay. An End of Therapy OMRA is performed with ARD on Day 22 and the Medicare Non-Therapy RUG (Z0150A) is billed from Day 21 (day after the last day therapy provided) to the end of the current payment period of Day 30.

4. Consider Example 4 where a scheduled PPS assessment has set the payment rate for the next payment period and then an End of Therapy OMRA is conducted before the beginning of that payment period.

   - EXAMPLE 4. The PPS 30-day assessment is performed with ARD on Day 27 to establish a Medicare RUG (Z0100A) for the Day 31 to Day 60 payment period. Rehabilitation therapy ends on Day 26 and an End of Therapy OMRA is performed with ARD on Day 29. The Medicare Non-Therapy RUG (Z0150A) from the End of Therapy OMRA is billed for the remainder of the current payment period, Day 27 through Day 30. The Medicare *Non-Therapy* RUG from the 30-day assessment is then billed for the next payment period. The Non-Therapy RUG from the 30-day assessment is used since all therapy had previously ended.

5. Consider Example 5 where an End of Therapy OMRA is performed and followed within a few days by a scheduled PPS assessment.

   - EXAMPLE 5. The End of Therapy OMRA assessment is performed with an ARD on Day 25 since therapy ended on Day 24. The PPS 30-day assessment is then performed with ARD on Day 28 to establish a Medicare RUG for the Day 31 to Day 60 payment period. The Medicare Non-Therapy RUG (Z0150A) from the End of Therapy OMRA is billed for the remainder of the current payment period, Day 25 through Day 30. The Medicare *Non-Therapy* RUG (Z150A) from the 30-day assessment is then billed for the next payment period, Day 31 through Day 60. The Non-Therapy RUG from the 30-day assessment is used since all therapy has previously ended. The normal Medicare RUG (Z0100A) should not be used since it may contain a Rehabilitation Plus Extensive or Rehabilitation group RUG, because the 7-day reference period extends back before therapy had ended.

6. Consider Example 6, a complicated example where an End of Therapy OMRA is performed, followed shortly by a scheduled PPS assessment, and then therapy is resumed at the prior level and this is reported with the Resumption of Therapy items

(O0450A and O0450B) being added to the End of Therapy OMRA converting it to an End of Therapy OMRA reporting Resumption of Therapy (EOT-R).

- EXAMPLE 6. The End of Therapy OMRA has an ARD on Day 26 with the last day of therapy being Day 24. The PPS 30-Day assessment is then performed with an ARD on Day 27 (the first day of the ARD window) to establish payment with the Medicare RUG (Z0100A) for Days 31-60. Therapy then resumes at the prior level and the EOT-R items (O0450A, and O0450B) indicate a resumption of therapy date of Day 28. The EOT OMRA would establish payment at a Medicare Non-Therapy RUG (Z0150A) for Days 25-27 and Resumption of Therapy reporting would reestablish payment from Day 28 through Day 30 (the end of the payment period) at the same Medicare RUG (Z0100A) provided on the resident's most recent PPS assessment used to establish payment prior to Day 25. The PPS 30-day assessment would then set the payment at the Medicare RUG (Z0100A) for the standard Day 31 to 60 payment period.

When the most recent assessment used for PPS, excluding an End of Therapy OMRA, has a sufficient level of rehabilitation therapy to qualify for an Ultra High, Very High, High, Medium, or Low Rehabilitation category (even if the final classification index maximizes to a group below Rehabilitation), then a change in the provision of therapy services is evaluated in successive 7-day Change of Therapy observation periods until a new assessment used for PPS occurs.

The first Change of Therapy OMRA evaluation occurs on Day 7 after the most recent assessment ARD (except in cases where the last assessment is an EOT-R, as outlined in Chapter 2) and the provision of therapy services are evaluated for the first COT observation period (Day 1 through Day 7 after the assessment ARD). If the provision of therapy services during this 7 day period no longer reflects the RUG-IV classification category on the most recent PPS assessment (as described in Chapter 2), then a Change of Therapy OMRA must be performed with the ARD on Day 7 of the COT observation period.

If the provision of therapy services are reflective of the most recent PPS assessment RUG category classification, a Change of Therapy OMRA is not performed and changes in the provision of therapy services would next be evaluated on Day 14 after the most recent assessment ARD using the second COT observation period (Day 8 through Day 14 after the assessment ARD). If a different RUG-IV classification category results for Day 14, then a Change of Therapy OMRA must be performed with an ARD on Day 14, which is Day 7 of that COT observation period, and payment is set retroactively back to the beginning of that COT observation period.

If the provision of therapy services are reflective of the most recent PPS assessment RUG category classification, a Change of Therapy OMRA is not performed with an ARD on Day 14 and the evaluation of the change in therapy services provided would next be evaluated on Day 21 after the most recent assessment ARD using the third COT observation period (Day 15 through Day 21 after the assessment ARD). This process continues until the next scheduled or unscheduled PPS assessment used for payment. When a new PPS assessment is performed (Change of Therapy OMRA, any other unscheduled PPS assessment, or scheduled PPS assessment), then the COT OMRA evaluation process restarts the day following the ARD of that intervening assessment. If at any point, rehabilitation therapy ends before the last day of a COT observation period and an End of Therapy OMRA is performed with an ARD set for on or prior to Day 7 of the COT observation period, then the change of therapy evaluation process ends until the next PPS assessment used for payment reflecting the utilization of skilled therapy services.

7. Example 7 presents a case where a Change of Therapy OMRA is performed.

- EXAMPLE 7. The 30-day assessment is performed with the ARD on Day 30, and the provision of therapy services are evaluated on Day 37. It is determined that the therapy services provided were reflective of the RUG-IV classification category on the most recent PPS assessment and therefore, no Change of Therapy OMRA is performed with an ARD set for Day 37. When the provision of therapy services are next evaluated on Day 44, it is determined that a different Rehabilitation category results and a Change of Therapy OMRA is performed with an ARD set for Day 44. The Change of Therapy OMRA will change the RUG payment beginning on Day 38 (the first day of the COT observation period). The Change of Therapy OMRA evaluation process then restarts with this Change of Therapy OMRA.

8. If a new PPS assessment used for payment occurs with an ARD set for on or prior to the last day of a COT observation period, then a Change of Therapy OMRA is not required for that observation period. Example 8 illustrates this case.

- EXAMPLE 8. An SCSA is performed with an ARD of Day 10. An evaluation for the Change of Therapy OMRA would occur on Day 17 but the 14-Day assessment intervenes with ARD on Day 15. A Change of Therapy OMRA is not performed with an ARD on Day 17. Rather, the COT OMRA evaluation process is restarted with the 14-day assessment with ARD on Day 15. Day 1 of the next COT observation period is Day 16 and the new COT OMRA evaluation would be done on Day 22.

9. Example 9 illustrates that the COT OMRA evaluation process ends when all rehabilitation therapy ends before the end of a COT observation period.

- EXAMPLE 9. The 14-Day assessment is performed with the ARD on Day 14. The first COT OMRA evaluation would normally happen on Day 21. However, all therapy ends on Day 20. The ARD for an EOT OMRA is set for Day 21 to reflect the discontinuation of therapy services. No Change of Therapy OMRA is performed with an ARD on Day 21 and the change of therapy evaluation process is discontinued.

Table 3 presents the types of unscheduled assessments, the second AI digit associated with each assessment type, and the payment impact for standard payment periods.

Table 3. Assessment Indicator Second Digit Table

Second Digit Values	Assessment Type	Impact on Standard Payment Period
0	Either a scheduled PPS assessment not replaced by or combined with an unscheduled PPS assessment OR an OBRA assessment not coded as a PPS assessment	• No impact on the standard payment period (the assessment is not unscheduled). • If the second digit value is 0, then the first digit must be 1 through 6, indicating a scheduled PPS assessment or an OBRA assessment not coded as a PPS assessment. • If the first digit value is a 6, then the second digit value must be 0.
1	Either an unscheduled OBRA assessment **or** Swing Bed CCA Do NOT use if • Combined with any OMRA • Medicare Short Stay assessment	• If the ARD of the unscheduled assessment is not within the ARD window of any scheduled PPS assessment, including grace days (the first digit is 0): — Use the Medicare RUG (Z0100A) from the ARD of this unscheduled assessment through the end of standard payment period. • If the ARD of the unscheduled assessment is within the ARD window of a scheduled PPS assessment, not using grace days: — Use the Medicare RUG (Z0100A) from the ARD of this unscheduled assessment through the end of standard payment period. • If the ARD of the unscheduled assessment is a grace day of a scheduled PPS assessment: — Use the Medicare RUG (Z0100A) from the start of the standard payment period.
2	Start of Therapy OMRA Do NOT use if • Medicare Short Stay assessment • Combined with End of Therapy OMRA • Combined with unscheduled OBRA • Combined with Swing Bed CCA	• If the unscheduled assessment gives a therapy group in the Medicare RUG (Z0100A): — Use the Medicare RUG (Z0100A) from the unscheduled assessment's earliest start of therapy date (speech-language pathology services in O0400A5, occupational therapy in O0400B5, or physical therapy in O0400C5) through the end of standard payment period. • If the unscheduled assessment does not give a therapy group in the Medicare RUG (Z0100A), do not use the unscheduled assessment RUG for any part of standard payment period. This is not a valid assessment and it will not be accepted by CMS.
3	Start of Therapy OMRA combined with either an unscheduled OBRA assessment **or** a Swing Bed CCA Do NOT use if • Medicare Short Stay assessment • Combined with End of Therapy OMRA	• If unscheduled assessment gives a therapy group in the Medicare RUG (Z0100A): — Use the unscheduled assessment Medicare RUG (Z0100A) from the earliest start of therapy date through the end of standard payment period. • If unscheduled assessment does not give a therapy group in the Medicare RUG (Z0100A), do not use the unscheduled assessment RUG for any part of the standard payment period. This is not a valid assessment and it will not be accepted by CMS.

(continued)

Table 3. Assessment Indicator Second Digit Table (continued)

Second Digit Values	Assessment Type	Impact on Standard Payment Period
4	End of Therapy OMRA **not reporting** Resumption of Therapy; **whether or not** combined with unscheduled OBRA assessment and **whether or not** combined with Swing Bed CCA Do NOT use if • Combined with Start of Therapy OMRA • Medicare Short Stay assessment • End of Therapy OMRA **reporting** Resumption of Therapy (EOT-R)	Use the unscheduled assessment Medicare non-therapy RUG (Z0150A) from the day after the latest therapy end date (speech-language pathology services in O0400A6, occupational therapy in O0400B6, or physical therapy in O0400C6) through the end of current payment period.
5	Start of Therapy OMRA combined with End of Therapy OMRA **not reporting** Resumption of Therapy Do NOT use if • Medicare Short Stay assessment • Combined with unscheduled OBRA • Combined with Swing Bed CCA • End of Therapy OMRA **reporting** Resumption of Therapy (EOT-R)	• If unscheduled assessment gives a therapy group Medicare RUG (Z0100A): — Use the unscheduled assessment Medicare RUG (Z0100A) from the earliest start of therapy date through the latest therapy end date. — Use the unscheduled assessment Medicare non-therapy RUG (Z0150A) from the day after the latest therapy end date through the end of current payment period. • If unscheduled assessment does not give a therapy group Medicare RUG (Z0100A), do not use the unscheduled assessment RUG for any part of the standard payment period. This is not a valid assessment and it will not be accepted by CMS.
6	Start of Therapy OMRA combined with End of Therapy OMRA **not reporting** Resumption of Therapy and combined with either an unscheduled OBRA assessment **or** Swing Bed CCA Do NOT use if 1. Medicare Short Stay assessment 2. End of Therapy OMRA **reporting** Resumption of Therapy (EOT-R)	• If unscheduled assessment gives a therapy group Medicare RUG (Z0100A): — Use the unscheduled assessment Medicare RUG (Z0100A) from the earliest start of therapy date through the latest therapy end date. — Use the unscheduled assessment non-therapy RUG (Z0150A) from the day after the latest therapy end date through the end of current payment period. • If unscheduled assessment does not give a therapy group in the Medicare RUG (Z0100A), do not use the unscheduled assessment RUG for any part of the standard payment period. This is not a valid assessment and it will not be accepted by CMS.
7	Medicare Short Stay Assessment (see **Medicare Short Stay Assessment** below for the definition of this assessment.)	See **Medicare Short Stay Assessment** below for impact on payment periods.

(continued)

Table 3. Assessment Indicator Second Digit Table (continued)

Second Digit Values	Assessment Type	Impact on Standard Payment Period
A	End of Therapy OMRA **reporting** Resumption of Therapy (EOT-R); **whether or not** combined with unscheduled OBRA assessment and **whether or not** combined with Swing Bed CCA Do NOT use if • Combined with Start of Therapy OMRA • Medicare Short Stay assessment	• Use the unscheduled assessment Medicare non-therapy RUG (Z0150A) from the day after the latest therapy end date (speech-language pathology services in O0400A6, occupational therapy in O0400B6, or physical therapy in O0400C6) through the day before the resumption of therapy date (O0450B). • Use the Medicare RUG (Z0100A) from the assessment (used for SNF/PPS) immediately preceding this End of Therapy OMRA, and bill this RUG from the resumption of therapy date (O0450B) through the end of the standard payment period in which the resumption of therapy occurs.
B	Start of Therapy OMRA combined with End of Therapy OMRA **reporting** Resumption of Therapy (EOT-R) Do NOT use if • Medicare Short Stay assessment • Combined with unscheduled OBRA • Combined with Swing Bed CCA	• If unscheduled assessment gives a therapy group Medicare RUG (Z0100A): — Use the unscheduled assessment Medicare RUG (Z0100A) from the earliest start of therapy date through the latest therapy end date. — Use the unscheduled assessment Medicare non-therapy RUG (Z0150A) from the day after the latest therapy end date through the day before the resumption of therapy date (O0450B). — Use the unscheduled assessment Medicare RUG (Z0100A) from the resumption of therapy date through the end of the standard payment period. • If unscheduled assessment does not give a therapy group Medicare RUG (Z0100A), do not use the unscheduled assessment RUG for any part of the standard payment period. This is not a valid assessment and it will not be accepted by CMS.
C	Start of Therapy OMRA combined with End of Therapy OMRA **reporting** Resumption of Therapy (EOT-R) and combined with either an unscheduled OBRA assessment **or** Swing Bed CCA Do NOT use if • Medicare Short Stay assessment	• If unscheduled assessment gives a therapy group Medicare RUG (Z0100A): — Use the unscheduled assessment Medicare RUG (Z0100A) from the earliest start of therapy date through the latest therapy end date. — Use the unscheduled assessment non-therapy RUG (Z0150A) from the day after the latest therapy end date through the day before the resumption of therapy date (O0450B). — Use the unscheduled assessment Medicare RUG (Z0100A) from the resumption of therapy date through the end of the standard payment period. • If unscheduled assessment does not give a therapy group in the Medicare RUG (Z0100A), do not use the unscheduled assessment RUG for any part of the standard payment period. This is not a valid assessment and it will not be accepted by CMS.

(continued)

Table 3. Assessment Indicator Second Digit Table (continued)

Second Digit Values	Assessment Type	Impact on Standard Payment Period
D	Change of Therapy OMRA; **whether or not** combined with unscheduled OBRA assessment and **whether or not** combined with Swing Bed CCA	• Use the unscheduled assessment Medicare RUG (Z0100A) from the first day of the Change of Therapy OMRA observation period through the end of the standard payment period. • Note that a Change in Therapy OMRA cannot be combined with a 5-day or readmission/return assessment.

The information presented in the preceding table illustrates the impact of one unscheduled PPS assessment within a standard payment period. If there are additional unscheduled PPS assessments, then there may be additional impacts to the standard payment period. Refer to Medicare Claims Processing Manual and Chapter 2 of this manual for details.

When a Start of Therapy OMRA is combined with a scheduled PPS assessment, any OBRA assessment, or a Swing Bed CCA, and the index maximized RUG-IV classification (Item Z0100A) is not a Rehabilitation Plus Extensive Services or a Rehabilitation group, the assessment will not be accepted by CMS. In these instances, the provider must still complete and submit an assessment that is accepted by CMS in order to be in compliance with OBRA and/or Medicare regulations.

Additional AI Codes

There are also two additional AI Codes (shown in Table 6-4) when a Medicare SNF Part A claim is filed without a corresponding PPS assessment having been completed or the assessment has invalid reasons for assessment.

Table 4. Additional Assessment Indicator Codes

Additional Assessment Indicator (AI) Codes	Description
00	This is the AI required when billing the default RUG code of AAA for a missed assessment only when specific circumstances are met (see Section 6.8 of this chapter for greater detail). The default code is paid based upon the payment associated with the lowest resource utilization group (RUG), PA1.
X	The AI "error" code provided by the RUG-IV grouper when RUG-IV cannot be calculated for the type of record (e.g., the record is an entry record). This is not an appropriate billing code.

Medicare Short Stay Assessment

To be considered a Medicare Short Stay assessment and use the special RUG-IV short stay rehabilitation therapy classification, the assessment must be a Start of Therapy OMRA, the resident must have been discharged from Part A on or before day 8 of the Part A stay, and the resident must have completed only 1 to 4 days of therapy, with therapy having started during the last 4 days of the Part A stay. To be considered a Medicare Short Stay assessment and use the special RUG-IV short stay rehabilitation therapy classification, all eight of the following conditions must be met:

1. **The assessment must be a Start of Therapy OMRA (A0310C = 1).** This assessment may be performed alone or combined with any OBRA assessment or combined with a PPS 5-day or readmission/return assessment. The Start of Therapy OMRA may not be combined with a PPS 14-day, 30-day, 60-day, or 90-day assessment. The Start of Therapy OMRA should also be combined with a discharge assessment when the end of Part A stay is the result of discharge from the facility, but not combined with a discharge if the resident dies in the facility or is transferred to another payer source in the facility.

2. **A PPS 5-day (A0310B = 01) or readmission/return assessment (A0310B = 06) has been performed.** The PPS 5-day or readmission/return assessment may be performed alone or combined with the Start of Therapy OMRA.

3. **The ARD (A2300) of the Start of Therapy OMRA must be on or before the 8th day of the Part A Medicare stay.** The ARD minus the start of Medicare stay date (A2400B) must be 7 days or less.

4. **The ARD (A2300) of the Start of Therapy OMRA must be the last day of the Medicare Part A stay (A2400C).** See instructions for Item A2400C in Chapter 3 for more detail.

5. **The ARD (A2300) of the Start of Therapy OMRA may not be more than 3 days after the start of therapy date (Item O0400A5, O0400B5, or O0400C5, whichever is earliest) not including the start of therapy date.** This is an exception to the rules for selecting the ARD for a SOT OMRA, as it is not possible for the ARD for the Short stay Assessment to be 5-7 days after the start of therapy since therapy must have been able to be provided only 1-4 days.

6. **Rehabilitation therapy (speech-language pathology services, occupational therapy or physical therapy) started during the last 4 days of the Medicare Part A covered stay (including weekends).** The end of Medicare stay date (A2400C) minus the earliest start date for the three therapy disciplines (O0400A5, O0400B5, or O0400C5) must be 3 days or less.

7. **At least one therapy discipline continued through the last day of the Medicare Part A stay.** At least one of the therapy disciplines must have a dash-filled end of therapy date (O0400A6, O0400B6, or O0400C6) indicating ongoing therapy or an end of therapy date equal to the end of covered Medicare stay date (A2400C). Therapy is considered to be ongoing when:

    *   The resident was discharged and therapy was planned to continue had the resident remained in the facility, or
    *   The resident's SNF benefit exhausted and therapy continued to be provided, or
    *   The resident's payer source changed and therapy continued to be provided.

8. **The RUG group assigned to the Start of Therapy OMRA must be Rehabilitation Plus Extensive Services or a Rehabilitation group (Z0100A).** If the RUG group assigned is not a Rehabilitation Plus Extensive Services or a Rehabilitation group, the assessment will be rejected.

See below for Medicare Short Stay Assessment Algorithm.

If all eight of these conditions are met, then MDS Item Z0100C (Medicare Short Stay Assessment indicator) is coded "Yes." the assignment of the RUG-IV rehabilitation therapy classification is calculated based on average daily minutes actually provided (when there is a fraction, the total therapy minutes is not rounded and only the whole number is used), and the resulting RUG-IV group is recorded in MDS Item Z0100A (Medicare Part A HIPPS Code).

1. 15-29 average daily therapy minutes ▶ Rehabilitation Low category (RLx)

2. 30-64 average daily therapy minutes ▶ Rehabilitation Medium category (RMx)

3. 65-99 average daily therapy minutes ▶ Rehabilitation High category (RHx)

4. 100-143 average daily therapy minutes ▶ Rehabilitation Very High category (RVx)

5. 144 or greater average daily therapy minutes ▶ Rehabilitation Ultra High category (RUx)

See the RUG-IV Calculation Worksheet in Section 6.6 for details of the rehabilitation classification for a Medicare Short Stay Assessment.

Medicare Short Stay Assessment Algorithm

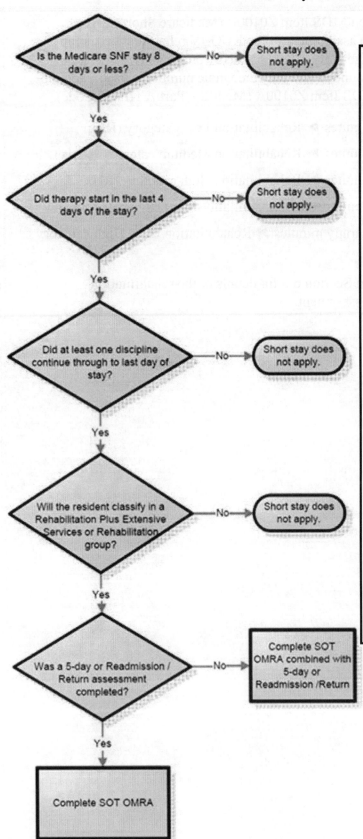

Medicare Short Stay Assessment Requirements:
All 8 must be true

Assessment Requirements:
1. Must be SOT OMRA
2. 5-day or readmission/return assessment must be completed (may be combined with the SOT OMRA)

ARD Requirements:
3. Must be Day 8 or earlier of Part A stay
4. Must be last day of Part A stay (see Item 2400 instructions)
5. Must be no more than 3 days after the start of therapy, not including the start of therapy date.

Rehabilitation Requirements:
6. Must have started in last 4 days of Part A stay
7. Must continue through last day of Part A stay

RUG Requirement:
8. Must classify resident into a Rehabilitation Plus Extensive Services or Rehabilitation group

Note: When the earliest start of therapy is 1st day of stay, then the Part A stay must be 4 days or less

The impacts on the payment periods for the Medicare Short Stay assessment are as follows:

1. If the earliest start of therapy date (Items O0400A5, O0400B5, or O0400C5) is the first day of the short stay, use the Medicare Short Stay assessment Medicare Part A RUG (Z0100) from the beginning of the short stay through the end of the stay (the Medicare stay must be 4 days or less).

2. If the earliest start of therapy date is after the first day of the short stay, the following apply:

    a. If a 5-day or readmission/return assessment was completed prior to Medicare Short Stay assessment, use the Medicare Part A RUG (Z0100A) from that assessment for the first day of the short stay through the day before therapy started; then use the Medicare Part A RUG (Z0100A) from the Medicare Short Stay assessment from the day therapy started through the end of the short stay; or

    b. If the Start of Therapy OMRA is combined with a 5-day or readmission/return assessment, use the Medicare Part A non-therapy RUG (Z0150A) for the first day of the short stay through the day before therapy started; then use the Medicare Part A RUG (Z0100A) from the day therapy started through the end of the short stay.

6.5   SNF PPS Eligibility Criteria

Under SNF PPS, beneficiaries must meet the established eligibility requirements for a Part A SNF-level stay. These requirements are summarized in this section. Refer to the **Medicare General Information, Eligibility, and Entitlement Manual**, Chapter 1 (Pub. 100-1), and the **Medicare Benefit Policy Manual**, Chapter 8 (Pub. 100-2), for detailed SNF coverage requirements and policies.

Technical Eligibility Requirements

The beneficiary must meet the following criteria:

- Beneficiary is Enrolled in Medicare Part A and has days available to use.
- There has been a three-day prior qualifying hospital stay (i.e., three midnights).
- Admission for SNF-level services is within 30 days of discharge from an acute care stay or within 30 days of discharge from a SNF level of care.

Clinical Eligibility Requirements

A beneficiary is eligible for SNF extended care if all of the following requirements are met:

- The beneficiary has a need for and receives medically necessary skilled care on a daily basis, which is provided by or under the direct supervision of skilled nursing or rehabilitation professionals.
- As a practical matter, these skilled services can only be provided in an SNF.
- The services provided must be for a condition:

— for which the resident was treated during the qualifying hospital stay, or

— that arose while the resident was in the SNF for treatment of a condition for which he/she was previously treated for in a hospital.

Physician Certification

The attending physician or a physician on the staff of the skilled nursing home who has knowledge of the case—or a nurse practitioner (NP), physician assistant (PA), or clinical nurse specialist (CNS) who does not have a direct or indirect employment relationship with the facility but who is working in collaboration with the physician—must certify and then periodically recertify the need for extended care services in the skilled nursing home.

- **Certifications** are required at the time of admission or as soon thereafter as is reasonable and practicable (42 CFR 424.20). The initial certification

    — affirms, per the required content found in 42 CFR 424.20, that the resident meets the existing SNF level of care definition, or

    — validates via written statement that the beneficiary's assignment to one of the upper RUG-IV (Top 52) groups is correct.

- **Re-certifications** are used to document the continued need for skilled extended care services.

    — The first re-certification is required no later than the 14th day.

    — Subsequent re-certifications are required at no later than 30 days intervals after the date of the first re-certification.

    — The initial certification and first re-certification may be signed at the same time.

6.6 RUG-IV 66-Group Model Calculation Worksheet for SNFs

The purpose of this RUG-IV Version 1.00 calculation worksheet for the 66-group model is to provide a step-by-step walk-through to manually determine the appropriate RUG-IV Classification based on the data from an MDS assessment. The worksheet takes the grouper logic and puts it into words. We have carefully reviewed the worksheet to ensure that it represents the standard logic.

In the RUG-IV 66-group model, there are 23 different Rehabilitation Plus Extensive Services and Rehabilitation groups, representing 10 different levels of rehabilitation services. In the 66-group model, the residents in the Rehabilitation Plus Extensive Services groups have the highest level of combined nursing and rehabilitation need, while residents in the Rehabilitation groups have the next highest level of need. Therefore, the 66-group model has the Rehabilitation Plus Extensive Services groups first followed by the Rehabilitation groups, the Extensive Services groups, the Special Care High groups, the Special Care Low groups, the Clinically Complex groups, the Behavioral Symptoms and Cognitive Performance groups, and the Reduced Physical Function groups.

There are two basic approaches to RUG-IV Classification: (1) hierarchical classification and (2) index maximizing classification. The current worksheet was developed for the hierarchical methodology. Instructions for adapting this worksheet to the index maximizing approach are included below (see "Index Maximizing Classification"). Note that the RUG classification used for Medicare PPS Part A billing is based on the index maximizing approach.

Hierarchical Classification. The present worksheet employs the hierarchical classification method. Hierarchical classification is used in some payment systems, in staffing analysis, and in many research projects. In the hierarchical approach, start at the top and work down through the RUG-IV model; the assigned classification is the first group for which the resident qualifies. In other words, start with the Rehabilitation Plus Extensive Services groups at the top of the RUG-IV model. Then go down through the groups in hierarchical order: Rehabilitation Plus Extensive Services, Rehabilitation, Extensive Services, Special Care High, Special Care Low, Clinically Complex, Behavioral Symptoms and Cognitive Performance, and Reduced Physical Function. When you find the first of the 66 individual RUG-IV groups for which the resident qualifies, assign that group as the RUG-IV classification.

If the resident qualifies in the Extensive Services group and a Special Care High group, always choose the Extensive Services classification because it is higher in the hierarchy. Likewise, if the resident qualifies for Special Care Low and Clinically Complex, always choose Special Care Low. In hierarchical classification, always pick the group nearest the top of the model.

Index Maximizing Classification. Index maximizing classification is used in Medicare PPS (and most Medicaid payment systems) to select the RUG-IV group for payment. There is a designated Case Mix Index (CMI) that represents the relative resource utilization for each RUG-IV group. For index maximizing, first determine all of the RUG-IV groups for which the resident qualifies. Then, from the qualifying groups, choose the RUG-IV group that has the highest CMI. For Medicare PPS, the index maximizing method uses the CMIs effective for the appropriate Federal Fiscal Year.

While the following worksheet illustrates the hierarchical classification method, it can be adapted for index maximizing. For index maximizing, evaluate all classification groups rather than assigning the resident to the first qualifying group. In the index maximizing approach, again start at the beginning of the worksheet. Then work down through all of the 66 RUG-IV Classification groups, ignoring instructions to skip groups and noting each group for which the resident qualifies. When finished, record the CMI for each of these groups. Select the group with the highest CMI. This group is the index-maximized classification for the resident.

Non-Therapy Classification. In some instances, the SNF provider may be required to report, on the SNF Medicare claim, a non-therapy RUG-IV classification according to the SNF PPS policies (as noted elsewhere in this chapter, Chapter 8 of the **Medicare Benefit Policy Manual**, and Chapter 6 of the **Medicare Claims Processing Manual**). The non-therapy classification uses all the RUG-IV payment items except the rehabilitation therapy Items (O0400A,B,C) to determine a non-therapy, clinical RUG. To obtain a non-therapy RUG with this worksheet, skip Category I (Rehabilitation Plus Extensive Services) and Category II (Rehabilitation) and start with Category III (Extensive Services). Both the standard Medicare Part A RUG reported in Item Z0100A and the Medicare Part A non-therapy RUG in Item Z0150A are recorded on the MDS 3.0. When rehabilitation services are not provided, the standard Medicare Part A RUG will match the Medicare Part A non-therapy RUG.

CALCULATION OF TOTAL "ADL" SCORE
RUG-IV, 66-GROUP HIERARCHICAL CLASSIFICATION

The ADL score is a component of the calculation for placement in all RUG-IV groups. The ADL score is based upon the four "late loss" ADLs (bed mobility, transfer, toilet use, and eating), and this score indicates the level of functional assistance or support required by the resident. It is a very important component of the classification process.

STEP # 1

To calculate the ADL score use the following chart for bed mobility (G0110A), transfer (G0110B), and toilet use (G0110I). **Enter the ADL score for each item.**

Self-Performance Column 1 =		Support Column 2 =	ADL Score =	SCORE
-, 0, 1, 7, or 8	and	(any number)	0	G0110A = ___
2	and	(any number)	1	G0110B = ___
3	and	-, 0, 1, or 2	2	G0110I = ___
4	and	-, 0, 1, or 2	3	
3 or 4	and	3	4	

STEP # 2

To calculate the ADL score for eating (G0110H), use the following chart. Enter ADL score.

Self-Performance Column 1 (G0110H) =		Support Column 2 =	ADL Score =	SCORE
-, 0, 1, 2, 7, or 8	and	-, 0, 1, or 8	0	G0110H = ___
-, 0, 1, 2, 7, or 8	and	2 or 3	2	
3 or 4	and	-, 0, or 1	2	
3	and	2 or 3	3	
4	and	2 or 3	4	

STEP # 3

Add the four scores for the total ADL score. This is the **RUG-IV TOTAL ADL SCORE.** The total ADL score ranges from 0 through 16.

TOTAL RUG-IV ADL SCORE _____

Other ADLs are also very important, but the research indicates that the late loss ADLs predict resource use most accurately. The early loss ADLs do not significantly change the classification hierarchy or add to the prediction of resource use.

CALCULATION OF TOTAL REHABILITATION THERAPY MINUTES
RUG-IV, 66-GROUP HIERARCHICAL CLASSIFICATION

For Speech-Language Pathology Services (Items at O0400A), Occupational Therapy (Items at O0400B), and Physical Therapy (Items at O0400C), the MDS 3.0 separately captures minutes that the resident was receiving individual, concurrent, and group therapy (see Chapter 3, Section O for definitions) during the last 7 days. For each therapy discipline, actual minutes the resident spent in treatments are entered on the MDS for each of the three modes of therapy. The total minutes used for RUG-IV classification include all minutes in individual therapy, one-half of the minutes in concurrent therapy, and all minutes in group therapy for non-Medicare classification. For Medicare Part A classification, the total minutes used for RUG-IV classification include all minutes in individual therapy, one-half the minutes in concurrent therapy, and the group time is allocated among 4 residents and only one-fourth of the minutes of group time are included for the resident in the total minutes for RUG-IV classification. For Medicare Part A there is a limitation that the group minutes cannot exceed 25% of the total minutes, a limitation that is applied by the grouper software. This limitation is applied after allocation of group minutes.

Skip this section if therapy is not provided.

In Steps #1 through #3 in calculating Rehabilitation Therapy Minutes, retain all decimal places in the calculated values. Values where decimal points are retained are indicated by an asterisk (*).

STEP # 1

Calculate the total minutes for speech-language pathology services as follows:

> Add the individual minutes (O0400A1) and one-half of the concurrent minutes (O0400A2). Add all of the group minutes (O0400A3) for non-Medicare classification or one-quarter of the group minutes for Medicare classification and record as Total Minutes.
> Total Minutes* = _____

For Medicare classification the 25% group therapy limitation applies as follows:

> If allocated group minutes (one-quarter of O0400A3) divided by Total Minutes is greater than 0.25, then add individual minutes (O0400A1) and one-half of concurrent minutes (O0400A2), multiply this sum by 4.0 and then divide by 3.0, and record as Adjusted Minutes.
> Adjusted Minutes* = _____

Record Total Minutes or Adjusted Minutes as appropriate:
> Speech-Language Pathology Services Minutes* = _____

STEP # 2

Calculate the total minutes for occupational therapy as follows:

Add the individual minutes (O0400B1) and one-half of the concurrent minutes (O0400B2). Add all of the group minutes (O0400B3) for non-Medicare classification or one-quarter of the group minutes for Medicare classification and record as Total Minutes.

Total Minutes* = _____

For Medicare classification, the 25% group therapy limitation applies as follows:

If allocated group minutes (one-quarter of O0400B3) divided by Total Minutes is greater than 0.25, then add individual minutes (O0400B1) and one-half of concurrent minutes (O0400B2), multiply this sum by 4.0 and then divide by 3.0, and record as Adjusted Minutes.

Adjusted Minutes* = _____

Record Total Minutes or Adjusted Minutes as appropriate:

Occupational Therapy Minutes* = _____

STEP # 3

Calculate the total minutes for physical therapy as follows:

Add the individual minutes (O0400C1) and one-half of the concurrent minutes (O0400C2). Add all of the group minutes (O0400C3) for non-Medicare classification or one-quarter of the group minutes for Medicare classification and record as Total Minutes.

Total Minutes* = _____

For Medicare classification, the 25% group therapy limitation applies as follows:

If allocated group minutes (one-quarter of O0400C3) divided by Total Minutes is greater than 0.25, then add individual minutes (O0400C1) and one-half of concurrent minutes (O0400C2), multiply this sum by 4.0 and then divide by 3.0, and record as Adjusted Minutes.

Adjusted Minutes* = _____

Record Total Minutes or Adjusted Minutes as appropriate:

Physical Therapy Minutes* = _____

STEP # 4

Sum the speech-language pathology services minutes, occupational therapy minutes, and physical therapy minutes and record as Total Therapy Minutes. These are the minutes that will be used for RUG-IV rehabilitation therapy classification (when there is a fraction, the total therapy minutes is not rounded and only the whole number is used).

TOTAL THERAPY MINUTES^ = _____

^Total Therapy Minutes is not rounded. Record only the whole number with all values after the decimal dropped.

Total Rehabilitation Therapy Minutes Calculation Example

Mrs. D., whose stay is covered under SNF PPS, received the following rehabilitation services during FY2012 (group therapy time is allocated) as follows:

Speech-language Pathology Services:

Individual minutes = 110 (Item O0400A1),
Concurrent minutes = 99 (Item O0400A2),
Group minutes = 100 (Item O0400A3).
Calculate total SLP minutes = 110 + 99/2 + 100/4 = <u>184.5</u> (retain the decimal).
Check group proportion (after group allocation) = (100/4)/184.5 = 0.136.
Do not adjust SLP minutes for Medicare Part A since group proportion is not greater than .25. Use unadjusted total SLP minutes.
Total Speech-Language Pathology Services Minutes = **184.5** (retain the decimal).

Occupational Therapy:

Individual minutes = 78 (Item O0400B1),
Concurrent minutes = 79 (Item O0400B2),
Group minutes = 320 (Item O0400B3).
Calculate total OT minutes = 78 + 79/2 + 320/4 = <u>197.5</u> (retain the decimal).
Check group proportion = (320/4)/197.5 = 0.405.
Adjust OT minutes for Medicare Part A since group proportion is greater than .25.
Adjusted Occupational Therapy Minutes = [(78 + 79/2) x 4]/3 = **156.6666** (retain the decimal).

Physical Therapy:

Individual minutes = 92 (Item O0400C1),
Concurrent minutes = 93 (Item O0400C2),
Group minutes = 376 (Item O0400C3).
Calculate total PT minutes = 92 + 93/2 + 376/4 = <u>232.5</u> (retain the decimal).
Check group proportion = (376/4)/232.5 = 0.404.
Adjust PT minutes for Medicare Part A since group proportion is greater than .25.
Adjusted Physical Therapy Minutes = [(92 + 93/2) x 4]/3 = **184.6666** (retain the decimal).

Total Adjusted Therapy Minutes:
Sum SLP, OT and PT minutes after any adjustment= 184.5 + 156.6666 + 184.6666 =
525.8332
Drop decimals = **525 minutes**
(this is the total therapy minutes value for RUG-IV classification).

MEDICARE SHORT STAY ASSESSMENT
RUG-IV, 66-GROUP HIERARCHICAL CLASSIFICATION

STEP # 1

Set the Medicare Short Stay Indicator (Z0100C) as follows:

RUG-IV uses an alternative rehabilitation therapy classification when an assessment is a Medicare Short Stay assessment. To be considered a Medicare Short Stay assessment and use the special RUG-IV short stay rehabilitation therapy classification, all eight of the following conditions must be met:

1. **The assessment must be a Start of Therapy OMRA (Item A0310C = 1).** This assessment may be performed alone or combined with any OBRA assessment or combined with a PPS 5-day or readmission/return assessment. The Start of Therapy OMRA may not be combined with a PPS 14-day, 30-day, 60-day, or 90-day assessment. The Start of Therapy OMRA should also be combined with a discharge assessment when the end of Part A stay is the result of discharge from the facility, but should not be combined with a discharge if the resident dies in the facility or is transferred to another payer source in the facility.

2. **A PPS 5-day (Item A0310B = 01) or readmission/return assessment (A0310B = 06) has been performed.** The PPS 5-day or readmission/return assessment may be performed alone or combined with the Start of Therapy OMRA.

3. **The ARD (Item A2300) of the Start of Therapy OMRA must be on or before the 8th day of the Part A Medicare covered stay.** The ARD minus the start of Medicare stay date (A2400B) must be 7 days or less.

4. **The ARD (Item A2300) of the Start of Therapy OMRA must be the last day of the Medicare Part A stay (A2400C).** See instructions for Item A2400C in Chapter 3 for more detail.

5. **The ARD (Item A2300) of the Start of Therapy OMRA may not be more than 3 days after the start of therapy date (Items O0400A5, O0400B5, or O0400C5, whichever is earliest) not including the start of therapy date.** This is an exception to the rules for selecting the ARD for a SOT OMRA, as it is not possible for the ARD for the Short Stay Assessment to be 5-7 days after the start of therapy since therapy must have been able to be provided only 1-4 days.

6. **Rehabilitation therapy (speech-language pathology services, occupational therapy or physical therapy) started during the last 4 days of the Medicare Part A stay (including weekends).** The end of Medicare stay date (Item A2400C) minus the earliest start date for the three therapy disciplines (Items O0400A5, O0400B5, or O0400C5) must be 3 days or less.

7. **At least one therapy discipline continued through the last day of the Medicare Part A stay.** At least one of the therapy disciplines must have a dash-filled end of therapy date (Items O0400A6, O0400B6, or O0400C6) indicating ongoing therapy or an end of therapy date equal to the end of covered Medicare stay date (Item A2400C). Therapy is considered to be ongoing when:

    - The resident was discharged and therapy was planned to continue had the resident remained in the facility, or

    - The resident's SNF benefit exhausted and therapy continued to be provided, or

    - The resident's payer source changed and therapy continued to be provided.

8. **The RUG group assigned to the Start of Therapy OMRA must be Rehabilitation Plus Extensive Services or a Rehabilitation group (Item Z0100A).** If the RUG group assigned is not a Rehabilitation Plus Extensive Services or a Rehabilitation group, the assessment will be rejected.

If all eight conditions are satisfied, record "Yes" in the Medicare Short Stay Assessment Indicator Z0100C); otherwise record "No."

MEDICARE SHORT STAY ASSESMENT INDICATOR Yes_____ No_____

STEP # 2

If the Medicare Short Stay Assessment Indicator is "Yes," then calculate the Medicare Short Stay Average Therapy Minutes as follows:

This average is the Total Therapy Minutes (calculated above in Calculation of Total Rehabilitation Therapy Minutes) divided by the number of days from the start of therapy (earliest date in O0400A5, O0400B5, and O0400C5) through the assessment reference date (A2300). For example, if therapy started on August 1 and the assessment reference date is August 3, the average minutes is calculated by dividing by 3 days. Discard all numbers after the decimal point and record the result.

MEDICARE SHORT STAY AVERAGE THERAPY MINUTES = _____

See Section 6.4 for Medicare Short Stay Assessment Algorithm.

CATEGORY I: REHABILITATION PLUS EXTENSIVE SERVICES
RUG-IV, 66-GROUP HIERARCHICAL CLASSIFICATION

Start the classification process beginning with the Rehabilitation Plus Extensive Services category. In order for a resident to qualify for this category, he/she must meet three requirements: (1) have an ADL score of 2 or more, (2) meet one of the criteria for the Extensive Services category, and (3) meet the criteria for one of the Rehabilitation categories.

STEP # 1

Check the resident's ADL score. If the resident's ADL score is 2 or higher, **go to Step #2.**

If the ADL score is less than 2, skip to Category II now.

STEP # 2

Determine whether the resident is coded for **one** of the following treatments or services:

O0100E2	Tracheostomy care while a resident
O0100F2	Ventilator or respirator while a resident
O0100M2	Infection isolation while a resident

If the resident does not receive one of these treatments or services, skip to Category II now.

STEP # 3

Determine if the resident's rehabilitation therapy services (speech-language pathology services, or occupational or physical therapy) satisfy the criteria for one of the RUG-IV Rehabilitation categories. **If the resident does not meet all of the criteria for a Rehabilitation category (e.g., Ultra High Intensity), then move to the next category (e.g., Very High Intensity).**

- **Ultra High Intensity Criteria** (the resident qualifies if either [1] or [2] is satisfied)

    1. In the past 7 days:
        Total Therapy Minutes (calculated on page 6-25 – 6-28) of 720 minutes or more
        and
        One discipline (O0400A4, O0400B4 or O0400C4) for at least 5 days
        and
        A second discipline (O0400A4, O0400B4 or O0400C4) for at least 3 days
    2. **If the Medicare Short Stay Assessment Indicator (determined on page 6-20) is "Yes":**
        Medicare Short Stay Average Therapy Minutes (see page 6-19) of 144 minutes or more

RUG-IV ADL Score	RUG-IV Class
11-16	RUX
2-10	RUL

- **Very High Intensity Criteria** (the resident qualifies if either [1] or [2] is satisfied)

  1. In the last 7 days:
     Total Therapy Minutes (calculated on page 6-25 - 6-28) of 500 minutes or more
     and
     At least 1 discipline (O0400A4, O0400B4 or O0400C4) for at least 5 days

  2. **If the Medicare Short Stay Assessment Indicator (determined on page 6-20) is "Yes":**
     Medicare Short Stay Average Therapy Minutes (see page 6-19) of between 100 and 143 minutes

RUG-IV ADL Score	RUG-IV Class
11-16	RVX
2-10	RVL

- **High Intensity Criteria** (the resident qualifies if either [1] or [2] is satisfied)

  1. In the last 7 days:
     Total Therapy Minutes (calculated on page 6-25 - 6-28) of 325 minutes or more
     and
     At least 1 discipline (O0400A4, O0400B4, or O0400C4) for at least 5 days

  2. **If the Medicare Short Stay Assessment Indicator (determined on page 6-20) is "Yes":**
     Medicare Short Stay Average Therapy Minutes (see page 6-19) of between 65 and 99 minutes

RUG-IV ADL Score	RUG-IV Class
11-16	RHX
2-10	RHL

- **Medium Intensity Criteria** (the resident qualifies if either [1] or [2] is satisfied)

  1. In the last 7 days:
     Total Therapy Minutes (calculated on page 6-25 - 6-28) of 150 minutes or more
     and
     At least 5 days of any combination of the three disciplines (O0400A4 plus O0400B4 plus O0400C4)

  2. **If the Medicare Short Stay Assessment Indicator (determined on page 6-20) is "Yes":**
     Medicare Short Stay Average Therapy Minutes (see page 6-19) of between 30 and 64 minutes

RUG-IV ADL Score	RUG-IV Class
11-16	RMX
2-10	RML

- **Low Intensity Criteria** (the resident qualifies if either [1] or [2] is satisfied):

  1. In the last 7 days:

     Total Therapy Minutes (calculated on page 6-25 - 6-28) of 45 minutes or more

     and

     At least 3 days of any combination of the 3 disciplines (O0400A4, plus O0400B4 plus O0400C4)

     and

     Two or more restorative nursing services* received for 6 or more days for at least 15 minutes a day

  2. **If the Medicare Short Stay Assessment Indicator (determined on page 6-20) is "Yes":**

     Medicare Short Stay Average Therapy Minutes (see page 6-19) of between 15 and 29 minutes

     *Restorative Nursing Services
      H0200C, H0500** Urinary toileting program and/or bowel toileting program
      O0500A,B** Passive and/or active ROM
      O0500C Splint or brace assistance
      O0500D,F** Bed mobility and/or walking training
      O0500E Transfer training
      O0500G Dressing and/or grooming training
      O0500H Eating and/or swallowing training
      O0500I Amputation/prostheses care
      O0500J Communication training

      **Count as one service even if both provided

RUG-IV ADL Score	**RUG-IV Class**
2-16	RLX

RUG-IV Classification _____

If the resident does not classify in the Rehabilitation Plus Extensive Services Category, proceed to Category II.

CATEGORY II: REHABILITATION
RUG-IV, 66-GROUP HIERARCHICAL CLASSIFICATION

Rehabilitation therapy is any combination of the disciplines of physical therapy, occupational therapy, or speech-language pathology services, and is located in Section O (Items at O0400A,B,C). Nursing rehabilitation is also considered for the low intensity classification level. It consists of urinary or bowel toileting program, providing active or passive range of motion, providing splint/brace assistance, training in bed mobility or walking, training in transfer, training in dressing/grooming, training in eating/swallowing, training in amputation/prosthesis care, and training in communication. This information is found in Sections H0200C, H0500, and O0500.

STEP # 1

Determine whether the resident's rehabilitation therapy services satisfy the criteria for one of the RUG-IV Rehabilitation categories. **If the resident does not meet all of the criteria for one Rehabilitation category (e.g., Ultra High Intensity), then move to the next category (e.g., Very High Intensity).**

A. **Ultra High Intensity Criteria** (the resident qualifies if either [1] or [2] is satisfied)

1. In the last 7 days:
   Total Therapy Minutes (calculated on page 6-25 - 6-28) of 720 minutes or more
   and
   One discipline (O0400A4, O0400B4 or O0400C4) for at least 5 days
   and
   A second discipline (O0400A4, O0400B4 or O0400C4) for at least 3 days

2. **If the Medicare Short Stay Assessment Indicator (determined on page 6-20) is "Yes":**
   Medicare Short Stay Average Therapy Minutes (see page 6-19) of 144 minutes or more

RUG-IV ADL Score	RUG-IV Class
11-16	RUC
6-10	RUB
0-5	RUA

B. **Very High Intensity Criteria** (the resident qualifies if either [1] or [2] is satisfied)

1. In the last 7 days:
   Total Therapy Minutes (calculated on page 6-25 - 6-28) of 500 minutes or more
   and
   At least 1 discipline (O0400A4, O0400B4 or O0400C4) for at least 5 days

2. **If the Medicare Short Stay Assessment Indicator (determined on page 6-20) is "Yes":**
   Medicare Short Stay Average Therapy Minutes (see page 6-19) of between 100 and 143 minutes

RUG-IV ADL Score	RUG-IV Class
11-16	RVC
6-10	RVB
0-5	RVA

C. **High Intensity Criteria** (the resident qualifies if either [1] or [2] is satisfied)

   1. In the last 7 days:

      Total Therapy Minutes (calculated on page 6-25 - 6-28) of 325 minutes or more
        and
      At least 1 discipline (O0400A4, O0400B4 or O0400C4) for at least 5 days

   2. **If the Medicare Short Stay Assessment Indicator (determined on page 6-20) is "Yes":**

      Medicare Short Stay Average Therapy Minutes (see page 6-19) of between 65 and 99 minutes

RUG-IV ADL Score	RUG-IV Class
11-16	RHC
6-10	RHB
0-5	RHA

D. **Medium Intensity Criteria** (the resident qualifies if either [1] or [2] is satisfied)

   1. In the last 7 days:

      Total Therapy Minutes (calculated on page 6-25 - 6-28) of 150 minutes or more
        and
      At least 5 days of any combination of the three disciplines (O0400A4, plus O0400B4 plus O0400C4)

   2. **If the Medicare Short Stay Assessment Indicator (determined on page 6-20) is "Yes":**

      Medicare Short Stay Average Therapy Minutes (see page 6-19) of between 30 and 64 minutes

RUG-IV ADL Score	RUG-IV Class
11-16	RMC
6-10	RMB
0-5	RMA

E. **Low Intensity Criteria** (the resident qualifies if either [1] or [2] is satisfied):

   1. In the last 7 days:

      Total Therapy Minutes (calculated on page 6-25 - 6-28) of 45 minutes or more
        and
      At least 3 days of any combination of the three disciplines (O0400A4 plus O0400B4 plus O0400C4)

        and
      Two or more restorative nursing services* received for 6 or more days for at least 15 minutes a day

2. **If the Medicare Short Stay Assessment Indicator (determined on page 6-20) is "Yes":**

    Medicare Short Stay Average Therapy Minutes (see page 6-19) of between 15 and 29 minutes

*Nursing Restorative Services

    H0200C, H0500** Urinary toileting program and/or bowel toileting program

    O0500A,B** Passive and/or active ROM

    O0500C Splint or brace assistance

    O0500D,F** Bed mobility and/or walking training

    O0500E Transfer training

    O0500G Dressing and/or grooming training

    O0500H Eating and/or swallowing training

    O0500I Amputation/prostheses care

    O0500J Communication training

    **Count as one service even if both provided

RUG-IV ADL Score	RUG-IV Class
11-16	RLB
0-10	RLA

RUG-IV Classification _____

If the resident does not classify in the Rehabilitation Category, proceed to Category III.

CATEGORY III: EXTENSIVE SERVICES
RUG-IV, 66-GROUP HIERARCHICAL CLASSIFICATION

The classification groups in this category are based on various services provided. Use the following instructions to begin the calculation:

STEP # 1

Determine whether the resident is coded for **one** of the following treatments or services:

O0100E2	Trachcostomy carc whilc a rcsidcnt
O0100F2	Ventilator or respirator while a resident
O0100M2	Infection isolation while a resident

If the resident does not receive one of these treatments or services, skip to Category IV now.

STEP # 2

If at least **one** of these treatments or services is coded and the resident has a total RUG-IV ADL score of 2 or more, he/she classifies as Extensive Services. **Move to Step #3. If the resident's ADL score is 0 or 1, s/he classifies as Clinically Complex. Skip to Category VI, Step #2.**

STEP # 3

The resident classifies in the Extensive Services category according to the following chart:

Extensive Service Conditions	RUG-IV Class
Tracheostomy care* **and** ventilator/respirator*	ES3
Tracheostomy care* **or** ventilator/respirator*	ES2
Infection isolation*	ES1
without tracheostomy care*	
without ventilator/respirator*	

*while a resident

RUG-IV Classification _____

If the resident does not classify in the Extensive Services Category, proceed to Category IV.

October 2011   **Page 6-37**

CATEGORY IV: SPECIAL CARE HIGH
RUG-IV, 66-GROUP HIERARCHICAL CLASSIFICATION

The classification groups in this category are based on certain resident conditions or services. Use the following instructions:

STEP # 1

Determine whether the resident is coded for **one** of the following conditions or services:

B0100, ADLs	Comatose and completely ADL dependent or ADL did not occur (G0110A1, G0110B1, G0110H1, and G0110I1 all equal 4 or 8)
I2100	Septicemia
I2900, N0350A,B	Diabetes with **both** of the following: Insulin injections (N0350A) for all 7 days Insulin order changes on 2 or more days (N0350B)
I5100, ADL Score	Quadriplegia with ADL score >= 5
I6200, J1100C	Chronic obstructive pulmonary disease **and** shortness of breath when lying flat
J1550A, others	Fever and one of the following; I2000 Pneumonia J1550B Vomiting K0300 Weight loss (1 or 2) K0510B1 or K0510B2 Feeding tube*
K0510A1 or K0510A2	Parenteral/IV feedings
O0400D2	Respiratory therapy for all 7 days

*Tube feeding classification requirements:
   (1) K0700A is 51% or more of total calories OR
   (2) K0700A is 26% to 50% of total calories and K0700B is 501 cc or more per day fluid enteral intake in the last 7 days.

If the resident does not have one of these conditions, skip to Category V now.

STEP # 2

If at least **one** of the special care conditions above is coded and the resident has a total RUG-IV ADL score of 2 or more, he or she classifies as Special Care High. **Move to Step #3. If the resident's ADL score is 0 or 1, he or she classifies as Clinically Complex. Skip to Category VI, Step #2.**

STEP # 3

Evaluate for depression. Signs and symptoms of depression are used as a third-level split for the Special Care High category. Residents with signs and symptoms of depression are identified by the Resident Mood Interview (PHQ-9$^{©}$) or the Staff Assessment of Resident Mood (PHQ-9-OV$^{©}$). Instructions for completing the PHQ-9$^{©}$ are in Chapter 3, Section D. The following items comprise the PHQ-9$^{©}$:

Resident	Staff	Description
D0200A	D0500A	Little interest or pleasure in doing things
D0200B	D0500B	Feeling down, depressed, or hopeless
D0200C	D0500C	Trouble falling or staying asleep, sleeping too much
D0200D	D0500D	Feeling tired or having little energy
D0200E	D0500E	Poor appetite or overeating
D0200F	D0500F	Feeling bad or failure or let self or others down
D0200G	D0500G	Trouble concentrating on things
D0200H	D0500H	Moving or speaking slowly or being fidgety or restless
D0200I	D0500I	Thoughts better off dead or hurting self
-	D0500J	Short-tempered, easily annoyed

These items are used to calculate a Total Severity Score for the resident interview at Item D0300 and for the staff assessment at Item D0600. The resident qualifies as depressed for RUG-IV classification in either of the two following cases:

The D0300 Total Severity Score is greater than or equal to 10 but not 99,

or

The D0600 Total Severity Score is greater than or equal to 10.

Resident Qualifies as Depressed Yes _____   No _____

STEP # 4

Select the Special Care High classification based on the ADL score and the presence or absence of depression record this classification:

RUG-IV ADL Score	Depressed	RUG-IV Class
15-16	Yes	HE2
15-16	No	HE1
11-14	Yes	HD2
11-14	No	HD1
6-10	Yes	HC2
6-10	No	HC1
2-5	Yes	HB2
2-5	No	HB1

RUG-IV CLASSIFICATION _____

CATEGORY V: SPECIAL CARE LOW
RUG-IV, 66-GROUP HIERARCHICAL CLASSIFICATION

The classification groups in this category are based on certain resident conditions or services. Use the following instructions:

STEP # 1

Determine whether the resident is coded for **one** of the following conditions or services:

I4400, ADL Score	Cerebral palsy, with ADL score >=5
I5200, ADL Score	Multiple sclerosis, with ADL score >=5
I5300, ADL Score	Parkinson's disease, with ADL score >=5
I6300, O0100C2	Respiratory failure and oxygen therapy while a resident
K0510B1 or K0510B2	Feeding tube*
M0300B1	Two or more stage 2 pressure ulcers with two or more selected skin treatments**
M0300C1,D1,F1	Any stage 3 or 4 pressure ulcer with two or more selected skin treatments**
M1030	Two or more venous/arterial ulcers with two or more selected skin treatments**
M0300B1, M1030	1 stage 2 pressure ulcer and 1 venous/arterial ulcer with 2 or more selected skin treatments**
M1040A,B,C; M1200I	Foot infection, diabetic foot ulcer or other open lesion of foot with application of dressings to the feet
O0100B2	Radiation treatment while a resident
O0100J2	Dialysis treatment while a resident

*Tube feeding classification requirements:
  (1) K0700A is 51% or more of total calories OR
  (2) K0700A is 26% to 50% of total calories and K0700B is 501 cc or more per day fluid enteral intake in the last 7 days.

**Selected skin treatments:
  M1200A,B# Pressure relieving chair and/or bed
  M1200C Turning/repositioning
  M1200D Nutrition or hydration intervention
  M1200E Ulcer care
  M1200G Application of dressings (not to feet)
  M1200H Application of ointments (not to feet)
#Count as one treatment even if both provided

If the resident does not have one of these conditions, skip to Category VI now.

STEP # 2

If at least **one** of the special care conditions above is coded and the resident has a total RUG-IV ADL score of 2 or more, he or she classifies as Special Care Low. **Move to Step #3. If the resident's ADL score is 0 or 1, he or she classifies as Clinically Complex. Skip to Category VI, Step #2.**

STEP # 3

Evaluate for depression. Signs and symptoms of depression are used as a third-level split for the Special Care Low category. Residents with signs and symptoms of depression are indentified by the Resident Mood Interview (PHQ-9©) or the Staff Assessment of Resident Mood (PHQ-9-OV©). Instructions for completing the PHQ-9© are in Chapter 3, Section D. The following items comprise the PHQ-9©:

Resident	Staff	Description
D0200A	D0500A	Little interest or pleasure in doing things
D0200B	D0500B	Feeling down, depressed, or hopeless
D0200C	D0500C	Trouble falling or staying asleep, sleeping too much
D0200D	D0500D	Feeling tired or having little energy
D0200E	D0500E	Poor appetite or overeating
D0200F	D0500F	Feeling bad or failure or let self or others down
D0200G	D0500G	Trouble concentrating on things
D0200H	D0500H	Moving or speaking slowly or being fidgety or restless
D0200I	D0500I	Thoughts better off dead or hurting self
-	D0500J	Short-tempered, easily annoyed

These items are used to calculate a Total Severity Score for the resident interview at Item D0300 and for the staff assessment at Item D0600. The resident qualifies as depressed for RUG-IV classification in either of the two following cases:

The D0300 Total Severity Score is greater than or equal to 10 but not 99,

or

The D0600 Total Severity Score is greater than or equal to 10.

Resident Qualifies as Depressed Yes _____   No _____

STEP # 4

Select the Special Care Low classification based on the ADL score and the presence or absence of depression; record this classification:

RUG-IV ADL Score	Depressed	RUG-IV Class
15-16	Yes	LE2
15-16	No	LE1
11-14	Yes	LD2
11-14	No	LD1
6-10	Yes	LC2
6-10	No	LC1
2-5	Yes	LB2
2-5	No	LB1

RUG-IV CLASSIFICATION _____

CATEGORY VI: CLINICALLY COMPLEX
RUG-IV, 66-GROUP HIERARCHICAL CLASSIFICATION

The classification groups in this category are based on certain resident conditions or services. Use the following instructions:

STEP # 1

Determine whether the resident is coded for **one** of the following conditions or services:

I2000	Pneumonia
I4900, ADL Score	Hemiplegia/hemiparesis with ADL score >=5
M1040D,E	Surgical wounds or open lesions with any selected skin treatment*
M1040F	Burns
O0100A2	Chemotherapy while a resident
O0100C2	Oxygen therapy while a resident
O0100H2	IV medications while a resident
O0100I2	Transfusions while a resident

*Selected Skin Treatments
 M1200F Surgical wound care
 M1200G Application of dressing (not to feet)
 M1200H Application of ointments (not to feet)

If the resident does not have one of these conditions, skip to Category VII now.

STEP # 2

Evaluate for depression. Signs and symptoms of depression are used as a third-level split for the Clinically Complex category. Residents with signs and symptoms of depression are indentified by the Resident Mood Interview (PHQ-9$^©$) or the Staff Assessment of Resident Mood (PHQ-9-OV$^©$). Instructions for completing the PHQ-9$^©$ are in Chapter 3, section D. The following items comprise the PHQ-9$^©$:

Resident	Staff	Description
D0200A	D0500A	Little interest or pleasure in doing things
D0200B	D0500B	Feeling down, depressed, or hopeless
D0200C	D0500C	Trouble falling or staying asleep, sleeping too much
D0200D	D0500D	Feeling tired or having little energy
D0200E	D0500E	Poor appetite or overeating
D0200F	D0500F	Feeling bad or failure or let self or others down
D0200G	D0500G	Trouble concentrating on things
D0200H	D0500H	Moving or speaking slowly or being fidgety or restless
D0200I	D0500I	Thoughts better off dead or hurting self
-	D0500J	Short-tempered, easily annoyed

These items are used to calculate a Total Severity Score for the resident interview at Item D0300 and for the staff assessment at Item D0600. A higher Total Severity Score is associated with more symptoms of depression. For the resident interview, a Total Severity Score of 99 indicates that the interview was not successful.

The resident qualifies as depressed for RUG-IV classification in either of the two following cases:

The D0300 Total Severity Score is greater than or equal to 10 but not 99,

or

The D0600 Total Severity Score is greater than or equal to 10.

Resident Qualifies as Depressed Yes _____   No _____

STEP # 3

Select the Clinically Complex classification based on the ADL score and the presence or absence of depression record this classification:

RUG-IV ADL Score	Depressed	RUG-IV Class
15-16	YES	CE2
15-16	NO	CE1
11-14	YES	CD2
11-14	NO	CD1
6-10	YES	CC2
6-10	NO	CC1
2-5	YES	CB2
2-5	NO	CB1
0-1	YES	CA2
0-1	NO	CA1

RUG-IV CLASSIFICATION _____

CATEGORY VII: BEHAVIORAL SYMPTOMS AND COGNITIVE PERFORMANCE
RUG-IV, 66-GROUP HIERARCHICAL CLASSIFICATION

Classification in this category is based on the presence of certain behavioral symptoms or the resident's cognitive performance. Use the following instructions:

STEP # 1

Determine the resident's ADL score. If the resident's ADL score is 5 or less, go to Step #2.

If the ADL score is greater than 5, skip to Category VIII now.

STEP # 2

If the resident interview using the Brief Interview for Mental Status (BIMS) was not conducted (indicated by a value of "0" for Item C0100), skip the remainder of this step and proceed to Step #3 to check staff assessment for cognitive impairment.

Determine the resident's cognitive status based on resident interview using the BIMS. Instructions for completing the BIMS are in Chapter 3, Section C. The BIMS items involve the following:

C0200	Repetition of three words
C0300	Temporal orientation
C0400	Recall

Item C0500 provides a BIMS Summary Score for these items and indicates the resident's cognitive performance, with a score of 15 indicating the best cognitive performance and 0 indicating the worst performance. If the resident interview is not successful, then the BIMS Summary Score will equal 99.

Determine whether the resident is cognitively impaired. **If the resident's Summary Score is less than or equal to 9, he or she is cognitively impaired and classifies in the Behavioral Symptoms and Cognitive Performance category. Skip to Step #5.**

If the resident's summary score is greater than 9 but not 99, proceed to Step #4 to check behavioral symptoms.

If the resident's Summary Score is 99 (resident interview not successful) or the Summary Score is blank (resident interview not attempted and skipped) or the Summary Score has a dash value (not assessed), proceed to Step #3 to check staff assessment for cognitive impairment.

STEP # 3

Determine whether the resident is cognitively impaired based on the staff assessment rather than on resident interview. The RUG-IV Cognitive Performance Scale (CPS) is used to determine cognitive impairment.

The resident is cognitively impaired if **one** of the three following conditions exists:

1. B0100   Coma (B0100 = 1) and completely ADL dependent or ADL did not occur (G0110A1, G0110B1, G0110H1, G0100I1 all = 4 or 8)
2. C1000   Severely impaired cognitive skills (C1000 = 3)
3. B0700, C0700, C1000   Two or more of the following impairment indicators are present:

   B0700 > 0   Problem being understood
   C0700 = 1   Short-term memory problem
   C1000 > 0   Cognitive skills problem
   and
   One or more of the following severe impairment indicators are present:
   B0700 >= 2 Severe problem being understood
   C1000 >= 2 Severe cognitive skills problem

If the resident meets the criteria for being cognitively impaired, then he or she classifies in Behavioral Symptoms and Cognitive Performance. Skip to Step #5. If he or she does not present with a cognitive impairment as defined here, proceed to Step #4.

STEP # 4

Determine whether the resident presents with **one** of the following behavioral symptoms:

E0100A	Hallucinations
E0100B	Delusions
E0200A	Physical behavioral symptoms directed toward others (2 or 3)
E0200B	Verbal behavioral symptoms directed toward others (2 or 3)
E0200C	Other behavioral symptoms not directed toward others (2 or 3)
E0800	Rejection of care (2 or 3)
E0900	Wandering (2 or 3)

If the resident presents with one of the symptoms above, then he or she classifies in Behavioral Symptoms and Cognitive Performance. Proceed to Step #5. If he or she does not present with behavioral symptoms or a cognitive impairment, skip to Category VIII.

STEP # 5

Determine Restorative Nursing Count

Count the number of the following services provided for 15 or more minutes a day for 6 or more of the last 7 days:

H0200C, H0500**	Urinary toileting program and/or bowel toileting program
O0500A,B**	Passive and/or active ROM
O0500C	Splint or brace assistance
O0500D,F**	Bed mobility and/or walking training
O0500E	Transfer training
O0500G	Dressing and/or grooming training
O0500H	Eating and/or swallowing training
O0500I	Amputation/prostheses care
O0500J	Communication training

**Count as one service even if both provided

Restorative Nursing Count _____

STEP # 6

Select the final RUG-IV Classification by using the total RUG-IV ADL score and the Restorative Nursing Count.

RUG-IV ADL Score	Restorative Nursing	RUG-IV Class
2-5	2 or more	BB2
2-5	0 or 1	BB1
0-1	2 or more	BA2
0-1	0 or 1	BA1

RUG-IV CLASSIFICATION _____

CATEGORY VIII: REDUCED PHYSICAL FUNCTION
RUG-IV, 66-GROUP HIERARCHICAL CLASSIFICATION

STEP # 1

Residents who do not meet the conditions of any of the previous categories, including those who would meet the criteria for the Behavioral Symptoms and Cognitive Performance category but have a RUG-IV ADL score greater than 5, are placed in this category.

STEP # 2

Determine Restorative Nursing Count

Count the number of the following services provided for 15 or more minutes a day for 6 or more of the last 7 days:

H0200C, H0500**	Urinary toileting program and/or bowel toileting program
O0500A,B**	Passive and/or active ROM
O0500C	Splint or brace assistance
O0500D,F**	Bed mobility and/or walking training
O0500E	Transfer training
O0500G	Dressing and/or grooming training
O0500H	Eating and/or swallowing training
O0500I	Amputation/prostheses care
O0500J	Communication training

**Count as one service even if both provided

Restorative Nursing Count _____

STEP # 3

Select the RUG-IV Classification by using the RUG-IV ADL score and the Restorative Nursing Count.

RUG-IV ADL Score	Restorative Nursing	RUG-IV Class
15-16	2 or more	PE2
15-16	0 or 1	PE1
11-14	2 or more	PD2
11-14	0 or 1	PD1
6-10	2 or more	PC2
6-10	0 or 1	PC1
2-5	2 or more	PB2
2-5	0 or 1	PB1
0-1	2 or more	PA2
0-1	0 or 1	PA1

RUG-IV CLASSIFICATION _____

ADJUSTMENT FOR START OF THERAPY OMRA
RUG-IV, 66-GROUP HIERARCHICAL CLASSIFICATION

A Start of Therapy (SOT) OMRA is a Medicare assessment used to initiate a Medicare payment level in either a Rehabilitation Plus Extensive or Rehabilitation group after rehabilitation therapy starts. The SOT OMRA is an abbreviated assessment that does not contain all of the items used for RUG-IV classification. The SOT OMRA only contains the RUG-IV items necessary for a Rehabilitation Plus Extensive or Rehabilitation classification. Classifications below the Rehabilitation category cannot be determined from an SOT OMRA unless it is combined with an assessment that contains all of the RUG-IV items (i.e., an OBRA assessment or other type of PPS assessment).

MEDICARE ADJUSTMENTS

Adjustments are performed for Medicare classification (Item Z0100A) on an SOT OMRA. There are three different situations relevant to Medicare classification adjustments as follows:

Situation 1

If an assessment is an SOT OMRA, indicated by MDS Item A0310C = 1 or 3, whether or not it is combined with other types of assessments, then the Medicare Index Maximized RUG-IV classification in item Z0100A must be a Rehabilitation Plus Extensive Services group or a Rehabilitation group. Lower classifications are not valid for Z0100A on an SOT OMRA.

If the Z0100A classification for any SOT OMRA (Item A0310C = 1 or 3) *is not* in a Rehabilitation Plus Extensive Services group or a Rehabilitation group, then the following adjustment should be made:

1. The Medicare RUG-IV group reported in Item Z0100A should be *adjusted to AAA* (the default group), the assessment should marked as invalid, and the assessment should be barred from submission. The Quality Improvement Evaluation System (QIES) Assessment Submission and Processing (ASAP) system will *reject the assessment* if submitted.

Situation 2

If the Z0100A classification for an SOT OMRA (Item A0310C = 1), *not combined* with an OBRA assessment or other PPS assessment, *is* in a Rehabilitation Plus Extensive Services group or a Rehabilitation group, then the following adjustment applies:

1. The Medicare Non-Therapy RUG-IV group reported in Item Z0150A should be *adjusted to AAA* (the default group).

Situation 3

If the Z0100A classification for an SOT OMRA, *combined* with an OBRA assessment or other PPS assessment, *is* in a Rehabilitation Plus Extensive Services group or a Rehabilitation group, then *no adjustment* is necessary.

OTHER PAYER ADJUSTMENT

This other payer adjustment is applied when performing the Medicaid RUG-IV classification for Items Z0200A and Z0250A or for classification for other payers.

1. When an SOT OMRA (MDS Item A0310C = 1) is *not combined* with an OBRA assessment or other type of PPS assessment, then an RUG-IV classification below the Rehabilitation Plus Extensive and Rehabilitation categories should be *adjusted to AAA* (the default group).

6.7 SNF PPS Policies

Requirements and policies for SNF PPS are described in greater detail in the **Medicare Benefit Policy Manual**. Here are some situations that the SNF may encounter that may impact Medicare Part A SNF coverage for a resident, affect the PPS assessment schedule, or impact the reimbursement received by the SNF.

Delay in Requiring and Receiving Skilled Services (30-Day Transfer)

There are instances in which the beneficiary does not require SNF level of care services when initially admitted to the SNF. When the beneficiary requires and receives SNF level of care services within 30 days from the hospital discharge, Day 1 for the Medicare assessment schedule is the day on which SNF level of care services begins. For example, if a beneficiary is discharged from the hospital on August 1 and the SNF determines on August 31 that the beneficiary requires skilled service for a condition that was treated during the qualifying hospital stay, then the SNF would start the Medicare assessment schedule with a 5-day Medicare-required assessment, with August 31 as Day 1 for scheduling purposes. However, if the beneficiary requires and receives a SNF level of care 31 or more days after the hospital discharge, the beneficiary does not qualify for a SNF Part A stay (see Medical Appropriateness Exception below).

Medical Appropriateness Exception (Deferred Treatment)

An elapsed period of more than 30 days is permitted for starting SNF Part A services when a resident's condition makes it inappropriate to begin an active course of treatment in a SNF immediately after a qualifying hospital stay discharge. It is applicable only where, under accepted medical practice, the established pattern of treatment for a particular condition indicates that a covered level of SNF care will be required within a predeterminable time frame, and it is medically predictable at the time of hospital discharge that the beneficiary will require SNF level of care within a predetermined time period (for more detailed information see Chapter 8 of the **Medicare Benefit Policy Manual**). For example, a beneficiary is admitted to the SNF after a qualifying hospital stay for an open reduction and internal fixation of a hip. It is determined upon hospital discharge that the beneficiary is not ready for weight-bearing activity but will most likely be ready in 4-6 weeks. The physician writes an order to start therapy when the beneficiary is able to tolerate weight bearing. Once the resident is able to start therapy, the Medicare Part A stay begins, and the Medicare-required 5-day assessment will be performed. Day 1 of the stay will be the first day on which the resident starts therapy services.

Resident Discharged from Part A Skilled Services and Returns to SNF Part A Skilled Level Services

In the situation in which a beneficiary is discharged from SNF Medicare Part A services and later requires SNF Part A skilled level of care services, the resident may be eligible for Medicare Part A SNF coverage if the following criteria are met:

1. Less than 30 days have elapsed since the last day on which SNF level of care services were required and received,

2. SNF-level services required by the resident are for a condition that was treated during the qualifying hospital stay or for a condition that arose while receiving care in the SNF for a condition for which the beneficiary was previously treated in the hospital,

3. Services must be reasonable and necessary,

4. Services can only be provided on an inpatient basis,

5. Resident must require and receive the services on a daily basis, and

6. Resident has remaining days in the SNF benefit period.

For greater detail, refer to the **Medicare Benefit Policy Manual**, Chapter 8.

6.8 Non-compliance with the SNF PPS Assessment Schedule

To receive payment under the SNF PPS, the SNF must complete scheduled and unscheduled assessments as described in Chapter 2.

According to 42 CFR 413.343, an assessment that does not have an ARD within the prescribed ARD window will be paid at the default rate for the number of days the ARD is out of compliance. Frequent early or late assessment scheduling practices may result in a review. The default rate (AAA) takes the place of the otherwise applicable Federal rate. It is equal to the rate paid for the RUG group reflecting the lowest acuity level, and would generally be lower than the Medicare rate payable if the SNF had submitted an assessment in accordance with the prescribed assessment schedule.

Early Assessment

An assessment must be completed according to the designated Medicare PPS assessment schedule. **If a scheduled Medicare-required assessment or an OMRA is performed earlier than the schedule indicates (the ARD is not in the defined window), the provider will be paid at the default rate for the number of days the assessment was out of compliance.** For example, a Medicare-required 14-day assessment with an ARD of Day 12 (1 day early) would be paid at the default rate for the first day of the payment period that begins on day 15.

In the case of an early COT OMRA, the early COT would reset the COT calendar such that the next COT OMRA, if deemed necessary, would have an ARD set for 7 days from the early COT ARD. For example, a facility completes a 30-day assessment with an ARD of November 1 which classifies a resident into a therapy RUG. A COT OMRA is completed for this resident with an ARD set for November 6, which is Day 5 of the COT observation period as opposed to November 8 which is Day 7 of the COT observation period. This COT OMRA would be considered an early assessment and, based on the ARD set for this early assessment would be paid at the default rate for the two days this assessment was out of compliance. The next seven day COT observation period would begin on November 7, and end on November 13.

Late Assessment

If the SNF fails to set the ARD within the defined ARD window for a Medicare-required assessment, including the grace days, and the resident is still on Part A, the SNF must complete a late assessment. The ARD can be no earlier than the day the error was identified.

If the ARD on the late assessment is set for **prior to the end of the period during which the late assessment would have controlled the payment,** had the ARD been set timely, and/or **no intervening assessments have occurred, the SNF will bill the default rate for the number of days that the assessment is out of compliance.** This is equal to the number of days between the day following the last day of the available ARD window (including grace days when appropriate) and the late ARD (including the late ARD). **The SNF would then bill the Health Insurance Prospective Payment System (HIPPS) code established by the late assessment for the remaining period of time that the assessment would have controlled payment.** For example, a Medicare-required 30-day assessment with an ARD of Day 41 is out of compliance for 8 days and therefore would be paid at the default rate for 8 days and the HIPPS code from the late 30-day assessment until the next scheduled or unscheduled assessment that controls payment.   In this example, if there are no other assessments until the 60-day assessment, the remaining 22 days are billed according to the HIPPS code on the late assessment.

A second example, involving a late unscheduled assessment would be if a COT OMRA was completed with an ARD of Day 39, while Day 7 of the COT observation period was Day 37. In this case, the COT OMRA would be considered 2 days late and the facility would bill the default rate for 2 days and then bill the HIPPS code from the late COT OMRA until the next scheduled or unscheduled assessment controls payment, in this case, for at least 5 days. NOTE: In such cases where a late assessment is completed and no intervening assessments occur, the late assessment is used to establish the COT calendar.

If the ARD of the late assessment is set **after the end of the period during which the late assessment would have controlled payment,** had the assessment been completed timely, or in cases where **an intervening assessment** has occurred and the resident is still on Part A, the provider must still complete the assessment. The ARD can be no earlier than the day the error was identified. **The SNF must bill all covered days during which the late assessment would have controlled payment had the ARD been set timely at the default rate regardless of the HIPPS code calculated from the late assessment**. For example, a Medicare-required 14-day assessment with an ARD of Day 32 would be paid at the default rate for Days 15 through 30. A late assessment cannot be used to replace a different Medicare-required assessment. In the example above, the SNF would also need to complete the 30-day Medicare-required assessment within Days 27-33, which includes grace days. The 30-day assessment would cover Days 31 through 60 as long as the beneficiary has SNF days remaining and is eligible for SNF Part A services. In this example, the late 14-day assessment would not be considered an assessment used for payment and would not impact the COT calendar, as only an assessment used for payment can affect the COT calendar (see section 2.8).

A second example involving an unscheduled assessment would be the following. A 30-day assessment is completed with an ARD of Day 30. Day 7 of the COT observation period is Day 37. An EOT OMRA is performed timely for this resident with an ARD set for Day 42 and the resident's last day of therapy was Day 39. Upon further review of the resident's record on Day 52, the facility determines that a COT should have been completed with an ARD of Day 37 but was not. The ARD for the COT OMRA is set for Day 52. The late COT OMRA should have controlled payment from Day 31 until the next assessment used for payment. Because there was an intervening assessment (in this case the EOT OMRA) prior to the ARD of the late COT OMRA, the facility would bill the default rate for 9 days (the period during which the COT OMRA would have controlled payment). The facility would bill the RUG from the EOT OMRA as per normal beginning the first non-therapy day, in this case Day 40, until the next scheduled or unscheduled assessment used for payment.

Missed Assessment

If the SNF fails to set the ARD of a scheduled PPS assessment prior to the end of the last day of the ARD window, including grace days, and the resident is no longer a SNF Part A resident, and as a result a Medicare-required assessment does not exist in the QIES ASAP for the payment period, the provider may not usually bill for days when an assessment does not exist in the QIES ASAP. When an assessment does not exist in the QIES ASAP, there is not an assessment based RUG the provider may bill. In order to bill for Medicare SNF Part A services, the provider must submit a valid assessment that is accepted into the QIES ASAP. The provider must bill the RUG category that is verified by the system. If the resident was already discharged from Medicare Part A when this is discovered, an assessment may not be performed.

However, there are instances when the SNF may bill the default code when a Medicare-required assessment does not exist in the QIES ASAP system. These exceptions are:

1. The stay is less than 8 days within a spell of illness,
2. The SNF is notified on an untimely basis of or is unaware of a Medicare Secondary Payer denial,
3. The SNF is notified on an untimely basis of a beneficiary's enrollment in Medicare Part A,
4. The SNF is notified on an untimely basis of the revocation of a payment ban,
5. The beneficiary requests a demand bill, or
6. The SNF is notified on an untimely basis or is unaware of a beneficiary's disenrollment from a Medicare Advantage plan.

In situations 2-6, the provider may use the OBRA Admission assessment to bill for all days of covered care associated with Medicare-required 5-day and 14-day assessments, even if the beneficiary is no longer receiving therapy services that were identified under the most recent clinical assessment. The ARD of the OBRA Admission assessment may be before or during the Medicare stay and does not have to fall within the ARD window of the 5-day or 14-day assessment.

When an OBRA Admission assessment does not exist, the SNF must have a valid OBRA assessment (except a stand-alone discharge assessment) in the QIES ASAP system that falls within the ARD window of the 5-day or the 14-day (including grace days) in order to receive full payment at the RUG category in which the resident grouped for days 1-14 **or** days 15-30. This assessment may only cover **one** payment period. If the ARD of the valid OBRA assessment falls outside the ARD window of the 5-day and 14-day PPS assessments (including grace days), the

SNF must bill the default code for the applicable payment period. For covered days associated with the Medicare-required 30-day, 60-day, or 90-day assessments, the SNF must have a valid OBRA assessment (except a stand-alone discharge assessment) in the QIES ASAP system that falls within the ARD window of the PPS assessment (including grace days) in order to receive full payment at the RUG category in which the resident grouped. If the ARD of the valid OBRA assessment falls outside the ARD window of the PPS assessment (including grace days), the SNF must bill the default code.

Under all situations other than exceptions 1-5, the following apply when the SNF failed to set the ARD prior to the end of the last day of the ARD window, including grace days, or later and the resident was already discharged from Medicare Part A when this was discovered:

1. If a valid OBRA assessment (except a stand-alone discharge assessment) exists in the QIES ASAP system with an ARD that is within the ARD window of the PPS assessment (including grace days), the SNF may bill the RUG category in which the resident classified.
2. If a valid OBRA assessment (except a stand-alone discharge assessment) exists in the QIES ASAP system with an ARD that is outside the ARD window of the Medicare-required assessment (including grace days), the SNF may not bill for any days associated with the missing PPS assessment.
3. If a valid OBRA assessment (except a stand-alone discharge assessment) does not exist in the QIES ASAP system, the SNF may not bill for any days associated with the missing PPS assessment.

In the case of an unscheduled assessment if the SNF fails to set the ARD for an unscheduled PPS assessment within the defined ARD window for that assessment, and the resident has been discharged from Part A, the assessment is missed and cannot be completed. All days that would have been paid by the missed assessment (had it been completed timely) are considered provider-liable. However, as with late unscheduled assessment policy, the provider-liable period only lasts until the point when an intervening assessment controls the payment.

ARD Outside the Medicare Part A SNF Benefit

A SNF may not use a date outside the SNF Part A Medicare Benefit (i.e., 100 days) as the ARD for a PPS assessment. For example, the resident returns to the SNF on December 11 following a hospital stay, requires and receives SNF skilled services (and meets all other required coverage criteria), and has 3 days left in his/her SNF benefit period. The SNF must set the ARD for the PPS assessment on December 11, 12, or 13 to bill for the RUG category associated with the assessment.

APPENDIX A: GLOSSARY AND COMMON ACRONYMS

Glossary

Term	Abbreviation	Definition
Ability to Understand Others		Comprehension of direct person-to-person communication whether spoken, written, or in sign language or Braille. Includes the resident's ability to process and understand language.
Active Assisted Range of Motion		A type of active range of motion in which assistance is provided by an outside force, either manually or mechanically because the prime mover muscles need assistance to complete the motion. This type of range of motion may be used when muscles are weak or when joint movement causes discomfort; or for example, if the resident is able to move his or her limbs, but requires help to perform entire movement.
Active Disease Diagnosis		An illness or condition that is currently causing or contributing to a resident's complications and/or functional, cognitive, medical and psychiatric symptoms or impairments.
Active Range of Motion		Movement within the unrestricted range of motion for a segment, which is produced by active contraction of the muscles crossing that joint is completed without assistance by the resident. This type of range of motion occurs when a resident can move his or her limbs without assistance.
Activities of Daily Living	ADLs	Activities of daily living are those needed for self-care: bathing, dressing, mobility, toileting, eating, and transferring. The late-loss ADLs (eating, toileting, bed mobility, and transferring) are used to classify a patient into a RUG-IV group.
Acute Change in Mental Status		Alteration in mental status (e.g., orientation, inattention, organization of thought, level of consciousness, psychomotor behavior, change in cognition) that was new or worse for this resident, usually over hours to days.
ADL Aspects		Components of ADL activities. These are listed next to each ADL in the item set. For example, the aspects of G0110H (Eating) are eating, drinking, and intake of nourishment or hydration by other means, including tube feeding, total parenteral nutrition, and IV fluids for hydration.

(continued)

Term	Abbreviation	Definition
ADL Self-Performance Items		Measures what the resident actually did (not what he or she might be capable of doing) within each ADL category according to a performance-based scale.
ADL Support Provided		Measures the highest level of support provided by staff, even if that level of support only occurred once, according to a support-based scale.
Adverse Consequence		An unpleasant symptom or event that is caused by or associated with a medication, impairment or decline in an individual's physical condition, mental, functional or psychosocial status. It may include various types of adverse drug reactions (ADR) and interactions (e.g., medication-medication, medication-food, and medication-disease).
Adverse Drug Reaction (ADR)		ADR is a form of adverse consequence. It may be either a secondary effect of a medication that is usually undesirable and different from the therapeutic effect of the medication, or any response to a medication that is noxious and unintended and occurs in doses for prophylaxis, diagnosis or treatment. The term "side effect" is often used interchangeably with ADR; however, side effects are but one of five ADR categories, the others being hypersensitivity, idiosyncratic response, toxic reactions, and adverse medication interactions. A side effect is an expected, well-known reaction that occurs with a predictable frequency and may or may not constitute an adverse consequence.
Assessment Period		The time period during which the assessment coordinator starts the assessment until it is signed as complete.
Assessment Reference Date	ARD	The specific end point for look-back periods in the MDS assessment process. This look-back period is also called the observation or assessment period.
Assessment Submission and Processing System	ASAP	The CMS system that receives submissions of MDS 3.0 data files, validates records for accuracy and appropriateness, and stores validated records in the CMS database.
Assessment Window		The period of time defined by Medicare regulations that specifies when the ARD must be set.

(continued)

Term	Abbreviation	Definition
Audiology Services		Audiology services include the testing of hearing and balance; recommending assistive listening equipment; managing hearing screening programs; providing education regarding the effects of noise on hearing and the prevention of hearing loss; managing cochlear implants; and providing counseling and aural rehabilitation. Audiologist is defined in regulation (42 CFR 484).
Autism		A developmental disorder that is characterized by impaired social interaction, problems with verbal and nonverbal communication, and unusual, repetitive, or severely limited activities and interests.
Baseline		An individual's usual, customary, initial, or most common (depending on the item) range or level of something; for example, behavior, laboratory values, mood, endurance, function, vital signs, etc. "Baseline" information is often used as a basis for comparing findings or results over time.
Bladder Rehabilitation/ Bladder Retraining		A behavioral technique that requires the resident to resist or inhibit the sensation of urgency (the strong desire to urinate), to postpone or delay voiding, and to urinate according to a timetable rather than to the urge to void.
Body Mass Index	BMI	Number calculated from a person's weight and height. BMI is a reliable indicator of body fat. BMI is used as a screening tool to identify possible weight problems for adults.
Brief Interview for Mental Status	BIMS	The BIMS is a brief screener that aids in detecting cognitive impairment. It does not assess all possible aspects of cognitive impairment.
Broken Tooth		A tooth with a crack, chip, or other loss of structural integrity.
Browser		A program that allows access to the Internet or a private intranet site. A browser with 128-bit encryption is necessary to access the Centers for Medicare & Medicaid Services (CMS) intranet to submit data or report retrieval.
Care Area Assessment	CAA	The review of one or more of the twenty conditions, symptoms, and other areas of concern that are commonly identified or suggested by MDS findings. Care areas are triggered by responses on the MDS item set.

(continued)

Term	Abbreviation	Definition
Care Area Triggers	**CAT**	A set of items and responses from the MDS that are indicators of particular issues and conditions that affect nursing facility residents.
Case Mix Index	**CMI**	Weight or numeric score assigned to each Resource Utilization Group (RUG-III, RUG IV) that reflects the relative resources predicted to provide care to a resident. The higher the case mix weight, the greater the resource requirements for the resident.
Case Mix Reimbursement System		A payment system that measures the intensity of care and services required for each resident, and translates these measures into the amount of reimbursement given to the facility for care of a resident. Payment is linked to the intensity of resource use.
Cavity		A tooth with a hole due to decay or other erosion.
CMS Certification Number	**CCN**	Replaces the term "Medicare/Medicaid Provider Number" in survey and certification, and assessment-related activities.
Centers for Medicare & Medicaid Services	**CMS**	CMS is the Federal agency that administers the Medicare, Medicaid, and Child Health Insurance Programs.
Check and Change		Involves checking the resident's dry/wet status at regular intervals and using incontinence devices and products.
Code of Federal Regulations	**CFR**	A codification of the general and permanent rules published in the Federal Register by the Executive departments and agencies of the Federal Government.
Colostomy		A surgical procedure that brings the end of the large intestine through the abdominal wall.

(continued)

Term	Abbreviation	Definition
Comatose (Coma)		Pathological state in which neither arousal (wakefulness, alertness) nor awareness exists. The person is unresponsive and cannot be aroused; he or she may or may not open his or her eyes, does not speak, and does not move his or her extremities on command or in response to noxious stimuli (e.g., pain).
Comprehensive Assessment		Requires completion of the MDS and review of CAAs, followed by development and/or review of the comprehensive care plan.
Confusion Assessment Method	CAM	An instrument that screens for overall cognitive impairment as well as features to distinguish delirium or reversible confusion from other types of cognitive impairments.
Constipation		A condition of more than short duration where someone has fewer than three bowel movements a week or stools that are usually hard, dry, and difficult and/or painful to eliminate.
Continence		Any void into a commode, urinal, or bedpan that occurs voluntarily, or as the result of prompted toileting, assisted toileting, or scheduled toileting.
Daily Decision Making		Includes: choosing clothing; knowing when to go to scheduled meals; using environmental cues to organize and plan (e.g., clocks, calendars, posted event notices); in the absence of environmental cues, seeking information appropriately (i.e. not repetitively) from others in order to plan the day; using awareness of one's own strengths and limitations to regulate the day's events (e.g., asks for help when necessary); acknowledging need to use appropriate assistive equipment such as a walker.
Delirium		Acute onset or worsening of impaired brain function resulting in cognitive and behavioral symptoms such as worsening confusion, disordered expression of thoughts, frequent fluctuation in level of consciousness, and hallucinations.
Delusion		A fixed, false belief not shared by others that the resident holds even in the face of evidence to the contrary.

(continued)

Term	Abbreviation	Definition
Designated Local Contact Agency		Each state has designated a local contact agency responsible for contacting the individual with information about community living options. This local contact agency may be a single entry point agency, an Aging/Disabled Resource Center, an Area Agency on Aging, a Center for Independent Living, or other state contractor.
Disorganized Thinking		Having thoughts that are fragmented or not logically connected.
Dose		Total amount/strength/concentration of a medication given at one time or over a period of time. The individual dose is the amount/strength/concentration received at each administration. The amount received over a 24-hour period may be referred to as the "daily dose."
Down Syndrome		A common genetic disorder in which a child is born with 47 rather than 46 chromosomes, resulting in developmental delays, intellectual disability, low muscle tone, and other possible effects.
Dually Certified Facilities		Nursing facilities that participate in both the Medicare and Medicaid programs.
Duplicate Assessment Error		A fatal record error that results from a resubmission of a record previously accepted into the CMS MDS database. A duplicate record is identified as having the same target date, reason for assessment, resident, and facility. This is the only fatal record error that does not require correction and resubmission.
Entry Date		The initial date of admission/entry to the nursing home, or the date on which the resident most recently re-entered the nursing home after being discharged (whether or not the return was anticipated).
Epilepsy		A chronic neurological disorder that is characterized by recurrent unprovoked seizures, as a result of abnormal neuronal activity in the brain.
External Condom Catheter		Device attached to the shaft of the penis like a condom and connected to a drainage bag.

(continued)

Term	Abbreviation	Definition
Facility ID	**FAC_ID**	The facility identification number is assigned to each nursing facility by the State agency. The FAC_ID must be placed in the individual MDS and tracking form records. This normally is completed as a function within the facility's MDS data entry software.
Fall		Unintentional change in position coming to rest on the ground or onto the next lower surface (e.g., onto a bed, chair, or bedside mat), but not as a result of an overwhelming external force.
Fatal File Error		An error in the MDS file format that causes the entire file to be rejected. The individual records are not validated or stored in the database. The facility must contact its software support to resolve the problem with the submission file.
Fatal Record Error		An error in MDS record that is severe enough to result in record rejection. A fatal record is not saved in the CMS database. The facility must correct the error that caused the rejection and resubmit a corrected original record.
Fecal Impaction		A mass of dry, hard stool that can develop in the rectum due to chronic constipation. Watery stool from higher in the bowel or irritation from the impaction may move around the mass and leak out, causing soiling, often a sign of a fecal impaction.
Federal Register		The official daily publication for rules, proposed rules, and notices of Federal agencies and organizations, as well as Executive Orders and other Presidential Documents. It is a publication of the National Archives and Records Administration, and is available by subscription and online.
Feeding Tube		Presence of any type of tube that can deliver food/nutritional substances/fluids directly into the gastrointestinal system. Examples include, but are not limited to: nasogastric tubes, gastrostomy tubes, jejunostomy tubes, percutaneous endoscopic gastrotomy (PEG) tubes.
Fever		A fever is present when the resident's temperature (°F) is 2.4 degrees greater than the baseline temperature.

(continued)

Term	Abbreviation	Definition
Final Validation Report	**FVR**	A report generated after the successful submission of MDS 3.0 assessment data. This report lists all of the residents for whom assessments have been submitted in a particular submission batch, and displays all errors and/or warnings that occurred during the validation process. An FVR with a submission type of "production" is a facility's documentation for successful file submission. An individual record listed on the FVR marked as "accepted" is documentation for successful record submission.
First Time in This Facility		Newly admitted resident who has not been admitted to this facility before.
Fiscal Intermediary	**FI**	In the past, an organization designated by CMS to process Medicare claims for payment that are submitted by a nursing facility. Fiscal intermediaries (FIs) are now called Medicare Administrative Contractors (MACs).
F-Tag		Numerical designations for criteria reviewed during the nursing facility survey.
Functional Limitation in Range of Motion		Limited ability to move a joint that interferes with daily functioning (particularly with activities of daily living) or places the resident at risk of injury.
Grace Days		Predetermined additional days that may be added to the assessment window for Medicare scheduled assessments without incurring financial penalty. These may be used in situations such as an absence/illness or reassignment of the registered nurse (RN) assessment coordinator, or an unusually large number of assessments due at approximately the same time. Grace days may also be used to more fully capture therapy minutes or other treatments.
Gradual Dose Reduction (GDR)		Step-wise tapering of a dose to determine whether or not symptoms, conditions, or risks can be managed by a lower dose or whether or not the dose or medication can be discontinued.
Habit Training/ Scheduled Voiding		A behavior technique that calls for scheduled toileting at regular intervals on a planned basis to match the resident's voiding habits or needs.

(continued)

Term	Abbreviation	Definition
Hallucination		A perception in a conscious and awake state, of something in the absence of external stimuli. May be auditory or visual or involve smells, tastes, or touch.
Healthcare Common Procedure Coding System	HCPCS	A uniform coding system that describes medical services, procedures, products, and supplies. These codes are used primarily for billing.
Health Insurance Portability and Accountability Act of 1996	HIPAA	Federal law that gives the Department of Health and Human Services (DHHS) the authority to mandate regulations that govern privacy, security, and electronic transactions standards for health care information.
Health Insurance Prospective Payment System	HIPPS	Billing codes used when submitting claims to the MACs (previously FIs) for Medicare payment. Codes comprise the RUG category calculated by the assessment followed by an indicator to indicate which assessment was completed.
Hierarchy		The ordering of groups within the RUG Classification system is a hierarchy. The RUG hierarchy begins with groups with the highest resource use and descends to those groups with the lowest resource use. The RUG-IV Classification system has eight hierarchical levels or categories: Rehabilitation Plus Extensive Services, Rehabilitation, Extensive Services, Special Care High, Special Care Low, Clinically Complex, Behavioral Symptoms and Cognitive Performance, and Reduced Physical Function.
Hospice Services		A program for terminally ill persons where an array of services is provided for the palliation and management of terminal illness and related conditions. The hospice must be licensed by the state as a hospice provider and/or certified under the Medicare program as a hospice provider.
Ileostomy		A stoma that has been constructed by bringing the end or loop of small intestine (the ileum) out onto the surface of the skin.
Inactivation		A type of correction allowed under the MDS Correction Policy. When an invalid record has been accepted into the CMS database, a correction record is submitted with inactivation selected as the type of correction. An inactivation will remove the invalid record from the database.

(continued)

Term	Abbreviation	Definition
Inattention		Reduced ability to maintain attention to external stimuli and to appropriately shift attention to new external stimuli.
Indwelling Catheter		A catheter that is maintained within the bladder for the purpose of continuous drainage of urine.
Intermittent Catheterization		Sterile insertion and removal of a catheter through the urethra into the bladder for bladder drainage.
Internal Assessment ID		A sequential numeric identifier assigned to each record submitted to QIES ASAP.
International Classification of Diseases – Clinical Modification	ICD-CM	Official system of assigning codes to diagnoses and procedures associated with hospital utilization in the United States. The ICD-CM contains a numerical list of the disease code numbers in tabular form, an alphabetical index to the disease entries, and a classification system for surgical, diagnostic, and therapeutic procedures.
Invalid Record		As defined by the MDS Correction Policy, a record that was accepted into QIES ASAP that should not have been submitted. Invalid records are defined as: a test record submitted as production, a record for an event that did not occur, a record with the wrong resident identified or the wrong reason for assessment, or submission of an inappropriate non-required record.
Item Set Code	ISC	A code based upon combinations of reasons for assessment (A0310 items) that determines which items are active on a particular type of MDS assessment or tracking record.
Java-Based Resident Assessment Validation and Entry System	jRAVEN	Data entry software supplied by CMS for nursing facilities and hospital swing beds to use to enter MDS assessment data.
Legal Name		Resident's name as it appears on the Medicare card. If the resident is not enrolled in the Medicare program, use the resident's name as it appears on a government-issued document (i.e., driver's license, birth certificate, social security card).

(continued)

Term	Abbreviation	Definition
Level of Consciousness		Alert: startles easily to any sound or touch.
		Drowsy/Lethargic: repeatedly dozes off when you are asking questions but responds to voice or touch.
		Stuporous: very difficult to arouse and keep aroused for the interview.
		Comatose: cannot be aroused despite shaking and shouting.
Login ID		A State-assigned facility identifier required to access QIES ASAP. This may or may not be the same as the Facility ID.
Look-Back Period		A timeframe defined by counting backwards from the ARD that is used when coding each item on the MDS.
Makes Self Understood		Able to express or communicate requests, needs, opinions, and to conduct social conversation in his or her primary language, whether in speech, writing, sign language, gestures, or a combination of these. Deficits in ability to make one's self understood (expressive communication deficits) can include reduced voice volume and difficulty in producing sounds, or difficulty in finding the right word, making sentences, writing, and/or gesturing.
MDS Completion Date		The date at which the RN assessment coordinator attests that all portions of the MDS have been completed. This is the date recorded at Z0500B.
Mechanically Altered Diet		A diet specifically prepared to alter the texture or consistency of food in order to facilitate oral intake. Examples include soft solids, pureed foods, ground meat, and thickened liquids.
Medicaid		A Federal and State program subject to the provisions of Title XIX of the Social Security Act that pays for specific kinds of medical care and treatment for low-income families.

(continued)

Term	Abbreviation	Definition
Medicare		A health insurance program administered by CMS under provisions of Title XVIII of the Social Security Act for people aged 65 and over, for those who have permanent kidney failure, and for certain people with disabilities. Medicare Part A: The part of Medicare that covers inpatient hospital services and services furnished by other institutional health care providers, such as nursing facilities, home health agencies, and hospices. Medicare Part B: The part of Medicare that covers services of doctors, suppliers of medical items and services, and various types of outpatient services.
Medicare Administrative Contractor	MAC	An organization designated by CMS to process Medicare claims for payment that are submitted by a nursing facility. MACs were previously called Fiscal Intermediaries (FIs).
Medicare Covered Stay		Skilled Nursing Facility stays billable to Medicare Part A when specific requirements and criteria are met for an individual.
Medicare Number (or Comparable Railroad Insurance Number)		A number assigned to an individual for participation in national health insurance program. The first 9 characters must be numbers. The Medicare Health Insurance number may be different from the resident's social security number (SSN). For example, many residents may receive Medicare benefits based on a spouse's Medicare eligibility.
Medication Interaction		The impact of medication or other substance (such as nutritional supplements including herbal products, food or substances used in diagnostic studies) upon another medication. The interactions may alter absorption, distribution, metabolism, or elimination. These interactions may decrease the effectiveness of the medication or increase the potential for adverse consequences.
Minimum Data Set	MDS	A core set of screening, clinical assessment, and functional status elements, including common definitions and coding categories that form the foundation of the comprehensive assessment for all residents of long-term care facilities certified to participate in Medicare and Medicaid and for patients receiving SNF services in non-critical access hospitals with a swing bed agreement.

(continued)

Term	Abbreviation	Definition
Modification		A type of correction allowed under the MDS Correction Policy. A modification is required when a valid MDS record has been accepted by the CMS MDS database, but the information in the record contains errors. The modification will correct the record in the CMS database. A modification is not done when a record has been rejected.
Monitoring		The ongoing collection and analysis of information (such as observations and diagnostic test results) and comparison to baseline and current data in order to ascertain the individual's response to treatment and care, including progress or lack of progress toward a goal. Monitoring can detect any improvements, complications or adverse consequences of the condition or of the treatments; and support decisions about adding, modifying, continuing, or discontinuing, any interventions.
Most Recent Medicare Stay		This is a Medicare Part A covered stay that has started on or after the most recent admission/entry or reentry to the nursing facility.
Music Therapy		Music therapy is an intervention that uses music to address physical, emotional, cognitive, and social needs of individuals of all ages. Music therapy interventions can be designed to promote wellness, manage stress, alleviate pain, express feelings, enhance memory, improve communication, and promote physical rehabilitation. In order for music therapy to be coded on the MDS, the service must be provided or directly supervised by a qualified staff.
National Drug Code	NDC	A unique 10-digit number assigned to each drug product listed under Section 510 of the Federal Food, Drug and Cosmetic Act. The NDC code identifies the vendor, drug name, dosage, and form of the drug.
National Provider Identifier	NPI	A unique federal number that identifies providers of health care services. The NPI applies to the nursing facility for all of its residents.
Nephrostomy Tube		A catheter inserted through the skin into the kidney or its collecting system.

(continued)

Term	Abbreviation	Definition
Non-medication Pain Intervention		An intervention, other than medication, used to try to manage pain which may include, but are not limited to: bio-feedback, application of heat/cold, massage, physical therapy, nerve block, stretching and strengthening exercises, chiropractic, electrical stimulation, radiotherapy, ultrasound, and acupuncture.
Non-pharmacological Intervention		Approaches that do not involve the use of medication to address a medical condition.
Nursing Facility	**NF**	A facility that is primarily engaged in providing skilled nursing care and related services to individuals who require medical or nursing care or rehabilitation services for the rehabilitation of injured, disabled, or sick persons, or on a regular basis, health related care services above the level of custodial care to other than mentally retarded individuals.
Nursing Monitoring		Nursing Monitoring includes clinical monitoring by a licensed nurse (e.g. serial blood pressure evaluations, medication management, etc.).
Nutrition or Hydration Intervention to Manage Skin Problems		Interventions related to diet, nutrients, and hydration that are provided to prevent or manage specific skin conditions (e.g., wheat-free diet to prevent dermatitis, increased calorie diets to meet basic standards for daily energy requirements, vitamin or mineral supplements for specifically identified deficiencies.)
Occupational Therapy	**OT**	Services that are provided or directly supervised by a licensed occupational therapist. A qualified occupational therapy assistant may provide therapy but not supervise others (aides or volunteers) giving therapy. Includes services provided by a qualified occupational therapy assistant who is employed by (or under contract to) the nursing facility only if he or she is under the direction of a licensed occupational therapist. Occupational therapist and occupational therapy assistant are defined in regulations (42 CFR 484.4). Occupational therapy interventions address deficits in physical, cognitive, psychosocial, sensory, and other aspects of performance in order to support engagement in everyday life activities that affect health, well-being, and quality of life.

(continued)

Term	Abbreviation	Definition
Omnibus Budget Reconciliation Act of 1987	OBRA '87	Law that enacted reforms in nursing facility care and provides the statutory authority for the MDS. The goal is to ensure that residents of nursing facilities receive quality care that will help them to attain or maintain the highest practicable, physical, mental, and psychosocial well-being.
On Admission		On admission is defined as: as close to the actual time of admission as possible.
Oral Lesions		An abnormal area of tissue on the lips, gums, tongue, palate, cheek lining, or throat. This may include ulceration, plaques or patches (e.g. candidiasis), tumors or masses, and color changes (red, white, yellow, or darkened).
Pain Medication Regimen		Pharmacological agent(s) prescribed to relieve or prevent the recurrence of pain. Include all medications used for pain management by any route and any frequency during the look-back period.
Passive Range of Motion		Movement within the unrestricted range of motion for a segment, which is provided entirely by an external force. There is no voluntary muscle contraction. This type of range of motion is often used when a resident is not able to perform the movement at all; no effort is required from them.
Patient Health Questionnaire 9-Item	PHQ-9©	A validated interview that screens for symptoms of depression. It provides a standardized severity score and a rating for evidence of a depressive disorder.
Persistent Vegetative State	PVS	PVS is an enduring situation in which an individual has failed to demonstrate meaningful cortical function but can sustain basic body functions supported by noncortical brain activity.

(continued)

Term	Abbreviation	Definition
Physical Therapy	**PT**	Services that are provided or directly supervised by a licensed physical therapist. A qualified physical therapy assistant may provide therapy but not supervise others (aides or volunteers) giving therapy. Includes services provided by a qualified physical therapy assistant who is employed by (or under contract to) the nursing facility only if he or she is under the direction of a licensed physical therapist. Physical therapist and physical therapist assistant are defined in regulation 42 CFR 484.4. Physical therapists (PTs) are licensed health care professionals who diagnose and manage movement dysfunction and enhance physical and functional status for people of all ages. PTs alleviate impairments and activity limitations and participation restrictions, promote and maintain optimal fitness, physical function, and quality of life, and reduce risk as it relates to movement and health. Following an evaluation of an individual with impairments, activity limitations, and participation restrictions or other health-related conditions, the physical therapist designs an individualized plan of physical therapy care and services for each patient. Physical therapists use a variety of interventions to treat patients. Interventions may include therapeutic exercise, functional training, manual therapy techniques, assistive and adaptive devices and equipment, physical agents, and electrotherapeutic modalities.
Physician Prescribed Weight-loss Regimen		A weight reduction plan ordered by the resident's physician with the care plan goal of weight reduction. May employ a calorie-restricted diet or other weight-loss diets and exercise. Also includes planned diuresis. It is important that weight loss is intentional.
Program Transmittal		Transmittal pages summarize the instructions to providers, emphasizing what has been changed, added, or clarified. They provide background information that would be useful in implementing the instructions. Program Transmittals can be found at the following Web site: http://www.cms.hhs.gov/Transmittals/2010Trans/list.asp
Prompted Voiding		Prompted voiding is a behavioral intervention to maintain or regain urinary continence and may include timed verbal reminders and positive feedback for successful toileting.

(continued)

Term	Abbreviation	Definition
Prospective Payment System	**PPS**	A payment system, developed for Medicare skilled nursing facilities, which pays facilities an all-inclusive rate for all Medicare Part A beneficiary services. Payment is determined by a case mix classification system that categorizes patients by the type and intensity of resources used.
Psychological Therapy		The treatment of mental and emotional disorders through the use of psychological techniques designed to encourage communication of conflicts and insight into problems, with the goal being relief of symptoms, changes in behavior leading to improved social and vocational functioning, and personality growth. Psychological therapy may be provided by a psychiatrist, psychologist, clinical social worker, or clinical nurse specialist in mental health as allowable under applicable state laws.
Psychomotor Retardation		Visibly slowed level of activity or mental processing in residents who are alert. Psychomotor retardation should be differentiated from altered level of consciousness (i.e. stupor) and lethargy.
Quality Improvement and Evaluation System	**QIES**	The umbrella system that encompasses the MDS and Swing Bed (SB)-MDS system, other systems for survey and certification, and home health providers.
Quality Improvement Organization	**QIO**	A program administered by CMS that is designed to monitor and improve utilization and quality of care for Medicare beneficiaries. The program consists of a national network of fifty-three QIOs responsible for each U.S. State, territory, and the District of Columbia. Their mission is to ensure the quality, effectiveness, efficiency, and economy of health care services provided to Medicare beneficiaries.
Quality Measure	**QM**	Information derived from MDS data, that provides a numeric value to quality indicators. These data are available to the public as part of the Nursing Home Quality Initiative (NHQI), and are intended to provide objective measures for consumers to make informed decisions about the quality of care in nursing facilities.

(continued)

Term	Abbreviation	Definition
Recreational Therapy		Services that are provided or directly supervised by a qualified recreational therapist who holds a national certification in recreational therapy, also referred to as a Certified Therapeutic Recreation Specialist." Recreational therapy includes, but is not limited to, providing treatment services and recreation activities to individuals using a variety of techniques, including arts and crafts, animals, sports, games, dance and movement, drama, music, and community outings. Recreation therapists treat and help maintain the physical, mental, and emotional well-being of their clients by seeking to reduce depression, stress, and anxiety; recover basic motor functioning and reasoning abilities; build confidence; and socialize effectively. Recreational therapists should not be confused with recreation workers, who organize recreational activities primarily for enjoyment.
Re-entry		When a resident returns to a facility following a temporary discharge (return anticipated) and returns within 30 days of the discharge.
Registered Nurse Assessment Coordinator	**RNAC**	An individual licensed as a registered nurse by the State Board of Nursing and employed by a nursing facility, and is responsible for coordinating and certifying completion of the resident assessment instrument.
Religion		Belief in and reverence for a supernatural power or powers regarded as creator and governor of the universe. Can be expressed in practice of rituals associated with various religious faiths, attendance and participation in religious services, or in private prayer or religious study.
Resource Use		The measure of the wage-weighted minutes of care used to develop the RUG classification system.
Resource Utilization Group, Version IV	**RUG-IV**	A category-based classification system in which nursing facility residents classify into one of 66 or 57 or 47 RUG-IV groups. Residents in each group utilize similar quantities and patterns of resource. Assignment of a resident to a RUG-IV group is based on certain item responses on the MDS 3.0. Medicare Part A uses the 66-group classification.

(continued)

Term	Abbreviation	Definition
Respiratory Therapy		Services that are provided by a qualified professional (respiratory therapists, respiratory nurse). Respiratory therapy services are for the assessment, treatment, and monitoring of patients with deficiencies or abnormalities of pulmonary function. Respiratory therapy services include coughing, deep breathing, heated nebulizers, aerosol treatments, assessing breath sounds and mechanical ventilation, etc., which must be provided by a respiratory therapist or trained respiratory nurse. A respiratory nurse must be proficient in the modalities listed above either through formal nursing or specific training and may deliver these modalities as allowed under the state Nurse Practice Act and under applicable state laws.
Respite		Short-term, temporary care provided to residents to allow family members to take a break from the daily routine of care giving.
Significant Error		An error in an assessment where the resident's clinical status is not accurately represented (i.e. miscoded) on the erroneous assessment and the error has not been corrected via submission of a more recent assessment.
Skilled Nursing Facility	**SNF**	A facility that is primarily engaged in providing skilled nursing care and related services to individuals who require medical or nursing care or rehabilitation services of injured, disabled, or sick persons.
Sleep Hygiene		Practices, habits, and environmental factors that promote and/or improve sleep patterns.
Social Security Number		A tracking number assigned to an individual by the U.S. Federal government for taxation, benefits, and identification purposes.

(continued)

Term	Abbreviation	Definition
Speech-Language Pathology and Audiology Services		Services that are provided by a licensed speech-language pathologist and/or audiologist. Rehabilitative treatment addresses physical and/or cognitive deficits/disorders resulting in difficulty with communication and/or swallowing (dysphagia). Communication includes speech, language (both receptive and expressive) and non-verbal communication such as facial expression and gesture. Swallowing problems managed under speech therapy are problems in the oral, laryngeal, and/or pharyngeal stages of swallowing. Depending on the nature and severity of the disorder, common treatments may range from physical strengthening exercises, instructive or repetitive practice and drilling, to the use of audio-visual aids and introduction of strategies to facilitate functional communication. Speech therapy may also include sign language and the use of picture symbols. Speech-language pathologist is defined in regulation 42 CFR 484.4.
State Operations Manual	**SOM**	A manual provided by CMS that provides information regarding the how the State comes into compliance with Medicare and Medicaid requirements for survey and certification of all entities and appendices that provides regulatory requirements and related guidance.
State Provider Number		Medicaid Provider Number established by a state.
State Resident Assessment Instrument (RAI) Coordinator		A state agency person who provides information regarding RAI requirements and MDS coding instructions (See Appendix B).
Submission Confirmation Page		The initial feedback generated by the CMS MDS Assessment Submission and Processing System (ASAP) after an MDS data file is electronically submitted. This page acknowledges receipt of the submission file, but does not examine the file for any warnings and/or errors. Warnings and/or errors are provided on the Final Validation Report.
Submission Requirement	**SUB_REQ**	A field in the MDS electronic record that identifies the authority for data collection. CMS has authority to collect assessments for all residents (regardless of their payer source) who reside in Medicare- and/or Medicaid-certified units. States may or may not have regulatory authority to collect assessments for residents in non-certified units.

(continued)

Term	Abbreviation	Definition
Suprapubic Catheter		An indwelling catheter that is placed into the bladder through the abdominal wall above the pubic symphysis.
Swing Bed		A rural hospital with fewer than 100 beds that participates in the Medicare program that has CMS approval to provide post-hospital SNF care. The hospital may use its beds, as needed, to provide either acute or SNF care.
System of Records	**SOR**	Standards for collection and processing of personal information as defined by the Privacy Act of 1974.
Temporal Orientation		In general, the ability to place oneself in correct time. For BIMS, it is the ability to indicate correct date in current surroundings.
Therapeutic Diet		A therapeutic diet is a diet intervention ordered by a health care practitioner as part of the treatment for a disease or clinical condition manifesting an altered nutritional status, to eliminate, decrease, or increase certain substances in the diet (e.g., sodium, potassium) (ADA, 2011)
Tooth Fragment		A remnant of a tooth.
Total Severity Score		A summary of the Patient Health Questionnaire frequency scores that indicates the extent of potential depression symptoms. The score does not diagnose a mood disorder, but provides a standard of communication between clinicians and mental health specialists.
Urostomy		A stoma for the urinary system, intended to bypass the bladder or urethra.
Utilization Guidelines		Instructions concerning when and how to use the RAI. These include instructions for completion of the RAI as well as structured frameworks for synthesizing MDS and other clinical information.
V Codes		A supplementary classification of ICD codes used to describe the circumstances that influence a resident's health status and identify the reasons for medical visits resulting from circumstances other than a disease or injury.

(continued)

Term	Abbreviation	Definition
Vomiting		The forceful expulsion of stomach contents through the mouth or nose.
Worsening in Pressure Ulcer Status		Pressure ulcer "worsening" is defined as a pressure ulcer that has progressed to a deeper level of tissue damage and is therefore staged at a higher number using a numerical scale of 1-4 (using the staging assessment determinations assigned to each stage; starting at the stage 1, and increasing in severity to stage 4) on an assessment as compared to the previous assessment. For the purposes of identifying the absence of a pressure ulcer, zero pressure ulcers is used when there is no skin breakdown or evidence of damage.

Common Acronyms

Acronym	Definition
ADLs	Activities of Daily Living
ADR	Adverse Drug Reaction
AHEs	Average Hourly Earnings
ARD	Assessment Reference Date
ASAP	Assessment Submission and Processing System
BBA-97	Balanced Budget Act of 1997
BBRA	Medicare, Medicaid, and SCHIP Balanced Budget Refinement Act of 1999
BEA	(U.S) Bureau of Economic Analysis
BIMS	Brief Interview for Mental Status
BIPA	Medicare, Medicaid, and SCHIP Benefits Improvement and Protection Act (BIPA) of 2000
BLS	(U.S.) Bureau of Labor Statistics
BMI	Body mass index
CAA	Care Area Assessment
CAH	Critical Access Hospital
CAM	Confusion Assessment Method
CAT	Care Area Trigger
CBSA	Core-Based Statistical Area
CFR	Code of Federal Regulations
CLIA	Clinical Laboratory Improvements Amendments (1998)
CMI	Case Mix Index
CMS	Centers for Medicare and Medicaid Services
CNN	CMS Certification Number
COTA	Certified Occupational Therapist Assistant
CPI	Consumer Price Index
CPI-U	Consumer Price Index for All Urban Consumers
CPS	Cognitive Performance Scale (MDS)
CPT	(Physicians) Current Procedural Terminology
CR	Change Request
CWF	Common Working File
DME	Durable Medical Equipment
DMERC	Durable Medical Equipment Regional Carrier
DOS	Dates of Service
ECI	Employment Cost Index
ESRD	End Stage Renal Disease

Acronym	Definition
FAC_ID	Facility ID (for MDS submission)
FI	Fiscal Intermediary
FMR	Focused Medical Review
FR	Final Rule
FVR	Final Validation Report (MDS submission)
FY	Fiscal Year
HCPCS	Healthcare Common Procedure Coding System
HIPAA	Health Insurance Portability and Accountability Act of 1996
HIPPS	Health Insurance PPS (Rate Codes)
ICD	International Classification of Diseases
ICD-CM	International Classification of Diseases, Clinical Modification
IFC	Interim Final Rule with Comment
IOM	Internet-Only Manual
ISC	Item Set Code
jRAVEN	Java-Based Resident Assessment Validation and Entry System
LOA	Leave of Absence
MAC	Medicare Administrative Contractor
MDCN	Medicare Data Communications Network
MDS	Minimum Data Set
MEDPAR	Medicare Provider Analysis and Review (File)
MIM	Medicare Intermediary Manual
MRI	Magnetic Resonance Imaging
NCS	National Supplier Clearinghouse
NDC	National Drug Code
NDM	Network Data Mover
NF	Nursing Facility
NPI	National Provider Identifier
NSC	National Supplier Clearinghouse
OBRA	Omnibus Budget Reconciliation Act of 1987
OMB	Office of Management and Budget
OMRA	Other Medicare-required Assessment
OT	Occupational Therapy/Therapist
PCE	Personal Care Expenditures
PHQ-9	Patient Health Questionnaire 9-Item
PIM	Program Integrity Manual
POS	Point of Service

Acronym	Definition
PPI	Producer Price Index
PPS	Prospective Payment System
PRM	Provider Reimbursement Manual
PT	Physical Therapy/Therapist
PTA	Physical Therapist Assistant
Pub.100-1	Medicare General Information, Eligibility, and Entitlement IOM
Pub.100-2	Medicare Benefit IOM
Pub.100-4	Medicare Claims Processing IOM
Pub.100-7	Medicare State Operation IOM
Pub.100-8	Medicare Program Integrity IOM
Pub.100-12	State Medicaid IOM
PVS	Persistent Vegetative State
QI	Quality Indicator
QM	Quality Measure
QIES	Quality Improvement and Evaluation System
QIO	Quality Improvement Organization
RAI	Resident Assessment Instrument
RNAC	Registered Nurse Assessment Coordinator
RUG	Resource Utilization Group
SB-PPS	Swing Bed Prospective Payment System
SCSA	Significant Change in Status Assessment
SNF	Skilled Nursing Facility
SNF PPS	Skilled Nursing Facility Prospective Payment System
SLP (or ST)	Speech Language Pathology Services
SOM	State Operations Manual
SOR	Systems of Records
STM	Staff Time Measure
SUB_REQ	Submission Requirement

APPENDIX B: STATE AGENCY AND CMS REGIONAL OFFICE RAI/MDS CONTACTS

Appendix B: State Agency and CMS Regional Office RAI/MDS Contacts is located on the following website: http://www.cms.gov/Medicare/Quality-Initiatives-Patient-Assessment-Instruments/NursingHomeQualityInits/Downloads/MDS30Appendix_B.pdf

APPENDIX C

CARE AREA ASSESSMENT (CAA) RESOURCES

Chapter 4 of this manual provides information on specific care areas triggered and the CAA process. This appendix contains both specific and general resources that nursing homes may choose to use to further assess care areas triggered from the MDS 3.0 resident assessment instrument. The resources include the care area specific tools beginning in this section and the general resource list at the end of this appendix.

It is important to note that the resources provided in this appendix are provided solely as a courtesy for use by nursing homes, should they choose to, in completing the RAI CAA process. **It is also important to reiterate that CMS does not mandate, nor does it endorse, the use of any particular resource(s), including those provided in this appendix.** However, nursing homes should ensure that the resource(s) used are current, evidence-based or expert-endorsed research and clinical practice guidelines/resources.

DISCLAIMER: **The list of resources in this appendix is neither prescriptive nor all-inclusive. References to non-U.S. Department of Health and Human Services (HHS) sources or sites on the Internet are provided as a service and do not constitute or imply endorsement of these organizations or their programs by CMS or HHS. CMS is not responsible for the content of pages found at these sites. URL addresses were current as of the date of this publication.**

CARE AREA SPECIFIC RESOURCES

The specific resources or tools contained on the next several pages are provided by care area. The general instructions for using them include:

Step 1: After completing the MDS, review <u>all</u> MDS items and responses to determine if any care areas have been triggered.

Step 2: For any triggered care area(s), conduct a thorough assessment of the resident using the care area-specific resources.

Step 3: Check the box in the left column if the item is present for this resident. *Some of this information will be on the MDS - some will not.*

Step 4: In the right column the facility can provide a summary of supporting documentation regarding the basis or reason for checking a particular item or items. This could include the location and date of that information, symptoms, possible causal and contributing factor(s) for item(s) checked, etc.

Step 5: Obtain and consider input from resident and/or family/resident's representative regarding the care area.

Step 6: Analyze the findings in the context of their relationship to the care area and standards of practice. This should include a review of indicators and supporting documentation, including symptoms and causal and contributing factors, related to this care area. Draw conclusions about the causal/contributing factors and effect(s) on the resident, and document these conclusions in the Analysis of Findings section.

Step 7: Decide whether referral to other disciplines is warranted and document this decision.

Step 8: In the Care Plan Considerations section, document whether a care plan for the triggered care area will be developed and the reason(s) why or why not.

Step 9: Information in the *Supporting Documentation* column can be used to populate the *Location and Date of CAA Documentation* column in Section V, Item V0200A (CAA Results) – for e.g. "See Delirium CAA 4/30/11, H&P dated 4/18/11."

NOTE: An optional Signature/Date line has been added to each checklist. This was added if the facility wants to document the staff member who completed the checklist and date completed.

DISCLAIMER: **The checklists of care area specific resources in this appendix are not mandated, prescriptive, or all-inclusive and are provided as a service to facilities. They do not constitute or imply endorsement by CMS or HHS.**

TABLE OF CONTENTS

1. DELIRIUM

Review of Indicators of Delirium

✓	Changes in vital signs compared to baseline	Supporting Documentation (Basis/reason for checking the item, including the location, date, and source (if applicable) of that information)
☐	Temperatures 2.4^{0}F higher than baseline or a temperature of 100.4^{0}F (38^{0}C) on admission prior to establishment of baseline. (J1550A)	
☐	Pulse rate less than 60 or greater than 100 beats per minute	
☐	Respiratory rate over 25 breaths per minute or less than 16 per minute (J1100)	
☐	Hypotension or a significant decrease in blood pressure: (I0800)	
☐	• Systolic blood pressure of less than 90 mm Hg, OR	
☐	• Decline of 20 mm Hg or greater in systolic blood pressure from person's usual baseline, OR	
☐	• Decline of 10 mm Hg or greater in diastolic blood pressure from person's usual baseline, OR	
☐	Hypertension - a systolic blood pressure above 160 mm Hg, OR a diastolic blood pressure above 95 mm Hg (I0700)	

✓	Abnormal laboratory values (from clinical record)	
☐	• Electrolytes, such as sodium	
☐	• Kidney function	
☐	• Liver function	
☐	• Blood sugar	
☐	• Thyroid function	
☐	• Arterial blood gases	
☐	• Other	

✓	Pain	
☐	• Pain CAA triggered (J0100, J0200) [review findings for relationship to delirium (C1300)]	
☐	• Pain frequency, intensity, and characteristics (time of onset, duration, quality) (J0400, J0600, J0800, J0850 and clinical record) indicate possible relationship to delirium (C1300)	
☐	• Adverse effect of pain on function (J0500A, J0500B) may be related to delirium (C1300)	

✓	Diseases and conditions (diagnosis/signs/symptoms)	Supporting Documentation (Basis/reason for checking the item, including the location, date, and source (if applicable) of that information)
☐	• Circulatory/Heart — Anemia (I0200) — Cardiac dysrhythmias (I0300) — Angina, Myocardial Infarction (MI) (I0400) — Atherosclerotic Heart Disease (ASHD) (I0400) — Congestive Heart Failure (CHF) pulmonary edema (I0600) — Cerebrovascular Accident (CVA) (I4500) — Transient Ischemic Attack (TIA) (I4500)	
☐	• Respiratory — Asthma (I6200) — Emphysema/Chronic Obstructive Pulmonary Disease (COPD) (I6200) — Shortness of breath (J1100) — Ventilator or respirator (O0100F) — Respiratory Failure (I6300)	
☐	• Infectious — Infections (I1700-I2500) — Wound infection other than on foot or lower extremity (M) (I2500) — Isolation or quarantine for active infectious disease (O0100M)	
☐	• Metabolic — Diabetes (I2900) — Thyroid disease (I3400) — Hyponatremia (I3100)	
☐	• Gastrointestinal bleed (clinical record)	
☐	• Renal disease (I1500), Dialysis (O0100J)	
☐	• Hospice care (O0100K)	
☐	• Cancer (I0100)	
☐	• Dehydration (J1550C, clinical record)	

✓	Signs of Infection (from observation, clinical record)	
☐	• Fever (J1550A)	
☐	• Cloudy or foul smelling urine	
☐	• Congested lungs or cough	
☐	• Dyspnea (J1100)	
☐	• Diarrhea	
☐	• Abdominal pain	
☐	• Purulent wound drainage	
☐	• Erythema (redness) around an incision	

✓	Indicators of Dehydration	Supporting Documentation (Basis/reason for checking the item, including the location, date, and source (if applicable) of that information)
☐	• Dehydration CAA triggered, indicating signs or symptoms of dehydration are present (J1550C)	
☐	• Recent decrease in urine volume or more concentrated urine than usual (I and O) (clinical record)	
☐	• Recent decrease in eating habits – skipping meals or leaving food uneaten, weight loss (K0300)	
☐	• Nausea, vomiting (J1550B), diarrhea, or blood loss	
☐	• Receiving intravenous drugs (O0100H)	
☐	• Receiving diuretics or drugs that may cause electrolyte imbalance (medication administration record)(N0410G)	

✓	Functional Status	
☐	• Recent decline in ADL status (Section G0110) (may be related to delirium) (C1300)	
☐	• Increased risk for falls (J1700) (may be related to delirium) (See Falls CAA)	

✓	Medications (that may contribute to delirium)	
☐	• New medication(s) or dosage increase(s)	
☐	• Drugs with anticholinergic properties (for example, some antipsychotics (N0410A), antidepressants (N0410C), antiparkinsonian drugs, antihistamines)	
☐	• Opioids (narcotic pain drug)	
☐	• Benzodiazepines, especially long-acting agents (N0410B)	
☐	• Analgesics, cardiac and GI medications, anti-inflammatory drugs	
☐	• Recent abrupt discontinuation, omission, or decrease in dose of a short or long acting benzodiazepines (N0410B)	
☐	• Drug interactions (pharmacist review may be required)	
☐	• Resident taking more than one drug from a particular class of drugs	
☐	• Possible drug toxicity, especially if the person is dehydrated (J1550C) or has renal insufficiency (I1500). Check serum drug levels	

✓	Associated or progressive signs and symptoms	Supporting Documentation (Basis/reason for checking the item, including the location, date, and source (if applicable) of that information)
☐	• Sleep disturbances (for example, up and awake at night/asleep during the day) (D0100C, D0500C)	
☐	• Agitation and inappropriate movements (for example, unsafe climbing out of bed or chair, pulling out tubes) (E0500)	
☐	• Hypoactivity (for example, low or lack of motor activity, lethargy or sluggish responses) (D0200D, D0500D)	
☐	• Perceptual disturbances such as hallucinations (E0100A) and delusions (E0100B)	

✓	Other Considerations	
☐	Psychosocial • Recent change in mood; sad or anxious (for example, crying, social withdrawal) (D0200, D0500) • Recent change in social situation (for example, isolation, recent loss of family member or friend) • Use of restraints (P0100, clinical record)	
☐	Physical or environmental factors • Hearing or vision impairment (B0200, B1000) - may have an impact on ability to process information (directions, reminders, environmental cues) • Lack of frequent reorientation, reassurance, reminders to help make sense of things • Recent change in environment (for example, a room or unit change, new admission, or return from hospital) (A1700) • Interference with resident's ability to get enough sleep (for example, light, noise, frequent disruptions) • Noisy or chaotic environment (for example, calling out, loud music, constant commotion, frequent caregiver changes)	

Input from resident and/or family/representative regarding the care area. (Questions/Comments/Concerns/Preferences/Suggestions)

Analysis of Findings		**Care Plan Considerations**
Review indicators and supporting documentation, and draw conclusions. Document: • Description of the problem; • Causes and contributing factors; and • Risk factors related to the care area.	Care Plan Y/N	Document reason(s) care plan will/ will not be developed.

Referral(s) to another discipline(s) is warranted (to whom and why): _____

_____

Information regarding the CAA transferred to the CAA Summary (Section V of the MDS):
☐ Yes   ☐ No

Signature/Title:_____   Date:_____

2. COGNITIVE LOSS/DEMENTIA

<u>Review of Indicators of Cognitive Loss/Dementia</u>

✓	Reversible causes of cognitive loss	Supporting Documentation (Basis/reason for checking the item, including the location, date, and source (if applicable) of that information)
☐	• Delirium (C1300) CAA triggered (Immediate follow-up required. Perform the Delirium CAA to determine possible causes, contributing factors, etc., and go directly to care planning for those issues. Then continue below.)	

✓	Neurological factors	
☐	• Intellectual disability/Developmental Disability (A1550)	
☐	• Alzheimer's Disease or other dementias (I4200, I4800)	
☐	• Parkinson's Disease (I5300)	
☐	• Traumatic brain injury (I5500)	
☐	• Brain tumor (clinical record)	
☐	• Normal pressure hydrocephalus	
☐	• Other (clinical record, I8000)	

✓	Observable characteristics and extent of this resident's cognitive loss	
☐	• Analyze component of Brief Interview for Mental Status (BIMS) (C0200-C0500) (V0100D)	
☐	• If unable to complete BIMS, analyze components of Staff Assessment for Mental Status (C0700, C0800, C0900,C1000)	
☐	• Identify components of Delirium assessment (C1300) that are present and not new onset or worsening	
☐	• Confusion, disorientation, forgetfulness (observation, clinical record) (C0200, C0300, C0400, C0500,C0700, C0800, C0900, C1300, C1600)	
☐	• Decreased ability to make self understood (B0700) or to understand others (B0800)	
☐	• Impulsivity (observation, clinical record)	
☐	• Other (observation, clinical record)	

✓	Mood and behavior	Supporting Documentation (Basis/reason for checking the item, including the location, date, and source (if applicable) of that information)
☐	• Mood State (D0100) CAA triggered. Analysis of Findings indicates possible impact on cognition – important to consider when drawing conclusions about cognitive loss	
☐	• Behavioral Symptoms (E0200) CAA triggered: Analysis of Findings points to cause(s), contributing factors, etc. – important to consider when drawing conclusions about cognitive loss	

✓	Medical problems that can impact cognition	
☐	• Constipation (H0600), fecal impaction, diarrhea	
☐	• Diabetes (I2900)	
☐	• Thyroid Disorder (I3400)	
☐	• Congestive heart failure (I0600)/other cardiac diseases (I0300, I0400)	
☐	• Respiratory problems (I6200, I6300, I2000, I2200, I8000)/decreased oxygen saturation	
☐	• Cancer (I0100)	
☐	• Liver disease (I1100, I2400, I8000, clinical record)	
☐	• Renal failure (I1500)	
☐	• Psychiatric or mood disorder (I5700-I6100)	
☐	• Electrolyte imbalance (clinical record)	
☐	• Poor nutrition (I5600) or hydration status (J1550C) (clinical record)	
☐	• End of life (Hospice O0100K and clinical record)	
☐	• Alcoholism (I8000)	
☐	• Failure to thrive (I8000)	

✓	Pain and its relationship to cognitive loss and behavior	
☐	• Indications that pain is present (J0100, J0300, J0400, J0500, J0600 , J0700, J0800, J0850)	
☐	• Pain CAA triggered. Determine relationship between pain and cognitive status via observation and assessment.	

✓	Functional status and its relationship to cognitive loss	Supporting Documentation (Basis/reason for checking the item, including the location, date, and source (if applicable) of that information)
☐	• Activities of Daily Living (ADL) status (Section G) — ADL Care Area triggered (G0110). Analysis of Findings provides important information about relationship of ADL decline to cognitive loss (C0500, C0700, C0800, C0900, C1000, V0100D) — Resident has potential for more independence with cueing, restorative nursing program, and/or task segmentation or other programs (G0600, O0100 – O0500)	
☐	• Decline in continence (H0300, H0400, clinical record)	
☐	• Impaired daily decision-making (C1000, clinical record)	
☐	• Participates better in small group programs (F0800P, observation, clinical record)	
☐	• Staff and/or resident believe resident is capable of doing more (G0900)	

✓	Other Considerations	
☐	• Cognitive decline occurred slowly over time (V0100D)	
☐	• Unexplainable behavior may be attempt at communication about pain, toileting needs, uncomfortable position, etc.	
☐	• Use of physical restraints (P0100)	
☐	• Hearing or vision impairment (B0200, B0300, B1000, B1200) - may have an impact on ability to process information (directions, reminders, environmental cues)	
☐	• Lack of frequent reorientation, reassurance, reminders to help make sense of things (C0900, C1300)	
☐	• Interference with the resident's ability to get enough sleep (noise, light, etc.) (D0200C, D0500C)	
☐	• Noisy or chaotic environment (for example, calling out, loud music, constant commotion, frequent caregiver changes)	

Input from resident and/or family/representative regarding the care area.
(Questions/Comments/Concerns/Preferences/Suggestions)

Analysis of Findings		**Care Plan Considerations**
Review indicators and supporting documentation, and draw conclusions. Document: • Description of the problem; • Causes and contributing factors; and • Risk factors related to the care area.	Care Plan Y/N	Document reason(s) care plan will/ will not be developed.

Referral(s) to another discipline(s) is warranted (to whom and why): _____

_____

Information regarding the CAA transferred to the CAA Summary (Section V of the MDS):
☐ Yes   ☐ No
Signature/Title:_____ Date:_____

3. VISUAL FUNCTION

Review of Indicators of Visual Function

✓	**Diseases and conditions** of the eye (diagnosis OR signs/symptoms present)	**Supporting Documentation** (Basis/reason for checking the item, including the location, date, and source (if applicable) of that information)
☐	• Cataracts, Glaucoma, or Macular Degeneration (I6500)	
☐	• Diabetic retinopathy (I2900)	
☐	• Blindness (B1000 = 3 or 4)	
☐	• Decreased visual acuity (B1000, B1200 = 1)	
☐	• Visual field deficit (B1200 = 1)	
☐	• Eye pain (J0800)	
☐	• Blurred vision	
☐	• Double vision	
☐	• Sudden loss of vision	
☐	• Itching/burning eye	
☐	• Indications of eye infection (I8000)	

✓	**Diseases and conditions** that can cause visual disturbances	
☐	• Cerebrovascular accident or transient ischemic attack (I4500)	
☐	• Alzheimer's Disease and other dementias (I4200, I4800)	
☐	• Myasthenia gravis (I8000, clinical record)	
☐	• Multiple sclerosis (I5200)	
☐	• Cerebral palsy (I4400)	
☐	• Mood ((I5800, I5900, I5950, I6000, I6100, D0300 or D0600) or anxiety disorder (I5700)	
☐	• Traumatic brain injury (I5500)	
☐	• Other (I8000)	

✓	Functional limitations related to vision problems (from clinical record, resident and staff interviews, direct observation)	Supporting Documentation (Basis/reason for checking the item, including the location, date, and source (if applicable) of that information)
☐	• Peripheral vision or other visual problem that impedes ability to eat, walk, or interact with others (B1000 = 3, 4)	
☐	• Ability to recognize staff limited by vision problem (B1000 = 3, 4)	
☐	• Difficulty negotiating the environment due to vision problem (B1000 = 3, 4)	
☐	• Balance problems (G0300) exacerbated by vision problem (B1000, B1200)	
☐	• Participation in self-care limited by vision problem (B1000)	
☐	• Difficulty seeing television, reading material of interest, or participating in activities of interest because of vision problem (B1000 = 2, 3, 4)	
☐	• Increased risk for falls due to vision problems or due to bifocals or trifocals (B1200 = 1)	

✓	Environment	
☐	• Is resident's environment adapted to his or her unique needs, such as availability of large print books, high wattage reading lamp, night light, etc.?	
☐	• Are there aspects the facility's environment that should be altered to enhance vision, such as low-glare floors, low glare tables and surfaces, large print signs marking rooms, etc.?	

✓	Medications that can impair vision (consultant pharmacist review of medication regimen can be very helpful)	
☐	• Narcotics	
☐	• Antipsychotics (N0410A)	
☐	• Antidepressants (N0410C)	
☐	• Anticholinergics	
☐	• Hypnotics (N0410D)	
☐	• Other	

✓	Use of visual appliances (B1200)	
☐	• Reading glasses	
☐	• Distance glasses	
☐	• Contact lenses	
☐	• Magnifying glass	

Input from resident and/or family/representative regarding the care area. (Questions/Comments/Concerns/Preferences/Suggestions)

Analysis of Findings		**Care Plan Considerations**
Review indicators and supporting documentation, and draw conclusions. Document: • Description of the problem; • Causes and contributing factors; and • Risk factors related to the care area.	Care Plan Y/N	Document reason(s) care plan will/ will not be developed.

Referral(s) to another discipline(s) is warranted (to whom and why): _____

_____

Information regarding the CAA transferred to the CAA Summary (Section V of the MDS):
☐ Yes   ☐ No
Signature/Title:_____ Date:_____

4.   COMMUNICATION

Review of Indicators of Communication

✓	**Diseases and conditions** that may be related to communication problems	**Supporting Documentation** (Basis/reason for checking the item, including the location, date, and source (if applicable) of that information)
☐	• Alzheimer's Disease or other dementias (I4200, I4800, I8000)	
☐	• Aphasia (I4300) following a cerebrovascular accident (I4500)	
☐	• Parkinson's disease (I5300)	
☐	• Mental health problems (I5700 – I6100)	
☐	• Conditions that can cause voice production deficits, such as	
☐	— Asthma (I6200)	
☐	— Emphysema/COPD (I6200)	
☐	— Cancer (I0100)	
	— Poor-fitting dentures (L0200)	
☐	• Transitory conditions, such as	
☐	— Delirium (C1300, I8000, clinical record)	
☐	— Infection (I1700 – I2500)	
	— Acute illness (I8000, clinical record)	
☐	• Other (I8000, clinical record)	

✓	**Medications** (consultant pharmacist review of medication regimen can be very helpful)	
☐	• Narcotic analgesics (medication administration record)	
☐	• Antipsychotics (N0410A)	
☐	• Antianxiety (N0410B)	
☐	• Antidepressants (N0410C)	
☐	• Parkinson's medications (medication administration record)	
☐	• Hypnotics (N0410D)	
☐	• Gentamycin (N0410F) (medication administration record)	
☐	• Tobramycin(N0410F) (medication administration record)	
☐	• Aspirin (medication administration record)	
☐	• Other (clinical record)	

✓	Characteristics of the communication impairment (from clinical record)	Supporting Documentation (Basis/reason for checking the item, including the location, date, and source (if applicable) of that information)
☐	• Expressive communication (B0700)	
☐	— Speaks different language (A1100)	
☐	— Disruption in ability to speak (B0600, clinical record)	
☐	— Problem with voice production, low volume (B0600, clinical record)	
☐	— Word-finding problems (clinical record)	
☐	— Difficulty putting sentence together (B0700, C1300B, clinical record)	
☐	— Problem describing objects and events (B0700, clinical record)	
☐	— Pronouncing words incorrectly (B0600, clinical record)	
☐	— Stuttering (B0700, clinical record)	
☐	— Hoarse or distorted voice (clinical record)	
☐	• Receptive communication (B0800)	
☐	— Does not understand English (A1100)	
☐	— Hearing impairment (B0200, B0300 = 1, B0800)	
☐	— Speech discrimination problems (clinical record)	
☐	— Decreased vocabulary comprehension (clinical record) (A1100A-B)	
☐	— Difficulty reading and interpreting facial expressions (clinical record, direct observation)	
☐	• Communication is more successful with some individuals than with others. Identify and build on the successful approaches (clinical record, interviews, observation)	
☐	• Limited opportunities for communication due to social isolation or need for communication devices (clinical record, interviews)	
☐	• Communication problem may be mistaken as cognitive impairment	

✓	**Confounding problems** that may need to be resolved before communication will improve	**Supporting Documentation** (Basis/reason for checking the item, including the location, date, and source (if applicable) of that information)
☐	• Decline in cognitive status (clinical record) and BIMS decline (C0500, V0100D)	
☐	• Mood problem, increase in PHQ-9 score (D0300, D0600, V0100E)	
☐	• Increased dependence in Activities of Daily Living (ADLs) (clinical record, changes in G0110, G0120)	
☐	• Deterioration in respiratory status (clinical record)	
☐	• Oral motor function problems, such as swallowing, clarity of voice production (B0600, K0100, clinical record)	

✓	**Use of communication devices** (from clinical record, observation)	
☐	• Hearing aid (B0300)	
☐	• Written communication	
☐	• Sign language	
☐	• Braille	
☐	• Signs, gestures, sounds	
☐	• Communication board	
☐	• Electronic assistive devices	
☐	• Other	

Input from resident and/or family/representative regarding the care area. (Questions/Comments/Concerns/Preferences/Suggestions)

Analysis of Findings	Care Plan Y/N	Care Plan Considerations
Review indicators and supporting documentation, and draw conclusions. Document: • Description of the problem; • Causes and contributing factors; and • Risk factors related to the care area.		Document reason(s) care plan will/ will not be developed.

Referral(s) to another discipline(s) is warranted (to whom and why): _____

_____

Information regarding the CAA transferred to the CAA Summary (Section V of the MDS):
☐ Yes   ☐ No

Signature/Title:_____   Date:_____

5. ACTIVITIES OF DAILY LIVING (ADLs) – FUNCTIONAL STATUS/REHABILITATION POTENTIAL

Review of Indicators of ADLs - Functional Status/Rehabilitation Potential

✓	**Possible underlying problems** that may affect function. Some may be reversible.	**Supporting Documentation** (Basis/reason for checking the item, including the location, date, and source (if applicable) of that information)
☐	• Delirium (C1300) (clinical record and Delirium CAA)	
☐	• Acute episode or flare-up of chronic condition (I8000, clinical record)	
☐	• Changing cognitive status (C0100) (see Cognitive Loss CAA)	
☐	• Mood decline (D0100)(clinical record and Mood State CAA)	
☐	• Daily behavioral symptoms/decline in behavior(E0200) (see Behavioral Symptoms CAA)	
☐	• Use of physical restraints(P0100) (See Physical Restraints CAA)	
☐	• Pneumonia (I2000)	
☐	• Fall(J1700) (from record and Falls CAA)	
☐	• Hip fracture (I3900)	
☐	• Recent hospitalization (clinical record) (A1700, A1800= 3, 4)	
☐	• Fluctuating ADLs (G0110A-J, G0120, G0300A-E, G0900) (observation, clinical record)	
☐	• Nutritional problems (K0510A1, K0510A2) (clinical record and Nutrition CAA)	
☐	• Pain(J0700) (See Pain CAA)	
☐	• Dizziness	
☐	• Communication problems (B0200, B0700, B0800) (clinical record and Communication CAA)	
☐	• Vision problems(B1000) (observation, interview, clinical record, and Vision CAA)	

✓	**Abnormal laboratory values** (from clinical record)	
☐	• Electrolytes	
☐	• Complete blood count	
☐	• Blood sugar	
☐	• Thyroid function	
☐	• Arterial blood gases	
☐	• Other	

		Supporting Documentation (Basis/reason for checking the item, including the location, date, and source (if applicable) of that information)
✓	**Medications** that can contribute to functional decline	
☐	• Psychoactive medications (N0410A-D)	
☐	• Other medications – ask consultant pharmacist to review medication regimen to identify these medications	

✓	**Limiting factors** resulting in need for assistance with any of the ADLs (observation, interview, clinical record)	
☐	• Mental errors such as sequencing problems, incomplete performance, or anxiety limitations	
☐	• Physical limitations such as weakness (G0110A–J.1 = 2,3, 4) (G0110 A-J.2 = 2, 3), limited range of motion (G0400A = 1, 2, G0400B = 1, 2), poor coordination, poor balance (G0300A-E =2), visual impairment (B1000 = 1-4), or pain (J0300 = 1, J0700 =1)	
☐	• Facility conditions such as policies, rules, or physical layout	

✓	**Problems resident is at risk for** because of functional decline (from observation, assessment, clinical record)	
☐	• Falls (J1700)	
☐	• Weight loss (K0300)	
☐	• Unidentified pain (J0700)	
☐	• Social isolation	
☐	• Restraint use (P0100)	
☐	• Depression(D0100)	
☐	• Complications of immobility, such as — Pressure ulcers (M0210) — Muscular atrophy — Contractures (G0400 A, B = 1, 2) — Incontinence (H0300, H0400) — Urinary (I2300) and respiratory infections	

Input from resident and/or family/representative regarding the care area.
(Questions/Comments/Concerns/Preferences/Suggestions)

Analysis of Findings		**Care Plan Considerations**
Review indicators and supporting documentation, and draw conclusions. Document: • Description of the problem; • Causes and contributing factors; and • Risk factors related to the care area.	Care Plan Y/N	Document reason(s) care plan will/ will not be developed.

Referral(s) to another discipline(s) is warranted (to whom and why): _____

_____

Information regarding the CAA transferred to the CAA Summary (Section V of the MDS):
☐ Yes   ☐ No

Signature/Title:_____ Date:_____

Where rehabilitation goals are envisioned, use of the ***ADL Supplement*** will help care planners to focus on those areas that might be improved, allowing them to choose from among a number of basic tasks in designated areas. Part 1 of the supplement can assist in the evaluation of all residents that trigger this care area. Part 2 of the supplement can be helpful for residents with rehabilitation potential (ADL Triggers A), to help plan a treatment program.

ADL SUPPLEMENT
(Attaining maximum possible Independence)

PART 1: ADL Problem Evaluation

INSTRUCTIONS:
For those triggered -
In areas physical help provided, indicate reason(s) for this help.

	DRESSING	BATHING	TOILETING	LOCOMOTION	TRANSFER	EATING
Mental Errors: Sequencing problems, incomplete performance, anxiety limitations, etc.						
Physical Limitations: Weakness, limited range of motion, poor coordination, visual impairment, pain, etc.						
Facility Conditions: Policies, rules, physical layout, etc.						

PART 2: Possible ADL Goals

INSTRUCTIONS:
For those considered for rehabilitation or decline prevention treatment -

If wheelchair, check: ☐

Indicate specific type of ADL activity that might require:
1. Maintenance to prevent decline.
2. Treatment to achieve highest practical self-sufficiency (selecting ADL abilities that are just above those the resident can now perform or participate in).

DRESSING	BATHING	TOILETING	LOCOMOTION	TRANSFER	EATING
Locates/ selects/ obtains clothes	Goes to tub/ shower	Goes to toilet (include commode/ urinal at night)	Walks in room/ nearby ☐	Positions self in preparation	Opens/ pours/ unwraps/ cuts etc.
Grasps/puts on upper lower body	Turns on water/ adjusts temperature	Removes/ opens clothes in preparation	Walks on unit ☐	Approaches chair/bed	Grasps utensils and cups
Manages snaps, zippers, etc.	Lathers body (except back)	Transfers/ positions self	Walks throughout building (uses elevator) ☐	Prepares chair/bed (locks pad, moves covers)	Scoops/ spears food (uses fingers when necessary)
Puts on in correct order	Rinses body	Eliminates into toilet	Walks outdoors ☐	Transfers (stands/sits/ lifts/turns)	Chews, drinks, swallows
Grasps, removes each item	Dries with towel	Tears/uses paper to clean self	Walks on uneven surfaces ☐	Repositions/ arranges self	Repeats until food consumed
Replaces clothes properly	Other	Flushes	Other ☐	Other	Uses napkins, cleans self
Other		Adjusts clothes, washes hands			Other

6.   URINARY INCONTINENCE AND INDWELLING CATHETER

Review of Indicators of Urinary Incontinence and Indwelling Catheter

✓	Modifiable factors contributing to transitory urinary incontinence	Supporting Documentation (Basis/reason for checking the item, including the location, date, and source (if applicable) of that information)
☐	• Delirium (C1300) (See Delirium CAA)	
☐	• Urinary Tract Infection (I2300)	
☐	• Atrophic vaginitis in postmenopausal women (I8000)	
☐	• Medications (see below)	
☐	• Psychological or psychiatric problems (I5700-I6100)	
☐	• Constipation/impaction (H0600, clinical record)	
☐	• Caffeine use	
☐	• Excessive fluid intake	
☐	• Pain (J0300)	
☐	• Environmental factors	
☐	— Restricted mobility (G0110.1.A-F. = 2, 3,4)(G0110.2.A-F.=2, 3) (See ADL CAA)	
☐	— Lack of access to a toilet	
☐	— Other environmental barriers (such as pads or briefs)	
☐	— Restraints (P0100)	

✓	Other factors that contribute to incontinence or catheter use	
☐	• Excessive or inadequate urine output	
☐	• Urinary urgency AND need for assistance in toileting (G0110.1.I = 2, 3, 4)	
☐	• Bladder cancer (I0100) or stones (I8000)	
☐	• Spinal cord or brain lesions (I8000)	
☐	• Tabes dorsalis (I8000)	
☐	• Neurogenic bladder (I1550)	

✓	Laboratory tests	
☐	• High serum calcium	
☐	• High blood glucose	
☐	• Low B12	
☐	• High BUN or creatinine	

✓	Diseases and conditions	Supporting Documentation (Basis/reason for checking the item, including the location, date, and source (if applicable) of that information)
☐	• Benign prostatic hypertrophy (I1400)	
☐	• Congestive Heart Failure (CHF), pulmonary edema (I0600)	
☐	• Cerebrovascular Accident (CVA) (I4500)	
☐	• Transient Ischemic Attack (TIA) (I4500)	
☐	• Diabetes (I2900)	
☐	• Depression (I5800)	
☐	• Parkinson's disease (I5300)	
☐	• Prostate cancer (I0100)	

✓	Type of incontinence	
☐	• Stress (occurs with coughing, sneezing, laughing, lifting heavy objects, etc.)	
☐	• Urge (overactive or spastic bladder)	
☐	• Mixed (stress incontinence with urgency)	
☐	• Overflow (due to blocked urethra or weak bladder muscles)	
☐	• Transient (temporary/occasional related to a potentially improvable/reversible cause)	
☐	• Functional (can't get to toilet in time due to physical disability, external obstacles, or problems thinking or communicating)	

✓	Medications (from medication administration record and preadmission records if new admission; review by consultant pharmacist)	
☐	• Diuretics(N0410G)– can cause urge incontinence	
☐	• Sedative hypnotics (N0410B, N0410D)	
☐	• Anticholinergics – can lead to overflow incontinence — Parkinson's medications (except Sinemet and Deprenyl) — Disopyramide — Antispasmodics — Antihistamines — Antipsychotics (N0410A) — Antidepressants (N0410C) — Narcotics	
☐	• Drugs that stimulate or block sympathetic nervous system	
☐	• Calcium channel blockers	

✓	Use of indwelling catheter (H0100 is checked): (Presence of situation in which catheter use *may* be appropriate intervention after consideration of risks/benefits and after efforts to avoid catheter use have been unsuccessful	Supporting Documentation (Basis/reason for checking the item, including the location, date, and source (if applicable) of that information)
☐	• Coma (B0100)	
☐	• Terminal illness (O0100K)	
☐	• Stage 3 or 4 pressure ulcer in area affected by incontinence	
☐	• Need for exact measurement of urine output	
☐	• History of inability to void after catheter removal	

Input from resident and/or family/representative regarding the care area. (Questions/Comments/Concerns/Preferences/Suggestions)

Analysis of Findings		Care Plan Considerations
Review indicators and supporting documentation, and draw conclusions. Document: • Description of the problem; • Causes and contributing factors; and • Risk factors related to the care area.	Care Plan Y/N	Document reason(s) care plan will/ will not be developed.

Referral(s) to another discipline(s) is warranted (to whom and why): _____

_____

Information regarding the CAA transferred to the CAA Summary (Section V of the MDS):
□ Yes   □ No

Signature/Title:_____ Date:_____

7.   PSYCHOSOCIAL WELL-BEING

Review of Indicators of Psychosocial Well-Being

✓	Modifiable factors for relationship problems (from resident, family, staff interviews and clinical record)	Supporting Documentation (Basis/reason for checking the item, including the location, date, and source (if applicable) of that information)
☐	• Resident says or indicates he or she feels lonely — Recent decline in social involvement and associated loneliness can be sign of acute health complications and depression	
☐	• Resident indicates he or she feels distressed because of decline in social activities	
☐	• Over the past few years, resident has experienced absence of daily exchanges with relatives and friends	
☐	• Resident is uneasy dealing with others	
☐	• Resident has conflicts with family, friends, roommate, other residents, or staff	
☐	• Resident appears preoccupied with the past and unwilling to respond to needs of the present	
☐	• Resident seems unable or reluctant to begin to establish a social role in the facility; may be grieving lost status or roles	
☐	• Recent change in family situation or social network, such as death of a close family member or friend	

✓	Customary lifestyle (from resident, family, staff interviews and clinical record) (Section F)	
☐	• Was lifestyle more satisfactory to the resident prior to admission to the nursing home?	
☐	• Are current psychosocial/relationship problems consistent with resident's long-standing lifestyle or is this relatively new for the resident?	
☐	• Has facility care plan to date been as consistent as possible with resident's prior lifestyle, preferences, and routines (F0400, F0600, F0800)?	

CMS's RAI Version 3.0 Manual

Appendix C: CAA Resources
7. Psychosocial Well-Being

✓	**Diseases and conditions** that may impede ability to interact with others	**Supporting Documentation** (Basis/reason for checking the item, including the location, date, and source (if applicable) of that information)
☐	• Delirium (C1300, C1600 = 1, Delirium CAA)	
☐	• Intellectual disability /developmental disability (A1550)	
☐	• Alzheimer's disease (I4200)	
☐	• Aphasia (I4300)	
☐	• Other dementia (I4800)	
☐	• Depression (I5800)	

✓	**Health status factors** that may inhibit social involvement	
☐	• Decline in activities of daily living (G0110)	
☐	• Health problem, such as falls (J1700, J1800), pain (J0300, J0800), fatigue, etc.	
☐	• Mood (D0200A1, D0300, D0500A1, D0600) or behavior (E0200) problem that impacts interpersonal relationships or that arises because of social isolation (See Mood State and Behavioral Symptoms CAAs)	
☐	• Change in communication (B0700, B0800), vision (B1000), hearing (B0200), cognition (C0100, C0600)	
☐	• Medications with side effects that interfere with social interactions, such as incontinence, diarrhea, delirium, or sleepiness	

✓	**Environmental factors** that may inhibit social involvement	
☐	• Use of physical restraints (P0100)	
☐	• Change in residence leading to loss of autonomy and reduced self-esteem (A1700)	
☐	• Change in room assignment or dining location or table mates	
☐	• Living situation limits informal social interaction, such as isolation precautions (O0100M)	

April 2012

Appendix C-30

✓	**Strengths** to build upon (from resident, family, staff interviews and clinical record)	**Supporting Documentation** (Basis/reason for checking the item, including the location, date, and source (if applicable) of that information)
☐	• Activities in which resident appears especially at ease interacting with others	
☐	• Certain situations appeal to resident more than others, such as small groups or 1:1 interactions rather than large groups	
☐	• Certain individuals who seem to bring out a more positive, optimistic side of the resident	
☐	• Positive traits that distinguished the resident as an individual prior to his or her illness	
☐	• What gave the resident a sense of satisfaction earlier in his or her life?	

Input from resident and/or family/representative regarding the care area. (Questions/Comments/Concerns/Preferences/Suggestions)	

Analysis of Findings		Care Plan Considerations
Review indicators and supporting documentation, and draw conclusions. Document: • Description of the problem; • Causes and contributing factors; and • Risk factors related to the care area.	Care Plan Y/N	Document reason(s) care plan will/ will not be developed.

Referral(s) to another discipline(s) is warranted (to whom and why): _____
_____

Information regarding the CAA transferred to the CAA Summary (Section V of the MDS):
☐ Yes   ☐ No

Signature/Title:_____ Date:_____

8.   MOOD STATE

Review of Indicators of Mood

✓	Psychosocial changes	Supporting Documentation (Basis/reason for checking the item, including the location, date, and source (if applicable) of that information)
☐	• Personal loss	
☐	• Recent move into or within the nursing home (A1700)	
☐	• Recent change in relationships, such as illness or loss of a relative or friend	
☐	• Recent change in health perception, such as perception of being seriously ill or too ill to return home (Q0300 - Q0600)	
☐	• Clinical or functional change that may affect the resident's dignity, such as new or worsening incontinence, communication, or decline	

✓	Clinical issues that can cause or contribute to a mood problem	
☐	• Relapse of an underlying mental health problem (I5700 – I6100)	
☐	• Psychiatric disorder (anxiety, depression, manic depression, schizophrenia, post-traumatic stress disorder) (I5700 – I6100)	
☐	• Alzheimer's disease (I4200)	
☐	• Delirium (C1600)	
☐	• Delusions (E0100B)	
☐	• Hallucinations (E0100A)	
☐	• Communication problems (B0700, B0800)	
☐	• Decline in Activities of Daily Living (ADLs) (G0110, clinical record)	
☐	• Infection (I1700 – I2500, clinical record)	
☐	• Pain (J0300 or J0800)	
☐	• Cardiac disease (I0200 – I0900)	
☐	• Thyroid abnormality (I3400)	
☐	• Dehydration (J1550C, clinical record)	
☐	• Metabolic disorder (I2900 – I3400)	
☐	• Neurological disease (I4200 – I5500)	
☐	• Recent cerebrovascular accident (I4500)	
☐	• Dementia, cognitive decline (I4800, clinical record)	
☐	• Cancer (I0100)	
☐	• Other (I8000)	

✓	Medications (from medication administration record and preadmission records if new admission)	Supporting Documentation (Basis/reason for checking the item, including the location, date, and source (if applicable) of that information)
☐	• Antibiotics (N0410F)	
☐	• Anticholinergics	
☐	• Antihypertensives	
☐	• Anticonvulsants	
☐	• Antipsychotics (N0410A)	
☐	• Cardiac medications	
☐	• Cimetidine	
☐	• Clonidine	
☐	• Chemotherapeutic agents	
☐	• Digitalis	
☐	• Other	
☐	• Glaucoma medications	
☐	• Guanethidine	
☐	• Immuno-suppressive medications	
☐	• Methyldopa	
☐	• Narcotics	
☐	• Nitrates	
☐	• Propranolol	
☐	• Reserpine	
☐	• Steroids	
☐	• Stimulants	

✓	Laboratory tests	
☐	• Serum calcium	
☐	• Thyroid function	
☐	• Blood glucose	
☐	• Potassium	
☐	• Porphyria	

Input from resident and/or family/representative regarding the care area.
(Questions/Comments/Concerns/Preferences/Suggestions)

Analysis of Findings		**Care Plan Considerations**
Review indicators and supporting documentation, and draw conclusions. Document: • Description of the problem; • Causes and contributing factors; and • Risk factors related to the care area.	Care Plan Y/N	Document reason(s) care plan will/ will not be developed.

Referral(s) to another discipline(s) is warranted (to whom and why): _____

_____

Information regarding the CAA transferred to the CAA Summary (Section V of the MDS):
☐ Yes ☐ No

Signature/Title:_____ Date:_____

9. BEHAVIORAL SYMPTOMS

Review of Indicators of Behavioral Symptoms

✓	Seriousness of the behavioral symptoms (E0300, E0800, E0900, E1100)	Supporting Documentation (Basis/reason for checking the item, including the location, date, and source (if applicable) of that information)
☐	• Resident is immediate threat to self – IMMEDIATE INTERVENTION REQUIRED (D0200I.1=1, D0500I.1=1, E1000 = 1)	
☐	• Resident is immediate threat to others – IMMEDIATE INTERVENTION REQUIRED (E0600A)	

✓	Nature of the behavioral disturbance (resident interview, if possible; staff observations)	
☐	• Provoked or unprovoked	
☐	• Offensive or defensive	
☐	• Purposeful	
☐	• Occurs during specific activities, such as bath or transfers	
☐	• Pattern, such as certain times of the day, or varies over time	
☐	• Others in the vicinity are involved	
☐	• Reaction to a particular action, such as being physically moved	
☐	• Resident appears to startle easily	

✓	**Medication side effects** that can cause behavioral symptoms (from medication records)	**Supporting Documentation** (Basis/reason for checking the item, including the location, date, and source (if applicable) of that information)
☐	• New medication	
☐	• Change in dosage	
☐	• Antiparkinsonian drugs - may cause hypersexuality, socially inappropriate behavior	
☐	• Sedatives, centrally active antihypertensives, some cardiac drugs, anticholinergic agents can cause paranoid delusions, delirium	
☐	• Bronchodilators or other respiratory drugs, which can increase agitation and cause difficulty sleeping	
☐	• Caffeine	
☐	• Nicotine	
☐	• Medications that impair impulse control, such as benzodiazepines, sedatives, alcohol (or any product containing alcohol, such as some cough medicine)	

✓	**Illness or conditions** that can cause behavior problems	
☐	• Long-standing mental health problem associated with the behavioral disturbances, such as schizophrenia, bipolar disorder, depression, anxiety disorder, post-traumatic stress disorder (I5700 – I6100)	
☐	• New or acute physical health problem or flare-up of a known chronic condition (I8000)	
☐	• Delusions (E0100B)	
☐	• Hallucinations (E0100A)	
☐	• Paranoia (from record)	
☐	• Constipation (H0600)	
☐	• Congestive heart failure (I0600)	
☐	• Infection (I1700 – I2500)	
☐	• Head injury (I5500, clinical record)	
☐	• Diabetes (I2900)	
☐	• Pain (J0300, J0800)	
☐	• Fever (J1550A, clinical record)	
☐	• Dehydration (J1550C, clinical record; see Dehydration CAA)	

✓	Factors that can cause or exacerbate the behavior (from observation, interview, record)	Supporting Documentation (Basis/reason for checking the item, including the location, date, and source (if applicable) of that information)
☐	• Frustration due to problem communicating discomfort or unmet need	
☐	• Frustration, agitation due to need to urinate or have bowel movement	
☐	• Fear due to not recognizing caregiver	
☐	• Fear due to not recognizing the environment or misinterpreting the environment or actions of others	
☐	• Major unresolved sources of interpersonal conflict between the resident and family members, other residents, or staff (see Psychosocial Well-Being CAA)	
☐	• Recent change, such as new admission (A1700) or a new unit, assignment of new care staff, or withdrawal from a treatment program	
☐	• Departure from normal routines	
☐	• Sleep disturbance (D0500C = 1)	
☐	• Noisy, crowded area	
☐	• Dimly lit area	
☐	• Sensory impairment, such as hearing or vision problem (B0200, B1000)	
☐	• Restraints (P0100)	
☐	• Fatigue (D0500D = 1)	
☐	• Need for repositioning (M1200)	

✓	Cognitive status problems (also see Cognitive Loss CAT/CAA)	
☐	• Delirium (C1300), clinical record (Delirium CAT)	
☐	• Dementia (I4800)	
☐	• Recent cognitive loss (clinical record, interviews with family, etc.)	
☐	• Alzheimer's disease (I4200)	
☐	• Effects of cerebrovascular accident (I4500)	

✓	Other Considerations	Supporting Documentation (Basis/reason for checking the item, including the location, date, and source (if applicable) of that information)
☐	• May be communicating discomfort, personal needs, preferences, fears, feeling ill	
☐	• Persons exhibiting long-standing problem behaviors related to psychiatric conditions may place others in danger of physical assault, intimidation, or embarrassment and place themselves at increased risk of being stigmatized, isolated, abused, and neglected by loved ones or care givers	
☐	• The actions and responses of family members and caregivers can aggravate or even cause behavioral outbursts	

Input from resident and/or family/representative regarding the care area.
(Questions/Comments/Concerns/Preferences/Suggestions)

Analysis of Findings		**Care Plan Considerations**
Review indicators and supporting documentation, and draw conclusions. Document: • Description of the problem; • Causes and contributing factors; and • Risk factors related to the care area.	Care Plan Y/N	Document reason(s) care plan will/ will not be developed.

Referral(s) to another discipline(s) is warranted (to whom and why): _____

_____

Information regarding the CAA transferred to the CAA Summary (Section V of the MDS):
☐ Yes   ☐ No

Signature/Title:_____ Date:_____

10.   ACTIVITIES

Review of Indicators of Activities

✓	Activity preferences prior to admission (from interviews and clinical record)	Supporting Documentation (Basis/reason for checking the item, including the location, date, and source (if applicable) of that information)
☐	• Passive	
☐	• Active	
☐	• Outside the home	
☐	• Inside the home	
☐	• Centered almost entirely on family activities	
☐	• Centered almost entirely on non-family activities	
☐	• Group (F0500E) activities	
☐	• Solitary activities	
☐	• Involved in community service, volunteer activities	
☐	• Athletic	
☐	• Non-athletic	

✓	Current activity pursuits (from interviews and clinical record)	
☐	• Resident identifies leisure activities of interest	
☐	• Self-directed or done with others and/or planned by others	
☐	• Activities resident pursues when visitors are present	
☐	• Scheduled programs in which resident participates	
☐	• Activities of interest not currently available or offered to the resident	

✓	**Health issues** that result in reduced activity participation	**Supporting Documentation** (Basis/reason for checking the item, including the location, date, and source (if applicable) of that information)
☐	• Indicators of depression or anxiety (D0200, D0300, D0500, D0600)	
☐	• Use of psychoactive medications (N0410A-N0410D)	
☐	• Functional/mobility (G0110) or balance (G0300) problems; physical disability (G0300, G0400)	
☐	• Cognitive deficits (C0500, C0700-C1000), including stamina, ability to express self (B0700), understand others (B0800), make decisions (C1000)	
☐	• Unstable acute/chronic health problem (clinical record, O0100, J0100, J1100, J0700, J1400, J1550, I8000, M1040, M1200)	
☐	• Chronic health conditions, such as incontinence (H0300, H0400) or pain (J0300)	
☐	• Embarrassment or unease due to presence of equipment (O0100D, E, F), such as tubes, oxygen tank (O0100C), or colostomy bag (H0100) (observation, clinical record)	
☐	• Receives numerous treatments (O0100, O0400) that limit available time/energy (clinical record)	
☐	• Performs tasks slowly due to reduced energy reserves (observation, clinical record)	

✓	**Environmental or staffing issues** that hinder participation	
☐	• Physical barriers that prevent the resident from gaining access to the space where the activity is held (observation)	
☐	• Need for additional staff responsible for social activities (observation)	
☐	• Lack of staff time to involve residents in current activity programs (observation)	
☐	• Resident's fragile nature results in feelings of intimidation by staff responsible for the activity (from observation, interviews, clinical record)	

✓	**Unique skills or knowledge** the resident has that he or she could pass on to others (from interviews and clinical record)	**Supporting Documentation** (Basis/reason for checking the item, including the location, date, and source (if applicable) of that information)
☐	• Games	
☐	• Complex tasks such as knitting, or computer skills	
☐	• Topic that might interest others	

✓	**Issues** that result in reduced activity participation	
☐	• Resident is new to facility or has been in facility long enough to become bored with status quo (interview, clinical record)	
☐	• Psychosocial well-being issues, such as shyness, initiative, and social involvement	
☐	• Socially inappropriate behavior (E0200)	
☐	• Indicators of psychosis (E0100A-E0100C)	
☐	• Feelings of being unwelcome, due to issues such as those already involved in an activity drawing boundaries that are difficult to cross (observation, interview, clinical record)	
☐	• Limited opportunities for resident to get to know others through activities such as shared dining, afternoon refreshments, monthly birthday parties, reminiscence groups (observation, facility activity calendar)	
☐	• Available activities do not correspond to resident's values, attitudes, expectations (interview, clinical record) (F0500, F0800)	
☐	• Long history of unease in joining with others (interview, clinical record)	

<table>
<tr><td colspan="2" align="center">**Input from resident and/or family/representative regarding the care area.**
(Questions/Comments/Concerns/Preferences/Suggestions)</td></tr>
<tr><td colspan="2">

</td></tr>
</table>

Analysis of Findings		Care Plan Considerations
Review indicators and supporting documentation, and draw conclusions. Document: • Description of the problem; • Causes and contributing factors; and • Risk factors related to the care area.	Care Plan Y/N	Document reason(s) care plan will/ will not be developed.

Referral(s) to another discipline(s) is warranted (to whom and why): _____

_____

Information regarding the CAA transferred to the CAA Summary (Section V of the MDS):
☐ Yes   ☐ No

Signature/Title:_____   Date:_____

11.   FALL(S)

Review of Indicators of Fall Risk

✓	History of falling (J1700, J1800, J1900)	Supporting Documentation (Basis/reason for checking the item, including the location, date, and source (if applicable) of that information)
☐	• Time of day, exact hour of the fall(s)	
☐	• Location of the fall(s), such as bedroom, bathroom, hallway, stairs, outside, etc.	
☐	• Related to specific medication	
☐	• Proximity to most recent meal	
☐	• Responding to bowel or bladder urgency	
☐	• Doing usual/unusual activity	
☐	• Standing still or walking	
☐	• Reaching up or reaching down	
☐	• Identify the conclusions about the root cause(s), contributing factors related to previous falls	

✓	Physical performance limitations: balance, gait, strength, muscle endurance (G0300A-G0300E)	
☐	• Difficulty maintaining sitting balance	
☐	• Need to rock body or push off on arms of chair when standing up from chair	
☐	• Difficulty maintaining standing position	
☐	• Impaired balance during transitions (G0300A-G0300E)	
☐	• Gait problem, such as unsteady gait, even with mobility aid or personal assistance, slow gait, takes small steps, takes rapid steps, or lurching gait	
☐	• One leg appears shorter than the other	
☐	• Musculoskeletal problem, such as kyphosis, weak hip flexors from extended bed rest, or shortening of a leg	

✓	Medications	Supporting Documentation (Basis/reason for checking the item, including the location, date, and source (if applicable) of that information)
☐	• Antipsychotics (N0410A)	
☐	• Antianxiety agents (N0410B)	
☐	• Antidepressants (N0410C)	
☐	• Hypnotics (N0410D)	
☐	• Cardiovascular medications (from medication administration record)	
☐	• Diuretics (N0410G) (from medication administration record)	
☐	• Narcotic analgesics (from medication administration record)	
☐	• Neuroleptics (from medication administration record)	
☐	• Other medications that cause lethargy or confusion (from medication administration record)	

✓	Internal risk factors (from diagnosis list and clinical indicators)	
☐	• Circulatory/Heart — Anemia (I0200) — Cardiac Dysrhythmias (I0300) — Angina, Myocardial Infarction (MI), Atherosclerotic Heart Disease (ASHD) (I0400) — Congestive Heart Failure (CHF) pulmonary edema (I0600) — Cerebrovascular Accident (CVA) (I4500) — Transient Ischemic Attack (TIA) (I4500) — Postural/Orthostatic hypotension (I0800)	

(continued)

✓	**Internal risk factors** (from diagnosis list and clinical indicators) (continued)	**Supporting Documentation** (Basis/reason for checking the item, including the location, date, and source (if applicable) of that information)
☐	• Neuromuscular/functional — Cerebral palsy (I4400) — Loss of arm or leg movement (G0400) — Decline in functional status (G0110) — Incontinence (H0300, H0400) — Hemiplegia/Hemiparesis (I4900) — Parkinson's disease (I5300) — Seizure disorder (I5400) — Paraplegia (I5000) — Multiple sclerosis (I5200) — Traumatic brain injury (I5500) — Syncope — Chronic or acute condition resulting in instability — Peripheral neuropathy — Muscle weakness	
☐	• Orthopedic — Joint pain — Arthritis (I3700) — Osteoporosis (I3800) — Hip fracture (I3900) — Missing limb(s) (G0600D)	
☐	• Perceptual — Visual impairment (B1000) — Hearing impairment (B0200) — Dizziness/vertigo	
☐	• Psychiatric or cognitive — Impulsivity or poor safety awareness — Delirium (C1300) — Wandering (E0900) — Agitation behavior (E0200) – describe the specific verbal or motor activity- e.g. screaming, babbling, cursing, repetitive questions, pacing, kicking, scratching, etc. — Cognitive impairment (C0500, C0700-C1000) — Alzheimer's disease (I4200) — Other dementia (I4800) — Anxiety disorder (I5700) — Depression (I5800) — Manic depression (I5900) — Schizophrenia (I6000)	

(continued)

✓	Internal risk factors (from diagnosis list and clinical indicators) (continued)	Supporting Documentation (Basis/reason for checking the item, including the location, date, and source (if applicable) of that information)
☐	• Infection (I1700 – I2500)	
☐	• Low levels of physical activity	
☐	• Pain (J0300)	
☐	• Headache	
☐	• Fatigue, weakness	
☐	• Vitamin D deficiency	

✓	Laboratory tests	
☐	• Hypo- or hyperglycemia	
☐	• Electrolyte imbalance	
☐	• Dehydration (J1550C)	
☐	• Hemoglobin and hematocrit	

✓	Environmental factors (from review of facility environment)	
☐	• Poor lighting	
☐	• Glare	
☐	• Patterned carpet	
☐	• Poorly arranged furniture	
☐	• Uneven surfaces	
☐	• Slippery floors	
☐	• Obstructed walkway	
☐	• Poor fitting or slippery shoes	
☐	• Proximity to aggressive resident	

Input from resident and/or family/representative regarding the care area. (Questions/Comments/Concerns/Preferences/Suggestions)

Analysis of Findings		**Care Plan Considerations**
Review indicators and supporting documentation, and draw conclusions. Document: • Description of the problem; • Causes and contributing factors; and • Risk factors related to the care area.	Care Plan Y/N	Document reason(s) care plan will/ will not be developed.

Referral(s) to another discipline(s) is warranted (to whom and why): _____

_____

Information regarding the CAA transferred to the CAA Summary (Section V of the MDS):
☐ Yes   ☐ No

Signature/Title:_____ Date:_____

12.   NUTRITIONAL STATUS

Review of Indicators of Nutritional Status

✓	Current eating pattern – resident leaves significant proportion of meals, snacks, and supplements daily for even a few days	Supporting Documentation (Basis/reason for checking the item, including the location, date, and source (if applicable) of that information)
☐	• Food offered or available is not consistent with the resident's food choices/needs — Food preferences not consistently honored — Resident has allergies or food intolerance (for example, needs lactose-free) — Food not congruent with religious or cultural needs — Resident complains about food quality (for example, not like what spouse used to prepare, food lacks flavor) — Resident doesn't eat processed foods — Food doesn't meet other special diet requirements	
☐	• Pattern re: food left uneaten (for example, usually leaves the meat or vegetables)	
☐	• Intervals between meals may be too long or too short	
☐	• Unwilling to accept food supplements or to eat more than three meals per day	

✓	Functional problems that affect ability to eat	Supporting Documentation (Basis/reason for checking the item, including the location, date, and source (if applicable) of that information)
☐	• Swallowing problem (K0100)	
☐	• Arthritis (I3700)	
☐	• Contractures (G0400)	
☐	• Functional limitation in range of motion (G0400)	
☐	• Partial or total loss of arm movement (G0400A)	
☐	• Hemiplegia/hemiparesis (I4900)(G0400 A and B = 1)	
☐	• Quadriplegia/paraplegia (I5100/I5000) (G0400 A and/or B =2)	
☐	• Inability to perform ADLs without significant physical assistance (G0110)	
☐	• Inability to sit up (G0300)	
☐	• Missing limb(s) (G0600D)	
☐	• Vision problems (B1000)	
☐	• Decreased ability to smell or taste food	
☐	• Need for special diet or altered consistency which might not appeal to resident	
☐	• Recent decline in Activities of Daily Living (ADLs) (G0110-G0600)	

✓	Cognitive, mental status, and behavior problems that can interfere with eating	
☐	• Review Cognitive Loss CAA	
☐	• Alzheimer's Disease (I4200)	
☐	• Other dementia (I4800)	
☐	• Intellectual disability/developmental \disability (A1550)	
☐	• Paranoid fear that food is poisoned	
☐	• Requires frequent/constant cueing	
☐	• Disruptive behaviors (E0200)	
☐	• Indicators of psychosis (E0100)	
☐	• Wandering (E0900)	
☐	• Pacing (E0200)	
☐	• Throwing food (E0200C)	
☐	• Resisting care (E0800)	
☐	• Very slow eating	
☐	• Short attention span	
☐	• Poor memory (C0500, C0700-C0900)	
☐	• Anxiety problems (I5700)	

✓	Communication problems	Supporting Documentation (Basis/reason for checking the item, including the location, date, and source (if applicable) of that information)
☐	• Review Communication CAA	
☐	• Comatose (B0100)	
☐	• Difficulty making self understood (B0700)	
☐	• Difficulty understanding others (B0800)	
☐	• Aphasia (I4300)	

✓	Dental/oral problems (from Section L and physical assessment)	
☐	• See Dental Care CAA	
☐	• Broken or fractured teeth (L0200D)	
☐	• Toothache (L0200F)	
☐	• Bleeding gums (L0200E)	
☐	• Loose dentures, dentures causing sores (L0200A)	
☐	• Lip or mouth lesions (for example, cold sores, fever blisters, oral abscess) (L0200C)	
☐	• Mouth pain (L0200F)	
☐	• Dry mouth	

✓	Other diseases and conditions that can affect appetite or nutritional needs	
☐	• Anemia (I0200)	
☐	• Arthritis (I3700)	
☐	• Burns (M1040F)	
☐	• Cancer (I0100)	
☐	• Cardiovascular disease (I0300-I0900)	
☐	• Cerebrovascular accident (I4500)	
☐	• Constipation (H0600)	
☐	• Delirium (C1600)	
☐	• Depression (I5800)	
☐	• Diabetes (I2900)	
☐	• Diarrhea	
☐	• Gastrointestinal problem (I1100-I1300)	
☐	• Hospice care (O0100K)	
☐	• Liver disease (I8000)	
☐	• Pain (J0300)	
☐	• Parkinson's disease (I5300)	
☐	• Pressure ulcers (M0300)	

(continued)

✓	**Other diseases and conditions** that can affect appetite or nutritional needs (continued)	**Supporting Documentation (Basis/reason for checking the item, including the location, date, and source (if applicable) of that information)**
☐	• Radiation therapy (O0100B)	
☐	• Recent acute illness (I8000)	
☐	• Recent surgical procedure (I8000) (M1200F)	
☐	• Renal disease (I1500)	
☐	• Respiratory disease (I6200)	
☐	• Thyroid problem (I3400)	
☐	• Weight loss (K0300)	
☐	• Weight gain (K0310)	

✓	**Abnormal laboratory values** (from clinical record)	
☐	• Electrolytes	
☐	• Pre-albumin level	
☐	• Plasma transferrin level	
☐	• Others	

✓	**Medications** (from medication administration record and preadmission records if new admission)	
☐	• Antipsychotics (N0410A)	
☐	• Chemotherapy (O0100A)	
☐	• Cardiac drugs	
☐	• Diuretics (N0410G)	
☐	• Anti-inflammatory drug	
☐	• Anti-Parkinson's drugs	
☐	• Laxatives	
☐	• Antacids	
☐	• Start of a new drug	

✓	**Environmental factors** (from direct observation and clinical record)	
☐	• Sufficient eating assistance	
☐	• Availability of adaptive equipment	
☐	• Dining environment fosters pleasant social experience	
☐	• Appropriate lighting	
☐	• Sufficient personal space during meals	
☐	• Proper positioning in wheelchair/chair for dining	

Input from resident and/or family/representative regarding the care area. (Questions/Comments/Concerns/Preferences/Suggestions)

Analysis of Findings		Care Plan Considerations
Review indicators and supporting documentation, and draw conclusions. Document: • Description of the problem; • Causes and contributing factors; and • Risk factors related to the care area.	Care Plan Y/N	Document reason(s) care plan will/ will not be developed.

Referral(s) to another discipline(s) is warranted (to whom and why): _____
_____

Information regarding the CAA transferred to the CAA Summary (Section V of the MDS):
☐ Yes   ☐ No

Signature/Title:_____ Date:_____

13. FEEDING TUBE(S)

<u>Review of Indicators of Feeding Tubes</u>

✓	Reason for tube feeding	Supporting Documentation (Basis/reason for checking the item, including the location, date, and source (if applicable) of that information)
☐	• Unable to swallow or to eat food and unlikely to eat within a few days due to — Physical problems in chewing or swallowing (for example, stroke or Parkinson's disease) (L0200F, K0100D) — Mental problems (I5700 – I6100) (for example, Alzheimer's (I4200), depression (I5800))	
☐	• Normal caloric intake is substantially impaired due to endotracheal tube or a tracheostomy (O0100E)	
☐	• Prevention of meal-induced hypoxemia (insufficient oxygen to blood), in resident with COPD (I6200) or other pulmonary problems that interfere with eating (I6200)	

✓	Complications of tube feeding	
☐	• Diagnostic conditions — Delirium (C1600) — Repetitive physical movements — Anxiety (I5700, clinical record) — Depression (I5800) — Lung aspiration, pneumonia (I2000, clinical record) — Infection at insertion site — Shortness of breath (J1100)	
☐	• Bleeding around insertion site	
☐	• Constipation (H0600)	
☐	• Abdominal distension or abdominal pain	
☐	• Diarrhea or cramping	
☐	• Nausea, vomiting (J1550B)	
☐	• Tube dislodgement, blockage, leakage	
☐	• Bowel perforation	
☐	• Dehydration (J1550C) or fluid overload	
☐	• Self-extubation	
☐	• Use of physical restraints (P0100)	

✓	Psychosocial issues related to tube feeding	Supporting Documentation (Basis/reason for checking the item, including the location, date, and source (if applicable) of that information)
☐	• Signs of depression ((D0300, D0600, I5800); see Mood State CAA)	
☐	• Ways to socially engage the resident with a feeding tube	
☐	• Emotional and social support from social workers, other members of the healthcare team	

✓	Periodic evaluations and consultations	
☐	• Weight check at least monthly (K0300, K0310)	
☐	• Lab tests to monitor electrolytes, serum albumin, hematocrit	
☐	• Periodic evaluations by nutritionist or dietitian	
☐	• Periodic evaluation of possibility of resuming oral feeding	
☐	• Regular changing and replacement of PEG tubes and J-tubes, per physician order and facility protocol (K0510B1, K0510B2)	

✓	Factors that may impede removal of feeding tube	
☐	• Comatose (B0100)	
☐	• Failure to eat and resists assistance in eating (E0800)	
☐	• Cerebrovascular accident (I4500)	
☐	• Gastric ulcers, gastric bleeding, or other stomach disorder (I1200, I1300)	
☐	• Chewing problems unresolvable (L0200F)	
☐	• Swallowing problems (K0100) unresolvable	
☐	• Mouth pain (L0200F)	
☐	• Anorexia (I8000)	
☐	• Lab values indicating compromised nutritional status	
☐	• Significant weight loss (K0300)	
☐	• Significant weight gain (K0310)	
☐	• Prolonged illness	
☐	• Neurological disorder (I4200 – I5500)	
☐	• Cancer or side effects of cancer treatment (I0100, clinical record)	
☐	• Advanced dementia (I4800)	

Input from resident and/or family/representative regarding the care area. (Questions/Comments/Concerns/Preferences/Suggestions)

Analysis of Findings		Care Plan Considerations
Review indicators and supporting documentation, and draw conclusions. Document: • Description of the problem; • Causes and contributing factors; and • Risk factors related to the care area.	Care Plan Y/N	Document reason(s) care plan will/ will not be developed.

Referral(s) to another discipline(s) is warranted (to whom and why): _____

_____

Information regarding the CAA transferred to the CAA Summary (Section V of the MDS):
☐ Yes   ☐ No

Signature/Title:_____ Date:_____

14.   DEHYDRATION/FLUID MAINTENANCE

Review of Indicators of Dehydration/Fluid Maintenance

✓	Symptoms of dehydration	Supporting Documentation (Basis/reason for checking the item, including the location, date, and source (if applicable) of that information)
☐	• Dizziness on sitting or standing	
☐	• Confusion or change in mental status (delirium) (C1600, V0100D)	
☐	• Lethargy (C1300C)	
☐	• Recent decrease in urine volume or more concentrated urine than usual	
☐	• Decreased skin turgor, dry mucous membranes (J1550)	
☐	• Newly present constipation (H0600), fecal impaction	
☐	• Fever (J1550A)	
☐	• Functional decline (G0110)	
☐	• Increased risk for falls (J1700)	
☐	• Fluid and electrolyte disturbance	

✓	Abnormal laboratory values (from clinical record)	
☐	• Hemoglobin	
☐	• Hematocrit	
☐	• Potassium chloride	
☐	• Sodium	
☐	• Albumin	
☐	• Blood urea nitrogen	
☐	• Urine specific gravity	

✓	Cognitive, communication, and mental status issues that can interfere with intake	Supporting Documentation (Basis/reason for checking the item, including the location, date, and source (if applicable) of that information)
☐	• Depression (I5800, D0300, D0600) or anxiety (I5700)	
☐	• Behavioral disturbance that interferes with intake (E0200, clinical record)	
☐	• Recent change in mental status (C1600)	
☐	• Alzheimer's or other dementia that interferes with eating due to short attention span, resisting assistance, slow eating/drinking, etc. (I4200, I4800)	
☐	• Difficulty making self understood (B0700)	
☐	• Difficulty understanding others (B0800)	

✓	Diseases and conditions that predispose to limitations in maintaining normal fluid balance	
☐	• Infection (I1700 – I2500)	
☐	• Fever (J1550A)	
☐	• Diabetes (I2900)	
☐	• Congestive heart failure (I0600)	
☐	• Swallow problem (K0100)	
☐	• Renal disease (I1500)	
☐	• Weight loss (K0300)	
☐	• Weight gain (K0310)	
☐	• New cerebrovascular accident (clinical record, I4500)	
☐	• Unstable acute or chronic condition (clinical record, I8000)	
☐	• Nausea or vomiting (J1550B)	
☐	• Diarrhea (clinical record)	
☐	• Excessive sweating (clinical record)	
☐	• Recent surgery (clinical record, I8000)	
☐	• Recent decline in activities of daily living (G0110), including body control or hand control problems, inability to sit up (G0300), etc. (observation, interview, clinical record)	
☐	• Parkinson's or other neurological disease that requires unusually long time to eat (I4200 – I5500)	
☐	• Abdominal pain, with or without diarrhea, nausea, or vomiting (clinical record, (J1550B)	

(continued)

✓	**Diseases and conditions** that predispose to limitations in maintaining normal fluid balance (continued)	**Supporting Documentation** (Basis/reason for checking the item, including the location, date, and source (if applicable) of that information)
☐	• Newly taking a diuretic or recent increase in diuretic dose (N0410G) (medication records)	
☐	• Takes excessive doses of a laxative (interview, clinical record)	
☐	• Hot weather (increases risk for elderly in absence of increased fluid intake)	

✓	**Oral intake** (from observation and clinical record)	
☐	• Recent change in oral intake	
☐	• Skips meals or consumes less than 25 percent of meals	
☐	• Fluid restriction	
☐	• Newly prescribed diet	
☐	• Decreased perception of thirst	
☐	• Limited fluid-drinking opportunities	
☐	• Fluid intake limited to try to control incontinence	
☐	• Dependence on staff for fluid intake	
☐	• Excessive output compared to fluid intake	

Input from resident and/or family/representative regarding the care area. (Questions/Comments/Concerns/Preferences/Suggestions)

Analysis of Findings		Care Plan Considerations
Review indicators and supporting documentation, and draw conclusions. Document: • Description of the problem; • Causes and contributing factors; and • Risk factors related to the care area.	Care Plan Y/N	Document reason(s) care plan will/ will not be developed.

Referral(s) to another discipline(s) is warranted (to whom and why): _____

_____

Information regarding the CAA transferred to the CAA Summary (Section V of the MDS):
☐ Yes   ☐ No

Signature/Title:_____ Date:_____

15. DENTAL CARE

Review of Indicators of Oral/Dental Condition/Problem

✓	**Cognitive problems** that contribute to oral/dental problems	**Supporting Documentation (Basis/reason for checking the item, including the location, date, and source (if applicable) of that information)**
☐	• Needs reminders to clean teeth	
☐	• Cannot remember steps to complete oral hygiene	
☐	• Decreased ability to understand others (B0800) or to perform tasks following demonstration	
☐	• Cognitive deficit (C0500, C0700 – C1000)	

✓	**Functional impairment** limiting ability to perform personal hygiene	
☐	• Loss of voluntary arm movement (G0400A)	
☐	• Impaired hand dexterity (G0400A)	
☐	• Functional limitation in upper extremity range of motion (G0400A)	
☐	• Decreased mobility (G0110)	
☐	• Resists assistance with activities of daily living (E0800)	
☐	• Lacks motivation or knowledge regarding adequate oral hygiene, dental care	
☐	• Requires adaptive equipment for oral hygiene	

✓	**Dry mouth** causing buildup of oral bacteria	
☐	• Dehydration (see Dehydration/Fluid Maintenance CAA)	
☐	• Medications (from MDS and medication administration record) — Antipsychotics (N0410A) — Antidepressants (N0410C) — Antianxiety agents (N0410B) — Sedatives/hypnotics (N0410D) — Diuretics (N0410G) — Antihypertensives — Antiparkinsons medications — Narcotics — Anticonvulsants — Antihistamines — Decongestants — Antiemetics	
☐	• Antineoplastics	

✓	**Diseases and conditions** that may be related to poor oral hygiene, oral infection	**Supporting Documentation** (Basis/reason for checking the item, including the location, date, and source (if applicable) of that information)
☐	• Recurrent pneumonia related to aspiration of saliva contaminated due to poor oral hygiene (I2000)	
☐	• Unstable diabetes related to oral infection (I2900)	
☐	• Endocarditis related to oral infection (I8000)	
☐	• Sores in mouth related to poor-fitting dentures (L0200C)	
☐	• Poor nutrition (I5600) (See Nutrition CAA)	

Input from resident and/or family/representative regarding the care area. (Questions/Comments/Concerns/Preferences/Suggestions)

Analysis of Findings		Care Plan Considerations
Review indicators and supporting documentation, and draw conclusions. Document: • Description of the problem; • Causes and contributing factors; and • Risk factors related to the care area.	Care Plan Y/N	Document reason(s) care plan will/ will not be developed.

Referral(s) to another discipline(s) is warranted (to whom and why): _____

_____

Information regarding the CAA transferred to the CAA Summary (Section V of the MDS):
☐ Yes   ☐ No

Signature/Title:_____ Date:_____

16. PRESSURE ULCER(S)
Review of Indicators of Pressure Ulcer(s)

✓	Existing pressure ulcer(s) (M0100)	Supporting Documentation (Basis/reason for checking the item, including the location, date, and source (if applicable) of that information)
☐	• Assess location, size, stage, presence and type of drainage, presence of odors, condition of surrounding skin (M0610) — Note if eschar or slough is present (M0300F, M0700 = 4) — Assess for signs of infection, such as the presence of a foul odor, increasing pain, surrounding skin is reddened (erythema) or warm, or there is a presence of purulent drainage — Note whether granulation tissue (required for healing) is present and the wound is healing as expected (M0700 = 2)	
☐	• If the ulcer does not show signs of healing despite treatment, consider complicating factors — Elevated bacterial level in the absence of clinical infection — Presence of exudate, necrotic debris or slough in the wound, too much granulation tissue, or odor in the wound bed — Underlying osteomyelitis (bone infection)	
✓	**Extrinsic risk factors**	
☐	• Pressure — Requires staff assistance to move sufficiently to relieve pressure over any one site — Confined to a bed or chair all or most of the time — Needs special mattress or seat cushion to reduce or relieve pressure (M1200A, M1200B) — Requires regular schedule of turning (M1200C)	
☐	• Friction and shear — Slides down in the bed — Moved by sliding rather than lifting	
☐	• Maceration — Persistently wet, especially from fecal incontinence, wound drainage, or perspiration — Moisture associated skin damage (M1040H)	

✓	Intrinsic risk factors	Supporting Documentation (Basis/reason for checking the item, including the location, date, and source (if applicable) of that information)
☐	• Immobility (G0110)	
☐	• Altered mental status — Delirium limits mobility (see Delirium CAA) — Cognitive loss (C0500, C0700-C1000) limits mobility (see Cognitive Loss CAA)	
☐	• Incontinence (H0300, H0400, M1040H) (see Incontinence CAA)	
☐	• Poor nutrition (see Nutrition CAA)	

✓	Medications that increase risk for pressure ulcer development	
☐	• Antipsychotics (N0410A)	
☐	• Antianxiety agents (N0410B)	
☐	• Antidepressants (N0410C)	
☐	• Hypnotics (N0410D)	
☐	• Steroids	
☐	• Narcotics	

✓	Diagnoses and conditions that present complications or increase risk for pressure ulcers	
☐	• Delirium (C1600)	
☐	• Comatose (B0100)	
☐	• Cancer (I0100)	
☐	• Peripheral Vascular Disease (I0900)	
☐	• Diabetes (I2900)	
☐	• Alzheimer's disease (I4200)	
☐	• Cerebrovascular Accident (I4500)	
☐	• Other dementia (I4800)	
☐	• Hemiplegia/hemiparesis (I4900)	
☐	• Paraplegia (I5000), Quadriplegia (I5100)	
☐	• Multiple sclerosis (I5200)	
☐	• Depression (D0300, D0600, I5800)	
☐	• Edema	
☐	• Severe pulmonary disease (I6200)	
☐	• Sepsis (I2100)	
☐	• Terminal illness (O0100K)	

(continued)

✓	Diagnoses and conditions that present complications or increase risk for pressure ulcers (continued)	Supporting Documentation (Basis/reason for checking the item, including the location, date, and source (if applicable) of that information)
☐	• Chronic or end-stage renal (I1500) , liver, or heart disease (I0400, I0600)	
☐	• Pain (J0300)	
☐	• Dehydration (J1500C, I8000)	
☐	• Shortness of breath (J1100)	
☐	• Recent weight loss (K0300)	
☐	• Recent weight gain (K0310)	
☐	• Malnutrition (I5600)	
☐	• Decreased sensory perception	
☐	• Recent decline in Activities of Daily Living (ADLs) (G0110-G0600)	

✓	Treatments and other factors that cause complications or increase risk	
☐	• Newly admitted or readmitted (A1700)	
☐	• History of healed pressure ulcer(s) (M0900)	
☐	• Chemotherapy (O0100A)	
☐	• Radiation therapy (O0100B)	
☐	• Ventilator or respirator (O0100F)	
☐	• Renal dialysis (O0100J)	
☐	• Functional limitation in range of motion (G0400)	
☐	• Head of bed elevated most or all of the time	
☐	• Physical restraints (P0100)	
☐	• Devices that can cause pressure, such as oxygen (O0100C) or indwelling catheter (H0100A) tubing, TED hose, casts, or splints	

Input from resident and/or family/representative regarding the care area. (Questions/Comments/Concerns/Preferences/Suggestions)

Analysis of Findings		Care Plan Considerations
Review indicators and supporting documentation, and draw conclusions. Document: • Description of the problem; • Causes and contributing factors; and • Risk factors related to the care area.	Care Plan Y/N	Document reason(s) care plan will/ will not be developed.

Referral(s) to another discipline(s) is warranted (to whom and why): _____

_____

Information regarding the CAA transferred to the CAA Summary (Section V of the MDS):
☐ Yes   ☐ No

Signature/Title:_____ Date:_____

17. PSYCHOTROPIC MEDICATION USE

Review of Indicators of Psychotropic Drug Use

✓	**Class(es) of medication** this resident is taking	**Supporting Documentation** (Basis/reason for checking the item, including the location, date, and source (if applicable) of that information)
☐	• Antipsychotic (N0410A)	
☐	• Antianxiety (N0410B)	
☐	• Antidepressant (N0410C)	
☐	• Sedative/Hypnotic (N0410D)	

✓	**Unnecessary drug evaluation** (from clinical record)	
☐	• Excessive dose, including duplicate medications	
☐	• Excessive duration and/or without gradual dose reductions	
☐	• Inadequate monitoring for effectiveness and/or adverse consequences	
☐	• Inadequate or inappropriate indications for use	
☐	• In presence of adverse consequences of the drug	

✓	**Treatable/reversible reasons for use** of psychotropic drug	
☐	• Environmental stressors such as excessive heat, noise, overcrowding, etc. (observation, clinical record)	
☐	• Psychosocial stressors such as abuse, taunting, not following resident's customary routine, etc. (observation, clinical record) (F0300 – F0800)	
☐	• Treatable medical conditions, such as heart disease (I0200 – I0900) , diabetes (I2900), or respiratory disease (from medical evaluation) (I6200, I6300)	

✓	Adverse consequences of ANTIDEPRESSANTS exhibited by this resident	Supporting Documentation (Basis/reason for checking the item, including the location, date, and source (if applicable) of that information)
☐	• Worsening of depression and/or suicidal behavior or thinking (D0350, D0650, V0100E, V0100F, clinical record)	
☐	• Delirium unrelated to medical illness or severe depression (C1600, clinical record)	
☐	• Hallucinations (E0100A)	
☐	• Dizziness (clinical record)	
☐	• Nausea (clinical record)	
☐	• Diarrhea (clinical record)	
☐	• Anxiety (I5700, clinical record)	
☐	• Nervousness, fidgety or restless (clinical record)	
☐	• Insomnia (clinical record)	
☐	• Somnolence (clinical record)	
☐	• Weight gain (K0310, clinical record)	
☐	• Anorexia or increased appetite (clinical record)	
☐	• Increased risk for falls (clinical record), falls (J1700-J1900)	
☐	• Seizures (I5400)	
☐	• Hypertensive crisis if combined with certain foods, cheese, wine (MAO inhibitors)	
☐	• Anticholinergic (tricyclics), such as constipation, dry mouth, blurred vision, urinary retention, etc. (clinical record)	
☐	• Postural hypotension (tricyclics) (I0800, clinical record)	

✓	Adverse consequences of ANTIPSYCHOTICS exhibited by this resident	
☐	• Anticholinergic effects, such as constipation, dry mouth, blurred vision, urinary retention, etc. (clinical record)	
☐	• Increase in total cholesterol and triglycerides (clinical record)	
☐	• Akathisia (inability to sit still) (clinical record)	
☐	• Parkinsonism (any combination of tremors, postural unsteadiness, muscle rigidity, pill-rolling of hands, shuffling gait, etc.) (clinical record)	

(continued)

✓	Adverse consequences of **ANTIPSYCHOTICS** exhibited by this resident	**Supporting Documentation** (Basis/reason for checking the item, including the location, date, and source (if applicable) of that information)
☐	• Neuroleptic malignant syndrome (high fever with severe muscular rigidity) (clinical record)	
☐	• Blood sugar elevation (clinical record)	
☐	• Cardiac arrhythmias (I0300)	
☐	• Orthostatic hypotension (I0800, clinical record)	
☐	• Cerebrovascular accident or transient ischemic attack (I4500)	
☐	• Falls (J1700-J1900)	
☐	• Tardive dyskinesia (persistent involuntary movements such as tongue thrusting, lip movements, chewing or puckering movements, abnormal limb movements, rocking or writhing trunk movements) (clinical record)	
☐	• Lethargy (D0200D, clinical record)	
☐	• Excessive sedation (clinical record)	
☐	• Depression (D0300, D0600, I5800)	
☐	• Hallucinations (E0100A)	
☐	• Delirium unrelated to medical illness or severe depression (C1600, clinical record)	

✓	Adverse consequences of **ANXIOLYTICS** exhibited by this resident	
☐	• Sedation manifested by short-term memory loss (C0500, C0700), decline in cognitive abilities, slurred speech (B0600), drowsiness, little/no activity involvement (clinical record)	
☐	• Delirium unrelated to medical illness or severe depression (C1600, clinical record)	
☐	• Hallucinations (E0100A)	
☐	• Depression (D0300, D0600, I5800)	
☐	• Disturbances of balance, gait, positioning ability (G0300, G0110C, G0110D, G0110A, clinical record)	

✓	Adverse consequences of **SEDATIVES/HYPNOTICS** exhibited by this resident	Supporting Documentation (Basis/reason for checking the item, including the location, date, and source (if applicable) of that information)
☐	• May increase the metabolism of many medications (for example, anticonvulsants, antipsychotics), which may lead to decreased effectiveness and subsequent worsening of symptoms or decreased control of underlying illness (clinical record)	
☐	• Hypotension (I0800, clinical record)	
☐	• Dizziness, lightheadedness (clinical record)	
☐	• "Hangover" effect (interview, clinical record)	
☐	• Drowsiness (observation, clinical record)	
☐	• Confusion, delirium unrelated to acute illness or severe depression (C1600, clinical record)	
☐	• Mental depression (I5800, I5900)	
☐	• Unusual excitement (clinical record)	
☐	• Nervousness (clinical record)	
☐	• Headache (interview, clinical record)	
☐	• Insomnia (clinical record)	
☐	• Nightmares (interview, clinical record)	
☐	• Hallucinations (E0100A)	
☐	• Falls (J1700-J1900)	

✓	**Drug-related discomfort** requiring treatment and/or prevention	
☐	• Dehydration (J1550C, I8000)	
☐	• Reduced dietary bulk (from observation of food intake)	
☐	• Lack of exercise (observation, clinical record)	
☐	• Constipation/fecal impaction (H0600, clinical record)	
☐	• Urinary retention (clinical record)	
☐	• Dry mouth (interview, clinical record)	

✓	**Overall status change** for relationship to psychotropic drug use (from clinical record)	
☐	• Major differences in a.m./p.m. performance	
☐	• Decline in cognition/communication (V0100D)	
☐	• Decline in mood (V0100E, V0100F)	
☐	• Decline in behavior	
☐	• Decline in Activities of Daily Living (ADLs) (G0110)	

Input from resident and/or family/representative regarding the care area. (Questions/Comments/Concerns/Preferences/Suggestions)

Analysis of Findings		**Care Plan Considerations**
Review indicators and supporting documentation, and draw conclusions. Document: • Description of the problem; • Causes and contributing factors; and • Risk factors related to the care area.	Care Plan Y/N	Document reason(s) care plan will/ will not be developed.

Referral(s) to another discipline(s) is warranted (to whom and why): _____

_____

Information regarding the CAA transferred to the CAA Summary (Section V of the MDS):
☐ Yes   ☐ No

Signature/Title:_____ Date:_____

18. PHYSICAL RESTRAINTS

Review of Indicators of Physical Restraints

✓	Evaluation of current restraint use (based on chart documentation, including care plan)	Supporting Documentation (Basis/reason for checking the item, including the location, date, and source (if applicable) of that information)
☐	• Does not meet regulatory definition of restraint (stop here and check accuracy of MDS item that triggered this CAA)	
☐	• Evidence of informed consent not evident on chart	
☐	• Medical symptom not identified for treatment via restraints	
☐	• Used for staff convenience	
☐	• Used for discipline purposes	
☐	• Multiple restraints in use	
☐	• Non-restraint interventions not attempted prior to restraining	
☐	• Less restrictive devices not attempted	
☐	• No regular schedule for removing restraints	
☐	• No schedule for frequency by hour of the day for checking on resident's well-being	
☐	• No plan for reducing/eliminating restraints	

✓	Medical conditions/treatments that may lead to restraint use	
☐	• Indwelling catheter (H0100A), external catheter (H0100B), or ostomy (H0100C)	
☐	• Parenteral/IV feeding (K0510A1, K0510A2)	
☐	• Feeding tube (K0510B1. K0510B2)	
☐	• Pressure ulcer (M0210) or pressure ulcer care (M1200E)	
☐	• Other skin ulcers, wounds, skin problems (M1040) or wound care (M1200F-M1200I)	
☐	• Oxygen therapy (O0100C)	
☐	• Tracheostomy (O0100E, clinical record)	
☐	• Ventilator or respirator (O0100F)	
☐	• IV medications (O0100H)	
☐	• Transfusions (O0100I)	
☐	• Functional decline, decreased mobility (clinical record)	
☐	• Other medical problem or equipment associated with restraint use (clinical record)	

✓	Cognitive impairment/behavioral symptoms that may lead to restraint use (also see Cognitive Loss and Behavior CAAs)	Supporting Documentation (Basis/reason for checking the item, including the location, date, and source (if applicable) of that information)
☐	• Inattention, easily distracted (C1300A)	
☐	• Disorganized thinking (C1300B)	
☐	• Fidgety, restless	
☐	• Agitation behavior (E0200) – describe the specific verbal or motor activity- e.g. screaming, babbling, cursing, repetitive questions, pacing, kicking, scratching, etc.	
☐	• Confusion (C0100, C0600)	
☐	• Psychosis (E0100A, E0100B)	
☐	• Physical symptoms directed toward others (E0200A)	
☐	• Verbal behavioral symptoms directed toward others (E0200B)	
☐	• Rejection of care (E0800)	
☐	• Wandering (E0900)	
☐	• Delirium (C1600), including side effects of medications (clinical record)	
☐	• Alzheimer's disease (I4200) or other dementia (I4800)	
☐	• Traumatic brain injury (I5500)	
☐	• Psychiatric disorder (I5700-I6100)	

✓	Risk for falls that may lead to restraint use (also see Falls CAA)	
☐	• Poor safety awareness, impulsivity (clinical record)	
☐	• Urinary urgency (clinical record)	
☐	• Incontinence of bowel and/or bladder (H0300, H0400)	
☐	• Side effect of medication, such as dizziness, postural/orthostatic hypotension (I0800), sedation, etc. (clinical record)	
☐	• Insomnia, fatigue (D0200D, D0500D)	
☐	• Need for assistance with mobility (G0110)	
☐	• Balance problem (G0300)	
☐	• Postural/orthostatic hypotension (I0800, clinical record)	
☐	• Hip or other fracture (I3900, I4000)	
☐	• Hemiplegia/hemiparesis (I4900), paraplegia (I5000), quadriplegia (I5100)	
☐	• Other neurological disorder (for example, Cerebral Palsy (I4400), Multiple Sclerosis (I5200), Parkinson's Disease (I5300))	
☐	• Respiratory problems (J1100, I6200, I6300, clinical record)	
	• History of falls (J1700 – J1900)	

✓	Adverse reaction to restraint use	Supporting Documentation (Basis/reason for checking the item, including the location, date, and source (if applicable) of that information)
☐	• Skin breakdown (Section M)	
☐	• Incontinence or increased incontinence (H0300, H0400, clinical record)	
☐	• Moisture associated skin damage (M1040H)	
☐	• Constipation (H0600)	
☐	• Increased agitation behavior (E0200, clinical record) – describe the specific verbal or motor activity- e.g. screaming, babbling, cursing, repetitive questions, pacing, kicking, scratching, etc.	
☐	• Depression, withdrawal, diminished dignity, social isolation (I5800, I5900, clinical record)	
☐	• Loss of muscle mass, contractures, lessened mobility (G0110, G0300, G0400) and stamina (clinical record)	
☐	• Infections, such as UTI or pneumonia (I1700 – I2500)	
☐	• Frequent attempts to get out of the restraints (P0100), falls (J1700 – J1900, clinical record)	

Input from resident and/or family/representative regarding the care area.
(Questions/Comments/Concerns/Preferences/Suggestions)

Analysis of Findings		**Care Plan Considerations**
Review indicators and supporting documentation, and draw conclusions. Document: • Description of the problem; • Causes and contributing factors; and • Risk factors related to the care area.	Care Plan Y/N	Document reason(s) care plan will/ will not be developed.

Referral(s) to another discipline(s) is warranted (to whom and why): _____

_____

Information regarding the CAA transferred to the CAA Summary (Section V of the MDS):
☐ Yes   ☐ No

Signature/Title:_____ Date:_____

19. PAIN

Review of Indicators of Pain

✓	Diseases and conditions that may cause pain (diagnosis OR signs/symptoms present)	Supporting Documentation (Basis/reason for checking the item, including the location, date, and source (if applicable) of that information)
☐	• Cancer (I0100)	
☐	• Circulatory/heart — Angina, Myocardial Infarction (MI), Atherosclerotic Heart Disease (ASHD) (I0400) — Deep Vein Thrombosis (I0500) — Peripheral Vascular Disease (I0900)	
☐	• Skin/Wound — Pressure ulcer (section M) — Other ulcers, wounds, incision, skin problems (M1040) — Moisture associated skin damage (M1040H)	
☐	• Infections — Urinary tract infection (I2300) — Pneumonia (I2000)	
☐	• Neurological (I4200 – I5500) — Head trauma (clinical record) — Headache — Neuropathy — Post-stroke syndrome	
☐	• Gastrointestinal — Gastroesophageal Reflux Disease/Ulcer (I1200) — Ulcerative Colitis/Crohn's Disease/Inflammatory Bowel Disease (I1300) — Constipation (H0600, clinical record, resident interview)	
☐	• Hospice care (O0100K)	
☐	• Musculoskeletal — Arthritis (I3700) — Osteoporosis (I3800) — Hip fracture (I3900) — Other fracture (I4000) — Back problems (I8000) — Amputation (O0500) — Other (I8000)	
☐	• Dental problems (section L) (L0200)	

✓	Characteristics of the pain	Supporting Documentation (Basis/reason for checking the item, including the location, date, and source (if applicable) of that information)
☐	• Location	
☐	• Type (constant, intermittent, varies over time, etc.)	
☐	• What makes it better	
☐	• What makes it worse	
☐	• Words that describe it (for example, aching, soreness, dull, throbbing, crushing) — Burning, pins and needles, shooting, numbness (neuropathic) — Cramping, crushing, throbbing, stabbing (musculoskeletal) — Cramping, tightness (visceral)	

✓	Frequency and intensity of the pain (J0400, J0600, J0850)	
☐	• How often it occurs	
☐	• Time or situation of onset	
☐	• How long it lasts	

✓	Non-verbal indicators of pain (particularly important if resident is stoic)	
☐	• Facial expression (frowning, grimacing, etc.) (J0800A, J0800C)	
☐	• Vocal behaviors (signing, moaning, groaning, crying, etc.) (J0800A, J0800B)	
☐	• Body position (guarding, distorted posture, restricted limb movement, etc.) (J0800D)	
☐	• Restlessness	

✓	Pain effect on function	
☐	• Disturbs sleep (J0500A)	
☐	• Decreases appetite (clinical record)	
☐	• Adversely affects mood (D0200, D0500, clinical record)	
☐	• Limits day-to-day activities (J0500B) (social events, eating in dining room, etc.)	
☐	• Limits independence with at least some Activities of Daily Living (ADLs) (G0110)	

✓	Associated signs and symptoms	Supporting Documentation (Basis/reason for checking the item, including the location, date, and source (if applicable) of that information)
☐	• Agitation or new or increased behavior problems (E0200) – describe the specific verbal or motor activity- e.g. screaming, babbling, cursing, repetitive questions, pacing, kicking, scratching, etc.	
☐	• Delirium (C1600)	
☐	• Withdrawal	

✓	Other Considerations	
☐	• Improper positioning (M1200C)	
☐	• Contractures (G0400)	
☐	• Immobility (G0110)	
☐	• Use of restraints (P0100)	
☐	• Recent change in pain (characteristics, frequency, intensity, etc.) (J0400, J0600)	
☐	• Insufficient pain relief (from resident/staff interview, clinical record, direct observation) (J0100 – J0850)	
☐	• Pain relief occurs, but duration is not sufficient, resulting in breakthrough pain (J0100 – J0850)	

Input from resident and/or family/representative regarding the care area. (Questions/Comments/Concerns/Preferences/Suggestions)

Analysis of Findings		**Care Plan Considerations**
Review indicators and supporting documentation, and draw conclusions. Document: • Description of the problem; • Causes and contributing factors; and • Risk factors related to the care area.	Care Plan Y/N	Document reason(s) care plan will/ will not be developed.

Referral(s) to another discipline(s) is warranted (to whom and why): _____

_____

Information regarding the CAA transferred to the CAA Summary (Section V of the MDS):
☐ Yes   ☐ No

Signature/Title:_____ Date:_____

20.   RETURN TO COMMUNITY REFERRAL

Review of Return to Community Referral

✓	Steps in the Process
☐	1. Document in the care plan whether the individual indicated a desire to talk to someone about the possibility of returning to the community or not (Q0500B).
☐	2. Discuss with the individual and his or her family to identify potential barriers to transition planning. The care planning/discharge planning team should have additional discussions with the individual and family to develop information that will support the individual's smooth transition to community living. (Q0100)
☐	3. Other factors to consider regarding the individual's discharge assessment and planning for community supports include: • Cognitive skills for decision making (C1000) and Cognitive deficits (C0500, C0700-C1000) • Functional/mobility (G0110) or balance (G0300) problems • Need for assistive devices and/or home modifications if considering a discharge home
☐	4. Inform the discharge planning team and other facility staff of the individual's choice.
☐	5. Look at the previous care plans of this individual to identify their previous responses and the issues or barriers they expressed. Consider the individual's overall goals of care and discharge planning from previous items responses (Q0300 and Q0400B). Has the individual indicated that his or her goal is for end-of-life-care (palliative or hospice care)? Or does the individual expect to return home after rehabilitation in your facility? (Q0300, Q0400)
☐	6. Initiate contact with the State-designated local contact agency within approximately 10 business days, and document (Q0600). Follow-up is expected in a "reasonable" amount of time, 10 business days is a recommendation and not a requirement.
☐	7. If the local contact agency does not contact the individual by telephone or in person within approximately 10 business days, make another follow-up call to the designated local contact agency as necessary. The level and type of response needed by a particular individual is determined on a resident-by-resident basis, so timeframes for response may vary depending on the needs of the resident and the supports available within the community.
☐	8. Communicate and collaborate with the State-designated local contact agency on the discharge process. Identify and address challenges and barriers facing the individual in their discharge process. Develop solutions to these challenges in the discharge/transition plan.
☐	9. Communicate findings and concerns with the facility discharge planning team, the individual's support circle, the individual's physician and the local contact agency in order to facilitate discharge/transition planning.

Input from resident and/or family/representative regarding the care area. (Questions/Comments/Concerns/Preferences/Suggestions)

Analysis of Findings		Care Plan Considerations
Review indicators and supporting documentation, and draw conclusions. Document: • Description of the problem; • Causes and contributing factors; and • Risk factors related to the care area.	Care Plan Y/N	Document reason(s) care plan will/ will not be developed.

Referral(s) to another discipline(s) is warranted (to whom and why): _____

_____

Information regarding the CAA transferred to the CAA Summary (Section V of the MDS):
☐ Yes ☐ No

Signature/Title:_____ Date:_____

CARE AREA GENERAL RESOURCES

The general resources contained on this page are not specific to any particular care area. Instead, they provide a general listing of known clinical practice guidelines and tools that may be used in completing the RAI CAA process.

NOTE: This list of resources is neither prescriptive nor all-inclusive. References to non-U.S. Department of Health and Human Services (HHS) sources or sites on the Internet are provided as a service and do not constitute or imply endorsement of these organizations or their programs by CMS or HHS. CMS is not responsible for the content of pages found at these sites. URL addresses were current as of the date of this publication.

- Advancing Excellence in America's Nursing Homes Resources: http://www.nhqualitycampaign.org/star_index.aspx?controls=resImplementationGuides;
- Agency for Health Care Research and Quality – Clinical Information, Evidence-Based Practice: http://www.ahrq.gov/clinic/;
- Alzheimer's Association Resources: http://www.alz.org/professionals_and_researchers_14899.asp#professional;
- American Dietetic Association – Individualized Nutrition Approaches for Older Adults in Health Care Communities (PDF Version): http://www.eatright.org/About/Content.aspx?id=8373;
- American Geriatrics Society Clinical Practice Guidelines and Tools: http://www.americangeriatrics.org/health_care_professionals/clinical_practice/featured_programs_products/;
- American Medical Directors Association (AMDA) Clinical Practice Guidelines and Tools: http://www.amda.com/tools;
- American Pain Society: http://www.ampainsoc.org/pub/cp_guidelines.htm;
- American Society of Consultant Pharmacists Practice Resources: http://www.ascp.com/articles/professional-development/clinical-practice-resources;
- Association for Professionals in Infection Control and Epidemiology Practice Resources: http://www.apic.org/AM/Template.cfm?Section=Practice;
- Centers for Disease Control and Prevention: Infection Control in Long-Term Care Facilities Guidelines: http://www.cdc.gov/HAI/settings/ltc_settings.html;
- CMS Pub. 100-07 State Operations Manual Appendix PP – Guidance to Surveyors for Long Term Care Facilities (federal regulations noted throughout; resources provided in endnotes): http://cms.gov/manuals/Downloads/som107ap_pp_guidelines_ltcf.pdf;
- Emerging Solutions in Pain Tools: http://www.emergingsolutionsinpain.com/;
- Hartford Institute for Geriatric Nursing Access to Important Geriatric Tools: http://www.hartfordign.org/resources;
- Hartford Institute for Geriatric Nursing Evidence-Based Geriatric Content: http://www.hartfordign.org/practice/consultgerirn/;
- Improving Nursing Home Culture (CMS Special Study): http://www.healthcentricadvisors.org/images/stories/documents/inhc.pdf
- Institute for Safe Medication Practices: http://www.ismp.org/;
- Quality Improvement Organizations: http://www.qualitynet.org/dcs/ContentServer?c=Page&pagename=QnetPublic%2FPage%2FQnetTier2&cid=1144767874793;

CARE AREA GENERAL RESOURCES (cont.)

- University of Missouri's Geriatric Examination Tool Kit: http://web.missouri.edu/~proste/tool/; and
- U.S. Department of Health and Human Services Agency for Healthcare Research and Quality's National Guideline Clearinghouse: http://www.guideline.gov/;

APPENDIX D: INTERVIEWING TO INCREASE RESIDENT VOICE IN MDS ASSESSMENTS

All residents capable of any communication should be asked to provide information regarding what they consider to be the most important facets of their lives. There are several MDS 3.0 sections that require direct interview of the resident as the primary source of information (e.g., mood, preferences, pain). Self-report is the single most reliable indicator of these topics. Staff should actively seek information from the resident regarding these specific topic areas; however, resident interview/inquiry should become part of a supportive care environment that helps residents fulfill their choices over aspects of their lives.

In addition, a simple performance-based assessment of cognitive function can quickly clarify a resident's cognitive status. The majority of residents, even those with moderate to severe cognitive impairment, are able to answer some simple questions about these topics.

Even simple scripted interviews like those in MDS 3.0 involve a dynamic, collaborative process. There are some basic approaches that can make interviews simpler and more effective.

- **Introduce yourself** to the resident.
- **Be sure the resident can hear what you are saying.**
    - Do not mumble or rush. Articulate words clearly.
    - Ask the resident if he or she uses or owns a hearing aid or other communication device.
    - Help him or her get the aid or device in place before starting the interview.
    - The assessor may need to offer an assistive device (headphones).
    - If the resident is using a hearing aid or other communication device make sure that it is operational.
- **Ask whether the resident would like an interpreter (language or signing)** if the resident does not appear to be fluent in English or continues to have difficulty understanding. Interpreters are people who translate oral or written language from one language to another. If an interpreter is used during resident interviews, he or she should not attempt to determine the intent behind what is being translated, the outcome of the interview, or the meaning or significance of the interviewee's responses. The resident should determine meaning based solely on his or her interpretation of what is being translated.
- **Find a quiet, private area where you are not likely to be interrupted or overheard.** This is important for several reasons:
    - Background noise should be minimized.
    - Some items are personal, and the resident will be more comfortable answering in private. The interviewer is in a better position to respond to issues that arise.
    - Decrease available distractions.

- **Sit where the resident can see you clearly and you can see his or her expressions.**
  — Have your face well lighted.
  — Minimize glare.
  — Ask the resident where you should sit so that he or she can see you best. Some residents have decreased central vision or limited ability to turn their heads.

- **Establish rapport and respect.**
  — The steps you have already taken to ensure comfort go a long way toward establishing rapport and demonstrating respect.
  — You can also engage the resident in general conversation to help establish rapport.
  — If the resident asks a particular question or makes a request, try to address the request or question before proceeding with the interview.

- **Explain the purpose of the questions to the resident.**
  — Start by introducing the topic and explain that you are going to ask a series of questions.
  — You can tell the resident that these questions are designed to be asked of everyone to make sure that nothing is missed.
  — Highlight what you will ask.
  — End by explaining that his or her answers will help the care team develop a care plan that is appropriate for the resident.
  — Suggested explanations and introductions are included in specific item instructions.

- **Say and show the item responses.**
  — It is helpful to many older adults to both hear and read the response options.
  — As you verbally review the response options, show the resident the items written in large, clear print on a piece of paper or card.
  — Residents may respond to questions verbally, by pointing to their answers on the visual aid or by writing out their answers.

- **Ask the questions** as they appear in the questionnaire.
  — Use a nonjudgmental approach to questioning.
  — Don't be afraid of what the resident might say; you are there to hear it.
  — Actively listen; these questions can provide insights beyond the direct answer.

- **Break the question apart if necessary.** If the resident has difficulty understanding, requests clarification, or seems hesitant, you can employ unfolding or disentangling techniques. (Do not, however, use these techniques for the memory test).

  1. **Unfolding** refers to the use of a general question about the symptom followed by a sequence of more specific questions if the symptom is reported as present. This approach walks the resident through the steps needed to think through the question.

Example: Read the item (or part of the item) to the resident, then ask, "Do you have this at all?" If yes, then ask, "Do you have it every day?" If no, then ask, "Did you have it at least half the days in the past 2 weeks?"

2. **Disentangling** refers to separating items with several parts into manageable pieces. The type of items that lend themselves to this approach are those that include a list and phrases such as "and" or "or." The resident is given a chance to respond to each piece separately. If a resident responds positively to more than one component of a complex item, obtain a frequency rating for each positive response and score that item using the frequency of the component that occurred most often.

   Example: An item asks about "Poor appetite or overeating." Disentangle this item by asking, "Poor appetite?"; pause for a response and then ask, "Or overeating?" If neither part is rated positively by the resident, mark no. If either or both are rated positively, then mark yes.

- **Clarify using echoing.** If the resident appears to understand but is having difficulty selecting an answer, try clarifying his or her response by first echoing what he or she told you and then repeating the related response options.

  — **Echoing** means simply restating part of the resident's response. This is often extremely helpful during clinical interviews. If the resident provides a related response but does not use the provided response scale or fails to directly answer the question, then help clarify the best response by repeating the resident's own comment and then asking the related response options again. This interview approach frequently helps the resident clarify which response option he or she prefers.

- **Repeat the response options** as needed. Some residents might need to have response choices repeated for each item on a given list.

- **Move on to another question** if the resident is unable to answer.

  — Even if the interview item cannot be completed the time spent is not wasted. The observation of resident behaviors and attention during the interview attempt provide important insights into delirium, cognition, mood, etc.

- **Break up the interview if the resident becomes tired or needs to leave for rehabilitation, etc.**

  — Try to complete the current item set and then offer to come back at another time to complete the remaining interview sections.

  — It is particularly important to complete the performance-based cognitive items in one sitting.

- **Do not try to talk a resident out of an answer.** If the resident expresses strong emotions, be nonjudgmental, and listen.

- **Record the resident's response,** not what you believe he or she should have said.

- **If the resident becomes deeply sorrowful or agitated,** sympathetically respond to his or her feelings.

  — Allowing emotional expression—even when it is uncomfortable for you as the interviewer—recognizes its validity and provides cathartic support to residents.

— If the resident remains agitated or overly emotional and does not want to continue, respond to his or her needs. This is more important than finishing the interview at that moment. You can complete this and other sections at a later point in time.

- **Resident preferences may be influenced by many factors in a resident's physical, psychological and environmental state, and can be challenging to truly discern.**

    — Residents should be encouraged to articulate their desires and not be strictly limited by their physical limitations and perceived environmental restrictions.

    — When a resident is unable to communicate information about his or her preferences, a family member, close friend, or other representative must be used to complete preference questions. In this case, it is important to emphasize that this person should try to answer based on what the resident would prefer. The resident's preferences while in the nursing home and the resident's current responses when the particular item is offered or provided should form the basis for these responses.

APPENDIX E: PHQ-9 SCORING RULES AND INSTRUCTION FOR BIMS (WHEN ADMINISTERED IN WRITING)

Scoring Rules: Resident Mood Interview Total Severity Score D0300

- Item D0300 is used to store the total severity score for the Resident Mood Interview. The score in item D0300 is based upon the sum of the values that are contained in the following nine items: D0200A2, D0200B2, D0200C2, D0200D2, D0200E2, D0200F2, D0200G2, D0200H2, D0200I2. These are referred to as the "items in Column 2", below.
- The following rules explain how to compute the score that is placed in item D0300. These rules consider the "number of missing items in Column 2" which is the number of items in Column 2 that are either skipped or are equal to dash. An item in Column 2 could be skipped if the corresponding item in Column 1 was equal to 9 (no response). An item in Column 2 could be equal to dash if the item could not be assessed for some other reason (e.g., if the resident was unexpectedly discharged before the assessment could be completed).
- If all of the items in Column 2 have a value of 0, 1, 2, or 3 (i.e., they all contain non-missing values), then item D0300 is equal to the simple sum of those values.
- If any of the items in Column 2 are skipped or equal to dash, then omit their values when computing the sum.
- If the number of missing items in Column 2 is equal to **one**, then compute the simple sum of the eight items in Column 2 that have non-missing values, multiply the sum by 9/8 (1.125), and place the result rounded to the nearest integer in item D0300.
- If the number of missing items in Column 2 is equal to **two,** then compute the simple sum of the seven items in Column 2 that have non-missing values, multiply the sum by 9/7 (1.286), and place the result rounded to the nearest integer in item D0300.
- If the number of missing items in Column 2 is equal to **three or more but at least one of the items in Column 2 is not equal to dash,** then item D0300 must equal [99].

If all of the items in Column 2 are equal to dash, then enter dash in item D0300.

Scoring Rules: Resident Mood Interview Total Severity Score: D0300 (cont.)

Example 1: All Items in Column 2 Have Non-missing Values

The following example shows how to score the resident interview when all of the items in Column 2 have non-missing values:

Item	Value
D0200A2	0
D0200B2	1
D0200C2	2
D0200D2	2
D0200E2	3
D0200F2	0
D0200G2	1
D0200H2	3
D0200I2	2
D0300	**14**

In this example, all of the items in Column 2 have non-missing values (i.e., none of the values are skipped or equal to dash). Therefore, the value of D0300 is equal to the simple sum of the values in Column 2, which is 14.

Example 2: One Missing Value in Column 2

The following example shows how to score the resident interview when one of the items in Column 2 has a missing value:

Item	Value
D0200A2	0
D0200B2	1
D0200C2	2
D0200D2	2
D0200E2	
D0200F2	0
D0200G2	1
D0200H2	3
D0200I2	2
0300	**12**

Scoring Rules: Resident Mood Interview Total Severity Score: D0300 (cont.)

In this example, one of the items in Column 2 (D0200E2) has a missing value (it is blank or skipped) and the other 8 items have non-missing values. D0300 is computed as follows:

1. Compute the sum of the 8 items with non-missing values. This sum is 11.
2. Multiply this sum by 1.125. In the example, 11 x 1.125 = 12.375.
3. Round the result to the nearest integer. In the example, 12.375 rounds to 12.
4. Place the rounded result in D0300.

Example 3: Two Missing Values in Column 2

The following example shows how to score the resident interview when two of the items in Column 2 have missing values:

Item	Value
D0200A2	0
D0200B2	1
D0200C2	2
D0200D2	2
D0200E2	
D0200F2	0
D0200G2	1
D0200H2	-
D0200I2	2
D0300	**10**

In this example, two of the items in Column 2 have missing values: D0200E2 is blank or skipped, and D0200H2 is equal to dash. The other 7 items have non-missing values. D0300 is computed as follows:

1. Compute the sum of the 7 items with non-missing values. This sum is 8.
2. Multiply this sum by 1.286. In the example, 8 x 1.286 = 10.288.
3. Round the result to the nearest integer. In the example, 10.288 rounds to 10.
4. Place the rounded result in D0300.

Scoring Rules: Resident Mood Interview Total Severity Score: D0300 **(cont.)**

Example 4: Three or More Missing Values in Column 2

The following example shows how to score the resident interview when three or more of the items in Column 2 have missing values and at least one of the values is not equal to dash:

Item	Value
D0200A2	0
D0200B2	1
D0200C2	2
D0200D2	2
D0200E2	
D0200F2	
D0200G2	1
D0200H2	-
D0200I2	2
D0300	**99**

In this example, three of the items in Column 2 have missing values: D0200E2 and D0200F2 are blank or skipped, and D0200H2 is equal to dash. The other 6 items have non-missing values and at least one of these items is not equal to dash. Because three or more items have missing values, D0300 is equal to 99.

Example 5: All Items in Column 2 Have Dashes

The following example shows how to score the resident interview when all of the items in Column 2 have dashes:

Item	Value
D0200A2	-
D0200B2	-
D0200C2	-
D0200D2	-
D0200E2	-
D0200F2	-
D0200G2	-
D0200H2	-
D0200I2	-
D0300	-

Scoring Rules: Resident Mood Interview Total Severity Score: D0300 **(cont.)**

In this example, all of the items in Column 2 contain dashes. In this special case, enter a dash in D0300 (enter a single dash in the leftmost space of D0300 and leave the second space blank).

Scoring Rules: Staff Assessment of Resident Mood Total Severity Score: D0600

- Item D0600 is used to store the total severity score for the Staff Assessment of Resident Mood. The score in item D0600 is based upon the sum of the values that are contained in the following ten items: D0500A2, D0500B2, D0500C2, D0500D2, D0500E2, D0500F2, D0500G2, D0500H2, D0500I2, D0500J2. These are referred to as the "items in Column 2", below.

- The following rules explain how to compute the score that is placed in item D0600. These rules consider the "number of missing items in Column 2" which is the number of items in Column 2 that are equal to dash (an item could be equal to dash if the it could not be assessed – for example, if the resident was unexpectedly discharged before the assessment could be completed).

- If all of the items in Column 2 have a value of 0, 1, 2, or 3 (i.e., they all contain non-missing values), then item D0600 is equal to the simple sum of those values.

- If any of the items in Column 2 are equal to dash, then omit their values when computing the sum.

- If the number of missing items in Column 2 is equal to one, then compute the simple sum of the nine items in Column 2 that have non-missing values, multiply the sum by 10/9 (1.111), and place the result rounded to the nearest integer in item D0600.

- If the number of missing items in Column 2 is equal to two, then compute the simple sum of the eight items in Column 2 that have non-missing values, multiply the sum by 10/8 (1.250), and place the result rounded to the nearest integer in item D0600.

- If the number of missing items in Column 2 is equal to three or more, then enter a dash in item D0600.

Scoring Rules: Staff Assessment of Resident Mood Total Severity Score: D0600 (cont.)

Example 1: All Items in Column 2 Have Non-missing Values

The following example shows how to score the resident interview when all of the items in Column 2 have non-missing values:

Item	Value
D0500A2	0
D0500B2	1
D0500C2	2
D0500D2	2
D0500E2	3
D0500F2	0
D0500G2	1
D0500H2	3
D0500I2	2
D0500J2	1
D0600	**15**

In this example, all of the items in Column 2 have non-missing values (i.e., none of the values are skipped or equal to dash). Therefore, the value of D0600 is equal to the simple sum of the values in Column 2, which is 15.

Example 2: One Missing Value in Column 2

The following example shows how to score the resident interview when one of the items in Column 2 has a missing value:

Item	Value
D0500A2	0
D0500B2	1
D0500C2	2
D0500D2	2
D0500E2	-
D0500F2	0
D0500G2	1
D0500H2	3
D0500I2	2
D0500J2	1
D0600	**13**

Scoring Rules: Staff Assessment of Resident Mood Total Severity Score: D0600 (cont.)

In this example, one of the items in Column 2 (D0500E2) has a missing value (it is equal to dash) and the other 9 items have non-missing values. D0600 is computed as follows:

1. Compute the sum of the 9 items with non-missing values. This sum is 12.

2. Multiply this sum by 1.111 (See bullet 5 on page E-5 for calculation of multiplier). In the example, the sum of non-missing values is 12. Therefore, the calculation is: 12 x 1.111 = 13.332.

3. Round the result to the nearest integer. In the example, 13.332 rounds to 13.

4. Place the rounded result in D0600.

Example 3: Two Missing Values in Column 2

The following example shows how to score the resident interview when two of the items in Column 2 have missing values:

Item	Value
D0500A2	0
D0500B2	1
D0500C2	2
D0500D2	2
D0500E2	-
D0500F2	0
D0500G2	1
D0500H2	-
D0500I2	2
D0500J2	1
D0600	**11**

In this example, two of the items in Column 2 have missing values: D0500E2 and D0500H2 are equal to dash. The other 8 items have non-missing values. D0600 is computed as follows:

1. Compute the sum of the 8 items with non-missing values. This sum is 9.

2. Multiply this sum by 1.250 (See bullet 6 on page E-5 for calculation of multiplier). In the example, the sum of non-missing values is 9. Therefore, the calculation is: 9 x 1.250 = 11.250.

3. Round the result to the nearest integer. In the example, 11.250 rounds to 11.

4. Place the rounded result in D0600.

Scoring Rules: Staff Assessment of Resident Mood Total Severity Score: D0600 (cont.)

Example 4: Three or More Missing Values in Column 2

The following example shows how to score the resident interview when three or more of the items in Column 2 have missing values:

Item	Value
D0500A2	0
D0500B2	1
D0500C2	2
D0500D2	2
D0500E2	-
D0500F2	-
D0500G2	1
D0500H2	-
D0500I2	2
D0500J2	1
D0600	-

In this example, three of the items in Column 2 have missing values: D0500E2, D0500F2, and D0500H2 are equal to dash. Because three or more items have missing values, enter a dash in D0600 (enter a single dash in the leftmost space of D0600 and leave the second space blank).

Instructions for BIMS When Administered in Writing

When staff identify that the resident's primary method of communication is in written format, the BIMS and Category Cues can be administered in writing. **The administration of the BIMS in writing should be limited only to this circumstance.**

1. Interview any resident not screened out by **Should Brief Interview for Mental Status Be Conducted?** item (C0100).
2. Conduct the interview in a private setting.
3. Residents with visual impairment should be tested using their usual visual aids.
4. Minimize glare by directing light sources away from the resident's face and from written materials.
5. Provide a written introduction before starting the interview.

   Suggested language: "I would like to ask you some questions, which I will show you in a moment. We ask everyone these same questions. This will help us provide you with better care. Some of the questions may seem very easy, while others may be more difficult. We ask these questions of everyone so we can make sure that our care will meet your needs."

6. Directly provide the written questions for each item in C0200 through C0400 at one sitting and in the order provided.

   - For each BIMS question, show the resident a sheet of paper or card with the instruction for that question from the form clearly written in a large enough font to be easily seen.

   - The resident may respond to any of the BIMS questions in writing.

   - Show separate sheets or cards for each question or statement.

   - For C0200 items, instructions should be written as:

     — I have written 3 words for you to remember. Please read them. Then I will remove the card and ask you repeat or write down the words as you remember them.

     — Category cues should be provided to the resident in writing after the resident's first attempt to answer. Written category cues should state: "sock, something to wear; blue, a color; bed, a piece of furniture."

   - For C0300 items, instructions should be written as:

     — C0300A: "Please tell me what year it is right now."

     — C0300B: "What month are we in right now?"

     — C0300C: "What day of the week is today?"

   - For C0400 items, instructions should be written as:

     — "Let's go back to an earlier question. What were those three words that I asked you to repeat?"

     — If the resident is unable to remember a word, provide Category cues again, but without using the actual word. Therefore, Category cues for:

       o   C0400A should be written as "something to wear,"
       o   C0400B should be written as "a color," and
       o   C0500C should be written as "a piece of furniture."

7. If the resident chooses not to answer a particular item, accept his or her refusal and move on to the next questions. For C0200 through C0400, code refusals as incorrect.

8. Rules for stopping the interview are the same as if for administering the BIMS verbally.

The following resources may be used, or the facility may develop their own. If the facility develops their own, they must use the exact language as in these resources.

Written Introduction Card – BIMS – Items C0200 – C0400

I would like to ask you some questions, which I will show you in a moment.

We ask everyone these same questions.

This will help us provide you with better care.

Some of the questions may seem very easy, while others may be more difficult.

We ask these questions so that we can make sure that our care will meet your needs.

Written Instruction Cards – Item C0200 – Repetition of Three Words

I have written 3 words for you to remember.

Please read them.

Then, I will remove the card and ask you repeat or write down the words as you remember them.

Word Card – Item C0200

SOCK

BLUE

BED

Category Cue Card – Item C0200

SOCK, something to wear

BLUE, a color

BED, a piece of furniture

Written Instruction Cards – Item C0300 – Temporal Orientation

Statement Card – C0300A - Year

Please tell me what year it is right now.

Question Card – C0300B - Month

What month are we in right now?

Question Card – Item C0300C - Day

What day of the week is today?

Written Instruction Card – Item C0400 - Recall

Let's go back to an earlier question.

What were those three words that I asked you to repeat?

Category Cue Card – Item C0400A - Sock

Something to wear

Category Cue Card – Item C0400B - Blue

A color

Category Cue Card – Item C0400C

A piece of furniture

APPENDIX F

MDS ITEM MATRIX

MDS Item	Description	Skip trigger items	NOA item	Submitted Item	NC - Comp	NQ - Quart	NP - PPS	NS - OMRA SOT	NSD-OMRA SOT+DC	NO - OMRA other	NOD - OMRA other + DC	ND - Disch	NT - Tracking	SP - PPS	SS - OMRA SOT	SSD-OMRA SOT+DC	SO - OMRA other	SOD - OMRA other + DC	SD - Disch	ST - Tracking	XX - Inactivation	Demog/Admin	QI items	QM items	CAA items	RUG rehab grp	RUG non-rehab	RUG-III items	S&C items	PDC - Planned D/C	UPD - Unplanned D/C
A0050	Type of Record	×		×	×	×	×	×	×	×	×	×	×	×	×	×	×	×	×	×	×	×								×	×
A0100A	Facility National Provider Identifier (NPI)			×	×	×	×	×	×	×	×	×	×	×	×	×	×	×	×	×	×	×								×	×
A0100B	Facility CMS Certification Number (CCN)			×	×	×	×	×	×	×	×	×	×	×	×	×	×	×	×	×	×	×								×	×
A0100C	State provider number			×	×	×	×	×	×	×	×	×	×	×	×	×	×	×	×	×	×	×								×	×
A0200	Type of provider	×		×	×	×	×	×	×	×	×	×	×	×	×	×	×	×	×	×	×	×	×	×				×		×	×
A0310A	Type of assessment: OBRA	×		×	×	×	×	×	×	×	×	×	×	×	×	×	×	×	×	×	×	×	×	×	×		×		×	×	×
A0310B	Type of assessment: PPS			×	×	×	×	×	×	×	×	×	×	×	×	×	×	×	×	×	×	×	×	×	×	×	×	×	×	×	×
A0310C	Type of assessment: OMRA			×	×	×	×	×	×	×	×	×	×	×	×	×	×	×	×	×	×	×				×	×	×		×	×
A0310D	Swing bed clinical change assessment			×	×	×	×	×	×	×	×	×	×	×	×	×	×	×	×	×	×	×				×	×			×	×
A0310E	First assessment since most recent entry	×		×	×	×	×	×	×	×	×	×	×	×	×	×	×	×	×	×	×	×	×							×	×
A0310F	Entry/discharge reporting	×		×	×	×	×	×	×	×	×	×	×	×	×	×	×	×	×	×	×	×	×	×						×	×
A0310G	Planned/unplanned discharge	×		×	×	×	×	×	×	×	×	×	×	×	×	×	×	×	×	×	×	×								×	×
A0410	Submission requirement			×	×	×	×	×	×	×	×	×	×	×	×	×	×	×	×	×	×	×								×	×
A0500A	Resident first name			×	×	×	×	×	×	×	×	×	×	×	×	×	×	×	×	×		×								×	×
A0500B	Resident middle initial			×	×	×	×	×	×	×	×	×	×	×	×	×	×	×	×	×		×								×	×
A0500C	Resident last name			×	×	×	×	×	×	×	×	×	×	×	×	×	×	×	×	×		×								×	×
A0500D	Resident name suffix			×	×	×	×	×	×	×	×	×	×	×	×	×	×	×	×	×		×								×	×
A0600A	Social Security Number			×	×	×	×	×	×	×	×	×	×	×	×	×	×	×	×	×		×								×	×
A0600B	Resident Medicare/railroad insurance number			×	×	×	×	×	×	×	×	×	×	×	×	×	×	×	×	×		×								×	×
A0700	Resident Medicaid number			×	×	×	×	×	×	×	×	×	×	×	×	×	×	×	×	×		×								×	×
A0800	Gender			×	×	×	×	×	×	×	×	×	×	×	×	×	×	×	×	×		×								×	×
A0900	Birthdate	×		×	×	×	×	×	×	×	×	×	×	×	×	×	×	×	×	×		×								×	×
A1000A	Ethnicity: American Indian or Alaska Native			×	×	×	×	×	×	×	×	×	×	×	×	×	×	×	×	×		×								×	×
A1000B	Ethnicity: Asian			×	×	×	×	×	×	×	×	×	×	×	×	×	×	×	×	×		×								×	×
A1000C	Ethnicity: Black or African American			×	×	×	×	×	×	×	×	×	×	×	×	×	×	×	×	×		×								×	×
A1000D	Ethnicity: Hispanic or Latino			×	×	×	×	×	×	×	×	×	×	×	×	×	×	×	×	×		×								×	×
A1000E	Ethnicity: Native Hawaiian/Pacific Islander			×	×	×	×	×	×	×	×	×	×	×	×	×	×	×	×	×		×								×	×
A1000F	Ethnicity: White			×	×	×	×	×	×	×	×	×	×	×	×	×	×	×	×	×		×								×	×
A1100A	Does the resident need or want an interpreter	×		×	×	×	×	×	×	×	×	×	×	×	×	×	×	×	×	×		5								×	×
A1100B	Preferred language			×	×	×	×	×	×	×	×	×	×	×	×	×	×	×	×	×		5								×	×
A1200	Marital status			×	×	×	×	×	×	×	×	×	×	×	×	×	×	×	×	×		×								×	×
A1300A	Medical record number			×	×	×	×	×	×	×	×	×	×	×	×	×	×	×	×	×		×								×	×
A1300B	Room number			×	×	×	×	×	×	×	×	×	×	×	×	×	×	×	×	×		×								×	×
A1300C	Name by which resident prefers to be addressed			×	×	×	×	×	×	×	×	×	×	×	×	×	×	×	×	×		×								×	×
A1300D	Lifetime occupation(s)			×	×	×	×	×	×	×	×	×	×	×	×	×	×	×	×	×		×								×	×
A1500	Resident evaluated by PASRR			×	×		×	×	×	×	×	×											×								×	×
A1510A	Level II PASRR conditions: Serious Mental Illness			×	×								×							×											×	×
A1510B	Level II PASRR conditions: Mental Retardation			×	×								×							×											×	×
A1510C	Level II PASRR conditions: Other related conditions			×	×								×							×											×	×
A1550A	MR/DD status: Down syndrome			×	×								×							×										×	×	×
A1550B	MR/DD status: Autism			×	×								×							×										×	×	×
A1550C	MR/DD status: Epilepsy			×	×								×							×										×	×	×

Item matrix for April 2012

MDS Item	Description	Item Info: Skip trigger items	NOA item	Submitted Item	Nursing Home Item Subsets: NC - Comp	NQ - Quart	NP - PPS	NS - OMRA SOT	NSD-OMRA SOT+DC	NO - OMRA other	NOD - OMRA other + DC	ND - Disch	NT - Tracking	Swing Bed Item Subsets: SP - PPS	SS - OMRA SOT	SSD-OMRA SOT+DC	SO - OMRA other	SOD - OMRA other + DC	SD - Disch	ST - Tracking	XX - Inactivation	Item Groups: Demog/Admin	QI items	QM items	CAA items	RUG rehab grp	RUG non-rehab	RUG-III items	S&C items	New D/C: PDC - Planned D/C	UPD - Unplanned D/C
A1550D	MR/DD status: other organic MR/DD condition			x	x	x	x	x	x	x	x	x			x	x	x	x	x	x									x	x	x
A1550E	MR/DD status: MR/DD with no organic condition			x	x	x	x	x	x	x	x	x			x	x	x	x	x	x									x	x	x
A1550Z	MR/DD status: none of the above			x	x	x	x	x	x	x	x	x			x	x	x	x	x	x										x	x
A1600	Entry date (date of admission/reentry in facility)	x	x	x	x	x	x	x	x	x	x	x	x	x	x	x	x	x	x	x		x	x	x					x	x	x
A1700	Type of entry			x	x	x	x	x	x	x	x	x	x	x	x	x	x	x	x	x		x	x	x							x
A1800	Entered from			x	x	x	x	x	x	x	x	x	x	x	x	x	x	x	x	x		x								x	x
A2000	Discharge date			x	x	x	x	x	x	x	x	x			x	x	x	x	x			x	x	x						x	x
A2100	Discharge status			x	x	x	x	x	x	x	x	x			x	x	x	x	x			x								x	x
A2200	Previous asmt reference date for signif correction			x									x								x	1	x	x							
A2300	Assessment reference date	x		x	x	x	x	x	x	x	x	x		x	x	x	x	x	x			2	x	x			x			x	x
A2400A	Has resident had Medicare-covered stay	x		x	x	x	x	x	x	x	x			x	x	x	x	x				x	x								x
A2400B	Start date of most recent Medicare stay			x	x	x	x	x	x	x	x			x	x	x	x	x				x				x				x	x
A2400C	End date of most recent Medicare stay			x	x	x	x	x	x	x	x			x	x	x	x	x				x				x				x	x
B0100	Comatose	x		x	x	x	x	x	x	x	x	x			x	x	x	x	x					x				x	x		x	x
B0200	Hearing			x	x	x	x								x										x	x					x	
B0300	Hearing aid			x	x	x	x								x															x	
B0600	Speech clarity			x	x	x	x																								
B0700	Makes self understood			x	x	x	x			x	x							x	x						x			x	x		
B0800	Ability to understand others			x	x	x	x																		x						
B1000	Vision			x	x	x	x								x										x					x	
B1200	Corrective lenses			x	x	x	x								x										x					x	
C0100	BIMS: should resident interview be conducted	x		x	x	x	x			x	x		x		x	x	x	x	x	x										x	
C0200	BIMS res interview: repetition of three words			x	x	x	x			x	x		x		x	x	x	x	x	x				+				+	+	x	x
C0300A	BIMS res interview: able to report correct year			x	x	x	x			x	x		x			x	x	x	x	x				+				+	+	x	x
C0300B	BIMS res interview: able to report correct month			x	x	x	x			x	x		x			x	x	x	x	x				+				+	+	x	x
C0300C	BIMS res interview: can report correct day of week			x	x	x	x			x	x		x			x	x	x	x	x				+				+	+	x	x
C0400A	BIMS res interview: able to recall "sock"			x	x	x	x			x	x		x			x	x	x	x	x				+				+	+	x	x
C0400B	BIMS res interview: able to recall "blue"			x	x	x	x			x	x		x			x	x	x	x	x				+				+	+	x	x
C0400C	BIMS res interview: able to recall "bed"			x	x	x	x			x	x		x			x	x	x	x	x				+				+	+	x	x
C0500	BIMS res interview: summary score			x	x	x	x			x	x		x			x	x	x	x	x				+				+	x	x	x
C0600	Staff asmt mental status: conduct asmt	x		x	x	x	x																							x	x
C0700	Staff asmt mental status: short-term memory OK			x	x	x	x								x	x	x	x	x	x				x				x	x	x	x
C0800	Staff asmt mental status: long-term memory OK			x	x	x	x								x									x	x	x		x		x	
C0900A	Staff asmt mental status: recall current season			x	x	x	x								x																
C0900B	Staff asmt mental status: recall location of room			x	x	x	x								x																
C0900C	Staff asmt mental status: recall staff names/faces			x	x	x	x								x																
C0900D	Staff asmt mental status: recall in nursing home			x	x	x	x								x																
C0900Z	Staff asmt mental status: none of above recalled		x	x	x	x	x								x																

MDS Item	Description	Skip trigger items	NOA item	Submitted Item	NC - Comp	NQ - Quart	NP - PPS	NS - OMRA SOT	NSD-OMRA SOT+DC	NO - OMRA other	NOD - OMRA other + DC	ND - Disch	NT - Tracking	SP - PPS	SS - OMRA SOT	SSD-OMRA SOT+DC	SO - OMRA other	SOD - OMRA other + DC	SD - Disch	ST - Tracking	XX - Inactivation	Demog/Admin	QI items	QM items	CAA items	RUG rehab grp	RUG non-rehab	RUG-III items	S&C items	PDC - Planned D/C	UPD - Unplanned D/C
C1000	Cognitive skills for daily decision making			x	x	x	x	x	x	x	x	x	x	x	x	x	x	x	x	x					x		x	x	x	x	x
C1300A	Signs of delirium: inattention			x	x	x	x	x	x	x	x	x	x	x	x	x	x	x	x	x					x		+	+	x	x	x
C1300B	Signs of delirium: disorganized thinking			x	x	x	x	x	x	x	x	x	x	x	x	x	x	x	x	x					x		+	+	x	X	x
C1300C	Signs of delirium: altered level of consciousness			x	x	x	x	x	x	x	x	x	x	x	x	x	x	x	x	x					x		+	+	x	x	x
C1300D	Signs of delirium: psychomotor retardation			x	x	x	x	x	x	x	x	x	x	x	x	x	x	x	x	x					x		+	+	x	x	x
C1600	Acute onset mental status change			x	x	x	x	x	x	x	x	x	x	x	x	x	x	x	x	x					x		+	+	x	x	x
D0100	PHQ: should resident mood interview be conducted	x		x	x	x	x	x	x	x	x	x	x	x	x	x	x	x	x	x							+	+	x	x	
D0200A1	PHQ res: little interest or pleasure - presence	x		x	x	x	x	x	x	x	x	x	x	x	x	x	x	x	x	x					x		+	+		x	
D0200A2	PHQ res: little interest or pleasure - frequency			x	x	x	x	x	x	x	x	x	x	x	x	x	x	x	x	x				x			+	+	x	x	
D0200B1	PHQ res: feeling down, depressed - presence	x		x	x	x	x	x	x	x	x	x	x	x	x	x	x	x	x	x							+	+		x	
D0200B2	PHQ res: feeling down, depressed - frequency			x	x	x	x	x	x	x	x	x	x	x	x	x	x	x	x	x				x			+	+	x	x	
D0200C1	PHQ res: trouble with sleep - presence	x		x	x	x	x	x	x	x	x	x	x	x	x	x	x	x	x	x							+	+		x	
D0200C2	PHQ res: trouble with sleep - frequency			x	x	x	x	x	x	x	x	x	x	x	x	x	x	x	x	x				x			+	+	x	x	
D0200D1	PHQ res: feeling tired/little energy - presence	x		x	x	x	x	x	x	x	x	x	x	x	x	x	x	x	x	x							+	+		x	
D0200D2	PHQ res: feeling tired/little energy - frequency			x	x	x	x	x	x	x	x	x	x	x	x	x	x	x	x	x				x			+	+	x	x	
D0200E1	PHQ res: poor appetite or overeating - presence	x		x	x	x	x	x	x	x	x	x	x	x	x	x	x	x	x	x							+	+		x	
D0200E2	PHQ res: poor appetite or overeating - frequency			x	x	x	x	x	x	x	x	x	x	x	x	x	x	x	x	x				x			+	+	x	x	
D0200F1	PHQ res: feeling bad about self - presence	x		x	x	x	x	x	x	x	x	x	x	x	x	x	x	x	x	x							+	+		x	
D0200F2	PHQ res: feeling bad about self - frequency			x	x	x	x	x	x	x	x	x	x	x	x	x	x	x	x	x				x			+	+	x	x	
D0200G1	PHQ res: trouble concentrating - presence	x		x	x	x	x	x	x	x	x	x	x	x	x	x	x	x	x	x							+	+		x	
D0200G2	PHQ res: trouble concentrating - frequency			x	x	x	x	x	x	x	x	x	x	x	x	x	x	x	x	x				x			+	+	x	x	
D0200H1	PHQ res: slow, fidgety, restless - presence	x		x	x	x	x	x	x	x	x	x	x	x	x	x	x	x	x	x							+	+		x	
D0200H2	PHQ res: slow, fidgety, restless - frequency			x	x	x	x	x	x	x	x	x	x	x	x	x	x	x	x	x				x			+	+	x	x	
D0200I1	PHQ res: thoughts better off dead - presence	x		x	x	x	x	x	x	x	x	x	x	x	x	x	x	x	x	x					x		+	+		x	
D0200I2	PHQ res: thoughts better off dead - frequency			x	x	x	x	x	x	x	x	x	x	x	x	x	x	x	x	x				x			+	+	x	x	
D0300	PHQ res: total mood severity score			x	x	x	x	x	x	x	x	x	x	x	x	x	x	x	x	x				x	x		x	x	x	x	
D0350	PHQ res: safety notification			x	x	x	x	x	x	x	x	x	x	x	x	x	x	x	x	x							+	+	x	x	
D0500A1	PHQ staff: little interest or pleasure - presence			x	x	x	x	x	x	x	x	x	x	x	x	x	x	x	x	x					x		+	+		x	
D0500A2	PHQ staff: little interest or pleasure - frequency			x	x	x	x	x	x	x	x	x	x	x	x	x	x	x	x	x				x			+	+	x	x	
D0500B1	PHQ staff: feeling down, depressed - presence			x	x	x	x	x	x	x	x	x	x	x	x	x	x	x	x	x							+	+	x	x	
D0500B2	PHQ staff: feeling down, depressed - frequency			x	x	x	x	x	x	x	x	x	x	x	x	x	x	x	x	x				x			+	+	x	x	
D0500C1	PHQ staff: trouble with sleep - presence			x	x	x	x	x	x	x	x	x	x	x	x	x	x	x	x	x							+	+	x	x	
D0500C2	PHQ staff: trouble with sleep - frequency			x	x	x	x	x	x	x	x	x	x	x	x	x	x	x	x	x				x			+	+	x	x	
D0500D1	PHQ staff: feeling tired/little energy - presence			x	x	x	x	x	x	x	x	x	x	x	x	x	x	x	x	x							+	+	x	x	
D0500D2	PHQ staff: feeling tired/little energy - frequency			x	x	x	x	x	x	x	x	x	x	x	x	x	x	x	x	x				x			+	+	x	x	
D0500E1	PHQ staff: poor appetite or overeating - presence			x	x	x	x	x	x	x	x	x	x	x	x	x	x	x	x	x							+	+	x	x	
D0500E2	PHQ staff: poor appetite or overeating - frequency			x	x	x	x	x	x	x	x	x	x	x	x	x	x	x	x	x				x			+	+	x	x	
D0500F1	PHQ staff: feeling bad about self - presence			x	x	x	x	x	x	x	x	x	x	x	x	x	x	x	x	x							+	+	x	x	

April 2012 item matrix

Item matrix for April 2012		Item Info			Nursing Home Item Subsets									Swing Bed Item Subsets									Item Groups							New D/C	
MDS Item	Description	Skip trigger items	NOA item	Submitted Item	NC - Comp	NQ - Quart	NP - PPS	NS - OMRA SOT	NSD-OMRA SOT+DC	NO - OMRA other	NOD - OMRA other + DC	ND - Disch	NT - Tracking	SP - PPS	SS - OMRA SOT	SSD-OMRA SOT+DC	SO - OMRA other	SOD - OMRA other + DC	SD - Disch	ST - Tracking	XX - Inactivation	Demog/Admin	QI items	QM items	CAA items	RUG rehab grp	RUG non-rehab	RUG-III items	S&C items	PDC - Planned D/C	UPD - Unplanned D/C
D0500F2	PHQ staff: feeling bad about self - frequency			X	X	X	X	X	X	X	X	X		X	X	X	X	X	X					X			+	+		X	
D0500G1	PHQ staff: trouble concentrating - presence			X	X	X	X	X	X	X	X	X		X	X	X	X	X	X								+	+	X	X	
D0500G2	PHQ staff: trouble concentrating - frequency			X	X	X	X	X	X	X	X	X		X	X	X	X	X	X					X			+	+		X	
D0500H1	PHQ staff: slow, fidgety, restless - presence			X	X	X	X	X	X	X	X	X		X	X	X	X	X	X								+	+	X	X	
D0500H2	PHQ staff: slow, fidgety, restless - frequency			X	X	X	X	X	X	X	X	X		X	X	X	X	X	X					X			+	+		X	
D0500I1	PHQ staff: thoughts better off dead - presence	X		X	X	X	X	X	X	X	X	X		X	X	X	X	X	X					X	X		+	+	X	X	
D0500I2	PHQ staff: thoughts better off dead - frequency			X	X	X	X	X	X	X	X	X		X	X	X	X	X	X								+	+		X	
D0500J1	PHQ staff: short-tempered - presence			X	X	X	X	X	X	X	X	X		X	X	X	X	X	X					X			+	+	X	X	
D0500J2	PHQ staff: short-tempered - frequency			X	X	X	X	X	X	X	X	X		X	X	X	X	X	X								+	+		X	
D0600	PHQ staff: total mood severity score			X	X	X	X	X	X	X	X	X		X	X	X	X	X	X					X	X		+	+	X	X	
D0650	PHQ staff: safety notification			X	X	X	X	X	X	X	X	X		X	X	X	X	X	X											X	
E0100A	Psychosis: hallucinations			X	X	X	X	X	X	X	X	X		X	X	X	X	X	X				X				x	x		X	X
E0100B	Psychosis: delusions			X	X	X	X	X	X	X	X	X		X	X	X	X	X	X				X				x	x		X	X
E0100Z	Psychosis: none of the above		x	X	X	X	X	X	X	X	X	X		X	X	X	X	X	X								+	+		X	X
E0200A	Physical behav symptoms directed toward others	X		X	X	X	X	X	X	X	X	X		X	X	X	X	X	X				X		X		x	x	X	X	X
E0200B	Verbal behavioral symptoms directed toward others	X		X	X	X	X	X	X	X	X	X		X	X	X	X	X	X				X		X		x	x	X	X	X
E0200C	Other behav symptoms not directed toward others	X		X	X	X	X	X	X	X	X	X		X	X	X	X	X	X				X		X		x	x		X	X
E0300	Overall presence of behavioral symptoms	X		X	X	s	s	s	s	s	s	s											X		X				X		
E0500A	Behav symptoms put res at risk for illness/injury			X	X	s	s	s	s	s	s	s																			
E0500B	Behav symptoms interfere with resident care			X	X	s	s	s	s	s	s	s																			
E0500C	Behav symptoms interfere with social activities			X	X	s	s	s	s	s	s	s																			
E0600A	Behav symptoms put others at risk for injury			X	X	s	s	s	s	s	s	s																			
E0600B	Behav symptoms intrude on privacy of others			X	X	s	s	s	s	s	s	s																			
E0600C	Behav symptoms disrupt care or living environment			X	X	s	s	s	s	s	s	s																			
E0800	Rejection of care: presence and frequency			X	X	X	X	X	X	X	X	X		X	X	X	X	X	X				X		X		x	x	X	X	X
E0900	Wandering: presence and frequency	X		X	X	X	X	X	X	X	X	X		X	X	X	X	X	X				X		X		x	x	X	X	X
E1000A	Wandering: risk of getting to dangerous place			X	X	s	s	s	s	s	s	s																			
E1000B	Wandering: intrude on privacy of others			X	X	s	s	s	s	s	s	s																			
E1100	Change in behavioral or other symptoms			X	X	s	s	s	s	s	s	s														X					
F0300	Conduct res interview for daily/activity prefs	X		X	X	s	s	s	s	s	s	s																			
F0400A	Res interview: choose clothes to wear			X	X	s	s	s	s	s	s	s																			
F0400B	Res interview: take care of personal belongings			X	X	s	s	s	s	s	s	s																			
F0400C	Res interview: choose tub, bath, shower, sponge			X	X	s	s	s	s	s	s	s																			
F0400D	Res interview: have snacks between meals			X	X	s	s	s	s	s	s	s																			
F0400E	Res interview: choose own bedtime			X	X	s	s	s	s	s	s	s																			
F0400F	Res interview: discuss care with family/friend			X	X	s	s	s	s	s	s	s																			
F0400G	Res interview: use phone in private			X	X	s	s	s	s	s	s	s																			
F0400H	Res interview: lock things to keep them safe			X	X	s	s	s	s	s	s	s																			

MDS Item	Description	Skip trigger items	NOA item	Submitted Item	NC - Comp	NQ - Quant	NP - PPS	NS - OMRA SOT	NSD - OMRA SOT+DC	NO - OMRA other	NOD - OMRA other + DC	ND - Disch	NT - Tracking	SP - PPS	SS - OMRA SOT	SSD - OMRA SOT+DC	SO - OMRA other	SOD - OMRA other + DC	SD - Disch	ST - Tracking	XX - Inactivation	Demog/Admin	QI items	QM items	CAA items	RUG rehab grp	RUG non-rehab	RUG-III items	S&C items	PDC - Planned D/C	UPD - Unplanned D/C
F0500A	Res interview: have books, newspaper, mags to read			x	x	s	s																			x						
F0500B	Res interview: listen to music			x	x	s	s																			x						
F0500C	Res interview: be around animals/pets			x	x	s	s																			x						
F0500D	Res interview: keep up with news			x	x	s	s																			x						
F0500E	Res interview: do things with groups of people			x	x	s	s																			x						
F0500F	Res interview: do favorite activities			x	x	s	s																			x						
F0500G	Res interview: go outside when good weather			x	x	s	s																			x						
F0500H	Res interview: participate in religious practices			x	x	s	s																			x						
F0600	Primary respondent: daily/activities prefs			x	x	s	s																			x						
F0700	Conduct staff assessment for daily/activity prefs	x		x	x	s	s																			x						
F0800A	Staff assessment: choosing clothes to wear			x	x	s	s																									
F0800B	Staff assessment: caring for personal belongings			x	x	s	s																									
F0800C	Staff assessment: receiving tub bath			x	x	s	s																									
F0800D	Staff assessment: receiving shower			x	x	s	s																									
F0800E	Staff assessment: receiving bed bath			x	x	s	s																									
F0800F	Staff assessment: receiving sponge bath			x	x	s	s																									
F0800G	Staff assessment: snacks between meals			x	x	s	s																									
F0800H	Staff assessment: staying up past 8PM			x	x	s	s																									
F0800I	Staff assessment: discuss care with family/other			x	x	s	s																									
F0800J	Staff assessment: use phone in private			x	x	s	s																									
F0800K	Staff assessment: place to lock personal things			x	x	s	s																									
F0800L	Staff assessment: reading books, newspapers, mags			x	x	s	s																			x						
F0800M	Staff assessment: listening to music			x	x	s	s																			x						
F0800N	Staff assessment: being around animals/pets			x	x	s	s																			x						
F0800O	Staff assessment: keeping up with news			x	x	s	s																			x						
F0800P	Staff assessment: doing things with groups			x	x	s	s																			x						
F0800Q	Staff assessment: participate favorite activities			x	x	s	s																			x						
F0800R	Staff assessment: spend time away from nursng home			x	x	s	s																			x						
F0800S	Staff assessment: spend time outdoors			x	x	s	s																			x						
F0800T	Staff assessment: participate religious activities			x	x	s	s																			x						
F0800Z	Staff assessment: none of above activities		x	x	x	s	s																									
G0110A1	Bed mobility: self-performance			x	x	s	x	x	x	x	x	x		x	x	x	x	x	x					x	x	x	x	x			x
G0110A2	Bed mobility: support provided			x	x	s	x	x	x	x	x	x		x	x	x	x	x	x					x		x	x	x			
G0110B1	Transfer: self-performance			x	x	s	x	x	x	x	x	x		x	x	x	x	x	x					x		x	x	x	x		x
G0110B2	Transfer: support provided			x	x	s	x	x	x	x	x	x		x	x	x	x	x	x							x	x	x			
G0110C1	Walk in room: self-performance			x	x		x	x	x	x	x	x		x	x	x	x	x	x					x	x				x		x
G0110C2	Walk in room: support provided			x	x		x		x		x	x		x		x		x	x										x		
G0110D1	Walk in corridor: self-performance			x	x		x	x	x	x	x	x		x	x	x	x	x	x					x	x				x		x

April 2012 item matrix

Item matrix for April 2012

MDS Item	Description	Skip trigger items	NOA item	Submitted Item	NC-Comp	NQ-Quart	NP-PPS	NS-OMRA SOT	NSD-OMRA SOT+DC	NO-OMRA other	NOD-OMRA other+DC	ND-Disch	NT-Tracking	SP-PPS	SS-OMRA SOT	SSD-OMRA SOT+DC	SO-OMRA other	SOD-OMRA other+DC	SD-Disch	ST-Tracking	XX-Inactivation	Demog/Admin	QI items	QM items	CAA items	RUG rehab grp	RUG non-rehab	RUG-III items	S&C items	PDC-Planned D/C	UPD-Unplanned D/C
G0110D2	Walk in corridor: support provided			X	X	X	X							X																		
G0110E1	Locomotion on unit: self-performance			X	X	X	X	X	X	X	X	X		X	X	X	X	X	X						CAA					X	X
G0110E2	Locomotion on unit: support provided			X	X	X	X		X		X	X		X		X		X	X											X	X
G0110F1	Locomotion off unit: self-performance			X	X	X	X	X	X	X	X	X		X	X	X	X	X	X						CAA					X	X
G0110F2	Locomotion off unit: support provided			X	X	X	X		X		X	X		X		X		X	X											X	X
G0110G1	Dressing: self-performance			X	X	X	X	X	X	X	X	X		X	X	X	X	X	X						CAA				X	X	X
G0110G2	Dressing: support provided			X	X	X	X		X		X	X		X		X		X	X											X	X
G0110H1	Eating: self-performance			X	X	X	X	X	X	X	X	X		X	X	X	X	X	X					X	CAA	X	X	X	X	X	X
G0110H2	Eating: support provided			X	X	X	X		X		X	X		X		X		X	X							X	X	X		X	X
G0110I1	Toilet use: self-performance			X	X	X	X	X	X	X	X	X		X	X	X	X	X	X					X	CAA	X	X	X	X	X	X
G0110I2	Toilet use: support provided			X	X	X	X		X		X	X		X		X		X	X							X	X	X		X	X
G0110J1	Personal hygiene: self-performance			X	X	X	X	X	X	X	X	X		X	X	X	X	X	X					X	CAA				X	X	X
G0110J2	Personal hygiene: support provided			X	X	X	X		X		X	X		X		X		X	X											X	X
G0120A	Bathing: self-performance			X	X	X	X	X	X	X	X	X		X	X	X	X	X	X					X	CAA				X	X	X
G0120B	Bathing: support provided			X	X	X	X							X																	
G0300A	Balance: moving from seated to standing position			X	X									X											CAA						
G0300B	Balance: walking (with assistive device if used)			X	X									X											CAA						
G0300C	Balance: turning around while walking			X	X									X											CAA						
G0300D	Balance: moving on and off toilet			X	X									X											CAA						
G0300E	Balance: surface-to-surface transfer			X	X									X											CAA						
G0400A	ROM limitation: upper extremity			X	X	X	X							X															X		
G0400B	ROM limitation: lower extremity			X	X	X	X							X															X		
G0600A	Mobility devices: cane/crutch			X	X	X	X							X															X		
G0600B	Mobility devices: walker			X	X	X	X							X															X		
G0600C	Mobility devices: wheelchair (manual or electric)			X	X	X	X							X																	
G0600D	Mobility devices: limb prosthesis			X	X	X	X							X																	
G0600Z	Mobility devices: none of the above		X	X	X	X	X							X																	
G0900A	Resident believes capable of increased independ			X	X						X	X		X					X	X					CAA						
G0900B	Staff believes res capable of increased independ			X	X						X	X		X					X	X					CAA						
H0100A	Appliances: indwelling catheter			X	X	X	X	X	X	X	X	X		X	X	X	X	X	X					X	CAA				X	X	X
H0100B	Appliances: external catheter			X	X	X	X	X	X	X	X	X		X	X	X	X	X	X						CAA					X	X
H0100C	Appliances: ostomy			X	X	X	X	X	X	X	X	X		X	X	X	X	X	X					X	CAA				X	X	X
H0100D	Appliances: intermittent catheterization			X	X	X	X	X	X	X	X	X		X	X	X	X	X	X						CAA					X	X
H0100Z	Appliances: none of the above		X	X	X	X	X							X																X	X
H0200A	Urinary toileting program: has been attempted	X		X	X	s	s							X																	
H0200B	Urinary toileting program: response			X	X	s	s							X																	
H0200C	Urinary toileting program: current program/trial			X	X	X	X	X	X	X	X	X		X	X	X	X	X	X							X		X	X		X
H0300	Urinary continence			X	X	X	X	X	X	X	X	X		X	X	X	X	X	X					X	CAA		X		X	X	X

Item matrix for April 2012

MDS Item	Description	Skip trigger items	NOA item	Submitted item	NC - Comp	NQ - Quart	NP - PPS	NS - OMRA SOT	NSD - OMRA SOT+DC	NO - OMRA other	NOD - OMRA other + DC	ND - Disch	NT - Tracking	SP - PPS	SS - OMRA SOT	SSD - OMRA SOT+DC	SO - OMRA other	SOD - OMRA other + DC	SD - Disch	ST - Tracking	XX - Inactivation	Demog/Admin	QI items	QM items	CAA items	RUG rehab grp	RUG non-rehab	RUG-III items	S&C items	PDC - Planned D/C	UPD - Unplanned D/C
H0400	Bowel continence			X	X	X	X	X	X	X	X	X		X	X	X	X	X	X					X	X				X	X	X
H0500	Bowel toileting program being used			X	X	X	X	X	X	X	X			X	X	X	X	X								X	X	X	X		
H0600	Constipation			X	X	s	s																			X						
I0100	Cancer (with or without metastasis)			X	X	s	s							X																		
I0200	Anemia			X	X	X	X							X																		
I0300	Atrial fibrillation and other dysrhythmias			X	X	s	s																									
I0400	Coronary artery disease (CAD)			X	X	s	s																									
I0500	Deep venous thrombosis (DVT), PE, or PTE			X	X	s	s																									
I0600	Heart failure			X	X	X	X							X																		
I0700	Hypertension			X	X	X	X							X																		
I0800	Orthostatic hypotension			X	X	X	X							X																		
I0900	Peripheral vascular disease (PVD) or PAD			X	X	X	X		X	X	X	X		X		X	X	X	X					X						X	X
I1100	Cirrhosis			X	X	s	s																									
I1200	Gastroesophageal reflux disease (GERD) or ulcer			X	X	s	s																									
I1300	Ulcerative colitis, Chrohn's, inflam bowel disease			X	X	s	s																									
I1400	Benign prostatic hyperplasia (BPH)			X	X	s	s																									
I1500	Renal insufficiency, renal failure, ESRD			X	X	s	s																									
I1550	Neurogenic bladder			X	X	X	X		X	X	X	X		X		X	X	X	X					X							X	X
I1650	Obstructive uropathy			X	X	X	X		X	X	X	X		X		X	X	X	X					X							X	X
I1700	Multidrug resistant organism (MDRO)			X	X	X	X		X	X	X	X		X		X	X	X	X						X					X		
I2000	Pneumonia			X	X	X	X		X	X	X	X		X		X	X	X	X						X	X		X	X	X		
I2100	Septicemia			X	X	X	X		X	X	X	X		X		X	X	X	X						X	X		X	X	X		
I2200	Tuberculosis			X	X	X	X		X	X	X	X		X											X					X		
I2300	Urinary tract infection (UTI) (LAST 30 DAYS)			X	X	X	X		X	X	X	X		X		X	X	X	X					X	X					X	X	X
I2400	Viral hepatitis (includes type A, B, C, D, and E)			X	X	X	X																		X					X		
I2500	Wound infection (other than foot)			X	X	X	X							X											X					X		
I2900	Diabetes mellitus (DM)			X	X	X	X		X	X	X	X		X		X	X	X	X					X				X	X		X	X
I3100	Hyponatremia			X	X	X	X							X																		
I3200	Hyperkalemia			X	X	X	X							X																		
I3300	Hyperlipidemia (e.g., hypercholesterolemia)			X	X	s	s							X																		
I3400	Thyroid disorder			X	X	s	s							X																		
I3700	Arthritis			X	X	s	s																									
I3800	Osteoporosis			X	X	s	s							X																X		
I3900	Hip fracture			X	X	X	X																							X		
I4000	Other fracture			X	X	X	X																							X		
I4200	Alzheimer's disease			X	X	X	X		X	X	X	X		X		X	X	X	X							X		X	X	X		
I4300	Aphasia			X	X	X	X		X	X	X	X		X		X	X	X	X									X	X			
I4400	Cerebral palsy			X	X	X	X		X	X	X	X		X				X		X								X	X			

April 2012 item matrix

MDS item matrix for APR 2012 (v13) 10-27-2011

Item matrix for April 2012

MDS Item	Description	Skip trigger items	NOA item	Submitted Item	NC-Comp	NQ-Quart	NP-PPS	NS-OMRA SOT	NSD-OMRA SOT+DC	NO-OMRA other	NOD-OMRA other+DC	ND-Disch	NT-Tracking	SP-PPS	SS-OMRA SOT	SSD-OMRA SOT+DC	SO-OMRA other	SOD-OMRA other+DC	SD-Disch	ST-Tracking	XX-Inactivation	Demog/Admin	QI items	QM items	CAA items	RUG rehab grp	RUG non-rehab	RUG-III items	S&C items	PDC-Planned D/C	UPD-Unplanned D/C
I4500	Cerebrovascular accident (CVA), TIA, or stroke			x	x	x	x							x																	
I4800	Non-Alzheimer's Dementia			x	x	x	x							x											x				x		
I4900	Hemiplegia or hemiparesis			x	x	x	x			x	x			x			x	x									x	x			x
I5000	Paraplegia			x	x	x	x							x																	
I5100	Quadriplegia			x	x	x	x			x	x			x			x	x									x	x			
I5200	Multiple sclerosis			x	x	x	x			x	x			x			x	x									x	x			
I5250	Huntington's disease			x	x	x	x		x			x		x		x			x				x							x	x
I5300	Parkinson's disease			x	x	x	x			x	x			x			x	x									x				
I5350	Tourette's syndrome			x	x	x	x		x			x		x		x			x				x							x	x
I5400	Seizure disorder or epilepsy			x	x	x	x							x																	
I5500	Traumatic brain injury (TBI)			x	x	x	x							x																	
I5600	Malnutrition (protein, calorie), risk of malnutrit			x	x	x	x		x			x		x		x			x					x						x	x
I5700	Anxiety disorder			x	x	x	x		x			x		x		x			x				x						x	x	x
I5800	Depression (other than bipolar)			x	x	x	x							x															x		
I5900	Manic depression (bipolar disease)			x	x	x	x		x			x		x		x			x				x						x	x	x
I5950	Psychotic disorder (other than schizophrenia)			x	x	x	x		x	x		x		x		x	x		x				x						x	x	x
I6000	Schizophrenia			x	x	x	x		x	x		x		x		x	x		x				x						x	x	x
I6100	Post-traumatic stress disorder PTSD			x	x	x	x		x			x		x		x			x				x							x	x
I6200	Asthma (COPD) or chronic lung disease			x	x	x	x			x	x			x			x	x									x			x	x
I6300	Respiratory failure			x	x	x	x			x	x			x			x	x									x				
I6500	Cataracts, glaucoma, or macular degeneration			x	x	x	x							x											x						
I7900	None of above active diseases within last 7 days		x	x	x	s	s					x		x					x												
I8000A	Additional active ICD diagnosis 1			x	x	x	x	x	x	x	x	x		x	x	x	x	x	x			3		x						x	x
I8000B	Additional active ICD diagnosis 2			x	x	x	x	x	x	x	x	x		x	x	x	x	x	x			3		x						x	x
I8000C	Additional active ICD diagnosis 3			x	x	x	x	x	x	x	x	x		x	x	x	x	x	x			3		x						x	x
I8000D	Additional active ICD diagnosis 4			x	x	x	x	x	x	x	x	x		x	x	x	x	x	x			3		x						x	x
I8000E	Additional active ICD diagnosis 5			x	x	x	x	x	x	x	x	x		x	x	x	x	x	x			3		x						x	x
I8000F	Additional active ICD diagnosis 6			x	x	x	x	x	x	x	x	x		x	x	x	x	x	x			3		x						x	x
I8000G	Additional active ICD diagnosis 7			x	x	x	x	x	x	x	x	x		x	x	x	x	x	x			3		x						x	x
I8000H	Additional active ICD diagnosis 8			x	x	x	x	x	x	x	x	x		x	x	x	x	x	x			3		x						x	x
I8000I	Additional active ICD diagnosis 9			x	x	x	x	x	x	x	x	x		x	x	x	x	x	x			3		x						x	x
I8000J	Additional active ICD diagnosis 10			x	x	x	x	x	x	x	x	x		x	x	x	x	x	x			3		x						x	x
J0100A	Pain: Received scheduled pain med regimen			x	x	x	x	x	x			x		x	x	x			x										x	x	x
J0100B	Pain: received PRN pain medications			x	x	x	x	x	x			x		x	x	x			x										x	x	x
J0100C	Pain: received non-medication intervention			x	x	x	x	x	x			x		x	x	x			x										x	x	x
J0200	Should pain assessment interview be conducted			x	x	x	x	x	x	x	x	x		x	x	x	x	x	x					+						x	x
J0300	Res pain interview: presence	x		x	x	x	x		x			x		x		x			x					x						x	x
J0400	Res pain interview: frequency	x		x	x	x	x		x			x		x		x			x					x	x						

Column groups: **Item Info** (Skip trigger items, NOA item, Submitted Item) · **Nursing Home Item Subsets** (NC - Comp, NQ - Quart, NP - PPS, NS - OMRA SOT, NSD-OMRA SOT+DC, NO - OMRA other, NOD - OMRA other + DC, ND - Disch, NT - Tracking) · **Swing Bed Item Subsets** (SP - PPS, SS - OMRA SOT, SSD-OMRA SOT+DC, SO - OMRA other, SOD - OMRA other + DC, SD - Disch, ST - Tracking) · **Item Groups** (XX - Inactivation, Demog/Admin, QI items, QM items, CAA items, RUG rehab grp, RUG non-rehab, RUG-III items, S&C items) · **New D/C** (PDC - Planned D/C, UPD - Unplanned D/C)

MDS Item	Description	Skip	NOA	Sub	NC	NQ	NP	NS	NSD	NO	NOD	ND	NT	SP	SS	SSD	SO	SOD	SD	ST	XX	Demog	QI	QM	CAA	RUGreh	RUGnon	RUG3	S&C	PDC	UPD
J0500A	Res pain interview: made it hard to sleep			X	X	X	X		X		X	X		X		X		X	X						X					X	X
J0500B	Res pain interview: limited daily activities			X	X	X	X		X		X	X		X		X		X	X						X					X	X
J0600A	Res pain interview: intensity rating scale			X	X	X	X		X		X	X		X		X		X	X					X	X					X	X
J0600B	Res pain interview: verbal descriptor scale			X	X	X	X		X		X	X		X		X		X	X					X	X					X	X
J0700	Should staff assessment for pain be conducted	X		X	X	X	X							X											+						
J0800A	Staff pain asmt: non-verbal sounds			X	X	X	X							X											X						
J0800B	Staff pain asmt: vocal complaints of pain			X	X	X	X							X											X						
J0800C	Staff pain asmt: facial expressions			X	X	X	X							X											X						
J0800D	Staff pain asmt: protective movements/postures			X	X	X	X							X											X						
J0800Z	Staff pain asmt: none of these signs observed	X		X	X	X	X							X											+						
J0850	Staff pain asmt: frequency of pain			X	X	X	X							X																	
J1100A	Short breath/trouble breathing: with exertion			X	X	X	X		X		X	X		X		X		X	X											X	X
J1100B	Short breath/trouble breathing: sitting at rest			X	X	X	X		X		X	X		X		X		X	X											X	X
J1100C	Short breath/trouble breathing: lying flat			X	X	X	X		X	X	X	X		X		X	X	X	X								X			X	X
J1100Z	Short breath/trouble breathing: none of above		X	X	X	X	X		X	X	X	X		X		X	X	X	X											X	X
J1300	Current tobacco use		X	X	X	s	s			X	X	X					X	X	X											X	X
J1400	Prognosis: life expectancy of less than 6 months			X	X	X	X		X		X	X		X		X		X	X				X		X					X	X
J1550A	Problem conditions: fever			X	X	X	X		X		X	X		X		X		X	X						X		X	X		X	X
J1550B	Problem conditions: vomiting			X	X	X	X		X		X	X		X		X		X	X								X	X		X	X
J1550C	Problem conditions: dehydrated			X	X	X	X		X	X	X	X		X		X	X	X	X						X			X	X	X	X
J1550D	Problem conditions: internal bleeding			X	X	X	X		X	X	X	X		X		X	X	X	X						X			X	X	X	X
J1550Z	Problem conditions: none of the above		X	X	X	X	X		X	X	X	X		X		X	X	X	X						+			+	X	X	X
J1700A	Fall history: fall during month before admission			X	X		X		X		X	X		X		X		X	X						X				X	X	X
J1700B	Fall history: fall 2-6 months before admission			X	X		X		X		X	X		X		X		X	X						X					X	X
J1700C	Fall history: fracture from fall 6 month pre admit			X	X		X		X		X	X		X		X		X	X											X	X
J1800	Falls since admit/prior asmt: any falls	X		X	X	X	X		X		X	X		X		X		X	X				X		X				X	X	X
J1900A	Falls since admit/prior asmt: no injury			X	X	X	X		X		X	X		X		X		X	X											X	X
J1900B	Falls since admit/prior asmt: injury (not major)			X	X	X	X		X		X	X		X		X		X	X					X					X	X	X
J1900C	Falls since admit/prior asmt: major injury			X	X	X	X		X		X	X		X		X		X	X										X	X	X
K0100A	Swallow disorder: loss liquids/solids from mouth			X	X	X	X		X		X	X		X		X		X	X										X	X	X
K0100B	Swallow disorder: holds food in mouth/cheeks			X	X	X	X		X		X	X		X		X		X	X											X	X
K0100C	Swallow disorder: cough/choke with meals/meds			X	X	X	X		X		X	X		X		X		X	X											X	X
K0100D	Swallow disorder: difficulty or pain swallowing			X	X	X	X		X		X	X		X		X		X	X											X	X
K0100Z	Swallow disorder: none of the above		X	X	X	X	X		X		X	X		X		X		X	X											X	X
K0200A	Height (in inches)			X	X	X	X		X		X	X		X		X		X	X					X	X				X	X	X
K0200B	Weight (in pounds)			X	X	X	X		X	X	X	X		X		X	X	X	X					X	X		X	X	X	X	X
K0300	Weight loss		X	X	X	X	X		X	X	X	X		X		X	X	X	X					X	X		X	X	X	X	X
K0310	Weight Gain			X	X	X	X		X	X	X	X		X		X	X	X	X					X	X			X	X	X	X

April 2012 item matrix

Item matrix for April 2012

MDS Item	Description	Skip trigger items	NOA item	Submitted Item	NC - Comp	NQ - Quart	NP - PPS	NS - OMRA SOT	NSD-OMRA SOT+DC	NO - OMRA other	NOD - OMRA other + DC	ND - Disch	NT - Tracking	SP - PPS	SS - OMRA SOT	SSD-OMRA SOT+DC	SO - OMRA other	SOD - OMRA other + DC	SD - Disch	ST - Tracking	XX - Inactivation	Demog/Admin	QI items	QM items	CAA items	RUG rehab grp	RUG non-rehab	RUG-III items	S&C items	PDC - Planned D/C	UPD - Unplanned D/C
K0510A1	Nutrition approach: Not Res: parenteral /IV feeding	x		x	x	x	x		x	x	x	x		x		x	x	x	x						x		x	x	x	x	x
K0510A2	Nutrition approach: Res: parenteral /IV feeding	x		x	x	x	x		x	x	x	x		x		x	x	x	x						x		x	x	x	x	x
K0510B1	Nutrition approach: Not Res: feeding tube	x		x	x	x	x		x	x	x	x		x		x	x	x	x						x		x	x	x	x	x
K0510B2	Nutrition approach: Res: feeding tube	x		x	x	x	x		x	x	x	x		x		x	x	x	x						x		x	x	x	x	x
K0510C1	Nutrition approach: Not Res: mechanically altered diet			x	x	x	x		x	x	x	x		x		x	x	x	x						x					x	
K0510C2	Nutrition approach: Res: mechanically altered diet			x	x	x	x		x	x	x	x		x		x	x	x	x						x				x	x	
K0510D1	Nutrition approach: Not Res: therapeutic diet			x	x	x	x		x	x	x	x		x		x	x	x	x						x					x	
K0510D2	Nutrition approach: Res: therapeutic diet			x	x	x	x		x	x	x	x		x		x	x	x	x						x				x	x	
K0510Z1	Nutrition approach: Not Res: none of the above		x	x	x	x	x		x	x	x	x		x		x	x	x	x						+				x	x	
K0510Z2	Nutrition approach: Res: none of the above		x	x	x	x	x		x	x	x	x		x		x	x	x	x						+				+	x	
K0700A	Proportion total calories via parenteral/tube feed			x	x	x	x		x	x	x	x				x	x	x									x	x			
K0700B	Average fluid intake per day by IV or tube			x	x	x	x		x	x	x	x				x	x	x									x	x			
L0200A	Dental: broken or loosely fitting denture			x	x	s	s																		x						
L0200B	Dental: no natural teeth or tooth fragment(s)			x	x	s	s																		x						
L0200C	Dental: abnormal mouth tissue			x	x	s	s																		x						
L0200D	Dental: cavity or broken natural teeth			x	x	s	s																		x						
L0200E	Dental: inflamed/bleeding gums or loose teeth			x	x	s	s																		x						
L0200F	Dental: pain, discomfort, difficulty chewing			x	x	s	s																		x						
L0200G	Dental: unable to examine		x	x	x	x	x																								
L0200Z	Dental: none of the above	x		x	x	x	x																								
M0100A	Risk determination: has ulcer, scar, or dressing			x	x	x	x		x			x	x		x		x			x					x		x	x			x
M0100B	Risk determination: formal assessment			x	x	x	x								x																
M0100C	Risk determination: clinical assessment			x	x	x	x								x																
M0100Z	Risk determination: none of the above		x	x	x	x	x								x																
M0150	Is resident at risk of developing pressure ulcer			x	x	x	x		x		x	x	x		x		x		x	x					x		x	x		x	x
M0210	Resident has Stage 1 or higher pressure ulcers	x		x	x	x	x																								
M0300A	Stage 1 pressure ulcers: number present			x	x	x	x		x		x	x	x		x		x		x	x					x		x	x		x	x
M0300B1	Stage 2 pressure ulcers: number present	x		x	x	x	x		x		x	x	x		x		x		x	x				x	x		x	x	x	x	x
M0300B2	Stage 2 pressure ulcers: number at admit/reentry			x	x	x	x						x		x					x									x		
M0300B3	Stage 2 pressure ulcers: date of oldest			x	x	x	x								x																
M0300C1	Stage 3 pressure ulcers: number present	x		x	x	x	x		x		x	x	x		x		x		x	x				x	x		x	x	x	x	x
M0300C2	Stage 3 pressure ulcers: number at admit/reentry			x	x	x	x						x		x					x									x		
M0300D1	Stage 4 pressure ulcers: number present	x		x	x	x	x		x		x	x	x		x		x		x	x				x	x		x	x	x	x	x
M0300D2	Stage 4 pressure ulcers: number at admit/reentry			x	x	x	x						x		x					x									x		
M0300E1	Unstaged due to dressing: number present	x		x	x	x	x		x		x	x	x		x		x		x	x					x		x		x	x	x
M0300E2	Unstaged due to dressing: number at admit/reentry			x	x	x	x						x		x					x											
M0300F1	Unstaged slough/eschar: number present	x		x	x	x	x		x		x	x	x		x		x		x	x					x		x		x	x	x
M0300F2	Unstaged slough/eschar: number at admit/reentry			x	x	x	x						x		x					x											

MDS Item	Description	Skip trigger items	NOA item	Submitted Item	NC-Comp	NQ-Quart	NP-PPS	NS-OMRA SOT	NSD-OMRA SOT+DC	NO-OMRA other	NOD-OMRA other+DC	ND-Disch	NT-Tracking	SP-PPS	SS-OMRA SOT	SSD-OMRA SOT+DC	SO-OMRA other	SOD-OMRA other+DC	SD-Disch	ST-Tracking	XX-Inactivation	Demog/Admin	QI items	QM items	CAA items	RUG rehab grp	RUG non-rehab	RUG-III items	S&C items	PDC-Planned D/C	UPD-Unplanned D/C
M0300G1	Unstageable - deep tissue: number present	x		x	x	x	x		x		x	x		x		x		x	x						x					x	x
M0300G2	Unstageable - deep tissue: number at admit/reentry			x	x	x	x		x		x	x		x		x		x	x											x	x
M0610A	Stage 3 or 4 pressure ulcer longest length			x	x	x	x		x		x	x		x		x		x	x											x	x
M0610B	Stage 3 or 4 pressure ulcer width (same ulcer)			x	x	x	x		x		x	x		x		x		x	x											x	x
M0610C	Stage 3 or 4 pressure ulcer depth (same ulcer)			x	x	x	x		x		x	x		x		x		x	x											x	x
M0700	Tissue type for ulcer at most advanced	x		x	x	x	x		x		x	x		x		x		x	x											x	x
M0800A	Worsened since prior asmt: Stage 2 pressure ulcers			x	x	x	x		x		x	x		x		x		x	x					x	x					x	x
M0800B	Worsened since prior asmt: Stage 3 pressure ulcers			x	x	x	x		x		x	x		x		x		x	x					x	x					x	x
M0800C	Worsened since prior asmt: Stage 4 pressure ulcers			x	x	x	x		x		x	x		x		x		x	x					x	x					x	x
M0900A	Pressure ulcers on prior assessment	x		x	x	x	x		x		x	x		x		x		x	x											x	x
M0900B	Healed pressure ulcers: Stage 2			x	x	x	x		x		x	x		x		x		x	x											x	x
M0900C	Healed pressure ulcers: Stage 3			x	x	x	x		x		x	x		x		x		x	x											x	x
M0900D	Healed pressure ulcers: Stage 4			x	x	x	x		x		x	x		x		x		x	x											x	x
M1030	Number of venous and arterial ulcers			x	x	x	x	x	x	x	x	x		x	x	x	x	x	x								x	x		x	x
M1040A	Other skin probs: infection of the foot			x	x	x	x	x	x	x	x	x		x	x	x	x	x	x						x		x	x	x	x	x
M1040B	Other skin probs: diabetic foot ulcer(s)			x	x	x	x	x	x	x	x	x		x	x	x	x	x	x								x	x		x	x
M1040C	Other skin probs: other open lesion(s) on the foot			x	x	x	x	x	x	x	x	x		x	x	x	x	x	x								x	x		x	x
M1040D	Other skin probs: lesions not ulcers, rashes, cuts			x	x	x	x	x	x	x	x	x		x	x	x	x	x	x								x	x		x	x
M1040E	Other skin probs: surgical wound(s)			x	x	x	x	x	x	x	x	x		x	x	x	x	x	x								x	x		x	x
M1040F	Other skin probs: burns (second or third degree)			x	x	x	x	x	x	x	x	x		x	x	x	x	x	x								x	x		x	x
M1040G	Skin Tear(s)			x	x	x	x	x	x	x	x	x		x	x	x	x	x	x											x	x
M1040H	Moisture Associated Skin Damage (MASD)			x	x	x	x	x	x	x	x	x		x	x	x	x	x	x						x					x	x
M1040Z	Other skin probs: none of the above		x	x	x	x	x	x	x	x	x	x		x	x	x	x	x	x						x				x	x	x
M1200A	Skin/ulcer treat: pressure reduce device for chair			x	x	x	x	x	x	x	x	x		x	x	x	x	x	x								x	x	x	x	x
M1200B	Skin/ulcer treat: pressure reducing device for bed			x	x	x	x	x	x	x	x	x		x	x	x	x	x	x								x	x	x	x	x
M1200C	Skin/ulcer treat: turning/repositioning			x	x	x	x	x	x	x	x	x		x	x	x	x	x	x								x	x	x	x	x
M1200D	Skin/ulcer treat: nutrition/hydration			x	x	x	x	x	x	x	x	x		x	x	x	x	x	x								x	x	x	x	x
M1200E	Skin/ulcer treat: pressure ulcer care			x	x	x	x	x	x	x	x	x		x	x	x	x	x	x								x	x	x	x	x
M1200F	Skin/ulcer treat: surgical wound care			x	x	x	x	x	x	x	x	x		x	x	x	x	x	x								x	x	x	x	x
M1200G	Skin/ulcer treat: application of dressings			x	x	x	x	x	x	x	x	x		x	x	x	x	x	x								x	x	x	x	x
M1200H	Skin/ulcer treat: apply ointments/medications			x	x	x	x	x	x	x	x	x		x	x	x	x	x	x								x	x	x	x	x
M1200I	Skin/ulcer treat: apply dressings to feet			x	x	x	x	x	x	x	x	x		x	x	x	x	x	x								x	x	x	x	x
M1200Z	Skin/ulcer treat: none of the above		x	x	x	x	x	x	x	x	x	x		x	x	x	x	x	x								+	+	+	x	x
N0300	Number of days injectable medications received	x		x																							+	+	x	x	x
N0350A	Insulin: insulin injections			x	x	x	x	x	x	x	x	x		x	x	x	x	x	x								x	x			
N0350B	Insulin: orders for insulin			x	x	x	x	x	x	x	x	x		x	x	x	x	x	x								x	x			
N0410A	Medication received: Days: antipsychotic			x	x	x	x	x	x	x	x	x		x	x	x	x	x	x				x		x				x	x	x
N0410B	Medication received: Days: antianxiety			x	x	x	x	x	x	x	x	x		x	x	x	x	x	x				x		x				x	x	x

April 2012 item matrix

MDS item matrix for APR 2012 (v13) 10-27-2011

Item matrix for April 2012

MDS Item	Description	Skip trigger items	NOA item	Submitted Item	NC - Comp	NQ - Quart	NP - PPS	NS - OMRA SOT	NSD - OMRA SOT+DC	NO - OMRA other	NOD - OMRA other + DC	ND - Disch	NT - Tracking	SP - PPS	SS - OMRA SOT	SSD - OMRA SOT+DC	SO - OMRA other	SOD - OMRA other + DC	SD - Disch	ST - Tracking	XX - Inactivation	Demog/Admin	QI items	QM items	CAA items	RUG rehab grp	RUG non-rehab	RUG-III items	S&C items	PDC - Planned D/C	UPD - Unplanned D/C
N0410C	Medication received: Days: antidepressant			X	X	X	X		X		X	X		X		X		X	X						X				X	X	X
N0410D	Medication received: Days: hypnotic			X	X	X	X		X		X	X		X		X		X	X				X		X				X	X	X
N0410E	Medication received: Days: anticoagulant			X	X	X	X		X		X	X		X		X		X	X											X	X
N0410F	Medication received: Days: antibiotic			X	X	X	X		X		X	X		X		X		X	X											X	X
N0410G	Medication received: Days: diuretic			X	X	X	X		X		X	X		X		X		X	X											X	X
O0100A1	Treatment: chemotherapy - while not resident			X	X	X	X		X		X			X		X		X										X	X		
O0100A2	Treatment: chemotherapy - while resident			X	X	X	X		X	X	X			X		X	X	X									X	X	X		
O0100B1	Treatment: radiation - while not resident			X	X	X	X		X		X			X		X		X										X	X		
O0100B2	Treatment: radiation - while resident			X	X	X	X		X	X	X			X		X	X	X									X	X	X		
O0100C1	Treatment: oxygen therapy - while not resident			X	X	X	X		X		X			X		X		X										X	X		
O0100C2	Treatment: oxygen therapy - while resident			X	X	X	X		X	X	X			X		X	X	X									X	X	X		
O0100D1	Treatment: suctioning - while not resident			X	X	X	X		X		X			X		X		X											X		
O0100D2	Treatment: suctioning - while resident			X	X	X	X		X	X	X			X		X	X	X										X	X		
O0100E1	Treatment: tracheostomy care - while not resident			X	X	X	X		X		X			X		X		X										X	X		
O0100E2	Treatment: tracheostomy care - while resident			X	X	X	X	X	X	X	X			X	X	X	X	X								X	X	X	X		
O0100F1	Treatment: vent/respirator - while not resident			X	X	X	X		X		X			X		X		X										X	X		
O0100F2	Treatment: vent/respirator - while resident			X	X	X	X	X	X	X	X			X	X	X	X	X								X	X	X	X		
O0100G1	Treatment: BiPAP/CPAP - while not resident			X	X	s	s		X		X			X		X		X										X	X		
O0100G2	Treatment: BiPAP/CPAP - while resident			X	X	s	s		X	X	X			X		X	X	X									X	X		
O0100H1	Treatment: IV medications - while not resident			X	X	X	X		X		X			X		X		X										X	X		
O0100H2	Treatment: IV medications - while resident			X	X	X	X		X	X	X			X		X	X	X									X	X	X		
O0100I1	Treatment: transfusions - while not resident			X	X	s	s		X		X			X		X		X										X	X		
O0100I2	Treatment: transfusions - while resident			X	X	s	s		X	X	X			X		X	X	X									X	X	X		
O0100J1	Treatment: dialysis - while not resident			X	X	s	s		X		X			X		X		X										X	X		
O0100J2	Treatment: dialysis - while resident			X	X	s	s		X	X	X			X		X	X	X									X	X	X		
O0100K1	Treatment: hospice care - while not resident			X	X	s	s		X		X			X		X		X						X				X	X		
O0100K2	Treatment: hospice care - while resident			X	X	s	s		X	X	X	X		X		X	X	X	X								X	X		
O0100L2	Treatment: respite care - while resident			X	X	s	s		X	X	X			X		X	X	X									X	X		
O0100M1	Treatment: isolate/quarantine - while not resident			X	X	s	s		X		X			X		X		X										X	X		
O0100M2	Treatment: isolate/quarantine - while resident			X	X	X	X	X	X	X	X			X	X	X	X	X								X	X	X	X		
O0100Z1	Treatment: none of above - while not resident		X	X	X	X	X		X		X			X		X		X								X		X			
O0100Z2	Treatment: none of above - while resident		X	X	X	X	X		X	X	X			X		X	X	X										X			
O0250A	Was influenza vaccine received	X		X	X	X	X	X	X	X	X	X		X	X	X	X	X	X					X					X	X	
O0250B	Date influenza vaccine received.			X	X	X	X		X		X	X		X		X		X	X										X	X	
O0250C	If influenza vaccine not received, state reason	X		X	X	X	X	X	X	X	X	X		X	X	X	X	X	X					X					X	X	
O0300A	Is pneumococcal vaccination up to date	X		X	X	X	X	X	X	X	X	X		X	X	X	X	X	X					X					X	X	
O0300B	If pneumococcal vacc not received, state reason			X	X	X	X	X	X	X	X	X		X	X	X	X	X	X					X					X	X	
O0400A1	Speech-language/audiology: individ minutes	X		X	X	X	X	X	X	X	X	X		X	X	X	X	X	X							X		X	X		

MDS Item	Description	Skip trigger items	NOA item	Submitted Item	NC - Comp	NQ - Quart	NP - PPS	NS - OMRA SOT	NSD-OMRA SOT+DC	NO - OMRA other	NOD - OMRA other + DC	ND - Disch	NT - Tracking	SP - PPS	SS - OMRA SOT	SSD-OMRA SOT+DC	SO - OMRA other	SOD - OMRA other + DC	SD - Disch	ST - Tracking	XX - Inactivation	Demog/Admin	QI items	QM items	CAA items	RUG rehab grp	RUG non-rehab	RUG-III items	S&C items	PDC - Planned D/C	UPD - Unplanned D/C
O0400A2	Speech-language/audiology: concur minutes	X		X	X	X	X	X	X	X	X			X	X	X	X	X								X			X		
O0400A3	Speech-language/audiology: group minutes	X		X	X	X	X	X	X	X	X			X	X	X	X	X								X		X	X		
O0400A4	Speech-language/audiology: number of days			X	X	X	X	X	X	X	X	X		X	X	X	X	X	X							X		X		X	X
O0400A5	Speech-language/audiology: start date			X	X	X	X	X	X	X	X	X		X	X	X	X	X	X							X				X	X
O0400A6	Speech-language/audiology: end date			X	X	X	X	X	X	X	X	X		X	X	X	X	X	X							X				X	X
O0400B1	Occupational therapy: individ minutes	X		X	X	X	X	X	X	X	X			X	X	X	X	X								X		X	X		
O0400B2	Occupational therapy: concur minutes	X		X	X	X	X	X	X	X	X			X	X	X	X	X								X		X	X		
O0400B3	Occupational therapy: group minutes	X		X	X	X	X	X	X	X	X			X	X	X	X	X								X			X		
O0400B4	Occupational therapy: number of days			X	X	X	X	X	X	X	X	X		X	X	X	X	X	X							X		X		X	X
O0400B5	Occupational therapy: start date			X	X	X	X	X	X	X	X	X		X	X	X	X	X	X							X				X	X
O0400B6	Occupational therapy: end date			X	X	X	X	X	X	X	X	X		X	X	X	X	X	X							X				X	X
O0400C1	Physical therapy: individ minutes	X		X	X	X	X	X	X	X	X			X	X	X	X	X								X		X	X		
O0400C2	Physical therapy: concur minutes	X		X	X	X	X	X	X	X	X			X	X	X	X	X								X		X	X		
O0400C3	Physical therapy: group minutes	X		X	X	X	X	X	X	X	X			X	X	X	X	X								X		X	X		
O0400C4	Physical therapy: number of days			X	X	X	X	X	X	X	X	X		X	X	X	X	X	X							X		X		X	X
O0400C5	Physical therapy: start date			X	X	X	X	X	X	X	X	X		X	X	X	X	X	X							X				X	X
O0400C6	Physical therapy: end date			X	X	X	X	X	X	X	X	X		X	X	X	X	X	X							X				X	X
O0400D1	Respiratory therapy: number of minutes	X		X	X	s	s	X	X	X	X			X	X	X	X	X								X			X		
O0400D2	Respiratory therapy: number of days			X	X	X	X			X	X			X			X	X									X	X			
O0400E1	Psychological therapy: number of minutes	X		X	X	s	s	X	X	X	X			X	X	X	X	X								X					
O0400E2	Psychological therapy: number of days			X	X	X	X			X	X			X			X	X									X					
O0400F1	Recreational therapy: number of minutes	X		X	X	s	s	X	X	X	X			X	X	X	X	X								X					
O0400F2	Recreational therapy: number of days			X	X	X	X			X	X			X			X	X									X					
O0450A	Resumption of Therapy: has it resumed	X		X	X	X	X	X	X	X	X			X	X	X	X	X								X					
O0450B	Resumption of Therapy: date resumed			X	X	X	X	X	X	X	X			X	X	X	X	X								X					
O0500A	Range of motion (passive): number of days			X	X	X	X	X	X	X	X			X			X	X								X	X	X			
O0500B	Range of motion (active): number of days			X	X	X	X	X	X	X	X			X			X	X								X	X	X			
O0500C	Splint or brace assistance: number of days			X	X	X	X	X	X	X	X			X			X	X								X	X	X	X		
O0500D	Bed mobility training: number of days			X	X	X	X	X	X	X	X			X			X	X								X	X	X			
O0500E	Transfer training: number of days			X	X	X	X	X	X	X	X			X			X	X								X	X	X			
O0500F	Walking training: number of days			X	X	X	X	X	X	X	X			X			X	X								X	X	X			
O0500G	Dressing and/or grooming training: number of days			X	X	X	X	X	X	X	X			X			X	X								X	X	X			
O0500H	Eating and/or swallowing training: number of days			X	X	X	X	X	X	X	X			X			X	X								X	X	X			
O0500I	Amputation/prosthesis training: number of days			X	X	X	X	X	X	X	X			X			X	X								X	X	X			
O0500J	Communication training: number of days			X	X	X	X	X	X	X	X			X			X	X								X	X	X			
O0600	Physician examinations: number of days			X	X	X	X			X	X	X		X			X	X										X			
O0700	Physician orders: number of days			X	X	X	X			X	X	X		X			X	X	X									X			
P0100A	Restraints used in bed: bed rail			X	X	X	X	X	X	X	X	X		X	X	X	X	X	X						X			X	X	X	X

April 2012 item matrix

MDS item matrix for APR 2012 (v13) 10-27-2011

MDS Item	Description	Skip trigger items	NOA item	Submitted Item	NC - Comp	NQ - Quart	NP - PPS	NS - OMRA SOT	NSD-OMRA SOT+DC	NO - OMRA other	NOD - OMRA other + DC	ND - Disch	NT - Tracking	SP - PPS	SS - OMRA SOT	SSD-OMRA SOT+DC	SO - OMRA other	SOD - OMRA other + DC	SD - Disch	ST - Tracking	XX - Inactivation	Demog/Admin	QI items	QM items	CAA items	RUG rehab grp	RUG non-rehab	RUG-III items	S&C items	PDC - Planned D/C	UPD - Unplanned D/C
P0100B	Restraints used in bed: trunk restraint			x	x	x	x		x		x	x		x		x		x	x					x	x				x	x	x
P0100C	Restraints used in bed: limb restraint			x	x	x	x		x		x	x		x		x		x	x					x	x				x	x	x
P0100D	Restraints used in bed: other			x	x	x	x		x		x	x		x		x		x	x						x				x	x	x
P0100E	Restraints in chair/out of bed: trunk restraint			x	x	x	x		x		x	x		x		x		x	x					x	x				x	x	x
P0100F	Restraints in chair/out of bed: limb restraint			x	x	x	x		x		x	x		x		x		x	x					x	x				x	x	x
P0100G	Restraints in chair/out of bed: chair stops rising			x	x	x	x		x		x	x		x		x		x	x					x	x				x	x	x
P0100H	Restraints in chair/out of bed: other			x	x	x	x		x		x	x		x		x		x	x						x				x	x	x
Q0100A	Resident participated in assessment			x	x	x	x	x	x	x	x	x		x	x	x	x	x	x			2									
Q0100B	Family/signif other participated in assessment			x	x	x	x	x	x	x	x			x	x	x	x	x				2									
Q0100C	Guardian/legal rep participated in assessment			x	x	x	x	x	x	x	x			x	x	x	x	x				2									
Q0300A	Resident's overall goal			x	x	x	x	x	x	x	x			x	x	x	x	x				3									
Q0300B	Information source for resident's goal			x	x	x	x	x	x	x	x			x		x		x				3									
Q0400A	Active discharge plan for return to community	x		x	x	x	x		x		x	x		x		x		x	x												
Q0490	Resident's preference to avoid being asked			x	x	x	x							x																	
Q0500B	Do you want to talk about returning to community			x	x	x	x							x																	
Q0550A	Reasking resident preference			x	x	x	x							x																	
Q0550B	Reasking resident preference source			x	x	x	x							x																	
Q0600	Referral been made to local contact agency			x	x	x	x		x		x	x		x		x		x	x						x					x	x
V0100A	Prior OBRA reason for assessment			x	x	s	s																								
V0100B	Prior PPS reason for assessment			x	x	s	s																								
V0100C	Prior assessment reference date			x	x	s	s																								
V0100D	Prior assessment BIMS summary score			x	x	s	s																								
V0100E	Prior asmt PHQ res: total mood severity score			x	x	s	s																								
V0100F	Prior asmt PHQ staff: total mood score			x	x	s	s																								
V0200A01A	CAA-Delirium: triggered			x	x	s	s																		x						
V0200A01B	CAA-Delirium: plan			x	x	s	s																		x						
V0200A02A	CAA-Cognitive loss/dementia: triggered			x	x	s	s																		x						
V0200A02B	CAA-Cognitive loss/dementia: plan			x	x	s	s																		x						
V0200A03A	CAA-Visual function: triggered			x	x	s	s																		x						
V0200A03B	CAA-Visual function: plan			x	x	s	s																		x						
V0200A04A	CAA-Communication: triggered			x	x	s	s																		x						
V0200A04B	CAA-Communication: plan			x	x	s	s																		x						
V0200A05A	CAA-ADL functional/rehab potential: triggered			x	x	s	s																		x						
V0200A05B	CAA-ADL functional/rehab potential: plan			x	x	s	s																		x						
V0200A06A	CAA-Urinary incont/indwell catheter: triggered			x	x	s	s																		x						
V0200A06B	CAA-Urinary incont/indwell catheter: plan			x	x	s	s																		x						
V0200A07A	CAA-Psychosocial well-being: triggered			x	x	s	s																		x						
V0200A07B	CAA-Psychosocial well-being: plan			x	x	s	s																		x						

Item matrix for April 2012

April 2012 item matrix

Column groups: **Item Info** (Skip trigger items, NOA item, Submitted Item) · **Nursing Home Item Subsets** (NC – Comp, NQ – Quart, NP – PPS, NS – OMRA SOT, NSD–OMRA SOT+DC, NO – OMRA other, NOD – OMRA other + DC, ND – Disch, NT – Tracking) · **Swing Bed Item Subsets** (SP – PPS, SS – OMRA SOT, SSD–OMRA SOT+DC, SO – OMRA other, SOD – OMRA other + DC, SD – Disch, ST – Tracking) · XX – Inactivation · **Item Groups** (Demog/Admin, QI items, QM items, CAA items, RUG rehab grp, RUG non-rehab, RUG-III items, S&C items) · **New D/C** (PDC – Planned D/C, UPD – Unplanned D/C)

MDS Item	Description	Skip trig	NOA	Subm	NC	NQ	NP	NS	NSD	NO	NOD	ND	NT	SP	SS	SSD	SO	SOD	SD	ST	XX	Dem/Adm	QI	QM	CAA	RUGreh	RUGnon	RUG-III	S&C	PDC	UPD
V0200A08A	CAA-Mood state: triggered			x	x	s	s																		x						
V0200A08B	CAA-Mood state: plan			x	x	s	s																		x						
V0200A09A	CAA-Behavioral symptoms: triggered			x	x	s	s																		x						
V0200A09B	CAA-Behavioral symptoms: plan			x	x	s	s																		x						
V0200A10A	CAA-Activities: triggered			x	x	s	s																		x						
V0200A10B	CAA-Activities: plan			x	x	s	s																		x						
V0200A11A	CAA-Falls: triggered			x	x	s	s																		x						
V0200A11B	CAA-Falls: plan			x	x	s	s																		x						
V0200A12A	CAA-Nutritional status: triggered			x	x	s	s																		x						
V0200A12B	CAA-Nutritional status: plan			x	x	s	s																		x						
V0200A13A	CAA-Feeding tubes: triggered			x	x	s	s																		x						
V0200A13B	CAA-Feeding tubes: plan			x	x	s	s																		x						
V0200A14A	CAA-Dehydration/fluid maintenance: triggered			x	x	s	s																		x						
V0200A14B	CAA-Dehydration/fluid maintenance: plan			x	x	s	s																		x						
V0200A15A	CAA-Dental care: triggered			x	x	s	s																		x						
V0200A15B	CAA-Dental care: plan			x	x	s	s																		x						
V0200A16A	CAA-Pressure ulcer: triggered			x	x	s	s																		x						
V0200A16B	CAA-Pressure ulcer: plan			x	x	s	s																		x						
V0200A17A	CAA-Psychotropic drug use: triggered			x	x	s	s																		x						
V0200A17B	CAA-Psychotropic drug use: plan			x	x	s	s																		x						
V0200A18A	CAA-Physical restraints: triggered			x	x	s	s																		x						
V0200A18B	CAA-Physical restraints: plan			x	x	s	s																		x						
V0200A19A	CAA-Pain: triggered			x	x	s	s																		x						
V0200A19B	CAA-Pain: plan			x	x	s	s																		x						
V0200A20A	CAA-Return to community referral: triggered			x	x	s	s																		x						
V0200A20B	CAA-Return to community referral: plan			x	x	s	s																		x						
V0200B1	CAA-Assessment process RN signature			x	x	s	s																								
V0200B2	CAA-Assessment process signature date			x	x	s	s																								
V0200C1	CAA-Care planning signature				x	s	s																								
V0200C2	CAA-Care planning signature date			x	x	s	s																								
X0150	Correction: type of provider	x			x	x	x	x	x	x	x	x	x	x	x	x	x	x	x	x	x	x								x	x
X0200A	Correction: resident first name			x	x	x	x	x	x	x	x	x	x	x	x	x	x	x	x	x	x	x								x	x
X0200C	Correction: resident last name			x	x	x	x	x	x	x	x	x	x	x	x	x	x	x	x	x	x	x								x	x
X0300	Correction: resident gender				x	x	x	x	x	x	x	x	x	x	x	x	x	x	x	x	x	x								x	x
X0400	Correction: resident birth date			x	x	x	x	x	x	x	x	x	x	x	x	x	x	x	x	x	x	x								x	x
X0500	Correction: resident social security number			x	x	x	x	x	x	x	x	x	x	x	x	x	x	x	x	x	x	x								x	x
X0600A	Correction: OBRA reason for assessment			x	x	x	x	x	x	x	x	x	x	x	x	x	x	x	x	x	x	x								x	x
X0600B	Correction: PPS reason for assessment			x	x	x	x	x	x	x	x	x	x	x	x	x	x	x	x	x	x	x								x	x

MDS item matrix for APR 2012 (v13) 10-27-2011

Item matrix for April 2012

MDS Item	Description	Skip trigger items	NOA item	Submitted Item	NC - Comp	NQ - Quart	NP - PPS	NS - OMRA SOT	NSD - OMRA SOT+DC	NO - OMRA other	NOD - OMRA other + DC	ND - Disch	NT - Tracking	SP - PPS	SS - OMRA SOT	SSD-OMRA SOT+DC	SO - OMRA other	SOD - OMRA other + DC	SD - Disch	ST - Tracking	XX - Inactivation	Demog/Admin	QI items	QM items	CAA items	RUG rehab grp	RUG non-rehab	RUG-III items	S&C items	PDC - Planned D/C	UPD - Unplanned D/C
X0600C	Correction: OMRA assessment			x	x	x	x	x	x	x	x	x	x	x	x	x	x	x	x	x	x	x								x	x
X0600D	Correction: Swing bed clinical change asmt			x	x	x	x	x	x	x	x	x	x	x	x	x	x	x	x	x	x	x								x	x
X0600F	Correction: entry/discharge reporting	x		x	x	x	x	x	x	x	x	x	x	x	x	x	x	x	x	x	x	x								x	x
X0700A	Correction: assessment reference date			x	x	x	x	x	x	x	x	x	x	x	x	x	x	x	x	x	x	x								x	x
X0700B	Correction: discharge date			x	x	x	x	x	x	x	x	x	x	x	x	x	x	x	x	x	x	x								x	x
X0700C	Correction: entry date			x	x	x	x	x	x	x	x	x	x	x	x	x	x	x	x	x	x	x								x	x
X0800	Correction: correction number			x	x	x	x	x	x	x	x	x	x	x	x	x	x	x	x	x	x	x								x	x
X0900A	Correction: modif reasons - transcription error			x	x	x	x	x	x	x	x	x	x	x	x	x	x	x	x	x	x	x								x	x
X0900B	Correction: modif reasons - data entry error			x	x	x	x	x	x	x	x	x	x	x	x	x	x	x	x	x	x	x								x	x
X0900C	Correction: modif reasons - software error			x	x	x	x	x	x	x	x	x	x	x	x	x	x	x	x	x	x	x								x	x
X0900D	Correction: modif reasons - item coding error			x	x	x	x	x	x	x	x	x	x	x	x	x	x	x	x	x	x	x								x	x
X0900E	Correction: Modif reasons - resume therapy			x	x	x	x	x	x	x	x	x	x	x	x	x	x	x	x	x	x	x								x	x
X0900Z	Correction: modif reasons - other error			x	x	x	x	x	x	x	x	x	x	x	x	x	x	x	x	x	x	x								x	x
X1050A	Correction: inact reasons - event did not occur			x	x	x	x	x	x	x	x	x	x	x	x	x	x	x	x	x	x	x								x	x
X1050Z	Correction: inact reasons - other reason			x	x	x	x	x	x	x	x	x	x	x	x	x	x	x	x	x	x	x								x	x
X1100A	Correction: attestor first name			x	x	x	x	x	x	x	x	x	x	x	x	x	x	x	x	x	x	x								x	x
X1100B	Correction: attestor last name			x	x	x	x	x	x	x	x	x	x	x	x	x	x	x	x	x	x	x								x	x
X1100C	Correction: attestor title				x	x	x	x	x	x	x	x	x	x	x	x	x	x	x	x	x	x								x	x
X1100D	Correction: attestor signature			x	x	x	x	x	x	x	x	x	x	x	x	x	x	x	x	x	x	x								x	x
X1100E	Correction: attestation date			x	x	x	x	x	x	x	x	x	x	x	x	x	x	x	x	x	x	x								x	x
Z0100A	Medicare Part A: HIPPS code			x	x	x	x	x	x	x	x			x	x	x	x	x								x	x			x	x
Z0100B	Medicare Part A: RUG version code			x	x	x	x	x	x	x	x			x	x	x	x	x								x	x			x	x
Z0100C	Medicare Part A: Medicare short stay asmt			x				x	x	x	x				x	x	x	x								x	x			x	x
Z0150A	Medicare Part A: non-therapy HIPPS code			x	x	x	x	x	x	x	x			x	x	x	x	x								x	x			x	x
Z0150B	Medicare Part A: non-therapy RUG version code			x	x	x	x	x	x	x	x			x	x	x	x	x								x	x			x	x
Z0200A	State case mix: RUG group			x	x	x	x	x	x	x	x											1									
Z0200B	State case mix: RUG version code			x	x	x	x	x	x	x	x											1									
Z0250A	State case mix: Alternate RUG group			x	x	x	x	x	x	x	x											1									
Z0250B	State case mix: Alternate RUG version code			x	x	x	x	x	x	x	x											1									
Z0300A	Insurance Billing: Billing Code				x	x	x	x	x	x	x	x		x	x	x	x	x	x			2								x	x
Z0300B	Insurance Billing: Billing Version				x	x	x	x	x	x	x	x		x	x	x	x	x	x			2								x	x
Z0400A	Attestation signature, title, sections, date				x	x	x	x	x	x	x	x	x	x	x	x	x	x	x	x		x								x	x
Z0400B	Attestation signature, title, sections, date				x	x	x	x	x	x	x	x	x	x	x	x	x	x	x	x		x								x	x
Z0400C	Attestation signature, title, sections, date				x	x	x	x	x	x	x	x	x	x	x	x	x	x	x	x		2								x	x
Z0400D	Attestation signature, title, sections, date				x	x	x	x	x	x	x	x	x	x	x	x	x	x	x	x		2								x	x
Z0400E	Attestation signature, title, sections, date				x	x	x	x	x	x	x	x	x	x	x	x	x	x	x	x		2								x	x
Z0400F	Attestation signature, title, sections, date				x	x	x	x	x	x	x	x	x	x	x	x	x	x	x	x		2								x	x
Z0400G	Attestation signature, title, sections, date				x	x	x	x	x	x	x	x	x	x	x	x	x	x	x	x		2								x	x

Item matrix for April 2012

MDS Item	Description	Skip trigger items	NOA item	Submitted Item	NC - Comp	NQ - Quart	NP - PPS	NS - OMRA SOT	NSD-OMRA SOT+DC	NO - OMRA other	NOD - OMRA other + DC	ND - Disch	NT - Tracking	SP - PPS	SS - OMRA SOT	SSD-OMRA SOT+DC	SO - OMRA other	SOD - OMRA other + DC	SD - Disch	ST - Tracking	XX - Inactivation	Demog/Admin	QI items	QM items	CAA items	RUG rehab grp	RUG non-rehab	RUG-III items	S&C items	PDC - Planned D/C	UPD - Unplanned D/C
					NC	NQ	NP	NS	NSD	NO	NOD	ND	NT	SP	SS	SSD	SO	SOD	SD	ST	XX	Demog/Admin	QI	QM	CAA	RUG reh	RUG non	RUG-III	S&C	PDC	UPD
Z0400H	Attestation signature, title, sections, date				x	x	x	x	x	x	x	x		x	x	x	x	x	x			2								x	x
Z0400I	Attestation signature, title, sections, date				x	x	x	x	x	x	x	x		x	x	x	x	x	x			2								x	x
Z0400J	Attestation signature, title, sections, date				x	x	x	x	x	x	x	x		x	x	x	x	x	x			2								x	x
Z0400K	Attestation signature, title, sections, date				x	x	x	x	x	x	x	x		x	x	x	x	x	x			2								x	x
Z0400L	Attestation signature, title, sections, date				x	x	x	x	x	x	x	x		x	x	x	x	x	x			2								x	x
Z0500A	Attestation signature, title, sections, date				x	x	x	x	x	x	x	x		x	x	x	x	x	x			2								x	x
Z0500B	Date RN signed assessment as complete			x	x	x	x	x	x	x	x	x		x	x	x	x	x	x			2								x	x
	Number of federally required items	71	19	600	619	482	482	137	333	258	374	295	72	445	137	323	258	364	285	72	29	72	26	85	182	55	95	110	171	295	231

Notes:

1 = Needed on nursing home comprehensive and quarterly for payment/administration.

2 = Needed on all assessments for documentation.

3 = Needed on all non-OMRA assessments for clinical and/or payment documentation.

4 = QM item not needed on discharge.

5 = Items needed on all assessments that include resident interview

+ = Supporting items (e.g., triggers for skip patterns, none-of-the-above items, component item for summary score)

s = State-optional item.

April 2012 item matrix

APPENDIX G: REFERENCES

American Psychiatric Association: <u>Diagnostic and Statistical Manual of Mental Disorders</u> (4th ed.). Washington, DC. American Psychiatric Association, 1994.

Baker, D.W., Cameron, K.A., Feinglass, J., Georgas, P., Foster, S., Pierce, D., Thompson, J.A., and Hasnain-Wynia, R.: Patients' attitudes toward health care providers collecting information about their race and ethnicity. <u>J. Gen. Intern. Med.</u> 20:895-900, 2005.

Bergstrom, N., Smout, R., Horn, S., Spector, W., Hartz, A., and Limcangco, M.R.: Stage 2 pressure ulcer healing in nursing homes. Journal of the American Geriatrics Society 56(7):1252-1258, 14 May 2008.

Centers for Disease Control and Prevention: <u>2007 Guideline for Isolation Precautions: Preventing Transmission of Infectious Agents in Healthcare Settings</u>. Available from <u>http://www.cdc.gov/ncidod/dhqp/pdf/guidelines/Isolation2007.pdf</u>.

Centers for Disease Control and Prevention: <u>The Pink Book: Chapters: Epidemiology and Prevention of Vaccine Preventable Diseases, 12th ed.</u> Available from <u>http://www.cdc.gov/vaccines/pubs/pinkbook/index.html#chapters</u>

Centers for Disease Control and Prevention: Prevention of pneumococcal disease: Recommendations of the Advisory Committee on Immunization Practices (ACIP). Recommended Adult Immunization Schedule – United States. <u>MMWR Recomm. Rep.</u> 57(53); Q1-Q-4, Jan. 9, 2009.

Centers for Medicare & Medicaid Services: <u>HIPPS Codes</u>. Jun. 22, 2009; retrieved Nov. 18, 2009, from <u>http://www.cms.hhs.gov/ProspMedicareFeeSvcPmtGen/02_HIPPSCodes.asp#TopOfPage</u>

Centers for Medicare & Medicaid Services: <u>MDS 3.0 Data Submission Specifications</u>. Available from <u>http://www.cms.gov/NursingHomeQualityInits/30_NHQIMDS30TechnicalInformation.asp#TopOfPage</u>

Centers for Medicare & Medicaid Services: <u>MDS 3.0 for Nursing Home</u>. Available from <u>http://www.cms.gov/NursingHomeQualityInits/30_NHQIMDS30TechnicalInformation.asp#TopOfPage</u>

Centers for Medicare & Medicaid Services: <u>Medicare Benefit Policy Manual</u> (Pub. 100-2). Available from <u>http://www.cms.hhs.gov/manuals/iom/List.asp</u>

Centers for Medicare & Medicaid Services: <u>Medicare Claims Processing Manual</u> (Pub. 100-4). <u>http://www.cms.hhs.gov/manuals/iom/List.asp</u>

Centers for Medicare & Medicaid Services: <u>Medicare General Information, Eligibility, and Entitlement Manual</u> (Pub. 100-1). Available from <u>http://www.cms.hhs.gov/manuals/iom/List.asp</u>

Centers for Medicare & Medicaid Services: <u>Memorandum to State Survey Agency Directors from CMS Director, Survey and Certification Group: Clarification of Terms Used in the Definition of Physical Restraints as Applied to the Requirements for Long Term Care Facilities</u>. Jun. 22, 2007; retrieved Oct. 16, 2009, from http://www.cms.hhs.gov/SurveyCertificationGenInfo/downloads/SCLetter07-22.pdf

Centers for Medicare & Medicaid Services: <u>Minimum Data Set (MDS) 3.0 Provider User's Guide</u>. Available from https://www.qtso.com/mds30.html

Centers for Medicare & Medicaid Services: <u>State Operations Manual, Appendix PP-Guidance to Surveyors for Long Term Care Facilities. Section 483.20(b) Utilization Guidelines for Completion of the RAI</u>. Available from http://cms.hhs.gov/manuals/Downloads/som107ap_pp_guidelines_ltcf.pdf

Folstein, M.F., Folstein, S.E., and McHugh, P.R.: "Mini-mental state." A practical method for grading the cognitive state of patients for the clinician. <u>J. Psychiatr. Res.</u> 12(3):189-198, Nov. 1975.

Healthcentric Advisors: <u>The Holistic Approach to Transformational Change</u> (HATCh). CMS NH QIOSC Contract. Providence, RI. 2006. Available from http://healthcentricadvisors.org/images/stories/documents/inhc.pdf.

Inouye, S.K., Van Dyck, C.H., Alessi, C.A., et al.: Clarifying confusion: the confusion assessment method. A new method for detection of delirium. <u>Ann. Intern. Med.</u> 113(12):941-948, 1990.

Institute of Medicine: <u>Improving the Quality of Care in Nursing Homes</u>. Washington, DC. National Academy Press, 1986.

National Institute of Mental Health: Suicide and the Elderly. n.d. Available from http://www.agingcare.com/Featured-Stories/125788/Suicide-and-the-Elderly.htm

National Pressure Ulcer Advisory Panel: <u>Suspected Deep Tissue Injury</u> [image of cross-sectioned suspected deep tissue injury]. Retrieved November 18, 2009, from http://www.npuap.org/images/NPUAP-SuspectDTI.jpg

National Pressure Ulcer Advisory Panel: <u>Unstageable</u> [image of cross-sectioned unstageable pressure ulcer]. Retrieved November 18, 2009, from http://www.npuap.org/images/NPUAP-Unstage2.jpg

Newman, D.K., and Wein, A.J.: <u>Managing and Treating Urinary Incontinence</u>. 2nd ed. Baltimore, MD. Health Professions Press, 2009.

Physicians' Desk Reference: Physicians' Desk Reference 2008. Montvale, NJ. Thomson PDR, 2007.

Quality Improvement and Evaluation System (QIES) Technical Support Office: QIES Technical Support Office Web site. Retrieved Nov. 18, 2009, from https://www.qtso.com/

Saliba, D., and Buchanan, J.: <u>Development and Validation of a Revised Nursing Home Assessment Tool: MDS 3.0 Final Report to CMS</u>. Contract No. 500-00-0027/Task Order #2. Santa Monica, CA. Rand Corporation, April 2008. Available from http://www.cms.hhs.gov/NursingHomeQualityInits/Downloads/MDS30FinalReport.pdf.

U.S. Department of Health and Human Services, Health Care Financing Administration: Medicare Program: Prospective Payment System and Consolidated Billing for Skilled Nursing Facilities; Final Rule. <u>Fed. Regist.</u> 63(91):26251-26316, May 12, 1998.

U.S. Department of Health and Human Services, Health Care Financing Administration: Medicare program; Prospective payment system and consolidated billing for skilled nursing facilities—Update; final rule and notice. <u>Fed. Regist.</u> 64(146):41644-41683, Jul. 30, 1999.

U.S. Department of Health and Human Services, Office of Disease Prevention and Health Promotion: <u>Healthy People 2020</u>. Available from http://www.healthypeople.gov/2020/default.aspx